CONNECTIONS
Nursing Research,
Theory, and Practice

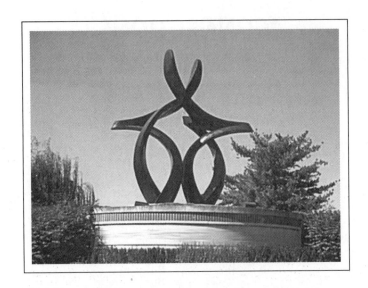

NEXUS statue, artist Larry Young
Courtesy Boone Hospital Center Board of Trustees
Columbia, Missouri

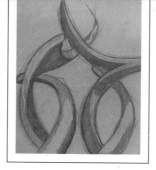

CONNECTIONS
Nursing Research, Theory, and Practice

ANNE YOUNG, RN, EdD

Associate Professor, Doctoral Program Coordinator,
College of Nursing—Houston Center,
Texas Woman's University,
Houston, Texas

SUSAN GEBHARDT TAYLOR, RN, PhD, FAAN

Professor Emerita, Sinclair School of Nursing,
University of Missouri—Columbia,
Columbia, Missouri

KATHERINE McLAUGHLIN-RENPENNING, RN, MScN

President and Chief Nursing Consultant,
MCL Education Services, Inc. and McLaughlin Associates,
White Rock, British Columbia, Canada

Illustrated

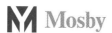 Mosby

A Harcourt Health Sciences Company

St. Louis   London   Philadelphia   Sydney   Toronto

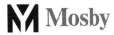

A Harcourt Health Sciences Company

Vice President, Nursing Division: Sally Schrefer
Executive Editor: June D. Thompson
Senior Developmental Editor: Linda Caldwell
Project Manager: Deborah L. Vogel
Associate Production Editor: Corinne Wohlford
Book Designer: Teresa Breckwoldt

Mosby, Inc.
A *Harcourt Health Sciences Company*
11830 Westline Industrial Drive
St. Louis, Missouri 63146

Printed in the United States of America

Library of Congress Cataloging in Publication Data

Young, Anne, RN
   Connections: nursing research, theory, and practice / Anne Young, Susan Gebhardt Taylor, Katherine McLaughlin-Renpenning.
      p. cm.
   Includes bibliographical references and index.
   ISBN 0-323-00948-4
   1. Nursing—Research. 2. Nursing. I. Taylor, Susan G. II. Renpenning, Kathie McLaughlin. III. Title.

RT81.5.Y68 2001
610.73'07'2—dc21   00-066858

00 01 02 03 04 05 TG/FF 9 8 7 6 5 4 3 2 1

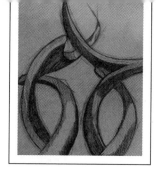

Reviewers

SALLY DECKER, PhD, RN
Professor of Nursing,
Saginaw Valley State University,
University Center, Michigan

SHARON A. DENHAM, DSN, RN
Associate Professor,
School of Nursing, Ohio University,
Athens, Ohio

DIANA D. HANKES, PhD, CS, RN
Professor,
Carroll College—Columbia College of Nursing,
Waukesha, Wisconsin

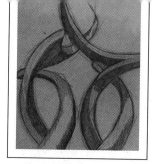

Preface

It is not enough simply to study. First one must determine what to study and what not to study; when to study and when not to study; and who to study under and who not to study with.

Peck, 1995

Discourse within a discipline occurs on many levels, from the philosophical to the theoretical and practical. In a practice discipline, discourse on the theoretical level must connect to the practice level. When these connections do not occur, discourse at the theoretical and philosophical levels is seen as so abstract that it has little meaning for practice. When discourse is limited to the practice level, it is heavily focused on the here-and-now, and it contributes little, if anything, to disciplinary knowledge.

In any mature discipline, scholars, scientists, and practitioners know the models that specify the phenomena and characteristics of the nature of the object or disciplinary focus. They also know the relationships between and among the phenomena of concern. They know the variables based on both universal and individual characteristics. They know what measures specific to phenomena are relevant or legitimate. They know how to use valid and reliable measures to ascertain the characteristics of the situation. They develop practice models that in turn enable practitioners to identify dimensions that are amenable to intervention or change. Expert practitioners use practice models in specific nursing situations to help them choose and understand their actions.

Not all nurses want to engage in discourse at the philosophical and theoretical levels. Many nurses see themselves as grounded in practice, yet they want to contribute to disciplinary knowledge. For these nurses, theory should be seen as a structure from which their research can gain meaning and within which that research can articulate with other works to fill in the disciplinary matrix. Many times theory is taught from a historical perspective. Although the student of nursing benefits from knowing who has done scholarly work and the nature of that work, its value is diminished if it does not guide research and practice.

This text offers an interactive view of nursing theoretical systems within which to position research and to serve as a basis for practice. *Theoretical system* refers to those theories, models, propositions, and cognitive methodologies or modes of inquiry within a common ontology or context. These make up the parameters of the system. The analogy used to describe the theoretical system is that of the nexus. This is depicted with Larry Young's sculpture NEXUS, used in the cover illustration and featured on page ii. Nexus is an irregular shape formed from a continuous line. The viewer's eye can move from one point to another, sometimes directly and sometimes by a more circuitous route. Likewise, one can move among theory, research, and practice in the development of the discipline. The movement is often from theory to research to practice. Other times, the movement is from research to theory to practice or, more simply, from theory to practice or practice to theory. The connections between and among the components of the theoretical system emerge over time. The term *modeling* is used to describe the process of development of these theoretical systems. Modeling is the process of developing and abstracting reality. The product of this process is called a theoretical system, which comprises philosophical premises and foundations, complexes of theories and models, empirical evidence, and models for use.

Diversity and even controversy figure into any discussion of theory. Therefore the terms and definitions used in this text to describe theoretical systems and their components may not be identical to those used by other authors. Nursing scholars do not yet agree on the definitions of these concepts and the terms used to label the concepts (King & Fawcett, 1997).

In Chapter 1 we make the point, supported by Harré (1998), that one selects an ontology that fits his or her beliefs and values about nursing. These beliefs and values are formed through formal education and experiences. Unit 2 presents an overview of each theoretical system to assist in determining which perspective or theoretical system is most congruent with one's personal beliefs about nursing practice and its place in the broader world. The types of scholarly work performed within each theoretical system are illustrated, and the principal research instruments are critiqued. In no way does this substitute for reading primary sources. After the theoretical system within which to frame practice, research, and scholarly endeavors has been chosen, the original sources must be consulted for full descriptions, information, and interpretation. As a scholar, a full understanding of the material, including knowing the unanswered questions, is necessary. In nursing, this means the theoretical system and the structures of clinical specialty knowledge within that framework. To determine an educational program, one might consider courses that will enable a better understanding of some of the foundational concepts or constructs of the selected theoretical system. For example, existential phenomenology courses would benefit a nurse practicing within Parse's theoretical system.

Unit 1 presents a knowledge base, structure, and process for nursing students, clinicians, and program administrators whose science and theory interests are based in specific clinical practice areas. This unit explicates for the clinical researcher the meanings of theory, research, and practice and the connections between and among them. Within each theoretical system, the representative models and theories are presented, and the relationships to the conduct of research and design of practice are identified.

Unit 2 presents nine theoretical systems of varying scope. Four are major theoretical systems that can serve as the disciplinary matrix for research and practice knowledge. These were developed by Orem, Rogers, Parse, and Roy, with contributions from other scholars. Three other theoretical systems—the works of King, Pender, and Peplau—are developed around a component of nursing that is more limited and focused in scope. These three theoretical systems are not linked to the broader disciplinary matrices described. The theoretical systems developed by Neuman and Watson began as specific to nursing but are now appropriate for all healthcare disciplines.

Of these nine systems, the major studies performed within each are reviewed. The instruments that have been developed to measure components of the particular theoretical system are critiqued, and related information is included. The ways in which the theory and research articulate with and inform practice are also considered.

Readers are encouraged to explore each of the units in a quest to discover a fit for themselves between theoretical perspectives and realities of practice. Consider the strengths and weaknesses of the instruments presented and the practical and theoretical implications of the research findings. Think about how these things might influence nursing conceptualizations, practice, and modes of discovery.

As Watson (1999) has noted,

One of the benefits of nursing theory and theory-guided practice (and reflective practice-guided theory) is that it helps clinicians and scholars alike to return to considering the ontological foundation of their practice. This ontological view assists in examining and critiquing basic values and premises about how one views person, humanity, environment, relationship, caring-healing, health and illness, suffering and wholeness. It helps one examine and reexamine the role and purpose of nursing (p. 186).

Anne Young
Susan Gebhardt Taylor
Katherine McLaughlin-Renpenning

REFERENCES

King, I. & Fawcett, J. (Eds.), *The language of nursing theory and metatheory*. Indianapolis: Sigma Theta Tau.
Harré, R. (1998). *The singular self*. Thousand Oaks, CA: Sage.
Peck, M.S. *In search of stones: A pilgrimage of faith, reason, and discovery*. New York: Hyperion.
Watson, J. (1999). *Postmodern nursing and beyond*. Edinburgh: Churchhill Livingstone.

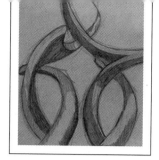

Contents

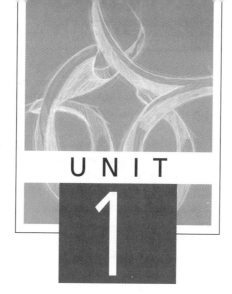

U N I T

1

NURSING RESEARCH, THEORY, and PRACTICE
Integrative Development

The links between and among nursing research, theory, and practice must be made explicit to interpret research findings, to establish the validity of theory, to articulate the outcomes of practice, and to continue to describe the discipline called nursing. The extensity of these relationships indicates the maturation of the discipline of nursing. As nursing researchers and scholars are able to join the individual bits of knowledge to a framework, the disciplinary matrix becomes more complete. Theory, research, and practice became disconnected as the discipline and profession of nursing were developing. Each of these areas developed into a specialty in its own right, and as the discipline matures, the contributions of each area to integrated systems of nursing knowledge are important.

This unit focuses on the components of the disciplinary matrix and the linkages with research and practice. Chapter 1 describes the components of theoretical systems. The nursing knowledge that fleshes out the disciplinary matrix includes empirics, ethics, aesthetics, and personal patterns of knowing. Integrated knowledge development using these four patterns will provide a complete picture of the discipline. This text focuses on empirics.

Nursing theoretical systems provide the object for nursing science and for research foundational to the practice of nursing. Research develops valid and reliable instruments for measuring theoretical and practice constructs and makes them available to other researchers and practitioners. The outcome is the development of nursing practice. These ideas are explained in Chapter 2 and are presented throughout the book.

Theory and research are important to the development of nursing practice. Theory considers how nursing practice should be constructed for intervention. Research informs practice. The implicit assumptions made by practice program designers about how to implement treatment suggest a major support for the use of theory in practice. Program theory includes the specification of what must be done to achieve desired goals, other anticipated outcomes, and how to generate these goals and impacts (Chen, 1990). The answers nursing research seeks are derived from theory and practice. The results of research are integrated into practice through the development of protocols, procedures, and practice programs. These ideas are developed in Chapter 3 and throughout the book.

Chapter 4 focuses on the integration of theory, research and practice. Collin (1992) described theoretical integration as the power of a theory or theoretical system to systematize and unify our knowledge within a particular field. Chapter 4 also summarizes the process for selecting a theoretical system.

Chen, H. (1990). *Theory-driven evaluations*. Newbury Park, CA: Sage.

Collin, F. (1992). Nursing science as an interpretive discipline: Problems and challenges. *Vard I Norden 12*(14) B23.

Developing the Discipline of Nursing Through Modeling

Objectives

- Describe the historical evolution of the nursing theoretical system.
- Examine the current state of nursing models, theories, and paradigms.
- Describe nursing as a discipline.
- Describe the overall process of the development of the discipline of nursing.
- Describe the value of the integral nature of nursing theoretical systems.
- Identify the importance of the object of a discipline to the development of theoretical systems.
- Discuss the role of philosophy in the development and analysis of nursing theoretical systems.
- Specify the structural elements of nursing theoretical systems.

Key Terms

The process of creating an abstraction of reality is called **modeling.** The product of this process is a theoretical system that comprises a philosophical foundation, a complex of conceptual models and theories, empirical evidence, and models. This chapter lays the foundation for understanding the process and elements of modeling for the discipline of nursing. **Discipline** refers to the structured body of knowledge that is unique to nursing and informs its profession and practice. Models and theories depict this structure. The subject matter, or body of knowledge, fleshes out this structure, giving the discipline substance or content. This chapter describes the overall development of the discipline of nursing. The chapter begins with a historical overview and later examines the current state of nursing models, theories, and paradigms.

HISTORICAL PERSPECTIVE
The Beginning of the Development of the Discipline

Nightingale's writings are considered the chronological beginning of modern nursing (Meleis, 1997). By laying out standards for nursing education, curriculum developers initated early work in structuring nursing knowledge (National League for Nursing Education, 1917, 1927, 1937). National League for Nursing Education documents from the first half of the twentieth century show that the knowledge content of nursing consisted of the tasks that nurses performed. This view of nursing and the idea that nursing knowledge is derived from other fields—notably, medicine—hampered the development of the body of nursing discipline-specific knowledge, until the 1950s, when the formal development of theoretical views of nursing began. At that point, nurses recognized that to meet the standards of a profession and gain a rightful place in academia, they needed to develop nursing science through research (Gunter, 1962).

Many authors, including Marriner-Tomey and Alligood (1998), Meleis (1997), the Nursing Development Conference Group (1973) and Nicoll (1992), have chronicled the history of nursing theory development. Although Nightingale typically is associated with early development of nursing practice, many other nurses contributed in earlier times and in different places; Theodore and Fredericke Fliedner in Germany and Louise de Marillac in France, for example, were pioneers. Meleis (1997) calls Roffaida Bent Saad Al-Islamiah, who accompanied the prophet Mohammed in his Islamic wars, the Eastern equivalent of Nightingale. Like Nightingale, she organized women to care for the wounded. Comparing the two women, Meleis states, "[t]hey both focused on caring, healing, promoting healthy environments, and on training other nurses" (1997, p. 27).

Nightingale's precepts became the structure for nurse education in Europe and the United States. The understanding that disease is a reparative process, that nursing ought to assist the reparative process, that the same laws of nursing pertain to the well and to the sick, and that special knowledge is needed by nurses (Nightingale, 1969) are some of the first theoretical statements in nursing. By 1917, the need for standardized education for nurses led the NLNE to develop the standard curriculum (1917), a curriculum for nursing education (1927), and a curriculum guide for nursing education (1937). The nursing leaders at that time accepted Nightingale's proposition that nursing handled illness and health both inside the hospital and at home. The nursing knowledge in books was based in the sciences as they were known at that time; the knowledge would not be accurate now (NLNE, 1917, 1927, 1937).

Nightingale's precepts remained unchanged throughout this period. Within the literature of the period, one can see that there were concerns about protecting or limiting the scope of nursing (NLNE, 1917, 1927, 1937). The need to protect the seedling profession of nursing likely delayed the development of the discipline of nursing.

As nursing moved into the second half of the twentieth century, the approach to the development of the discipline changed. Nursing began developing and articulating the purpose and nature of its contribution to health. Furthermore, the higher education community expected logically developed and justifiable curriculums for disciplines that sought academic affiliations. This spurred nurses' attempts to understand the knowledge structure and substance that make up their discipline. Justifying nursing education programs in academia required a conceptual and theoretical knowledge structure that could generate research and knowledge development. At the same time, the practice arena began to demand that scientific principles inform nursing practice. A process for making nursing judgments was adapted from the scientific method by Yura and Walsh (1967, 1973). It became apparent that although a process is necessary, knowing the end toward which that process is directed is even more crucial. Many nurses used the conceptualization of basic human needs as the end or objective for the process (Yura & Walsh, 1978). Maslow's hierarchy of human needs (1970) became the focus of curriculum for many nursing educators.

As the development of disciplinary knowledge and professional practice continued, several nursing scholars undertook the development of conceptual models and general theories of nursing. A **conceptual model** is "a network of concepts, in relationship, that accounts for broad nursing phenomena" (King & Fawcett, 1997, p. 93). A theory is the narrative that accompanies a conceptual model. It includes a description of the elements of the model and their relationships expressed in propositions. It is considered a general theory if it takes into account all instances of nursing. This work began in the 1950s. The work of these scholars culminated in the publication of models or theories of nursing. Rogers (1961, 1970), Levine (1967, 1969), Roy (1970, 1976), Orem (1971), King (1971, 1981), and Johnson (1980) were the first to move beyond defining nursing to develop more formal models or to explain the basis from which nursing science could develop. They attempted to discover the uniqueness of nursing, the nursing patient, people's behavior on their own behalf and on behalf of others, and the particular set of actions, processes, or relationships of nursing.

Each of these theorists developed conceptualizations of nursing as a *human endeavor* or nursing science as a *human science* (as opposed to physical or natural science), but they approached naming the object or focus of nursing differently. Orem conceptualized the object as the human person experiencing actual or potential limitations in his or her ability to provide ongoing self-care (Orem, 1971). Roy (1970) viewed the object of nursing as the human as an adaptive system. Rogers (1990) proposed what has become known as the Science of Unitary Human Beings—that is, unitary, irreducible human beings and their respective environments. Levine (1967) expressed the object of nursing through four principles of conservation; for Johnson (1980) the person was a behavioral system. King (1971) identified the human being as the basic element in dynamic interacting systems.

After the publication of these works in the 1960s and 1970s, the analysis, evaluation, and development of nursing theory continued. Watson (1979), Parse (1981), Neuman (1982), and other theory developers offered new approaches for substantive theoretical work. Some of these approaches are described more fully in later chapters.

Stevens (1979), Chinn and Jacobs (1983), Fawcett (1984), Meleis (1985), and others assumed the important role of theory evaluators. Each presented perspectives on models, theory and theory development, and the methods of theory analysis and evaluation. They developed and applied their criteria to the existing nursing theories or to models such as those of Orem, Rogers, and Roy. They debated the nature of theory and models in practice, the meaning of discipline, and the value and appropriateness of certain models or types of models or theories (such as grand theory) (Walker, 1971; Dickoff & James, 1968, 1971; Hardy, 1978; Donaldson & Crowley, 1978). This discussion continues today.

The Present State of Development

Nursing scholars and practitioners today remain engaged in knowledge development through theorizing and researching the substance and the structure of nursing knowledge. The meaning of nursing theory and the relationship of theory or knowledge from other disciplines to nursing theory is often expressed in middle-range theory and receives much attention. One area of discussion focuses on the meaning of nursing theory and its relationship to theory or knowledge from other disciplines. Another position suggests developing middle-range theory by incorporating theory from other disciplines. Ongoing research will attempt to validate outcomes and produce evidence-based nursing. Another position is that the development of nursing science must be based in a discipline-specific model or theory of nursing (Orem, 1997; Fawcett, 1999). This idea is the focus of this text.

The Logical Middle

The evolution of theory can be examined from both chronological and logical perspectives. Descriptions of nursing theoretical systems typically are presented in a logical manner, beginning with the philosophical structures, which are followed by models, concepts, propositions, and developed knowledge (see Marriner-Tomey & Alligood, 1998 for an example). However, the development of a structured body of knowledge does not occur linearly. Richardson (1958) observed that the development of a theory or science typically begins "in the logical middle. It begins with observations pertaining to some limited aspects of reality. Then it is noticed that some of these observed statements are logical consequences of others" (p. 36). These elements of reality and the identified relationships are modeled in words or symbols. Development then moves in one direction (philosophical) to the identification of the assumptions and underlying philosophical worldview and in another direction (logical) to the description and measurement of variables. In Richardson's view, the ultimate logical development would be a mathematical model of a portion of reality. However, he noted that the likelihood of establishing such a model for all reality is "very far from attainable because of the complexity of reality. Thus we use different models, isolating and abstracting from various aspects of reality, for different purposes" (p. 36). Nursing theorists and researchers develop meaningful, purposeful models for nursing and hope that, over time, the elements will coalesce into a meaningful whole.

Orem's Self-Care Deficit Theory of Nursing illustrates this development. Orem began her work in the logical middle with the insight persons need nursing because they are unable to care for themselves. Next, she developed the conceptual model, theories, propositions, and descriptions of theoretical elements. Wallace (1979) called Orem's work representative of moderate realism. Moderate realism suggests that a world or reality exists independent of thought and that it is possible to acquire knowledge of this world. This philosophical perspective recognizes that the reality cannot be fully known and emphasizes analogical reasoning, often in the form of modeling. (See Chapter 5.) More recently, Banfield (1997) conducted a philosophical inquiry of Orem's theory, which confirmed and elaborated on the moderate realist view. Simultaneously, a great deal of research has confirmed and extended Orem's work. A nursing scholar can begin from an understanding of moderate realism, learn the views of persons and action within that philosophical tradition, move to study Orem's conceptualizations and general theory, explore the empirical evidence, generate new research, and finally apply this to practice.

NURSING AS A DISCIPLINE

A discipline is a structured body of knowledge about a particular segment of reality. The structure serves as the matrix for examining relationships between concepts and propositions. It presents to the researcher a view of gaps in knowledge in the field and of where new knowledge, developed through research, articulates with current knowledge. The discipline provides the practitioner and potential researcher with a framework for interpreting and gaining insights into questions about nursing phenomena and practices.

The focus of a discipline is constituted by its object. **Object** defines the discipline; it designates that particular aspect of reality that is the subject of the discipline as it is knowable and expressed. Many disciplines consider the person the subject, but the ways of knowing and the types of knowledge that can be obtained in each discipline makes them different. These differences facilitate discourses related to fields and boundaries of the discipline. This is necessary because a discipline is not global (Bekel, 1998). Each discipline has a distinctive outlook and style of thinking as well as distinctive organized ideas and concepts, methods of inquiry, and modes of understanding data (Orem, 1995). Bekel (1998) asserts that the description of the object builds the center of professional endeavor of a discipline. Professional endeavor can mean the development of science and the professional practice congruent with the disciplinary object. The object is important in that it indicates the differences in scientific disciplines, the methods for investigating and exploring knowledge, and the conclusions.

Kuhn (1976) believed that a scientific community, which consists of the practitioners of a scientific specialty, is necessary for the production and validation of knowledge. This scientific community possesses a common paradigm or disciplinary matrix—*disciplinary* because it is the common possession of the practitioners of a professional discipline, and *matrix* because it is composed of ordered elements of various sorts, each requiring further specification. Suppe (1976) modified this view. He suggests that the only things necessary in the development of a discipline are sufficient agreement on (1) what theory to use, (2) what counts as good science within a particular community, (3) the relevant questions, (4) application of theories to nature, (5) what examples from which to work, and (6) the ability to communicate freely enough so that researchers and scholars seriously consider only certain characteristic problems.

These descriptions indicate that developing nursing as a discipline requires identification of an object or focus, sufficient agreement on that object, and methods of inquiry congruent with the object. The explication of disciplinary boundaries, domains, and substantive knowledge is an evolutionary process. As discussion about the object continues, varying and sometimes opposing positions will emerge. The different ontologies or theoretical approaches described in Unit 2 reflect this.

MODELING NURSING: PHILOSOPHICAL PERSPECTIVES

Much of the early work in nursing theory development and evaluation emphasized the differentiation of theories from conceptual models. Theorists develop models by using existing knowledge about the nature of the object of the discipline. Models and the philosophical underpinnings precede and guide the development of research and practice programs. A nursing scholar must work from a nursing-specific theoretical system and model. Theory, research, and practice that are congruent with that model can then be developed. Fawcett (1999) observed that nursing will not survive as a distinct discipline if it does not end its romance with nonnursing disciplines. She emphasized the need for nurses to practice from a nursing discipline-specific perspective and to conduct nursing discipline-specific research.

This does not mean that only one model or theoretical system for the discipline of nursing exists but proposes that, regardless of the theoretical system the practitioner or researcher chooses, it should be nursing discipline-specific. The ability to interpret the findings of research, to establish the validity of theory, articulate the outcomes of practice, and to continue describing nursing relies on this specificity. The established theoretical systems and models can be examined in the sense of theory evaluation and comparison through the range of their statements regarding the object of the discipline. Bekel (1998) contends that the examination of nursing theories in the sense of the range of their statements regarding the object would retain the potential of each theoretical system. The descriptions of theoretical systems in Unit 2 demonstrate the range of objects for the discipline. Eventually, a coalescing and refinement into a limited number of nursing discipline-specific theoretical systems with agreement on the object of the discipline could be expected.

The development of theory is considered first in its philosophical context and then for its specific knowledge domains. The philosophical structure used in this text follows from the traditional Aristotelian classification of the various branches of philosophy, namely cosmology, ontology, and epistemology (Wallace, 1977). The basic structures of philosophy for the specific theoretical systems detailed in later chapters are described in the following sections. Many different approaches and terms can express concepts related to theory and philosophy of nursing, and definitions of these are included. Comparative analyses of these terms also can be found in other works, such as those of Chinn and Kramer (1999) and King and Fawcett (1997).

Cosmology

Cosmology is the study of the whole universe, including theories about its origin, evolution, structure, and future. This typically includes the meaning and place of human beings within this universe. Although cosmology has the widest view of reality, the beginning point of cosmology is the ontology, which is defined in the next section of this chapter. The development of a theoretical system begins in the center, grounded in human reality, and expands outward to the perspective of the whole of the universe.

The specification of a cosmology foundational to a particular nursing theoretical system is a recent development. However, all theorists work from or hold specific views of the universe, sometimes referred to as worldviews, that are foundational to their conceptualizations. In 1997 Roy presented the cosmology underpinning her theory (see Chapter 10). She speaks directly about a god or transcendent being as an essential part of nursing theory, research, and practice. Watson (1999) posits a cosmology and ontology of transpersonal caring in which "the sacred feminine archetype is considered to be the very basis of reality" (p. 286). Other theorists leave the cosmology that is foundational to their views of the world to be inferred. For example, Rogers posits a universe of open systems and energy fields. Although she offers no further explanation or speculation about the universe's origin, she describes a theory of expanding evolution. The specific views of theorists are described more fully in later chapters.

The meaning of cosmology to nursing is not well established in the literature; however, the extensive literature on spirituality suggests that the meaning of a transcendent reality is a part of many nurses' worldviews. The introduction of cosmology into the discussion of nursing philosophy leads to a deeper exploration of the meaning of being that surpasses traditional considerations of person or self.

Religion and Cosmology. Philosophy deals with what humans can know through experiential evidence and reason. Faith, by definition, is separated from reason; it does not rest on logical proof or material evidence. Klubertanz (1953) states that a faith "can be held and carried out in practice, even to a very high degree of perfection, without any philosophy (or theology) whatsoever" (p. 278). Likewise, philosophy can be carried out without faith. For many nurses, reality is a conjunction of philosophy and faith. One's faith informs one's philosophy—that is, it forms and shapes the questions and answers about reality; it reflects the "unity of personality" (Klubertanz, 1953, p. 280). A person's faith must be congruent with rationally held views of reality. This is an important consideration for exploring nursing theoretical systems. If one's philosophical and personal views conflict, which will direct beliefs and values about nursing?

Ontology

Ontology refers to the totality of assumptions about the nature of the world or the portion of reality in question. Ontology examines the nature of being. In nursing, the primary ontology is the nature of person. Roy identified the person as an adaptive system. For Orem, the basic nature of human beings is that of agent, and for Rogers, the human is an energy field. An ontology, according to Harré & Gillett (1994), is a "systematic exposition of the assumptions about basic categories being admitted to the universe in some scientific field" (p. 29). An ontology should involve a location system, a basic class or classes of entities, and some type of structured relations that hold all these entities together in a single world.

Why is it important to know the ontology from which theories and models are developed? Harré's description (1998) of ontology suggests the answer to this question. He states:

Ontologies are, in effect, grammars. They are specifications, some explicit, some implicit, of ways of identifying and marking the boundaries of particulars for some purpose or other. Sciences are created by choosing an ontology—or, more likely, finding oneself already committed to one in the way one has been thinking and acting—through the use of which phenomena are to be identified and ordered and explanations are to be constructed. Ontologies, as expressed in grammars, loosely fix the forms of discourse appropriate to this or that human project, including laying out the project. Ontologies also fix methods. Since ontologies are prior to phenomena there is always a choice. In the end the choice of ontology is largely justified pragmatically: how many of the phenomena of interest does it enable us to comprehend in a fruitful and constructive way? (p. 47)

The nursing knowledge develops within an ontology. The ontology provides the language for talking about nursing. It directs the methods that can answer questions about phenomena that interest nurses. Explanation involves identifying or linking independent phenomena with aspects of a common ontology. Furthermore, the ontology tells us how to "be" as nurses, directing the characteristics of the practice and the practitioner. Reed (1997) suggested that the ontology of the discipline of nursing be defined as an "inherent human process of well-being, manifested by complexity and integration of human systems" (p. 76). Rawnsley (1998) noted a need to distinguish the particular ontology being described, since these could differ radically or even contradict.

Nurses currently use a variety of ontologies. Unit 2 describes the ontology that is identified or that can be inferred for each of the included theoretical systems. Harré noted that the assumptions of the ontology constrain the type of hypotheses that can be constructed. The concepts used in stating a hypothesis must be in keeping with one's general picture of the world. In selecting a theoretical system to use for research or practice, the theorist must know the ontology and understand how to discuss a specific area of nursing.

Epistemology

Epistemology is the study of knowledge itself: what it is, what its properties are, and why it has these properties. Epistemology seeks answers about the properties of truth and falsity, the nature of evidence, and the certainty that evidence produces in scientific knowledge (Wallace, 1977). Knowledge can be speculative or practical. *Speculative* knowledge is knowledge for its own sake, whereas *practical* knowledge exists for the sake of *operation*, e.g., the arts of making things, or *conduct*, e.g., the arts of directing human activity. The development of knowledge occurs through reflective thought and through science. To the extent that a practical science engages in analysis, it can speculate and use analytical procedures similar to those of the speculative sciences. A practical science seeks to produce its object and needs scientific knowledge to do this. It also must be complemented by an art or habit (e.g., prudence) that has as a proper concern the individual act in all its concrete circumstances (Wallace, 1977).

MODELING NURSING: THEORETICAL PERSPECTIVES
Definition of a Model

There are two basic types of models: concrete and abstract. For the purposes of this discussion, the following considers only abstract models. The heart of any scientific treatment of a field of phenomena, according to Harré and Gillett (1994), is a central model that represents the ontology. A **model** is a virtual or imagined system that bears varying degrees of relevant similarity to aspects of the real world it represents. Models are essentially ambiguous in that they are capable of interpretation. They may be considered representations of ways of understanding (observable properties) or as pictures of things that cannot be observed (unobservable properties or processes). A model controls the abstraction of features from the complex phenomena observed in some field of interest (Harré and Gillett, 1994). It is a system of relations used to represent another system of relations. The model may be depicted in symbols, words, numbers, or a combination of these. In nursing, models that depict the ontology are often called general models or grand models. Some models show the relationships of variables under study. In practice, models can depict a process, an interaction, a practice program, or a segment of such a program. Unit 2 illustrates many of these types of models.

A model may be evaluated by its conformity to the part of reality it is supposed to predict (Chen, 1990). Wallace (1996) explained a model as "an analogue or analogy that assists or promotes the gradual understanding of something not readily grasped in sense experience" (p. 5). He explained that models or analogies are helpful because

> we learn from things around us by noting similarities and differences. When we encounter something new, we attempt to understand it by conceiving it after the fashion of what is already familiar to us. We thus use things we know, or at least think we know, to advance into the realm of the unknown (p. 5).

Many practitioners of nursing use models or analogies when instructing patients; educators use models and analogies extensively in the classroom to convey new ideas. When working with models, scientists compare properties of things and types of systems within particular contexts (Wallace, 1996).

Modeling is the process of developing and providing an abstraction of reality—that is, a model (Wallace, 1994). The character and result of this process depends on the model's intended use. If the model is to provide normative guidelines—what one ought to do—it will be deductive and may represent a very idealized view of reality. Conversely, if the model is to describe reality, various inductive techniques are used, the most prominent being statistical analysis (Wallace, 1994). The process of modeling typically goes through the stages of problem conceptualization or formulation, model formalization, and validation. The resulting model is then implemented in research or practice. Although models and modeling are helpful or essential in understanding the structure and relationships of concepts, some limitations remain. One of these is most models' inherent assumptions of normality in a situation. Another limitation is that a good model may be used for the wrong purpose or in the wrong situation. If the model is being used to design a clinical program, these errors can cause significant problems. Chapter 3 presents a more detailed discussion of the use of models in designing clinical programs.

Definition of a Theory

A **theory** simply describes the nature and workings of a model. Theory is a frame of reference that helps humans to understand their world and to function in it. Theory provides not only guidelines for analyzing a phenomenon but also a scheme for understanding the significance of research findings (Chen, 1990). Theory is generally defined as a set of interrelated assumptions, principles, and/or propositions to explain or guide action. Nursing literature contains many definitions of theory. One widely accepted definition is that theory is a purposeful systematic abstraction of reality (Chinn & Kramer, 1995). This definition is congruent with the views expressed in this text. A **general theory** in a practice field descriptively explains the dominant features and relationships that characterize the field's practice situations. General theories structure what is already known and provide foundations for the continued development, structuring, and validation of knowledge (Orem, 1991).

Other types of theories are based on the level of abstraction or scope of variables included in the theory. These are referred to as middle-range and micro theories. A general theory covers a broad scope, whereas these are narrower and include only a portion of the scope of the broader theory. King's Conceptual System includes the middle-range Theory of Goal Attainment. Chinn and Kramer (1999) identified and defined many types of theory on the basis of scope, focus, and level of specificity: grand, atomistic, wholistic, macro, meta, micro, middle-range, molar, molecular, empiric, ethical, armchair, and grounded. This listing points to the complexity of theory work and the need to specify the type of theory being used or developed.

For the purposes of this text, the important levels of nursing theory are general and middle-range. General theory, explaining a general model of nursing, represents a complete view of nursing, whereas midrange or **middle-range theories** explain conceptual models that represent a partial view of nursing practice. Middle-range theory consists of concepts, propositions, or relational statements from which testable hypotheses can be derived and empirically measured. The development of middle-range theory can use theory or concepts from other disciplines synthesized into a nursing discipline-specific theory to explain practice. Research validates outcomes and produces evidence-based nursing. Fawcett (1997) makes a distinction between models and theories that are based on level of abstraction, but she does not link conceptual models and grand theories in her description. However, the distinction between conceptual models and grand theories has limited value.

A **nursing theoretical system** comprises (1) a general model and theory of nursing that is placed within a particular philosophical tradition and structures the discipline, (2) the models and middle-range theories and empirical referents, and (3) the models that give direction to practice.

Definition of a Paradigm

In nursing theory literature, the term **paradigm** often refers to "a worldview or ideology, a medium within which the theory, knowledge, and processes for knowing find meaning and coherence and are expressed" (Chinn & Kramer, 1995, p. 76). This definition is similar to the definition of ontology in this text. For clarity, this text uses the term *paradigm* to mean only *paradigms of inquiry*—that is, the following:

> the operating rules about the appropriate relationship among theories, methods and evidence that constitute the actual practices of the members of a scientific community, research program or tradition. [They] are the combination of theoretical assumptions, methodological procedures and standards of evidence that are taken for granted in particular works, are in the foreground (Alford, 1998, p. 2).

Paradigms are described in Chapter 2.

The Meaning of Metaphor in Nursing Theory

Metaphor is a language structure used extensively in writing about nursing. The use of the metaphor as a tool is both common and essential as new ways of looking at nursing and nursing science develop. Metaphor, in the broadest sense, sees something from the viewpoint of something else; it is an attempt to integrate diverse phenomena without destroying their unique differences. Metaphor transfers a term from one system of dimensional level of meaning to another. It is the "conscious application of relationships between the knower and the known. Metaphor is a connection between our consciousness and some tangible or sensible phenomenon, whether it be in a poem or in the heuristics of a diagnostic procedure" (Wallace, 1996, p. 41). A worldview is a product of human reason and is presented and understood through metaphors. "Metaphors represent the ways in which many kinds of discourses are structured and powerfully influence how we conceive things" (Watson, 1996, p. 12) and "reflect the prevailing cosmology of the time" (Watson, 1996, p. 59). Much of what is written about nursing is metaphorical. Watson (1999) seeks to "deconstruct and reconstruct" metaphors in her conceptualizations and musings about nursing. All theories or writings about theory contain metaphors that communicate meaning, suggest paths for action, and enhance concept and theory development (Smith, 1992). It is important to distinguish metaphors from science. Both are important, but they are not the same.

OUTCOMES OF MODELING NURSING

Two major outcomes can be expected from the development of nursing theoretical systems. One is scientific, systematized knowledge for nursing practice that also can be used in designing research and curriculum. The second is a formalized statement of a philosophical worldview on which to base further understanding of nursing theory. The development of knowledge fluctuates between these ends, at one time using empirical methods to generate a particular type of knowledge known as science and at other time using modes of inquiry that clarify the philosophical assumptions underlying the theory. Carper (1978) defined four "patterns of knowing, namely, empirics, ethics, personal, and esthetics, each an aspect of the whole of knowing, each making a unique contribution to the whole and each equally vital to the whole of knowing" (Chinn & Kramer, 1995, p. 4). At any time, the development of knowledge moves dynamically between the philosophical and the scientific, the empirical and the ethical, the speculative and the practical, and the formal and the personal. Nursing scholars' work reflects diverse theoretical conceptualizations, methodologies, and meanings.

Marriner-Tomey and Alligood (1998) identified some characteristics of middle-range nursing theory as "specific to nursing practice" and to "the area of practice, age range of the client, the nursing action or intervention, and the proposed outcome" (p. 333). Fawcett (1999) described middle-range theories as "narrower in scope than grand theories, made up of a limited number of concepts and propositions written at a relatively concrete and specific level, and generated and tested by empirical research" (p. 5). It would seem that general theories beget middle-range theories, whereas middle-range theories beget more middle-range theories. Liehr and Smith (1999) clarified some of the issues regarding middle-range theory. Among other things, they proposed categorizing middle-range theory by level of abstraction (i.e., high middle, middle, low middle). They noted that all middle-range theories generated through research and published in nursing journals since 1995 included diagrammed models.

A number of general nursing theories have evolved into theoretical systems. More formal knowledge work is necessary to move the development of nursing as a science. The development of middle-range theories is a part of this work. Again, in addition to general theories and conceptual models, theoretical systems include middle-range theories and integrated knowledge. Fawcett (1999) refers to this substructure as the "conceptual-theoretical-empirical structure" (p. 31). Middle-range theory development typically begins with identifying a concept derived from the broader general nursing theory. Concepts or theories from other disciplines often complement the development of the concept under study. Philosophical and logical congruence between the general theory, the focal concept, complementary theory or theories, and empirical methods is essential. Ulbrich (1999) developed a middle-range theory of exercise through triangulation of Orem's Self-Care Deficit Nursing Theory, the transtheoretical model of exercise behavior, and characteristics of a population at risk for cardiovascular disease. (See Figure 4-1 later in the text for the model used by Ulbrich to develop this middle-range theory.)

Summary

- Nursing theoretical systems have evolved from early writings to well-developed formal systems. The development began in the logical middle and moved in a philosophical direction—toward identifying the assumptions and underlying philosophical worldview and in a logical direction—toward describing and measuring variables.
- The current state of nursing models, theories and paradigms has engaged nursing scholars and practitioners in knowledge development through theorizing and researching the substance and structure of knowledge that form the discipline of nursing and inform the practice of nursing. The meaning of nursing theory and the relationship of theory or knowledge from other disciplines to nursing theory through middle-range theory are receiving much attention.
- The discipline of nursing is the structured body of knowledge unique to nursing. It informs the profession and practice of nursing. The development of this knowledge moves dynamically between the philosophical and the scientific, the empirical and the ethical, the speculative and the practical, the formal and the personal. A discipline has a distinctive outlook and style of thinking as well as distinctive organized ideas and concepts, methods of inquiry, and modes of understanding data.
- For nursing to be described as a discipline, there must be identification of an object or focus, sufficient agreement on that object, and methods of inquiry that are congruent with the object within the discipline. Development of disciplinary boundaries, domains, and substantive knowledge is also necessary.
- The unity in nursing theoretical systems begins with identifying the object of the discipline, based in a formalized statement of a philosophical worldview. Next, scientific, systematized knowledge for nursing practice can design research and curricula for advancing nursing theory. Nursing theoretical systems provide the object for nursing science and research that is foundational to the practice of nursing.

- The focus of a discipline is constituted by its object. This facilitates discourses related to fields and boundaries of the discipline. The description of the object builds the center of professional endeavor of a discipline.
- Philosophy considers what humans can know through experiential evidence and reason. The development of theory is considered first in its philosophical context and then in terms of its specific knowledge domains and various branches of philosophy, namely, cosmology, ontology, and epistemology.
- The structural elements of nursing theoretical systems include models and theories of general and middle-range levels of abstraction.

REFERENCES

Alford, R.R. (1998). *The craft of inquiry.* New York: Oxford University Press.

Banfield, B. (1997). *A philosophical inquiry of Orem's self-care deficit nursing theory.* Unpublished doctoral dissertation, Wayne State University.

Bekel, G. (1998, February-March). *Statements on the object of science: A discussion paper.* Paper presented at the meeting of the Orem Study Group. Savannah, GA. Published in *IOS Newsletter, 7* (1999), 1-3.

Carper, B.A. (1978). Fundamental patterns of knowing in nursing. *Advances in Nursing Science, 1*(1), 13-23.

Chen, H. (1990). *Theory-driven evaluations.* Newbury Park, CA: Sage Publications.

Chinn, P. & Jacobs, M. (1983). *Theory and nursing: A systematic approach.* St. Louis: Mosby.

Chinn, P. & Kramer, M. (1995). *Theory and nursing: A systematic approach.* (4th ed.). St. Louis: Mosby.

Chinn, P. & Kramer, M. (1999). *Theory and nursing: Integrated knowledge development.* (5th ed.). St. Louis: Mosby.

Dickoff, J. & James, P. (1968). On theory development in nursing. A theory of theories. *Nursing Research, 17*(3), 197-203.

Dickoff, J. & James, P. (1971). Clarity to what end? *Nursing Research, 20*(6), 499-502.

Donaldson, S.K. & Crowley, D.M. (1978). The discipline of nursing. *Nursing Outlook, 26*(2), 113-120.

Fawcett, J. (1984). *Analysis and evaluation of conceptual models of nursing.* Philadelphia: F.A. Davis.

Fawcett, J. (1997). The structural hierarchy of nursing knowledge: Components and theory definitions. In I. King & J. Fawcett (Eds.), *The language of nursing theory and metatheory.* Indianapolis: Sigma Theta Tau.

Fawcett, J. (1999). The state of nursing science: Hallmarks of the 20th and 21st centuries. *Nursing Science Quarterly, 12*(4), 311-314.

Gunter, L.M. (1962). Notes on a theoretical framework for nursing research. *Nursing Research, 11*(4), 219-222.

Hardy, M. (1978). Perspectives on nursing theory. *Advances in Nursing Science, 1*(1), 37-48.

Harré, R. (1998). *The singular self.* Thousand Oaks, CA: Sage.

Harré, R. & Gillett, G. (1994). *The discursive mind.* Thousand Oaks, CA: Sage.

Johnson, D.E. (1980). The behavioral systems model for nursing. In J.P. Riehl & C. Roy (Eds.), *Conceptual models for nursing practice* (2nd ed.). New York: Appleton-Century-Crofts.

King, I.M. (1971). *Toward a theory for nursing.* New York: John Wiley & Sons, Inc.

King, I.M. (1981). *A theory for nursing.* New York: John Wiley & Sons.

King, I.M. & Fawcett, J. (Eds.), (1997). *The language of nursing theory and metatheory.* Indianapolis: Sigma Theta Tau.

Klubertanz, G.P. (1953). *The philosophy of human nature.* New York: Appleton-Century-Crofts.

Kuhn, T. (1976). Second thoughts on paradigms. In F. Suppe (Ed.), *The Structure of Scientific Theories,* (2nd ed.). Urbana: University of Illinois.

Levine, M.E. (1967). The four conservation principles of nursing. *Nursing Forum, 6*(1), 45.

Levine, M.E. (1969). *Introduction to clinical nursing.* Philadelphia: F.A. Davis.

Liehr, P. & Smith, M.J. (1999). Middle-range theory: Spinning research and practice to create knowledge for the new millennium. *Advances in Nursing Science, 21*(4), 81-91.

Marriner-Tomey, A. & Alligood, M. (1998). *Nursing theorists and their work.* (4th ed.). St. Louis: Mosby.

Maslow, A.H. (1970). *Motivation and personality.* New York: Harper & Row.

Meleis, A. (1985). *Theoretical nursing: Development and progress.* Philadelphia: Lippincott.

Meleis, A.I. (1997). *Theoretical nursing: Development and progress.* (3rd ed.). Philadelphia: Lippincott.

National League of Nursing Education. (1917, 1927, 1937). *A Curriculum Guide for Schools of Nursing.* New York: Author.

Neuman, B. (1982). *The Neuman systems model: Application to nursing education and practice.* Norwalk, CT: Appleton-Century-Crofts.

Nicoll, L. (1992). *Perspectives on nursing theory.* Philadelphia: Lippincott.

Nightingale, F. (1969). *Notes on nursing: What it is, and what it is not.* New York: Dover.

Nursing Development Conference Group. (1973). *Concept formalization in nursing.* Boston: Little, Brown.

Orem, D.E. (1997). Views of human beings specific to nursing. *Nursing Science Quarterly, 10*(1), 26-31.

Orem, D.E. (1971). *Nursing: Concepts of practice.* New York: McGraw-Hill.

Orem, D.E. (1991). *Nursing: Concepts of practice.* (3rd ed.). St. Louis: Mosby.

Orem, D.E. (1995). *Nursing: Concepts of practice.* (5th ed.). St. Louis: Mosby.

Parse, R.R. (1981). *Man-living-health: A theory of nursing.* New York: John Wiley & Sons.

Rawnsley, M. (1998). Ontology, epistemology, and methodology: A clarification. *Nursing Science Quarterly, 11*(1), 2-4.

Reed, P. (1997). Nursing: The ontology of the discipline. *Nursing Science Quarterly, 10*(2), 76-79.

Richardson, M. (1958). *Fundamentals of mathematics.* New York: Macmillan.

Rogers, M.E. (1961). *Educational revolution in nursing.* New York: Macmillan.

Rogers, M.E. (1970). An introduction to the theoretical basis of nursing. Philadelphia: F.A. Davis.

Rogers, M.E. (1990). Nursing: Science of unitary, irreducible, human beings: Update 1990. In E.A.M. Barrett (Ed.), *Visions of Rogers' science-based nursing.* New York: National League for Nursing.

Roy, C. (1970). Adaptation: A conceptual framework in nursing. *Nursing Outlook, 18*(3), 42-45.

Roy, C. (1976). *Introduction to nursing: An adaptation model.* Englewood Cliffs, NJ: Prentice-Hall.

Smith, M.C. (1992). Metaphor in nursing theory. *Nursing Science Quarterly, 5*(2), 48-49.

Stevens, B. (1979). *Nursing theory: Analysis, application, evaluation.* Philadelphia: Lippincott.

Suppe, F. (1976). *The structure of scientific theories.* (2nd ed.). Urbana: University of Illinois.

Ulbrich, S.L. (1999). Nursing practice theory of exercise as self-care. *Image, 31*(1), 65-70,

Walker, L.O. (1971). Toward a clearer understanding of the concept of nursing theory. *Nursing Research, 20*(5), 428-435.

Wallace, W.A. (1977). *The elements of philosophy.* New York: Alba House.

Wallace, W.A. (1979). *From a realist point of view: Essays on the philosophy of science.* Washington, DC: University Press of America.

Wallace, W.A. (1994). *Ethnics in modeling.* Tarrytown, NY: Pergamon.

Wallace, W.A. (1996). *The modeling of nature.* Washington, DC: The Catholic University of America.

Watson, J. (1979). *Nursing: The philosophy and science of caring.* Boston: Little, Brown.

Watson, J. (1999). *Postmodern nursing and beyond.* New York: Churchill Livingstone.

Yura, H. & Walsh, M.B. (1967). *The nursing process: Assessing, planning, implementing, evaluating.* New York: Appleton-Century-Crofts.

Yura, H. & Walsh, M.B. (1973). *The nursing process: Assessing, planning, implementing, evaluating.* (2nd ed.). New York: Appleton-Century-Crofts.

Yura, H. & Walsh, M.B. (1978). *Human needs and the nursing process.* New York: Appleton-Century-Crofts.

C H A P T E R

2

Nursing Theory and Research
UNDERSTANDING the CONNECTIONS

Objectives

- Compare and contrast key characteristics of paradigms of discovery, including positivism, postpositivism, critical theory, and constructivism.
- Depict the reciprocal interaction of theory and research.
- Specify how theory can be used to generate research questions.
- Examine similarities and differences between theory-generating and theory-testing research.
- Discuss mechanisms for evaluating research studies.
- Specify essential attributes for reliability and validity of research instruments.

Key Terms

Chapter 1 focused on the evolution of theory and the current state of theories within nursing. This chapter, which discusses the connection between theory and research, will extend the discussion of paradigms of discovery and examine the influence of specific scientific modes of discovery on nursing theory and research. As nursing theory evolves, understanding what is known and how it came to be known is important. Knowing is a continuing process in which new ways of thinking modify the conceptualization of reality. Through research, science provides a mechanism for knowing. Worldviews or belief systems about discovery influence research and the types of questions. Because nursing theory is intertwined with research, it is important to understand the connection between the two and the dynamics surrounding discovery.

This chapter contains two major sections. The first part of the chapter presents a philosophical discussion of the connections between research and theory mediated by their scientific underpinnings. The role of theory in generating research questions and of research in generating theory is discussed. The second portion of the chapter provides guidelines for evaluating research instruments.

UNDERSTANDING THE CONNECTION

Students of nursing theory and research courses often hear that nursing theory and research are connected. This raises questions of how they are connected and why the connection is important. The Preface introduced the *nexus*, an irregularly shaped continuous line that permits movement either directly or circuitously. The interaction of nursing theory, research, and practice demonstrates a mutual dynamic between practice and theory formation and generation of research questions with theory suggesting research, research supporting theory, and research influencing practice. This interconnectedness informs each aspect of nursing theory, research, and practice.

As Chapter 1 indicated, knowledge often begins in the logical middle. Observations in practice may lead to understanding consequences of action that in turn may lead to the conceptualization and measurement of variables or back to the identification of underlying assumptions and a philosophical worldview. The fluidity associated with this process is critical to connecting theory and research. Knowledge does not necessarily develop linearly. Rather, the process may be irregular, with discovery occurring from different directions and then coming together again to form a way of knowing or understanding a particular phenomenon of interest.

Paradigms of Discovery

Nursing's scientific roots have significantly influenced methods for discovery, which in turn influence connections between theory and research. In developing its science, nursing has used paradigms of inquiry from other sciences. Although several ways of classifying paradigms exist, this discussion is guided by the four alternative paradigms of inquiry identified by Guba and Lincoln (1994). These paradigms–positivism, post-positivism, critical theory, and constructivism–have been adopted in nursing to varying degrees. The key characteristics of these paradigms are presented in Table 2-1. Understanding these philosophical worldviews is important because they influence the choice of research questions and methods of discovery. This process, in turn, influences nursing theory.

Historically, nursing research, like the hard sciences, has embraced a form of scientific inquiry embedded in positivism. The foundational belief in **positivism** is that a discoverable

TABLE 2-1

Characteristics of Research Paradigms

	Positivism	Postpositivism	Critical Theory	Constructivism
Ontology	Realism	Critical realism	Historical realism	Relativism
Epistemology	Dualist	Modified dualist/objectivist	Transactional/subjectivist/value mediated	Transactional/subjectivist/created findings
Research Aims	Explain, predict, control	Explain, predict, control	Critique, transform	Understand, reconstruct
Nature of Knowledge	Verified hypotheses establish facts	Nonfalsified hypotheses establish probable facts	Structural/historical insights transform over time	Individual reconstructions, centered around consensus; subject to revision
Research Setting	Highly controlled	Less controlled	May use natural setting	May use natural setting
Research Methods	Quantitative—Experimental	Quantitative—modified experimental; qualitative permitted	Primarily qualitative Dialogical/dialectical	Primarily qualitative Hermeneutical/dialectical

Modified from Guba, E.G., & Lincoln, Y.S. (1994). Competing paradigms in qualitative research. In E.K. Denzin & Y.S. Lincoln (Eds.), *Handbook of qualitative research*. Thousand Oaks, CA: Sage.

reality exists (Guba & Lincoln, 1994). Positivism represents the "received view," in which researchers unquestioningly accepted recognized methods of scientific discovery. Positivism has dominated discovery in the physical and social sciences for the past 400 years. The ontology is sometimes labeled "realism" and is exemplified by the belief in the existence of a reality driven by natural laws or mechanisms. In this view, research seeks to discover reality or truth and aims to explain, predict, and control phenomena. The research process attempts to objectify experiences, formally testing propositions and hypotheses to verify reality. In the positivist model truth is discovered through methods that promote freedom from bias, have mechanisms for verification, and use reductionistic approaches. Positivist research is quantitative and carefully controlled so as to minimize the influence of confounding variables. Rigorously prescribed procedures of study are used to prevent influence from values or biases. Although positivism has a respected, longstanding history in the scientific community, these methods do not always capture some of the practice-oriented perspectives associated with nursing (Gortner, 1990).

A variation of the positivist model, **postpositivism** attempts to respond to some of the criticisms of positivism. Although it retains many positivist tenets, postpositivism holds that reality can only be imperfectly understood (Guba & Lincoln, 1994). In this instance the ontology is called critical realism. Postpositivism considers reality only incompletely knowable due to flawed human intellect and the difficulty in studying phenomena. The goal of research is to gain knowledge through attempts at falsifying hypotheses. Hypotheses that are not falsified are considered representations of reality, at least as accurately as it can be known. Objectivity, with sensitivity to how findings fit within existing knowledge and to critique by a community of peers, remains important. Inquiry occurs in less controlled settings, and situational information is perceived as more important. Interviews and observations may be significant sources of data. Research methods may include modified experimental designs and the use of qualitative methods.

Critical theory is a broad term describing several paradigms that can include neo-Marxism, feminism, materialism, and participatory inquiry (Guba & Lincoln, 1994). Three substrands of critical theory include poststructuralism, postmodernism, and a combination of both. Critical theory, ontologically called historical realism, holds that reality is shaped by social, political, cultural, economic, ethnic, and gender factors that become crystallized into structures (Guba & Lincoln, 1994). Critical theory aims to critique and transform structures that permit human exploitation. In critical theory the investigator and subjects are linked interactively, and the investigator's values influence the process.

The key to understanding any strand or variation of critical theory is that inquiry is value-mediated, which means that findings are value-dependent. For example, a feminist investigator interpreting research data filters data through a feminist lens that would ultimately influence interpretation of research findings. This process would assist in freeing the knower from other biases that might distort interpretation of findings. Critical theorists consider knowledge to be structural or historical insight that may change over time as more informed insights or ways of thinking about the structure become available. Barnum (1998) interprets this process as inviting the researcher "to exchange one interpretative lens for another" (p. 272). Critical theorists may use a variety of research techniques—both quantitative and qualitative—although the dialogue between researcher and respondent is considered a key to empowerment and change. Dialectical methods of inquiry incorporate a dialogue that challenges individuals to transform accepted ways of thinking to more informed ways of thinking. Researchers using feminist perspectives to guide the research process demonstrate one example of critical social theory in nursing.

The final paradigm, **constructivism,** is ontologically relativist; realities are known through mental constructions (Guba & Lincoln, 1994). Relativism implies that truth is relative and may vary depending on the individual or group. Mental constructions are the ways in which individuals perceive or construct reality. Knowledge stems from the interaction between the investigator and respondents and is composed of constructions (mental interpretations) in which a relative consensus exists. However, more than one relative consensus can exist—or even conflict—at any given time. Knowledge grows through a more sophisticated and informed worldview acquired when more information becomes known. Hermeneutics and dialectical interchange are techniques of discovery used with constructivist research.

Hermeneutics focus on interpretation. Derived from phenomenological research approaches, hermeneutic methods are used to discover how humans understand experience by highlighting what is and by uncovering hidden meanings (Barnum, 1998; Welch, 1999). **Dialectical interchange** compares and contrasts individual understandings and enables investigators to make sense of the collective constructions by wholistically merging them so that the whole is considered greater than the sum of the parts (Barnum, 1998; Guba & Lincoln, 1994).

Although these four views—positivism, postpositivism, critical theory, and constructivism—are characteristically different, they provide powerful paradigms for guiding the discovery of truth. Hence nurses need to examine how each of these mechanisms for discovery might be reflected in the connection between theory and research. For example, an investigator approaching a research problem from a positivist perspective would investigate a narrow aspect of a phenomenon in a highly controlled setting. Thus only a piece of a theoretical framework could be investigated within the context of one study. Knowledge from a successive series of studies would accumulate and add to the knowledge base, permitting generalization and establishing cause-and-effect linkages. A positivist mode appealingly offers extensive control and thus a sense of certainty about discoveries. However, one concern about this perspective is the 'blind man describing the elephant' problem. Connections between the individual pieces may be found, but the whole picture of the elephant may not be discovered. On the other hand, an investigator studying a phenomenon from a constructivist perspective would ask research questions in a broader context and study the phenomena in natural settings. Descriptions derived regarding phenomena of interest are more wholistic and remain interpretable as more information becomes known. However, researchers guided by more traditional scientific paradigms consider these methods of discovery suspect.

Chinn and Kramer (1995) compare the connection between theory and research to an interactive spiral. Fawcett (1978) envisioned the connection between theory and research as a double helix in which theory is inextricably bound to both theory generation and theory testing through research. How an investigator proceeds with a particular study may depend on the purpose of the research. In theory-generating research, the investigator may know specifics about the clinical nature of the problem under investigation. In theory-testing research, the investigator can call on an established theory to describe or predict the outcomes of relationships. Although both processes are theory-linked, the research activities may differ according to the designated purpose.

This reciprocal interaction of research and theory can occur in two directions. In one direction, research guided by theory can clarify and extend the theory or suggest needed modifications. This deductive approach begins with abstract propositions derived from theory and then moves toward more specific applications. In this manner, theory stimulates thinking and directs research, permitting theory testing. Positivist and postpositivist methods of inquiry usually can be used in this process. Thus theory is not formed in a vacuum but depends on research for concepts and propositions. Observation or measurement of selected phenomena through research generates theory. This is an inductive process; specific and concrete observations build more general or abstract ideas. Postpositivist, critical theoretical, or constructivist paradigms of inquiry may be useful to inductive theory generation. As practitioners, nurses have a rich resource of experience that can generate explanations of common phenomena. For theory to be relevant and useful, practitioners and scientists must collaborate in generating clinically applicable theories.

Phenomena of concern to nursing tend to be complex and multifaceted. Therefore programs of research, building on previous findings and hinging on a theoretical system, are essential for a research-based practice. Whether theory is used to generate research questions or to develop theory, research enables discovery and thus further theorization. Theory enriches the value and interpretability of research and helps link the work of multiple researchers so that unique and common aspects of research about a phenomenon can be recognized. This mechanism makes nursing research findings more broadly applicable. Theory cohesively guides the generation of research by assisting the conceptualization of variables and suggesting potential relationships among them. In turn, research findings help to support or refute theoretical concepts related to nursing. Although nursing does not have a unified theory, a variety of grand and middle-range theories can explain some of the complexities of practice.

Although theory-linked research offers many advantages over isolated research, Chinn and Kramer (1995) warn of some pitfalls. For example, inappropriate use of theories can cause errors in judgment or interpretation. A theory meant to describe a particular phenomenon within a particular context may not be automatically transferable to a related group. Theories can become barriers if investigators permit them to become blinders and fail to recognize deviations from theoretically proposed outcomes. Researchers need to ensure that theory is not permitted to limit thinking about the full range of possibilities found within a phenomenon. To do so would limit the needed extension of a theoretical explanation of the phenomenon. Finally, the mental range of possibilities offered by theory can potentially extend beyond those that can be ethically tested. The rights and dignity of research participants must always be protected to avoid unwarranted exposure to risk.

Using Theory to Generate Research Ideas

A well-developed theory is an accurate depiction of the real world useful for generating research questions. Fawcett (1995) suggests that good theories give researchers sufficient direction about research questions to ask and about the methodology to use. For example, a nurse familiar with the Neuman Systems Model might ask research questions regarding the stressors of illness or examine the impact of particular care strategies on reducing stressors or improving the flexible lines of defense. A study simply examining stressors might be descriptive, whereas one examining an intervention could be experimental. Chinn and Kramer (1995) indicate that in theory-linked research, the purpose, problem statements, and hypotheses need to show the relationship between a selected theory and a specific study.

Recognizing that the global nature of conceptual models precludes direct testing, Fawcett (1999) proposes a conceptual-theoretical-empirical structure schema that links conceptual models to grand or middle-range theories and then to research. In this schema, research begins with a broad conceptual model, such as Rogers' Science of Unitary Human Beings or Roy's Adaptation Model, which provides a frame of reference for viewing phenomena. From the conceptual model, either a grand theory or middle-range theory is developed. If grand theories are derived from the conceptual model, the grand theories can generate middle-range theories. Because they are narrower in scope than grand theories, middle-range theories are used to describe, explain, or predict specific phenomena. This narrowed scope facilitates identification of research variables to be tested, the nature of the problem, the setting and source of data, research designs and instruments, methods to be used for analysis, and the nature of the contributions that the research will make to knowledge advancement (Fawcett, 1999).

Literature review can also be valuable as research questions are developed. If a literature review reveals no information related to the phenomenon of study, the nature of the research design may need to be more descriptive or exploratory. In theory-linked research, the investigator should evaluate the theoretical background found in the literature and survey relevant research findings (Chinn & Kramer, 1995). Often theory-generating research demands additional review of the literature as concepts emerge from the data. With theory-testing research, the investigator should not only review literature from studies based on the theory but also should critique studies using alternative, related theories. The review should incorporate the theoretical ideas and clarify how and why specific relationships are tested.

Theory-Generating Research

Theory-generating research is derived from real world observations in which the phenomenon of interest suggests areas to be examined (Chinn & Kramer, 1995; Fawcett, 1999). As members of a practice-based profession, nurses can observe clinical phenomena and ask relevant research questions. In theory-generating research, methods using less structured techniques offer a window of discovery about a selected phenomenon. Descriptive quantitative research or an array of qualitative methods can investigate the aspect of interest. Central to theory-generating research is approaching the phenomenon without imposing preconceived ideas about the concept or possible outcomes of the study. Preconceptions can bias the investigator and limit full exploration of a phenomenon.

Meleis (1997) proposed a research-theory strategy that could be used for developing theories that are based on research. In this strategy, researchers select and list the characteristics of a commonly occurring phenomenon. The characteristics are measured in as many different situations as possible. Data from the studies are analyzed to ascertain systematic patterns, and any significant patterns are formalized into theoretical statements. For nursing to maximize the use of research for theory generation, the problems identified for study should be ones unanimously considered central to the discipline of nursing (Meleis, 1997).

The beginning point for theory-generating studies is a statement of the research problem and questions. When less is known about the phenomenon of study or when new directions are sought, the problem statements may not be as explicit as those found in theory-testing research (Chinn & Kramer, 1995). Additionally, the literature review may not be complete before the beginning of the study. As concepts emerge from the data, additional exploration of the literature to investigate the emerging concepts may be warranted. During the study, the investigator should be aware of the literature reviewed and the potential need to return for additional review. For example, the investigator may uncover serendipitous findings or lack a rationale for unexplained findings. Analysis of data may include descriptive and nonparametric statistics in quantitative descriptive studies; if data are qualitative, coding and categorizing of observations are performed.

It should be noted that research findings in themselves are not theory; however, these findings may motivate a scholar toward a more adequate explanation of findings within the context of a new theory (Barnum, 1998). Theory evolves as relevant phenomena are probed further. This offers insight and catalyzes new research questions. For example, in a qualitative study using a grounded theory technique, Breckenridge (1997) investigated perceptions of renal dialysis patients about choices regarding their dialysis treatment modality. The Neuman Systems Model guided the study process. However, the end product of the study was a grounded theory entitled "Patient's Choice of a Treatment Modality versus Selection of a Patient's Treatment Modality" (p. 313). This model reflected considerations surrounding decision making about dialysis.

Theory-Testing Research

The purpose of **theory-testing research** is "to develop evidence about hypotheses derived from theory" (Acton, Irvin, & Hopkins, 1991, p. 53). As such, theory testing is a deductive operation. Following theory generation, research techniques can test the theory for validation. It should be noted that a whole theory—particularly a grand theory—is not tested at one time. As investigators approach theory testing, they identify and select an area of theory to test. The area selected for testing may depend on investigator interest, may be particularly amenable to testing, and/or build on findings of previous research.

The process of theory testing offers opportunities for further theory refinement (Meleis, 1997). Following selection of a theory compatible with the domain of interest, the investigator selects one or more specific propositions or relational statements from the theory to be systematically tested. In this instance, the investigator begins with broad theoretic concepts and narrows them down to concepts measurable by specific observation. Once findings are generated, the investigator must return to the theory and ascertain whether the findings are congruent with the theoretical propositions. In some instances the findings will support the theoretical assertions. Situations in which the theory is not supported may call for modification of the theory. In light of consistent adverse evidence, some theories may need to be discarded, and a new theory that reflects data findings may need to be generated. In this manner, researchers gain further insights into the explanation of phenomena.

Fawcett (1999) suggested that three formats for theory can be associated with specific forms of research. Descriptive theory, which is basic theory consisting of naming or classifying characteristics of a phenomenon, should be tested using descriptive research techniques. Descriptive research can answer questions regarding the characteristics and prevalence of a phenomenon and the process by which the phenomenon is experienced. This descriptive process can be either quantitative or qualitative. Explanatory theory that specifies relationships among characteristics of a phenomenon should be studied with correlational techniques. Explanatory research helps to explain why a phenomenon exists. Finally, predictive theory that predicts relationships among characteristics of a phenomenon or differences between groups should be studied using experimental research. Research for predictive theories could examine whether an intervention resulted in an intended effect.

Fawcett (1999) offered a specific framework for evaluating the conceptual-theoretical-empirical structures for research that addresses concerns related to using middle-range theory and the research testing or generating the theory. She indicated that adequate conceptual-theoretical-empirical linkages exist when the model is specified and the linkages between the model, theory linkages, and propositions are stated explicitly. For example, Lowry and Anderson (1993) used the Neuman System Model as the theoretical framework for their study of ventilator dependency. First, the study addressed extrapersonal stressors as the concept and mechanical ventilation as the research variable. The empirical indicator or linkage was the number of failed weaning attempts. In this instance Neuman's concepts were clearly linked to the research variables and measurable indicators. Second, the study methodology—including sample choice, instrumentation, study design, and statistical techniques—must be related clearly to the conceptual model. The theory must be evaluated for significance, consistency, parsimony, and testability. The research design must be assessed for sample representativeness, validity and reliability of empirical indicators, appropriateness of research procedures, and the ability of hypotheses to be falsified. Research findings should be evaluated for empirical adequacy to ensure congruence with empirical evidence and consideration of alternative explanations for findings. The utility of the theory for practice is considered in relationship to its practicality and feasibility of implementation.

Finally, evidence regarding the model's credibility is demonstrated. For example, in a test of King's Theory of Goal Attainment, Froman (1995) hypothesized that "the greater the degree of perceptual congruency between nurse and patient related to the illness situation and nursing care required, the greater the degree of goal attainment or satisfaction with nursing care" (p. 225). This study tested the proposition derived from goal attainment theory that "the presence of perceptual congruency between nurse and client influences the occurrence of transaction leading to goal attainment or effective nursing care." Froman's design to test the hypothesis matched nurse-patient pairs and measured them for perceptual congruency—which incorporated perceptions of illness, perceptions of mutual goal setting, and perception of information communicated—and patient satisfaction. Both instruments were deemed reliable and valid measures congruent with the Theory of Goal Attainment. Statistical testing determined that greater perceptual congruency between nurses and patients regarding the illness and nursing care led patients to a greater sense of satisfaction or goal attainment. This finding supported the proposition derived from King's Theory of Goal Attainment.

Theory testing also can be achieved through path analysis. Path analysis develops and tests a hypothesized model based on the theory (Knapp, 1998). Lusk, Ronis, Kerr, and Atwood (1994) developed a causal model about the use of hearing protection by individuals in the workplace, based on Pender's Health Promotion Model. To test their model they designed measurements of each variable of interest and then statistically tested the data to discover whether the predicted relationships within the proposed model actually occurred. Investigators predicted that the use of hearing protection would be influenced by workers' perceived control over their health, their definitions of health, and their perceived benefits of using hearing protection. They further hypothesized that the use of hearing protection would be influenced indirectly by factors such as the work situation, gender, age, education, and job category. In this particular study, the model developed explained almost 53% of the variance in how workers used hearing protection. As a result of these findings, the investigators made recommendations about the usefulness of the Health Promotion Model.

Generating Hypotheses for Research. In theory-testing research, explicit statements regarding the purpose of research, the research problem, and the hypotheses or research questions should be stated before conducting the study. This process will assist in moving from the broad intent of a theory to a more direct linkage to specific study variables (Chinn & Kramer, 1995).

Following Fawcett's (1999) proposal for techniques of theory-testing research, the following kinds of research questions or hypotheses might be generated. In descriptive research studies, research questions may aim toward discovering what a phenomenon comprises. In correlational studies, the question or hypothesis generated focuses on the extent to which two or more variables are associated with one another. The decision whether to use research questions or hypotheses depends on the assurance with which the researcher can specify the anticipated relationships. When using predictive theory to generate research, the researcher questions whether, if the theory is true—or, considering the nature of grand theories, if the *relational statement* is true—particular outcomes can be anticipated. The resulting hypothesis might reflect a predicted outcome for a given situation. In this manner, specific hypotheses or research questions associated with the study variables are derived.

CONGRUENCE BETWEEN THEORY AND RESEARCH

For theories to be useful, they must guide and be guided by research (Meleis, 1997). Because theories are established on current knowledge, future findings provide evidence for supporting or refuting theoretical claims. Fawcett (1993) indicated that the theoretical assertions of theory must be congruent with empirical evidence. If research findings consistently conform to the theory, accepting the theoretical assertions is valid. Ascertaining congruence requires a systematic review of studies using a particular theory. Building a case for congruence takes more than one study. The more studies with findings that agree with the theoretical assertions, the stronger the case for judging a theory to be adequate. Of course, no theory is absolute; theories are always open to modification when better explanations of phenomena—supported with research data—become available.

KNOWLEDGE OF THEORY THROUGH RESEARCH

The connection between nursing research and theory should be integrated. Positivist models view knowledge as additive, whereas other paradigms indicate that ultimately a theory is never confirmed or refuted because the possibility of other explanations always exists (Fawcett, 1978). In reality, at least according to postpositivists, theories approximate the real world and best explain phenomena as it is currently known. In other words, knowledge is imperfect and is subject to change as new discoveries are made. This perspective offers nursing unlimited opportunities to investigate significant phenomena related to practice. As more is learned, phenomena are better explained, and practice hopefully is influenced.

Unfortunately, nursing draws criticism charging that theories only marginally guide research and that theory testing is limited. To more accurately assess use of nursing theory in research, Silva (1986) identified three different ways in which nursing theory had been incorporated in research studies. The first manner was minimal use of theory, in which the theory is explicitly identified as a research framework but is minimally integrated into the study. These studies characteristically mention the guiding theoretical framework but neglect incorporation of theory as a guide to testing or putting research variables into operation. In the second way, concepts from theories were used to organize the research, usually for descriptive rather than theory-testing purposes. Characteristic manuscripts from these studies include a nice overview of the theory and linkages between the research variables and the framework, but the discussion often neglects how findings were predicted by the theoretical framework or the findings' implications for the framework. In the third manner, adequate use of models for theory testing is characterized by explicit indication of model use along with a study purpose of determining the model's validity. Hypotheses are deducted clearly from assumptions or propositions and tested in an appropriate manner. Discussion of findings related back to the theoretical framework.

Acton, Irvin, and Hopkins (1991) built on Silva's work by suggesting 15 specific criteria useful for evaluating theory-testing research studies. These include the following:

- The statement of purpose specifies theoretical testing.
- The researcher makes explicit the underlying theory and summarizes it appropriately.
- The researcher defines the concepts or constructs in terms of the theory.
- Prior studies based on the selected theoretical framework are included in the literature review, or derivation of the concepts is clearly shown.

- The researcher uses the tenets of the theory to logically arrive at his or her research questions.
- By using sufficiently specific hypotheses, the study places the theory at risk to be falsified.
- The terms of the theory clearly generate the operational definitions of the study.
- The theory and research design are philosophically congruent.
- Instruments used to test the theory have been demonstrated adequate reliability and validity.
- The theory guides the choice of samples for the study.
- Researchers should incorporate the strongest statistics available into the study.
- In analyzing the data, the researcher should offer support for or against the theory and/or possible revisions to the theory.
- An interpretive analysis of findings related to the theory must appear in the research report.
- The research report considers the theory's impact on nursing.
- The researcher offers suggestions for more studies based on his or her theoretical findings.

One shortcoming of the evaluative mechanisms by Silva (1986) and Acton, Irvin, and Hopkins (1991) is the focus on quantitative methodologies from studies philosophically guided by positivist and postpositivist paradigms. Silva and Sorrell (1992) expanded on the evaluation criteria, incorporating three alternative approaches to theory testing. The evaluation criteria found in Silva's first article (1986) can be considered empirical testing. One of the three additionally proposed evaluation mechanisms called for testing theory through critical reasoning. In this instance, verification of nursing theory is achieved through critical reasoning. Although all methods of theory verification involve critical reasoning, Silva and Sorrell's particular context relies on critique that incorporates judicious evaluation of strengths and weaknesses of works within a discipline. These critiques may be integrative literature reviews in which research in a given area is evaluated. Silva and Sorrell (1992) suggest eight criteria to judge nursing theory. These include the following (p. 17):

- Underlying philosophic assumptions regarding what constitutes truth in the testing of the theory are explicitly stated.
- The testing of nursing theory is congruent with philosophic assumptions regarding truth.
- The method for testing of nursing theory is congruent with purpose for testing.
- The purpose for testing is clearly stated and advances nursing knowledge or method.
- The testing of nursing theory is based on the simplest method needed to obtain the most valid and powerful results.
- The testing of nursing theory is constructed so that comparable or similar verification can occur.
- The testing of nursing theory lays the groundwork for an applied outcome.
- The overall processes used in testing exhibit internal consistency, aesthetic unity, and ethical integrity.

Another method of testing theory is through description of personal experiences (Silva & Sorrell, 1992). In this mechanism, direct participation provides knowledge or insight that permits theory development and verification of theory through the inductive strategies of qualitative techniques. Silva and Sorrell proposed 10 evaluative criteria for these studies (pp. 18-19):

- The purpose of the study is to verify relationships of described personal experiences to philosophical beliefs and assumptions that underlie the developing nursing theory.
- Identification of the research question(s) is based on an attempt to provide elaboration of concepts related to the developing nursing theory.
- The primary data sources include sufficient in-depth descriptions of personal experiences to capture the essence of the phenomenon under investigation.
- Simplicity, ethical integrity, and aesthetic presentation are integral characteristics of the described personal experiences.
- Analysis of data incorporates a sense of wholeness of the described personal experiences.
- Formative hypotheses and/or theory are derived inductively from qualitative analysis of the described personal experiences.
- Multiple personal experiences of an individual and/or similar personal experiences of several individuals about a particular phenomenon are used to validate the derived hypotheses.
- Analytic procedures of data analysis and fit of the generated concepts to the personal experiences provide indirect evidence of the validity (or lack thereof) of the developed nursing theory.
- Findings are discussed in terms of how they related to the developed nursing theory.
- If an existing nursing theory is used to frame a theory that is to be developed and tested inductively, both the developing and existing theories must be internally consistent and congruent with one another.

The final mechanism for theory verification suggested by Silva and Sorrell (1992) is application through practice. These studies assess whether what is purported as truth is, in fact, experienced in practice. In this instance, the theory is evaluated in terms of its problem-solving effectiveness. Successful theories demonstrate usefulness in clinical problem solving. Silva and Sorrell (1992) identify seven criteria for evaluating this type of theory testing, which include the following (p. 20):

- The purpose of the application is to demonstrate problem-solving effectiveness.
- The nursing theory is stated explicitly.
- Specific problems are targeted for solutions in the implementation plan.
- Problems are interesting, important, and ethical for practice.
- Outcomes are measured in terms of the theory's problem-solving effectiveness.
- Problem-solving effectiveness is determined in comparison with applications in which the theory is not used.
- Findings are discussed in terms of the theory's instrumentality in defining and implementing problem-solving strategies.

These additional theory evaluation methods broaden the scope of evaluation for theory-testing research.

Over the past several years, researchers have evaluated nursing research in selected areas and specific time frames. Brown, Tanner, and Padrick (1984) analyzed the characteristics of nursing research over three decades and evaluated their findings using criteria proposed by Dickoff, James, and Semradek (1975). One hundred thirty-seven studies from 1952 to 1953, 1960, 1970, and 1980 were reviewed. Over this 30-year period, nursing research increased substantially and became more clinically focused. Studies began to demonstrate more theoretical orientations; more than half explicitly identified a conceptual perspective. Larger numbers of explanatory studies used increasingly sophisticated methods. It was recommended that scholars undertake more studies concerning the reliability and validity of measuring instruments and fewer studies on education and nurse characteristics to advance nursing research.

Although Brown, Tanner, and Padrick's 1984 study indicated improvement in nursing research, other investigators indicated that nursing needed to make stronger connections in the theory-research linkages. Moody, Wilson, Smyth, Schwartz, Tittle, and Van Cott (1988) analyzed 720 research studies published from 1977 to 1986 in six research journals. Investigators discovered that only 3% explicitly used and tested a conceptual or theoretical framework. Silva (1986) examined 62 nursing research studies using the models of Johnson (1980), Roy (1976), Rogers (1970), Orem (1980), and Newman (1979). She found only nine studies that could be categorized as adequate tests of some aspect of the identified theory.

Murphy and Freston (1991) examined the extent to which theory and research were related in 142 gerontological nursing studies. The randomly selected studies were published between 1983 to 1989 in six nursing journals and focused on clinical problems in gerontology. Investigators developed the Theory Linkage Research Inventory (TLRI) using Fawcett's interrelationship (1978) between research and theory. In 59% ($\underline{n}$ = 124) of the studies, the study and the literature review were linked explicitly, whereas 17% ($\underline{n}$ = 24) had no theoretical perspective. Sixty-six studies identified a specific theory or conceptual model used to guide research or testing. Of these articles, the theory-research linkage was most strongly demonstrated in the empirical phase, which was characterized by theoretically related designs, sampling, instrumentation, and data collection and analysis. The weakest theoretical linkages were found in the interpretive phase. Although interpretation of findings from the theoretical perspective and in light of the literature often occurred, implications for practice were rarely theory-linked.

Jaarsma and Dassen (1993) reviewed research articles published in five international research journals from 1986 to 1990 to discover how often nursing theoretical models guided research. Excluding studies concerning instrumentation, education, administration, nurses, blood pressure, and temperature measurement, the investigators found that 72% of the 428 studies reviewed did not identifiably link to theory. Of the 28% (121) of studies with an identifiable theory linkage, 26% (31) identified only the theory; 22% (26) actually linked theory concepts to the research variables; 17% (20) used the theory as an organizing framework for data collection; and 25% (30) tested the theory. Only 6% (7) actually tested an intervention. The remaining studies used the theory in other ways.

In a review of 20 years of pediatric nursing research published in four pediatric practice journals, Betz and Beal (1996) found that only 17 of the 302 articles used nursing theories. Using Silva's criteria (1986) for evaluating theory utilization in nursing research studies, Betz and Beal found that six studies used nursing theory minimally, eight insufficiently used theory, and three adequately applied nursing theory. The most common problem was inadequate conceptualization of the problem. This finding means that most of these studies failed to link the variables under investigation to the theoretical framework, thus negating the opportunity to link the specific project to a larger research endeavor. Further refinement of middle-range nursing theory could lead to more refined concepts for explaining nursing practice.

Nursing needs to concentrate on strengthening the linkages between theory and research. Silva (1986) suggested that a lack of investigator commitment, a perception that the abstractness of selected theories leads to methodological imperfections, and a lack of systematic retrieval strategies because model use is not adequately cited in publication titles and abstracts impedes theory use and testing. However, she does not leave nursing without hope. To correct these deficiencies, Silva recommends better delineation of research-based testing criteria. Commitment to theory testing should be fostered among researchers, and better systematic retrieval processes should be developed. Cluster studies should be used systematically to test assumptions and propositions from models. Finally, healthcare providers should be assisted in facilitating the incorporation of theory into their practice.

Perhaps these studies reflect the 'half empty' or 'half full' glass of water. Nursing could take the perspective that the theory and research glass is half empty because the nursing research enterprise fails to consistently use theoretical models or to test those models. However, the good news is that theory development and testing does occur—not as often as is desirable—but with increasing frequency. With time and the development of a more expansive methodological orientation that incorporates a broad worldview of science and research approaches, the knowledge base of nursing will expand and fit clinical reality.

PRACTICAL POINTERS FOR EVALUATING RESEARCH ON INSTRUMENTATION

This section is designed to facilitate the reader's understanding of information included in each of the theory chapters on instrumentation. The discussion of each research instrument evaluated through the text will include aspects related to reliability and validity. Each chapter will use these terms as research instruments are discussed. Suggested values that should be achieved will help the reader evaluate the merits of each instrument.

Reliability

Reliability is a measure of the accuracy and dependability of an instrument. Three types of reliability—consistency, stability, and equivalence—may be of concern. Internal consistency occurs when individual items or subscales actually measure the phenomenon of interest. When assessing internal consistency, researchers compare items within the scale to other items or to the total scale in order to determine whether the item or items are measuring a similar concept. Internal consistency might be estimated through a coefficient alpha, or Cronbach's alpha statistic, which assesses items to determine their congruence. Coefficient alpha measures the degree to which items correlate with others on the test.

A similar but slightly less precise measurement is split-half reliability, in which the instrument is divided in half. The two halves are then compared to determine whether the scores are similar. Estimating the split-half reliability tends to underestimate the strength of the association. A Spearman-Brown Prophecy formula that accounts for the underestimation may correct this. In both cases, the higher the correlation between items, the more internally consistent the instrument is considered. According to Nunnally and Bernstein (1994), a reliability estimation of 0.70 generally would indicate modest reliability for a new instrument, and a reliability of 0.80 or greater is considered adequate. Nunnally and Bernstein caution that satisfactory reliability depends on the instrument's use.

Stability refers to the capacity of the instrument to repeatedly measure the same phenomenon and arrive at similar scores on the instrument. Test-retest reliability assesses stability. Measurements are obtained on the same group of people for at least two testings and the scores correlated. The space of time between testings depends on the nature of the instrument. One consideration of test-retest reliability is the time interval between tests. The interval should be long enough to permit subjects to forget their responses to the first testing but not so long that the construct being measured changes. Often the interval is approximately 2 to 3 weeks. Waltz, Strickland, and Lenz (1991) indicate that an acceptable value for a test/retest reliability is 0.80.

Equivalence is achieved when different raters similarly rate or score the same event. This is necessary to ensure interrater reliability when multiple raters measure a phenomenon of interest or when there is concern as to whether one rater rates a phenomenon consistently (a question of intrarater reliability). Equivalence is also important when alternate forms of an instrument are used. Each form of the instrument should rate the event being measured in a similar manner. Equivalence can be determined through correlation or percentage agreement.

Validity

Validity indicates that an instrument actually performs the intended measures. Validity of an instrument is not established through a single study but rather is an accumulative process. Each confirmation of validity is like adding a brick to a building, further establishing the case for the instrument's validity. Researchers can establish several types of validity, including content validity, criterion-related validity, and construct validity.

Content validity is established by sending the instrument to experts in the field. These experts evaluate instrument items and indicate whether the items measure the intended phenomena. Waltz, Strickland, and Lenz (1991) suggest that to evaluate content validity, experts should work from a list of objectives that guided construction of the instrument, a definition of terms, and a list of items to measure the designated objectives. The experts are asked to link the objective with the respective item, assess the relevance of the item, and determine whether the items on the instrument adequately represent the content of the domain of interest. Sometimes a content validity index (CVI) may be calculated. The CVI is the proportion of items rated by experts as relevant or very relevant to the instrument. A CVI of at least 0.80 is desirable.

Criterion-related validity occurs when comparing two instruments measuring the same event. One form of criterion-related validity, concurrent validity, records two measures of the event at the same time. Two examples include comparing the performance of a shorter instrument to a longer, more complex instrument or comparing a new measure to a measure recognized as a gold standard. Another form of criterion-related validity is predictive validity, in which performance on one instrument predicts future performance on another measure. A major difference between concurrent validity and predictive validity is the timing of the two measures. In concurrent validity the two measures are completed at the same time; with predictive validity one measure is completed before the second. In each instance a correlation can be used to assess the relationship between the two instruments. Waltz, Strickland, and Lenz (1991) suggest that measures of criterion-related validity must be interpreted carefully and in light of several factors. For example, do changes that would modify instrument performance occur within the target population? Validity estimates may underestimate the true validity of the predictor in question. Thus definition of criteria within the study is critical. Measurement of variables must be obtained independently and free of bias. Unreliable predictor and criterion measures may result in lower levels of validity.

Construct validity is concerned with testing an instrument to check whether it performs correctly. Several methods—including known groups; factor analysis; and multitrait, multimethod techniques—may establish construct validity. For example, in the known groups technique, two different groups would be expected to perform on the instrument in a particular way. The scores on the instruments from the two groups would then be compared. Factor analysis, a statistical procedure that places similar items into categories, is sometimes used to determine whether the instrument items will group into measures of the underlying theoretical constructs. To evaluate a factor analysis, items should have a minimum factor loading of 0.50, although some consider 0.30 adequate (Waltz, Strickland, & Lenz, 1991). Factors should be named based on the nature of the items grouped within the factor. Since some items may not load into factors in an easily interpretable manner, factor analysis can prove difficult.

To assess validity, multitrait, multimethod validity evaluation measures two or more constructs with two or more methods for each construct. The underlying principle is that different measures of the same construct should be highly correlated (Waltz, Strickland, & Lenz, 1991). This is sometimes called convergent validity. Measures of different constructs should exhibit a low correlation, sometimes called divergent or discriminant validity. The multitrait, multimethod assessment of validity is preferred for validity estimation. However, because of the inherent difficulties in measuring this form of validity, it tends to occur less often than assessment that uses other techniques.

When selecting an instrument, the investigator should try to use instruments that demonstrate adequate levels of reliability and validity. It is difficult for an instrument to achieve a high degree of validity if it does not possess reliability. It is good practice to continue assessment of validity and reliability when using instruments in studies.

Summary

- Key characteristics of the paradigms of discovery influence how investigators ask questions and the research techniques used to uncover specific phenomenal aspects. The four paradigms discussed are positivism, postpositivism, critical theory, and constructivism.
- Research and theory inform one another. Research can suggest or support essential elements of theory, and theory can suggest research questions. The practice component generates research questions and is the basis for theory formation. Theory and research findings can guide practice. Each of these pieces is part of an integral, inseparable process.
- Investigators use theory to guide research questions. Propositions within theory suggest relationships that should exist within practice. Research can investigate the reality of these propositions.

- Theory-generating and theory-testing research are parts of the theory-research-practice interconnection. Research offering new insights regarding practice can be incorporated into theory, and theoretical propositions can be tested with research techniques.
- Mechanisms for evaluating the testing of nursing theory include empirical testing, critical reasoning, description of personal experiences, and application to nursing practice.
- Adequate reliability and validity need to be ascertained for research instruments. Investigators should ascertain the conditions under which these characteristics are obtained and should also assess reliability and validity of the instruments used in their investigations.

REFERENCES

Acton, G.J., Irvin, B.L., & Hopkins, B.A. (1991). Theory-testing research: Building the science. *Advances in Nursing Science, 14*(1), 52-61.

Barnum, B.S. (1998). *Nursing theory: Analysis, application, evaluation*. Philadelphia: Lippincott.

Betz, C.L. & Beal, J. (1996). Use of nursing models in pediatric nursing research: A decade of review. *Issues in Comprehensive Pediatric Nursing, 19*(3), 153-167.

Breckinridge, D. (1997). Patients' perceptions of why, how, and by whom dialysis treatment modality was chosen. *ANNA Journal, 24*(3), 313-319.

Brown, J.S., Tanner, C.A., & Padrick, K.P. (1984). Nursing's search for scientific knowledge. *Nursing Research, 33*(1), 26-32.

Chinn, P.L. & Kramer, M.K. (1995). *Theory and nursing research: A systematic approach* (4th ed.). St. Louis: Mosby.

Dickoff, J., James, P., Semradek, J. (1975). A stance for nursing research—tenacity or inquiry. *Nursing Research, 24*(2), 84-88.

Fawcett, J. (1978). The relationship between theory and research: A double helix. *Advances in Nursing Science, 1*(1): 49-62.

Fawcett, J. (1993). *Analysis and evaluation of nursing theories*. Philadelphia: Davis.

Fawcett, J. (1995). *Analysis and evaluation of conceptual models of nursing*. (3rd ed.). Philadelphia: Davis.

Fawcett, J. (1999). *The relationship of theory and research*. (3rd ed.). Philadelphia: Davis.

Froman, D. (1995). Perceptual congruency between clients and nurses. In M. Frey & C. Sieloff (Eds.), *Advancing King's Systems Framework and theory of nursing*. Thousand Oaks, CA: Sage.

Gortner, S.R. (1990). Nursing's syntax revisited: A critique of philosophies said to influence nursing theories. *International Journal of Nursing Studies, 30*(6), 477-488.

Guba, E.G., & Lincoln, Y.S. (1994). Competing paradigms in qualitative research. In E.K. Denzin & Y.S. Lincoln (Eds.), *Handbook of qualitative research*. Thousand Oaks, CA: Sage.

Jaarsma, T. & Dassen, T. (1993). The relationship of nursing theory and research: The state of the art. *Journal of Advanced Nursing, 18*(5), 783-787.

Johnson, D. (1980). The behavioral system model for nursing. In J. Riehl & C. Roy (Eds.), *Conceptual Models for Nursing Practice*. (2nd ed.). New York: Appleton-Century Crofts.

Knapp, T. (1998). *Quantitative nursing research*. Thousand Oaks, CA: Sage.

Lowry, L.W. & Anderson, B. (1993). Neuman's framework and ventilator dependency: A pilot study. *Nursing Science Quarterly, 6*(4), 195-200.

Lusk, S., Ronis, D., Kerr, M., & Atwood, J. (1994). Test of the health promotion model as a causal model of workers' use of hearing protection. *Nursing Research, 43*(3), 151-157.

Meleis, A.I. (1997). *Theoretical nursing: Development and progress*. (3rd ed.). Philadelphia: Lippincott.

Moody, L.E., Wilson, M.E., Smyth, K., Schwartz, R., Tittle, M., & Van Cott, M.L. (1988). Analysis of a decade of nursing practice research: 1977-1986. *Nursing Research, 37*(6), 374-379.

Murphy, E. & Freston, M. (1991). An analysis of theory-research linkages in published gerontologic nursing studies, 1983-1989. *Advances in Nursing Science, 13*(4), 1-13.

Newman, M.A. (1979). *Theory development in nursing*. Philadelphia: F.A. Davis.

Nunnally, J. & Bernstein, I. (1994). *Psychometric Theory.* (3rd ed.). New York: McGraw-Hill.

Orem, D. (1980). *Nursing: Concepts of Practice.* (2nd ed.). New York: McGraw Hill.

Rogers, M.E. (1970). *An introduction to the theoretical basis of nursing.* Philadelphia: F.A. Davis.

Roy, C. (1976). *Introduction to nursing: An adaptation model.* Englewood Cliffs, NJ: Prentice Hall.

Silva, M.C. (1986). Research testing nursing theory: State of the art. *Advances in Nursing Science, 9*(1), 1-11.

Silva, M.C. & Sorrell, J.M. (1992). Testing of nursing theory: Critique and philosophical expansion. *Advances in Nursing Science, 14*(4), 12-23.

Waltz, C., Strickland, O., & Lenz, E. (1991). *Measurement in nursing research.* (2nd ed.). Philadelphia: F.A. Davis.

Welch, M. (1999). Phenomenology and hermeneutics. In E.C. Polifroni & M. Welch (Eds.), *Perspectives on philosophy of science in nursing: An historical and contemporary anthology.* Philadelphia: Lippincott.

The Structuring
of Nursing Practice

"Theories without practices, like man without routes, may be empty, but practices without theories, like routes without maps, are blind."

J.W. Gertzels, 1960

Objectives

- Discuss the role of theory in structuring nursing practice.
- Describe the impact of varying philosophical perspectives on nursing practice.
- Define conceptualizing nursing as a program.
- Identify the processes associated with developing nursing practice within a nursing theoretical system.
- Describe the benefits of a nursing discipline-specific integrated theory, research, and practice program.

Key Terms

practice models, p. 46
process models, p. 45

Knowing and *doing* are complementary areas in nursing practice. Nursing, as a practice discipline, requires nurses to generate knowledge about what they do and to act on that knowledge. Structuring and sharing practical knowledge is essential to developing nursing as a discipline. Discipline-specific theoretical systems can facilitate organizing the knowing and doing of nursing practice.

PURSUING THE THEORY-RESEARCH-PRACTICE LINK

Strengthening the practice component depends on explicitly joining the iteratively related theory development, research, and practice. Researchers and theorists need to make this nexus relationship known to the practitioner. Denyes, O'Connor, Oakley, and Ferguson (1989) described a process for facilitating development of this reciprocal relationship. Clinical nurse specialists and academic researchers collaborated in practice-oriented research programs to facilitate the desired integration of the three components of nursing. This collaborative research project demonstrated that both the theory base for primary care and the practice bases for research and theory development were strengthened. Project participants also described an increased understanding of the theoretical constructs.

Reed (1996) strategized extending the interrelationship of practice and knowledge development with Peplau's Theory of Interpersonal Relations (see Chapter 12). The first step identifies the fundamental units of concern to nurses. This involves "assisting patients to develop knowledge about destructive patterns and processes, and about the means for enacting more healthy behaviors" (Reed, 1996, p. 30). The second step is to abstract concepts from clinical knowledge—that is, from existing scientific theories and conceptual frameworks that represent phenomena observed in practice. This develops nursing knowledge within the practice context "through syntheses of (a) existing scientific theories, clinical observation and judgment of nursing, and (b) knowledge and active participation of patients" (Reed, 1996, p. 31).

This book discusses a range of nursing theories useful to the practitioner. These include general theories such as Orem's Self-Care Deficit Nursing Theory (Chapter 5) and Parse's Theory of Human Becoming (Chapter 7), which broadly describe the concerns of nursing, to more limited theories such as Pender's health promotion model (Chapter 11). The broad theoretical systems can identify the object or purpose of nursing in order to structure nursing practice, and the more limited theories direct particular components of practice. Both influence practice-oriented research. Denyes states that the "value of nursing theory for practice is predicated upon the degree to which theory provides description, understanding, explanation, and prediction about relevant nursing phenomena, and provides solutions to relevant clinical nursing problems" (1993, p. 213).

Research is fundamental to improving practice, and embedding research in a nursing theoretical framework is essential to developing nursing knowledge in all dimensions, whether empirical, esthetic, ethical, or personal. Nursing handles the complex realities of human beings. Within this complexity, the nurse focuses on particular phenomena. Because human beings are so complex, it is impossible to specify all the laws that explain the behavior of the phenomena with which nursing is concerned. Theories to help describe, explain, predict, and/or control those phenomena (McKenna, 1997).

DEVELOPING PRACTICE WITHIN NURSING THEORETICAL SYSTEMS

Conceptualizing nursing as program rather than as a collection of tasks can facilitate the health-related outcomes of nursing practice. Nursing practice begins with a mental model of nursing and its goals. It asks the purpose of nursing in a particular situation and point in time. Designing nursing practice programs from a theory base clarifies nursing's objectives.

A program is a specific set of activities within a structure organized to achieve specific outcomes. The questions of how to structure organized efforts and why such efforts succeed implies that a program operates under some theory, whether implicit and unsystematic or explicit and systematic (Chen, 1990). Discipline-specific nursing theoretical systems can provide the theory base for conceptualizing nursing as a program or programs. The better developed the theoretical system, the more systematic and explicit the nursing practice programs developed from this perspective.

Chen defines program theory "as a specification of what must be done to achieve desired goals, what other important impacts may also be anticipated, and how these goals and impact would be generated" (1990, p. 43). Program theory thus consists of two aspects: what should be (prescriptive theory) and what is (descriptive theory). Both aspects of program theory are represented within the range of nursing theoretical systems. When viewed as a practice program, nursing practice includes a normative component—what should be—and a causative component that specifies the relationship between treatment or intervention variables and outcome variables. Nursing theory helps to direct both components. It directs examination of premises and assumptions and evaluation of the utility of customary procedures. Nurses incorporate into practice those components that facilitate the desired goals and eliminate those that interfere with goal achievement. Subsequent chapters will provide examples of conceptualizing nursing as a program from the perspectives of the various nursing theoretical systems that illustrate the contribution of this approach to the advancement of nursing knowledge and the improvement of practice.

In developing the practice of nursing, both process and content require consideration. The late 19th century emphasized completing tasks, and process was related to accomplishing those tasks. In the 1950s the emphasis changed to process. As nurses began to describe the essence of nursing as something other than a derivative of medical practice, the concept of nursing process appeared in the literature. Nurses were encouraged to determine necessary nursing services by using a problem-solving approach of collecting, recording, and analyzing subjective and objective data (Weed, 1968a & 1968b; Thoma, 1972). Little guidance for determining what data to collect or how to analyze it was offered. Abdellah, Beland, and Matheney (1960), in an early attempt to specify the content of nursing practice, described 21 patient problems.

Other descriptions of commonly recurring patient problems and concepts associated with nursing eventually began to appear in the literature (Nursing Development Conference Group, 1973; Mitchell, 1977). Nursing students and nurses in service delivery agencies were encouraged to use nursing care plans that included significant concepts and problems (Mayers, 1972). This was an early attempt to address both content and process components. The basis for structuring the content was derived inductively from nursing practice or from medicine and the behavioral sciences. Subsequently, critical paths and care mapping were introduced. These also tend to be inductively derived from specific practice situations or to address scheduling and outcomes of specific treatments. For the most part these developments occurred outside of and without benefit of nursing theoretical systems.

The first conference dedicated to formalizing a classification of nursing diagnoses took place in 1973 (Gebbie & Lavin, 1975). At this conference the participants decided "that theory development would not precede terminological development" (Gebbie, 1982, p. 9). Diagnostic labels were to be developed inductively from practice situations. Gebbie asserted that theoretical precision should not bar clinicians' need for basic diagnostic labels. At this point, theory development separated from the movement wanting to develop nursing diagnoses through practice. This split severely impacted theory development and the perceived utility of nursing theory in practice. Several nurse theorists participated in the conferences as consultants, and some tried to integrate the diagnostic categories into theory development (Roy, 1982). However, others criticized the theoretical inconsistency of trying to meld nursing diagnostic activities with a broad nursing theoretical system (Taylor, 1989).

While these developments were taking place, practitioners also tried defining nursing by describing various roles. As nurses tried to define nursing by describing what they did, terms such as *independent, dependent,* and *interdependent nursing functions, primary nursing, clinical specialist,* and *advanced practice nurse* appeared in the literature. These developments also focused on problem-solving process rather than on content, the development of which requires discipline-specific theory.

NURSING THEORETICAL SYSTEMS, MODELS, AND PRACTICE

Each practitioner and administrator, nurse or not, who is responsible for provision of nursing services has an implicit or explicit model of nursing. Nursing theories provide direction for making that conceptualization of nursing or mental model explicit. By clarifying the object and concerns of nursing, a theoretical system provides direction for differentiating nursing knowledge and practice from the knowledge bases and practices of related disciplines. It also provides direction for specifying the articulation between the nursing discipline and other health-related disciplines. For example, both family therapists and nurses provide services to families. Family therapists take direction from family theory and are concerned with the whole of family functioning and interrelationships. Nurses take direction from nursing theory that incorporates aspects of family theory. Taylor (1989) proposed that the focus of nursing of families is derived from the functions of the family that are associated with self-care. Similarly, Taylor and McLaughlin (1991) and Taylor and McLaughlin-Renpenning (1995, 2001) describe the articulation of public health, community, and nursing in proposing a model for community nursing practice in which the concern of nursing is derived from the functions of community in relation to self-care.

Nursing theoretical systems assist in describing the domain and boundaries of nursing and the relevant phenomena of concern within the interdisciplinary healthcare delivery system (Northrup & Cody, 1998). Nursing's ontology can be identified, and nurses can move beyond describing nurses' contributions as a collection of tasks. Fawcett (1992) suggested a reciprocal relationship between conceptual models and nursing practice. Conceptual models assist in the development of statements of practice purpose, identification of clinical problems, understanding the content of the nursing process, and framing development of clinical information systems (Allison & McLaughlin-Renpenning, 1998; Bliss-Holtz, Taylor, & McLaughlin, 1992). Patient classification systems, measurement of outcomes, and quality assurance programs also demonstrate the contribution of conceptual models (Walker, 1993; Riggs & Bliss-Holtz, 1994).

The practice arena, in turn, validates and facilitates continued development of the theoretical systems (Mitchell, 1995; Reed, 1996). Structuring nursing practice in this manner is referred to as theory-based nursing practice. Theory-based nursing practice is:

> designed and produced for individuals and groups by nurses who have insights about and have conceptualized the specific characteristics of the human health service named nursing. Valid conceptualizations are in the form of descriptive explanations of the relationships between (1) the human variables that are interactive in bringing about requirements for nursing, and (2) the human variables that are interactive in the production of nursing in interpersonal or group situations. The insights include knowing how given parameters of the variables affect nursing requirements of people and, in turn, to valid and reliable designs for appropriate and effective systems of nursing care (Orem, 1987, p. 3).

The American Academy of Nursing's Expert Panel on Nursing Theory-Guided Practice has defined nursing theory-guided practice as:

> a human health service to society based on the discipline-specific knowledge articulated in the nursing frameworks and theories. The discipline-specific knowledge reflects the philosophical perspectives embedded in the ontological, epistemological, and methodological processes that frame nursing's ethical approach to the human-universe-health process (*Nursing Science Quarterly,* 2000, p. 177).

THE IMPORTANCE OF THEORETICAL PERSPECTIVES TO PRACTICE

Knowing the philosophical foundation of a theoretical perspective is more than just scholarly musing (Carper, 1978: Silva, Sorrell, & Sorrell, 1995; Kikuchi & Simmons, 1999). Knowledge for nursing practice must be developed by nursing scholars and practitioners. Building on Carper's four patterns of knowing as end products of knowledge development, Silva, Sorrell, and Sorrell (1995) explored how one comes to know. They argue that the patterns are not mutually exclusive or exhaustive. They introduced two new terms: the *in between*, referring to "what exists or reveals itself through nonlinear, meditative thinking that moves in all directions and depths" (p. 3), and *the beyond*, referring to "those aspects of reality, meaning, and being that persons only come to know with difficulty or that they cannot articulate or ever know" (p. 3). These concepts enable nurses to address ontologically issues of reality, meaning, and being. Uncovering the ontology frames exploration of these issues. Researchers and practitioners can better understand the nurse-patient relationship and the potential roles of nursing within the healthcare system. Understanding ontology is key in evidence-based practice issues (Estabrooks, 1998) and in determining the best practices in nursing. The following discussion samples the influence of philosophical foundations and theoretical perspectives on practice. Subsequent chapters expand on this topic.

Human Becoming Theory

Human becoming theory is based in an existential-phenomenological worldview. The phenomenon of concern to nursing is the human-universe-health process (Parse, 1999). Nurses engage in dialogues with patients to understand the patients' perspectives without allowing their own opinions to intrude or interfere. Patients' subjective perspectives and judgments are the basis for their health-related decisions (Mitchell, 1995; Parse, 1992). Parse (1999) calls health "a continuously changing process chosen by the person" (p. 1385). Nurses are "with" individuals, families, or communities; they listen, answer questions, and refer as necessary. They follow no standard teaching plans, since teaching is specific to the patient's questions and curiosity. There are no diagnostic labels as in medicine or as developed by the North American Nursing Diagnosis Association (NANDA). This perspective considers the diagnostic process reductionistic and dehumanizing.

Moderate Realist Perspective

Kikuchi and Simmons' (1999) moderate realist perspective on practice and knowing is consistent with Orem's self-care deficit nursing theory (see Chapter 5). From the moderate realist perspective, it is possible to obtain an objective view of reality. One can know what "is probably true by testing our various subjective views against reality which common sense tells us exists, and is the way it is regardless of how any one of us views it" (p. 45). To greater or lesser degrees all persons have natural powers of perception, judgment, and reason. These powers allow comparison of various views and facilitate judgments based on available evidence and reason. Moderate realist nurses consider both their perceptions of situations and patients' views of nursing decisions to be grounded in "objectively true principles related to the pursuit of happiness" (p. 46).

Nursing requires a three-tiered concept of practical nursing judgment. On a universal level, prescriptive, moral, or artistic judgments take the form of objective nursing principles that apply to all nurses at any time and place. Secondly, on a general level, judgments apply to a specific group of nurses practicing at a particular time and place. The third level applies to an individual nurse practicing in a particular place at a particular time. Practical nursing judgments result in principle-based nursing rules and decisions that are objectively grounded in nursing principles but also subjectively influenced by contingent facts.

Critical Theory/Feminist Perspective

Practice also can be structured from a critical theoretical perspective such as feminism. Critical theory aims to transform structures that permit human exploitation, and critical theorists see the existing healthcare system as such a structure. Feminism focuses on the structures most directly related to women. Nursing is one model of feminism. Watson's work, described in Chapter 13, is developed from this perspective. The practitioner must transform her or his worldview and nurse from the view of the feminine, in which caring is a central focus.

NURSING AS A PROGRAM

Conceptualizing nursing as a program facilitates the development of practice within a nursing theoretical system. This leads the program developer to do the following:
- Specify the variables of concern
- Develop an understanding of these for practice

- Use those variables to describe a population for nursing purposes
- Establish the expected outcomes of nursing
- Develop process and practice models
- Undertake appropriate research and evaluation

Individual practitioners or nurses employed by organizations can accomplish these steps.

Individual Practitioners

Through formal study of the various theoretical systems and their components, individual nurses determine the congruence between their belief systems and the nursing theories and then model their practices accordingly. Both educational institutions and employers have roles in facilitating theory-based practice for individual nurses. Nurses may incorporate research findings into their nursing practices after participation in education programs or reading the literature. However, most nurses work in healthcare organizations that in large part structure their practice. Examples of how nurses practice theory-based nursing in relation to specific theories are described in Unit 2.

In her study of knowledge sources of registered nurses, Estabrooks (1997, 1998) found that nurses relied most often on experience, followed by nursing school, workplace sources, physician sources, intuitions, "what has worked for years," and, lastly, the literature. Because most nurses in the study were in their forties and thus were likely to have been educated during a time when nursing theory was less developed, the knowledge base underlying their practice could be considered outdated and ungrounded in nursing science. Their knowledge bases probably were not developed within a nursing theoretical system. As a result, the nurses in this study most commonly read the newsletters of their provincial associations or the *Canadian Nurse* journal, neither of which is a major source for information about research or advances in nursing knowledge. Conversely, literature has been the primary manner in which researchers have shared their findings with the nursing world at large. If it is valid, this study suggests that practitioners rarely are exposed to current research.

Organizations and Institutions

Although the literature reports organizations developing theory-based nursing practice programs, organizations and institutions need to provide specifically for incorporating current research into nursing theory-based practice. As with many innovations in the design and delivery of nursing services, anecdotal support is strong. Claims include improved quality of care, greater patient satisfaction, and improved job satisfaction—but little formal evaluation of these programs has been conducted. In one study, changes in practice occurred after implementing practice based in Parse's Theory of Human Becoming and a related education program (Northrup & Cody, 1998). Change related to "shifting views of human beings, altered ways of listening, altered foci of nurse-person discussions, and personal transformations" (p. 23). Mitchell (1995) found similar changes.

Because many foundational theoretical perspectives for nursing practice exist, not all nurses will arrive at organizations ready to practice according to a particular institution's mission statement and objectives. Thus they may be unprepared to perform appropriate patient care. For example, if a nurse has always practiced from a Rogerian perspective, his or her practice will be directed at pattern appraisal, mutual patterning, and evaluation, whereas as a self-care perspective requires knowledge of self-care, self-care demand, and self-care agency. The education program, an essential component of every healthcare organization, should include strategies that help nurses achieve the organization's goals, including adoption of a theoretical viewpoint. Improving nursing through theory-based practice requires administrative support for education programs and allocation of resources. This includes knowledgeable support persons (Northrup & Cody, 1998). Principles derived from innovation diffusion theory as well as protocols derived from other theories related to planned change have been demonstrated to be useful (Rogers, 1995). Horsley (1985) conceptualized knowledge as both process and product in order to link research findings and practice. The product is "the packaged research findings in the form of a protocol which once it is in that form can be treated both conceptually and empirically as an innovation and diffusion theory applied" (Horsley, 1985 p. 136).

Designing a Nursing Program. The mental model of nursing held by persons within an organization is the basis for design of a nursing program. The more explicit this mental model, the more congruent the implementation and the more likely an organization achieves goals related to quality service. The mental model is reflected in all of the structural components of an organization: the mission statement, the objectives, the policies, the procedures, the protocols, the clinical information system, the performance appraisal system, the quality assurance program, and the research and development program (Allison & McLaughlin-Renpenning, 1998). The mission statement should be congruent with the theoretical framework, and the staff should be familiar with the mental model underlying the nursing program. Translating theory into practice requires identification and development of operational descriptions of the variables of concern in addition to the development of nursing practice models and nursing process models. The role of nursing and the relationship of nurse variables to patient variables should be described clearly.

Developing the Variables of Concern for Practice Purposes. Each of the nursing theoretical systems identifies phenomena of concern. These phenomena must be studied against the requirements of nursing practice to determine whether they are complete and adequate for practice. This includes evaluating the state of development of the substantive structure of each—that is, have the specified variables been adequately described for purposes of nursing practice? Have they been moved from theoretical formulations to concrete reality? For example, Orem (see Chapter 5) refers to self-care agency, a theoretical construct. This concept has been further developed through the work of the Nursing Development Conference Group (1979) to include specification of the following:

- three operations for self-care (knowing, decision making, and acting) and their related abilities
- ten power components (identified sets of abilities) for self-care
- a set of foundational capabilities and dispositions for deliberate action

This development moved the theoretical concept of self-care agency to concrete reality, thereby providing a structure for nurses to look for evidence that informs them about the extent to which the abilities associated with self-care are developed and exercised. Similar work is required within each theoretical system if it is to provide direction for practice. This may be accomplished through specific research or deduction and validated by practice and future research. Variations in the phenomena of concern and the development for practice of the associated variables are discussed in reference to various nursing theories in Unit 2.

After identifying the variables of concern, the organization should include specific data collection and direction for action in relation to those variables in its procedures and processes. The clinical/patient record should provide for methods of recording information about those variables. The integration of mission statement, processes and procedures, and expected outcomes in relation to Self-Care Deficit Nursing Theory should be described (Allison & McLaughlin-Renpenning, 1998). This provides the basis for evaluation.

Organizations using Self-Care Deficit Nursing Theory as a basis for practice express self-care as a value in the mission statement. Patient assessment processes include identifying action to accomplish self-care and evaluating patient capability in relation to that action. Expected outcomes are expressed in relation to the extent to which self-care is accomplished and self-care agency is developed, regulated and exercised. Subsequent chapters provide additional examples of this type of linking with other theoretical systems.

Describing a Population for Nursing Purposes. Describing populations from a nursing perspective is the first step in designing programs or systems of nursing. A significant contribution of the nursing theoretical systems to nursing practice is providing a language and schema for describing the characteristics of a patient population from the nursing perspective. Without direction from nursing theory, nursing relies on other disciplines to describe its populations. For example, medicine describes populations by disease entity and medical specialty. Nursing has also used age groups, developmental stages, and groups considered epidemiologically "at risk." However, nursing knowledge and service delivery can be discussed from its own perspective, using the language of nursing. As Geden suggests (1997a):

> Defining your nursing population is a critical process in this phase of knowledge development. . . . a nursing population is a description of a subgroup of class in need of nursing. It's defining who you nurse by the way you THINK NURSING, not the site or place where you nurse (p. 9).

Defining a nursing population begins with determining the group of persons with whom nursing is concerned and then selecting the most meaningful and commonly recurring variable(s), as derived from nursing theory. These variables become the basis for the population description. For example, nurses using Roy's Adaptation Model might describe a population as persons with perceived stress using inadequate coping strategies with non-adaptive responses in the self-concept mode. Describing populations in this manner allows nurses within an organization to explore commonalties for nursing requirements among patients in various clinical specialties and to develop appropriate strategies. Robinson (1987) moved from thinking of herself as a surgical-clinical nurse specialist to a facilitator of self-care. This includes assisting in developing self-management systems and creating nursing systems in response to processes of elimination and maintaining skin integrity. With this redefinition she more accurately defined her role and could better describe and identify her consultation abilities in surgical as well as other specialties.

Allison and McLaughlin-Renpenning (1998) and Taylor and McLaughlin-Renpenning (2001) provide examples of population description based in operational variables of concern, and they illustrate the utility of this process in designing nursing systems. "Persons needing to develop new self-management systems because of a change in health state" commonly require a nursing system (Allison & McLaughlin-Renpenning, 1998, p. 70). Other factors "include age range, health state, health care system factors, conditions and patterns of living, self-care limitations and capabilities, self-care demand"

(p. 70). Such a population description's use in developing a nursing system emphasizes self-management systems, and expected outcomes refer to the effectiveness of the self-management system.

Establishing Expected Outcomes of Nursing. Conceptualizing nursing as a program based in some nursing theoretical system provides a broad perspective for developing expected outcomes and specifying evaluation procedures. Program theory and nursing theory can frame decisions about establishing expected outcomes. The nature and evaluation of the outcomes will vary with the nature and philosophical basis of the theoretical system. Evaluating the effectiveness of nursing requires that the product of nursing be known—that is, what do nurses produce? What patient-related variables are the concerns of nursing? What are the nurse-related variables? How do the patient-related variables and the nurse-related variables interact? What should result from such interaction? What treatment will produce the intended changes in the social system? How can results be measured within an interdisciplinary healthcare delivery system?

From the perspective of program theory, "normative theory provides the rationale and justification for the program structure and activities. Normative theory guides program planning, formulation and implementation" (Chen, 1990, p. 43). Empirically based causative theory elucidates the relationship between the treatment variable(s) and the outcome variables of the program. Figure 3-1 presents a suggested range of evaluation types in relation to variations in nursing theory.

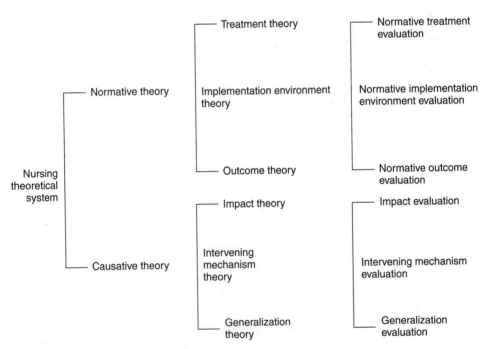

FIGURE 3-1   Relationship between nursing theoretical systems and basic evaluation types. (Modified from Chen, H. (1990). *Theory-driven evaluations.* Newbury Park, CA: Sage.)

Allison and McLaughlin-Renpenning (1998) suggest that nursing "has no consistent, identifiable mental model or framework by which to determine and evaluate the quality of nursing care" (p. 181). The literature rarely refers to the relationship between outcomes and nursing theory. Consequently, the variables reviewed tend to be vicarious measures of nursing activity. The American Nurses Association identified seven patient-related quality indicators of interest to nursing: nosocomial infections, patient injury rate, patient satisfaction, maintenance of skin integrity, nursing staff satisfaction, staff's mix of educational characteristics, and total nursing care hours per day (Canavan, 1996). These variables may or may not be primarily influenced by nursing action.

Maas, Johnson, and Morehead (1996) identified a set of nursing-sensitive outcomes as evidence of appropriate nursing care. A nursing-sensitive outcome is "a variable patient or family caregiver state, behavior, or perception that is responsive to nursing intervention and conceptualized at middle levels of abstraction (e.g., mobility level, nutritional status, health attitudes)" (p. 296). These outcomes presently are not linked to a nursing diagnosis classification system, a nursing intervention classification system, or a nursing theoretical system. This work remains to be completed. Currently these classification systems have no meaning to the nurse who structures practice from the perspective of the Theory of Human Becoming (Parse, 1999). That nurse has no nursing diagnosis *per se* and does not use the term *intervention*.

Critical paths are another way organizations have tried to specify expected outcomes of care over time. Interdisciplinary teams generally develop these outcomes, which pertain to specific populations often defined from a medical, rehabilitative, or developmental perspective. These include groups such as post-operative cholecystectomy patients, patients with spinal cord injuries, or preschool students. They identify time frames and milestones that patients should achieve for particular treatments and procedures. For the most part these critical paths lack nursing perspectives. Tasks for nursing may be identified, but they usually are related to therapeutic goals of related disciplines such as administration of medications. These outcome guidelines need direction from nursing theoretical systems and theoretical research to substantiate the nursing contribution and evaluate the effectiveness of nursing participation.

Development of Process Models. In addition to operationalizing the variables of concern, translating theory into practice requires developing nursing process models that specify the nature of the intervention—that is, the relationship of nursing to the patient variables. **Process models** represent the relationship between the nurse and patient variables and describe the actions, interactions, and interpersonal processes by which the goals of the relationship are achieved.

The process models referred to here are not synonymous with *the nursing process*, a term that began to appear in the nursing literature in the 1960s. That process paralleled the scientific problem-solving process of collecting data, analyzing it, determining the nature of the problem, intervening, and evaluating the effectiveness of the intervention. However, it was only a process. It did not direct what data to collect or how to analyze it, nor did it instruct how to know the nature of the problem, select appropriate interventions, and evaluate effectiveness. All of these factors require some theoretical basis. Lacking a nursing theory base, nurses borrowed from other disciplines; for example, the needs approach borrowed from the biological, social, and psychological sciences (Henderson, 1969).

Taylor (1998) distinguishes between *problem solving*, a means-end deliberation, and *problem setting*, which includes identifying, labeling, and understanding the problem from some theoretical perspective. Early works describing nursing process set the problems in theories of medicine, psychology, sociology, pathophysiology, and other disciplines related to but different from nursing. Advances in nursing theory development have allowed the problems to be framed in an explicit nursing perspective. Congruent with the stage of development of nursing theory, a tendency still exists to set nursing problems from the perspective of related disciplines. Many of the critical paths for managing patient care demonstrate this tendency.

The process models should cohere to the theoretical frameworks from which they are derived. A problem-solving process, for instance, is not congruent with Parse's Theory of Human Becoming. A process model consistent with this theory is described in Chapter 7. One theoretical perspective might seek to answer questions such as why a person needs a nurse, what nursing's concern is, what a nurse would do first, what continuing actions a nurse performs and why, what data a nurse needs, how data is collected, or what questions that data will be used to answer. Another theory might focus on the interaction and communication between nurse and patient. The development of the process model clarifies the domain and boundaries of nursing and the relationship of nursing to other disciplines. The developed model should specify the relationship between the nurse(s) and patient and direct their ongoing action, interaction, and interrelationships. The processes associated with the specific theoretical perspectives are discussed in detail in Unit 2.

Development of Practice Models. A nursing **practice model** is a "design for nursing action" (Orem, 1995, p. 180). It can represent what is or what should be. Derived from analysis and study of nursing practice situations, the practice model can address patient variables, nurse variables, and patient and nurse variables in interaction. Such a model can guide normative practice. The design for treating patients during the preoperative, intraoperative, and postoperative phases of surgery illustrates this type of model. Rules of nursing practice developed in association with these models guide nursing action within situations consistent with the range of variation expressed by the model. For example, preoperative instruction for surgical patients has become a norm of nursing care. Critical paths with the nursing contribution grounded in a nursing theoretical framework could be called a type of nursing practice model.

Theoretical systems can facilitate development of nursing practice models by systematically organizing knowledge derived from clinical experiences with theory. The advanced nurse practitioner contributes to the development of nursing knowledge when, as a scholar and researcher, he or she analyzes nursing cases from a nursing theoretical perspective. Such analysis reveals insights not generally perceived by nurses without a theoretical perspective (Geden, 1997b). For example, Anger, Crews, and other members of the Nursing Development Conference Group (NDCG, 1979) analyzed nursing cases of persons on anticoagulant therapy and formalized the notion of "the ideal general set" of actions necessary to regulate a therapy (Box 3-1). Moreover, a literature review and an analysis of cerebrovascular accident patient characteristics and needs reveals that Self-Care Nursing Deficit Theory variables served as a basis for descriptive nursing practice models and an organization of knowledge (NDCG, 1979). These models include a population description specific to the stage in time of a cerebrovascular accident, components of the therapeutic self-care demand, components of self-care agency, and the theoretical

BOX 3-1

General Ideal Set of Self-Care Actions

1. "Own" a self with an objectively established structural and/or functional state.
2. "Own" a self with a need for the use of a particular technology.
3. Perform the actions needed to make use of the technology and to move self to the structural or functional state possible by means of the technology.
4. Perform the actions necessary to keep self in the functional or structural state produced by the technology.
5. Refrain from actions that limit the achievement of results sought through the use of technology.
6. Take the actions needed to overcome undesirable responses that diminish therapeutic return.
7. Monitor self for structural or functional attributes that indicate an undesirable static state of response to the technology.
8. Monitor self for structural or functional attributes that indicate an undesirable regressive response in the presence of the use of the technology.
9. Control factors responsible for (or productive of) a regressive or static-state response to the technology.

From Nursing Development Conference Group. (1979). In D. Orem (Ed.), *Concept formalization in nursing: Process and product.* (2nd ed.). Boston: Little, Brown.

knowledge and skills required by nurses caring for that population. A seminal article by Backscheider (1974) describes the contribution the analysis of nursing situations that address some of these same variables can make to the development of nursing knowledge. The article also describes the linking of other theories, specifically Piaget's theories of cognitive development, to nursing theory as a basis for design of nursing systems for a particular patient population.

The classification of nursing outcomes as developed by Maas, Johnson, and Morehead (1996) and the classification of nursing indicators (Bowles & Naylor, 1996) are examples of components of practice models. The classification of nursing outcomes describes the desired results of nursing. The classification of nursing indicators, developed from a massive amount of data describing current nursing, describes what nurses should investigate. The classification of nursing outcomes and indicators structures practice but lacks the specific description and principles of nursing it represents. Although they were developed from practice, these models are not appropriate in all situations. For example, if a nurse practices from the perspective of the Theory of Human Becoming, neither the interventions nor the outcomes reflect that theory's ontology.

Evaluation and Research. Clear definitions of nursing and the interrelationships of nurse- and patient-related variables are fundamental to determining nursing success and for making appropriate changes in program design and delivery. Since nursing is a social program, the goals must include providing cost-effective, quality service. Research and development in nursing within an organization should be directed at the following areas:

- Constantly determining characteristics of the populations of specific interest to nursing

- Developing programs to meet the changing requirements of the population
- Determining the extent to which goals of nursing program(s) are being achieved
- Designing new strategies to meet goals
- Revising systems for collecting clinical data as basis for research and development programs
- Determining costs of nursing and effectiveness of nursing services within established budget
- Evaluating and adjusting staffing policies and budget to meet desired service quality

When the variables of concern to nursing have been identified in the mental model and integrated into the organization's documentation system, a basis for describing populations from a nursing perspective and for determining costs of nursing services emerges. The organization also can evaluate quality of service in relation to patient outcomes and service provided. Finally, a basis for designing research programs for validating or revising the theoretical framework underlying nursing practice, evaluating the achievement of patient outcomes, and implementing changes in nursing procedures and protocols to improve patient outcomes becomes available.

Summary

- Discipline-specific nursing theoretical systems frame descriptions of the domain and boundaries of nursing and the phenomena of concern. They guide the development of process and practice models.
- The understanding and ontology of the patient and of the relationships between the nurse and patient are derived from the philosophical perspectives from which nurses practice.
- Conceptualizing nursing as a program involves determining the theory under which nursing operates and making the mental model and the object of nursing explicit.
- Developing practice within a nursing program is based on understanding a particular nursing theoretical system and developing process and practice models within that system.
- As findings of nursing research are translated into procedures, protocols, and therapeutic regimens, they impact the conceptualization of nursing as well as its specific practices.
- Development of nursing knowledge and improvement of practice are the results of integrating nursing practice with research framed within the same nursing theoretical system.

REFERENCES

Abdellah, F.G., Beland, A.M. & Matheney, R.V. (1960). *Patient centered approaches to nursing.* New York: Macmillan.

Allison, S.E. & McLaughlin-Renpenning, K.E. (1998). *Nursing administration in the 21st century: A self-care theory approach.* Thousand Oaks, CA: Sage Publications.

Backscheider, J.E. (1974). Self-care requirements, self-care capabilities, and nursing systems in the diabetic nurse management clinic. *American Journal of Public Health, 64*(12), 1138-1146.

Bliss-Holtz, J., Taylor, S.G., McLaughlin, K. (1992). Nursing theory as a base for a computerized nursing information system. *Nursing Science Quarterly, 5*(3), 124-128.

Bowles K.H. & Naylor D. (1996). Nursing intervention classification. *Image, 28*(6), 303-308.

Canavan, K. (1996). ANA asserts attacks on practice threaten patient safety. *American Nurse, 28*(1), 1-9.

Carper, B.A. (1978). Fundamental patterns of knowing in nursing. *Advances in Nursing Science, 1*(1), 13-23.

Chen, H. (1990). *Theory-driven evaluations.* Newbury Park, CA: Sage.

Denyes, M.J., O'Connor, N.A., Oakley, D., Ferguson, S. (1989). Integrating nursing theory, practice and research through collaborative research. *Journal of Advanced Nursing, 14*(2), 141-145.

Denyes, M.J. (1993). Response to a predictor of children's self-care performance: Testing the theory of self-care deficit. *Scholarly Inquiry for Nursing Practice, 7*(3), 213-217.

Estabrooks, C.A. (1997). *Research utilization in nursing: An examination of formal structure and influencing factors.* Unpublished doctoral dissertation, University of Alberta, Edmonton, Alberta, Canada.

Estabrooks, C.A. (1998). Will evidence-based nursing practice make practice perfect? *Canadian Journal of Nursing Research, 30*(1), 15-36.

Fawcett, J. (1992). Conceptual models and nursing practice: The reciprocal relationship. *Journal of Advanced Nursing, 17*(2), 224-228.

Gebbie, K.M. & Lavin, M.A. (Eds.) (1975). *Classification of nursing diagnosis: Proceedings of the first national conference.* St. Louis: Mosby.

Gebbie, K.M. (1982). Toward the theory development for nursing diagnosis classification (1978). In M.J. King and D.A. Moritz (Eds.), *Classification of nursing diagnosis: Proceedings of the third and fourth national conferences.* New York: McGraw Hill.

Geden, E. (1997a). Theory-based research and defining populations. *The International Orem Society Newsletter, 5*(2) 6-9.

Geden, E. (1997b). How is nursing expressed by nurse practitioners in the primary health care setting. *The International Orem Society Newsletter, 5*(2), 9-11.

Gertzels, J.W. (1960.) A theory and practice in educational administration: An old question revisited. In R.F. Campbell & J.M. Lipman (Eds.), *Administrative theory as a guide to action.* Chicago: Midwest Administration Center, University of Chicago.

Henderson, V. (1969). *ICN Basic principles of nursing care.* Geneva: International Council of Nursing.

Horsley, J.A. (1985). Using research in practice: The current context. *Western Journal of Nursing Research, 7*(1), 135-139.

Kikuchi, J.F. & Simmons, H. (1999). Practical nursing judgment: A moderate realist conception. *Scholarly inquiry for nursing practice, 13*(1), 43-55.

Maas, M.L., Johnson, M. & Morehead, S. (1996). Classifying nursing sensitive patient outcomes. *Image, 28*(4), 295-301.

Mayers, M. (1972). *A systematic approach to nursing care planning.* New York: Appleton-Century-Crofts.

McKenna, H.P. (1997). Theory and research: a linkage to benefit practice. *International Journal of Nursing Studies, 34*(6), 431-437.

Mitchell, G.J. (1995). Evaluation of the human becoming theory in practice in an acute care setting. In R.R. Parse (Ed.), *Illuminations: The human becoming theory in practice and research.* New York: National League for Nursing Press.

Mitchell, P.H. (1977). *Concepts basic to nursing.* New York: McGraw-Hill.

Northrup, D.T., & Cody, W.K. (1998). Evaluation of the human becoming theory in practice in an acute care psychiatric setting. *Nursing Science Quarterly, 11*(1), 23-30.

Nursing Development Conference Group. (1973). In D. Orem (Ed.), *Concept formalization in nursing: Process and product.* Boston: Little, Brown.

Nursing Development Conference Group. (1979). In D. Orem (Ed.), *Concept formalization in nursing: Process and product.* (2nd ed.). Boston: Little, Brown.

Nursing Science Quarterly. (2000). Nursing theory guided by practice: A definition. *Nursing Science Quarterly, 13*(2), 177.

Orem, D.E. (1987). Why theory-based nursing. *Theory-based nursing process and product: Using Orem's self-care deficit theory of nursing in practice, education, and research.* Papers presented at the Fifth Annual Self-Care Deficit Theory Conference. School of Nursing, University of Missouri-Columbia. November 6-7, 1986. St. Louis, MO.

Orem, D.E. (1995). Nursing: *Concepts of practice.* (5th ed.). St. Louis: Mosby.

Parse, R.R. (1992). Human becoming: Parse's theory of nursing. *Nursing Science Quarterly, 5*(1), 35-42.

Parse, R.R. (1999). Nursing Science: the transformation of practice. *Journal of Advanced Nursing Science, 30*(6), 1383-1387.

Reed, P. (1996). Transforming practice knowledge into nursing knowledge–a revisionist analysis of Peplau. *Image, 28*(1), 29-33.

Riggs, J. & Bliss-Holtz, J. (1994). Competency-based assessment of theory-based practice. *The International Orem Society Newsletter, 2*(3), 6-7.

Robinson, V. (1987). Relationship of theory based nursing and defined populations in practice in *Theory-Based Nursing Process and Product: Using Orem's Self-Care Deficit Theory of Nursing in Practice, Education and Research.* Papers presented at the Fifth Annual Self-Care Deficit Theory Conference. School of Nursing, University of Missouri-Columbia. November 6-7, 1986. St. Louis, MO.

Rogers, E.M. (1995). *Diffusion of innovations.* (4th ed.). New York: The Free Press.

Roy, C. (1982). Theoretical framework for classification of nursing diagnosis (1978). In M.J. Kim and D.A. Moritz (Eds.), *Classification of Nursing Diagnosis: Proceedings of the third and fourth national conferences.* New York: McGraw-Hill.

Silva, M., Sorrell, J., & Sorrell, C. (1995). From Carper's patterns of knowing to ways of being: An ontological shift in nursing. *Advances in Nursing Science, 18*(1), 1-13.

Taylor, S.G. (1989). An interpretation of family within Orem's general theory of nursing. *Nursing Science Quarterly, 2*(3), 131-137.

Taylor, S.G. (1998). Clinical decision-making from the perspective of self-care deficit nursing theory. *The International Orem Society Newsletter, 6*(1), 2-6.

Taylor, S.G. & McLaughlin, K. (1991). Orem's general theory of nursing and community nursing. *Nursing Science Quarterly, 4*(4), 153-160.

Taylor, S.G. & McLaughlin-Renpenning, K. (1995). The practice of nursing in multi-person situations, family and community. In D.E. Orem (Ed). *Nursing: Concepts of practice.* (5th ed). St. Louis: Mosby.

Taylor, S.G. & McLaughlin-Renpenning, K. (2001). The practice of nursing in multiperson situations, family and community. In D.E. Orem (Ed.), *Nursing: Concepts of practice.* (6th ed). St. Louis: Mosby.

Thoma, D. (1972). Evaluation of problem-oriented nursing notes. *Journal of Nursing Administration. 2*(3): 50-58.

Walker, D. (1993). A nursing administrator's perspective of use of Orem's self-care deficit nursing theory. In M. Parker (Ed.), *Patterns of nursing theories in practice.* New York: National League for Nursing Press.

Weed, L. (1968a). Medical records that guide and teach. *New England Journal of Medicine, 278*(11), 593-600.

Weed, L. (1968b). Medical records that guide and teach. *New England Journal of Medicine, 278*(12), 652-657.

CHAPTER

4

Integration

Nursing's future will be created only as the discipline underlying nursing practices is identified, structured, and continuously updated by systematic inquiry…the kinds of knowledge contained within the discipline are identified and an approach to its structure is proposed.

Schlotfeldt, 1999

Objectives

- Describe the role of praxis in unifying theory and practice.
- Discuss the issues associated with viewing knowledge from other disciplines through a nursing perspective.
- Apply a systematic strategy for selecting a nursing theoretical system to use as a guide for practice and research.
- Compare and contrast the characteristics of quantitative and qualitative research methods, examining the appropriate use of each within different theoretical systems.
- Specify key attributes for evaluating quantitative research instruments.
- Describe criteria for selecting a theoretical system to guide nursing practice.
- Discuss the practice benefits derived by developing research and educational programs from the same theoretical perspective.

Key Terms

dialogical engagement, p. 60
emic, p. 58
ethnography, p. 58
etic, p. 58
grounded theory, p. 58
phenomenology, p. 57
praxiology, p. 52

Chapter 1 discussed the compartmentalized nature of nursing theory, research, and practice. Integrating these areas is the next step in the evolution of the discipline and profession of nursing. Nursing theoretical systems earn their integrity through adherence to a single object domain that is developed into a philosophically, conceptually, and logically coherent unity. It must remain integrated even as one changes position or perspective. Like the Nexus on the cover of this book, this integration relies on ideas and materials as well as thoughts and feelings. These are both abstract and conceptual. Although it is cast in bronze, the Nexus changes as one's viewing perspective changes. Yet it remains an ever-changing whole. Peck (1995) acknowledges the difficulty of achieving this type of integration. He states, "Compartmentalization is painless; integrity never is. Integrity requires that we fully experience the tensions of competing demands and conflicting ideas" (1995, p. 366). Competing demands and conflicting ideas have obscured the need for integration from many practicing nurses. Thus gaps between and among nursing's parts remain.

The theory-practice gap has been a topic of concern to nurse scientists and nurse theoreticians for many years. Fawcett (1999a) described a helical relationship between research and practice. Chinn and Kramer (1999) described a "whole of knowing" that comprises four patterns of knowing. Although it integrates knowledge development, this model, too, fails to completely integrate a nursing framework. Some nursing scholars consider doing research disconnected from theory unreasonable and argue that the gap occurs because theory and research have been neglected in structuring clinical practice. Nurses who have come to value theory through their exposure to nursing theory in their formal education often grow frustrated with task orientation in the workplace. Conversely, many practitioners deny the relevance of most theory and research to daily clinical practice. To resolve the debate and to develop nursing as a discipline and profession, the intertwining of theory, research, and practice is essential. Specialty nursing practice must embrace this nexus and ensure that their research and actions adhere to a nursing theoretical system. This long-standing gap will not be easily resolved, but it is an important challenge to face.

NURSING PRAXIS

Praxis, derived from the Greek word for *doing or action*, is a unifying concept that can help close this theory-practice gap. **Praxiology** is the study of human conduct or of efficient action—that is, sets of actions coordinated to achieve a common end (Kotarbinsky cited in Orem, 1995, p. 113). Within the nursing literature, praxis has taken on an additional meaning. According to Rolfe (1996), praxis indicates the inseparability of theory and practice. Practice spawns theory, and theory impacts practice. Chinn and Kramer (1999) labeled the "synchrony between thoughtful reflection and action" praxis (p. 1). Praxis requires approaching nursing as a practice discipline with both speculative and practical knowledge developed through research and philosophical inquiry. Nursing generated through research must be practical science—that is, science that leads to the synchrony Chinn and Kramer described.

KNOWLEDGE FROM OTHER DISCIPLINES

Viewing nursing science as a unique creative endeavor raises the question of its relationship to other disciplines. The current emphasis on middle-range theory, which integrates knowledge from other disciplines into nursing science, also highlights the need for discussion of this issue. Cody (1996, 1997) criticized continued use of theories from other disciplines and argued that using this outside knowledge impedes advancement of nursing discipline-specific knowledge. On the other hand, Rafferty (1995) advocates mutual exchange between nursing and related fields. She holds that instead of seeking a rarified view of nursing, nurses should embrace the work of other disciplines that helps explain the theoretical or speculative nursing sciences, usually by analogy. This can be achieved through identifying a nursing phenomenon, exploring a related concept or theory from another discipline, and reconstructing that concept into a model that generates research questions unique to nursing (Ulbrich, 1999). The development of middle-range theories with conceptual-theoretical-empirical structures bridges general theory and practice.

Fawcett (1999b) asserted nursing's need to end the romance with nonnursing disciplines and to focus on nursing discipline-specific knowledge. However, knowledge generated through other human sciences cannot be ignored. Such knowledge must be recognized for what it is—or for what it can be. For example, anatomy and physiology are foundational to discipline-specific nursing knowledge. Alternatively, philosophical knowledge elucidates the nature of the patient. Bekel's interpretation (1998) of Weingartner's conceptualization of object domains helpfully explains scientific disciplines' use of different objects for their scientific endeavors.

Appropriate to this discussion is the concept of the application domain. This domain describes the application of a discipline to another discipline such that the disciplines continue to exist in their original form. Moreover, specialized disciplines relevant to both disciplines sometimes emerge. Sentences or theoretical propositions of one discipline may be applied to another discipline, but each discipline has a different independent object. If the objects of the two disciplines were identical, one would be a genuine subdiscipline of the other. That is, if nursing were understood as an application domain of psychology, it would be a subdiscipline of psychology and not an independent discipline. Unfortunately, this is the direction many of the so-called middle-range theories are taking. The theories, principles, or sentences from a nonnursing discipline are held as primary and are applied to nursing, subordinating nursing to a subdiscipline. Using theory from other disciplines weakens the development of nursing as a discipline. The nursing theoretical system must be primary. Sentences from other disciplines may constitute a part of the domain of nursing if they are interpreted through a specific nursing theoretical system. Ulbrich's work exemplifies this (Figure 4-1).

SELECTING A NURSING THEORETICAL SYSTEM

The first three chapters of this book provided background information about theory, research, and practice and described links between and among these elements. The subsequent chapters present some of the integrated nursing theoretical systems. Nurses should find theoretical systems that meet their needs for developing nursing practice knowledge, but not all the theoretical systems have evolved to include explicit statements of the theoretical systems' foundational cosmologies. The movement from the logical middle occurs in varying ways and at varying speeds. To select an appropriate theoretical system, consider the following questions while reading and studying each chapter.

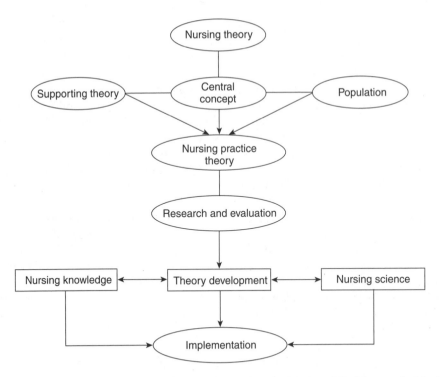

FIGURE 4-1   Exercise as self-care: A nursing practice model. (Modified from Ulbrich, S.L. (1999). Nursing practice theory of exercise as self-care. *Image, 31*(1), 65-70.)

Questions for the Selection of a Theoretical System as the Basis for Specialty Practice or Knowledge Development

One must first take into account one's current view of nursing practice or research. What do you consider important in a nursing theoretical system? That is, as a nurse, what must you know? About what do you inquire, and what research questions do you need to ask? What conclusions are valid? What practical meaning do you attach to the information obtained or to the judgments you make? Do you have a language to meaningfully express what you know to patients, other nurses, and other health workers? (Orem, 1995).

Conceptual-Theoretical Elements. To some degree, the selection of a particular theoretical system is a matter of preference for the ontological expression, the model depiction, and the theoretical expression. Perceived applicability to the specialty practice area or research question also shapes decisions. Thus you first should identify the cosmology and/or ontology congruent with your beliefs. What are your core values and beliefs? Are these captured in one or more of the theoretical systems?

Harré (1998) suggested a dual ontology for psychology—one that "permits a choice between founding the science of human thought and action on molecules as basic particulars, and founding it on people as the basic particulars" (p. 47). This might apply to nursing scholars as well. Adopting a dual or complex ontology rather than mutually exclusive categories could eliminate philosophical debates that have little if any meaning for research

---

BOX 4-1

Questions Guiding Theory Choice

COSMOLOGY/ONTOLOGY QUESTIONS

Is the object or focus of nursing specified? Is it specific to the discipline of nursing, or could it apply to any human science or helping service?

Do the statements about the object encompass all situations of nursing or situations of nursing within my specialty area?

What is my conceptualization of person?

Is my conceptualization of person consistent with that proposed by the theory?

What is the position of person in social and physical environment or contexts?

Does the language of the theory reflect my thinking about nursing practice?

Does the language provide me with a way in which I can "talk" about my specific area of nursing?

MODEL QUESTIONS

Is there a central model that represents the ontology?

Is the model relevant to the real world of nursing?

Are the variables specified by the model consistent with the phenomenon with which I am concerned?

Does the model help me understand the portion of reality it represents by showing the relationships of variables under study?

How well does the model conform to the part of reality it is supposed to predict?

THEORY QUESTIONS

Does the narrative accompanying the model help me understand the world of nursing and how nurses function within it?

Does the theory provide guidelines for analyzing a phenomenon?

METAPHOR QUESTIONS

Can I visualize my nursing specialty within this framework?

What are the metaphors used to describe nursing and nursing-specific concepts?

Are these metaphors congruent with my values and beliefs about nursing?

RESEARCH AND PRACTICE QUESTIONS

Can questions that arise in my practice be researched from this theoretical perspective?

With what phenomena am I concerned in my practice?

Which nursing theoretical framework reflects these phenomena?

Is there a scheme for understanding the significance of research findings?

Are nursing practice models derived from this theoretical framework adequate or sufficient for my practice?

---

and practice. As you review the theoretical systems presented in the following units, consider the possibility of selecting a dual ontology—for example, Peplau's interpersonal relations (Chapter 12) and Orem's general theory of nursing systems (Chapter 5). Then evaluate the philosophical and logical congruence between the two.

The questions presented in Box 4-1 can guide your thinking. In reviewing and reflecting on your responses, identify a theoretical system appropriate for you.

RESEARCH METHODS

Theory impacts research. Thus the theory selected should help the investigator visualize important research questions or hypotheses. As Chapter 2 mentions, research both tests and generates theory. Two major research approaches—quantitative and qualitative—are used for theory testing and generation. Guba and Lincoln (1994) suggest that these two approaches evolved from competing scientific paradigms that influence methods for discovery of truth (see Chapter 2). These competing paradigms are evident in several components of both types of research (Denzin & Lincoln, 1994). Quantitative researchers attempt to study and capture a knowable reality. Similarly, a positivist paradigm anticipates that research findings uncover the existence of truth. Thus positivist or postpositivist paradigms of inquiry shape much quantitative research, although a postpositivist paradigm approaches research findings a bit more tentatively, holding that reality can only be imperfectly known.

Qualitative researchers feel that reality can never be fully understood, only approximated. This perspective most reflects constructivism, but critical theory also applies. Critical theorists believe social, political, cultural, ethnic, or gender structures influence interpretation of reality. They are similar to postpositivists in their belief that reality can be only approximated. From a qualitative perspective, multiple realities might exist within a given context, whereas quantitative researchers believe in a singular reality (Haase & Myers, 1988). Both types of researchers are interested in capturing individual points of view. However, quantitative researchers attempt the process through empirical methods that focus on systematic and objective measurement. In contrast, qualitative researchers try to get closer approximations of individual perspectives through less structured interviews and observation. Qualitative research views subjective experiences as legitimate data sources.

Both quantitative and qualitative researchers consider the constraints of everyday life. However, quantitative researchers are less likely to study those constraints directly. The focus of quantitative research is reductionistic; the whole is broken into subparts so that each of the parts can be studied. To achieve control over the research setting, the researcher explicitly identifies the research problem and attempts to limit extraneous variables that might influence outcomes. In quantitative research, large numbers of randomly selected cases are used to draw conclusions based on the probability that these cases represent a larger population (Denzin & Lincoln, 1994). Researchers attempt to limit or at least account for data discrepancies by providing alternative explanations for the phenomenon (Haase & Myers, 1988). On the other hand, qualitative researchers are more concerned with describing the phenomenon as a whole, but they also deal with the specifics of particular cases, seeking to explain both the commonalties and differences among participants. Qualitative research may attribute discrepancies to the existence of multiple realities.

These differences direct investigators to different modes of discovery. Quantitative researchers use mathematical models and statistics. Instruments measuring selected aspects of the phenomena are constructed carefully to ensure reliability and validity. Qualitative researchers use a broader variety of data collection techniques, including prose narratives, first-person accounts, photographs, life histories, biographical and autobiographical materials, observation, and interviews.

Methods of Quantitative Research

Quantitative research approaches can include descriptive, correlational, and experimental techniques. Descriptive research uses structured or semi-structured interviews, observation, surveys, and questionnaires to describe phenomena of interest. Correlational research seeks to investigate systematic relationships between two or more variables of interest. Correlational research does not, however, measure cause and effect; rather, it determines association among variables. A variety of measuring instruments can assess the nature of variables of interest. Much nursing research has been descriptive or correlational. Although these studies are useful beginnings for describing the realities of nursing, they are insufficient for testing potential practice interventions.

When quantitative research moves beyond the descriptive or correlational realm, it becomes some form of experimental study. Experimental studies are systematic, highly controlled, and predictive. They manipulate an independent variable to determine to what degree the outcomes are influenced. The goal of these studies is to maximize the experimental variance while minimizing sources of error and controlling any extraneous variables (Kerlinger, 1973). Because the researcher maintains greater control over the research environment in experimental studies, these studies are the most powerful. The classification of experimental research is based on an investigators' control over the events in the study. The three elements factored into the structure of experimental studies are manipulation of an independent variable, use of controls (usually a control group), and subject assignment to groups (random assignment of subjects to groups is preferable). Including all these elements provides the investigator the most control over the study and greater certainty that the findings reflect reality. Experimental studies represent positivist and postpositivist approaches to testing theory and interventions.

True experimental designs, the strongest and most controlled of experimental design, include all three elements. Subjects are randomly assigned to groups; a control group is present; the independent variable is manipulated. However, sometimes an element may be missing. In quasi-experimental studies the investigator may have a control group and may be able to manipulate the independent variable but is unable to randomly assign subjects. In this situation, researchers have less control over the study events, which means the findings are less certain. Preexperimental studies use weak designs in which only the independent variable is manipulated. Although a preexperimental design may provide a mechanism for discovery, the study findings remain uncertain because poor study control may have allowed outside events to influence the outcome. Although true experimental studies are valuable, they are the most difficult to conduct and usually involve the most artificial settings.

Methods of Qualitative Research

Several modes of qualitative inquiry are useful for theory generation. Three types of qualitative research are phenomenology, ethnography, and grounded theory. Although the mechanisms for data collection in each of these types of research may overlap, the particular focus of each method varies.

Phenomenology focuses on experiential life in terms of individuals' views and interactions with the phenomena of concern in their everyday lives (Holstein & Gubrium, 1994). Investigators suspend judgment about the nature of the world and start from scratch, focusing on the ways individuals perceive their lives and life events. Expert and reliable informants are used to gather data. Informants interpret their experiences for the investigator, who then interprets the collective explanations of participants.

Ethnography stems from cultural anthropology. It offers a description of individuals living within cultural groups, whose members share a learned complex system of living (Boyle, 1994). Ethnography is concerned with the meaning of actions and events associated with the cultural group. Ethnography places group description data obtained through participant observations and individual interviews into a larger wholistic and contextual perspective (Boyle, 1994). Ethnography is called reflexive because the researcher, in the role of participant/observer, is a part of the world under study. An **emic** perspective offers an insider's view and is the goal of ethnography. An **etic,** or outsider's/investigator's perspective, helps scientifically view reality within the group under study.

The qualitative method of **grounded theory** specifically identifies theory generation regarding social and psychological phenomena as its purpose (Glaser & Strauss, 1967; Strauss & Corbin, 1990). Grounded theory, phenomenology, and ethnography share methods of discovery through observation and interviews. A major difference of grounded theory, however, is its focus on theory generation (Strauss & Corbin, 1994). Grounded theory involves a highly systematic set of procedures for discovery of information about a phenomenon of interest. From this, investigators inductively develop theory. Strauss and Corbin (1994) indicate that theory evolves through an interplay between data collection and analysis. Grounded theory considers relationships among the concepts and then produces relevant abstract concepts and propositions (Chenitz & Swanson, 1986). Constant comparative analysis, a central feature of grounded theory, continually seeks similarities and differences among participants, actions, or events. Data are coded, clustered into similar categories, and labeled. Collection of additional data may warrant recoding and reorganization. Relationships among categories are developed, and patterns among relationships are conceptualized. Ultimately, a general theory about relationships is produced.

Balance Between the Two Research Methods

One might ask which form of research is best for building a scientific knowledge base. Very practically, the answer is both. The goal of research and theory is an understanding that will ultimately influence practice. Addressing the cyclic interaction of theory and research, Benoliel (1977) established a case for nursing research derived both from traditional scientific models and more naturalistic models. Beck (1997) successfully incorporated both quantitative and qualitative research projects into a program of research on postpartum depression. She insisted that programs of research be knowledge-directed rather than limited by adherence to specific research methods. Silva (1977) indicated that although the use of the scientific methods is praiseworthy for its rigor, the narrow focus of some studies leads to trivial outcomes that fail to meaningfully advance nursing knowledge. Thus she argued for a more wholistic approach to the development of nursing knowledge. Haase and Myers (1988) suggested that because nurses must individualize care, multiple meanings can be associated realistically with individual experiences. Conversely, because phenomena of interest to nurses are complex, considering the component parts is also helpful. Often the choice of research model is based on the investigator's understanding of the world, which sometimes leads to exclusive use of either quantitative or qualitative research techniques.

However, both quantitative and qualitative research methods contribute to an understanding of reality useful for nursing theory development, testing, and practice.

Gortner and Schultz (1988) argued that good nursing science should be characterized by significance, theory-observation compatibility, generalizability, reproducibility, and precision. These characteristics—although sometimes identified with different terms—are present in both quantitative and qualitative research approaches. Of course, these characteristics also represent good science in other disciplines. Reed (1996) suggested that nursing scholarship should embrace a philosophical view in which each dimension—quantitative and qualitative—informs the other in knowledge development. If nursing attends to the contributions each can make, practice can significantly guide knowledge development, and scientific knowledge will become embedded in nursing practice.

Triangulation permits the use of multiple research methods, theories, data, and investigators for studying a common phenomenon. Duffy (1987) asserted that multiple research methods are useful in triangulating data gathered from a variety of sampling strategies. Triangulation assumes that the strengths of an alternate method might compensate for the weakness of one method. Therefore the methods selected must be based on common assumptions and must complement one another (Knafl & Breitmayer, 1991). A common type of methodological triangulation is the combination of quantitative and qualitative research methods in a single study. The data derived are then checked for mutual confirmation. Methodological triangulation incorporating qualitative and quantitative research approaches provides "richer and more insightful analyses of complex phenomena" (Duffy, 1987, p. 133) and permits verification and validation of findings. Triangulation can be a powerful tool for facilitating theory generation.

Selecting a Paradigm of Inquiry, Research Method, and Instrumentation

Earlier, this chapter provided guidance for selecting a theoretical system. Selecting a paradigm of scientific inquiry is a similarly important step. The choice of a theoretical system directly may influence the choice of a paradigm of inquiry. For example, some theoretical systems, such as those by Parse (1987) and Watson (1999), strongly reflect a constructivist paradigm of inquiry. Systems such as Orem's (1995) may reflect a more postpositivist paradigm. Therefore examining the theoretical system is crucial to selecting a paradigm of inquiry. Explore the ontological concerns mentioned earlier in this chapter and consider how the theorist posits them. What does the theorist say about persons? How is evidence supporting the theory accumulated? For example, Orem (see Chapter 5) suggests that theory changes when new knowledge becomes available—a belief congruent with a postpositivist paradigm. Rogers also believed that knowledge was an evolving process but felt it must be measured in a wholistic, acausal way.

Theoretical perspectives also influence the selection of research method to some degree. Box 4-2 presents questions to guide the selection of a research method. Some theorists rely primarily on quantitative approaches as mechanisms for discovery and model testing. Some advocate a combined approach of both quantitative and qualitative research. Many studies using frameworks developed by Orem, Roy, and Pender primarily use quantitative research coupled with a small amount of qualitative investigation. Research derived from Rogers' Science of Unitary Human Beings combines quantitative and qualita-

---

BOX 4-2

Developing Research from the Selected Theoretical System

RESEARCH QUESTIONS/HYPOTHESES

Can research questions or hypotheses be visualized with this theoretical perspective?
How can the phenomenon of interest within the perspective of this theory be
  conceptualized?

RESEARCH METHODS

Having derived the research question from the theoretical perspective, what
  method would be appropriate?
Are particular research methods more amenable to discovery within the selected
  theoretical context?
What is currently known about the phenomenon of interest?
What is the state of nursing knowledge regarding the phenomenon of interest?
Would the problem be best studied in a highly controlled environment or in a more
  naturalistic one?

Qualitative Methods	Quantitative Methods
What is the purpose of the investigation? • Description of life experiences? • Description of cultural groups? • Theory generation?	What is the purpose of the investigation? • To describe? • To look for associations? • To test interventions? **Quantitative Instrument Choice** Is there an instrument that measures the phenomenon of interest? Does the instrument possess adequate reliability? Does the instrument possess adequate validity? Is the instrument usable with the selected population?

---

tive approaches. Other theorists support using only qualitative approaches. For example, Parse would suggest that evidence be gathered only if the investigator is truly present with the participant and conducts the research investigation through a process termed **dialogical engagement.** Dialogical engagement is a process in which researchers are truly present with participants and are open to discussion of the phenomenon of study. All studies using Parse's Theory of Human Becoming as a framework are qualitative. In some ways selection of a theoretical system and a paradigm of inquiry can be a chicken-and-egg phenomenon. Individuals may already have opinions that will influence their choice of a paradigm of inquiry. For others, the theoretical system may be a driving factor.

Research methods also should be selected on the basis of what is currently known and of what needs to be discovered. If theory related to the phenomenon of study does not exist, the descriptive processes of either quantitative or qualitative research might be a good beginning point. Valuable nursing research stems from practice observations and can stimulate theory development or extension. Unfortunately, nursing sometimes neglects the process of description in the effort to deal with practice-associated problems. Other times, nursing research seems to describe a phenomenon "to death" before proceeding with explanatory or intervention studies. Evaluating the state of the nursing knowledge base, including a review of potentially relevant theory, is an important initial step in the research process.

The nature of the problem to be studied may also be a driving factor in selecting a research method. Use of a naturalistic environment may be desirable for broad, in-depth description. For other studies, using narrower foci and environments in which extraneous variation can be controlled at least to some extent is essential to answering the concern. For studies seeking in-depth description, a qualitative approach may serve the purpose best. When greater controls are needed, quantitative studies provide more adequate answers.

Once a qualitative or quantitative method is selected, more decisions remain (see Box 4-2). If investigators use qualitative research, they must determine the type of approach. For example, a phenomenological approach best serves the purpose if the investigator wants an in-depth understanding about the lived experience of a phenomenon. Ethnography would be most effective in studies of cultural practices. Grounded theory is valuable for theory generation. Once again, the purpose of study is important in quantitative investigations. A study with the primary purpose of description warrants a descriptive study. A correlational study would be used to investigate associations. Testing interventions requires some form of experimental study.

In quantitative studies, instrumentation is also an important issue (see Box 4-2). Investigators must look for instruments that will measure the phenomenon of interest. Alternatively, they must develop new instruments if none are available. Instruments should be evaluated for their reliability to ensure the accurate and dependable measurement. Because the instrument needs to measure what it says it measures, validity is also a concern. Chapter 2 reviews mechanisms for evaluating reliability and validity. Finally, one must consider the usability of the instrument in the population of interest. For example, an instrument that works well in young and middle-aged populations may not work well with older adults.

PRACTICE APPLICATIONS

All nursing practice can be called theory-based. The question is whether the theory on which practice is based is nursing discipline-specific. The advantage of structuring practice within a nursing theoretical system is that the practitioner's questions can use the language and perspective of nursing, and the related research can address the specific concerns of nursing. Survival of the profession depends on furthering the discipline through integrated programs of theory development, research and practice. Without such development, nursing becomes merely a collection of tasks. Examples of theory-research-practice programs in relation to specific theories are presented in subsequent chapters. Such programs are the products of researchers who deliberately set out to practice and research from a particular nursing theoretical perspective. Individual nurses, educators, or the collective nurses in a healthcare agency can also achieve integration of theory, research, and practice by practicing from particular nursing theoretical perspectives. Theory becomes eyeglasses through which to view the dilemmas of practice and identify related research questions (Denyes, O'Connor, Oakley, & Ferguson, 1989).

BOX 4-3

Developing Practice from Selected Nursing Theoretical System

INDIVIDUAL PRACTICE

What is the proper object or focus of concern of nursing within this theoretical system?

Can variables reflecting the concern of nursing practice be defined in operational terms?

What are the characteristics of my patient population?

What should be the outcomes of my nursing practice?

What are the processes of nursing through which I can achieve the desired outcomes?

What variations should be made to the nursing practice model in relation to my specific patient populations?

ORGANIZATIONAL PERSPECTIVE

Is the selected theoretical system's conceptualization of person and beliefs about nursing congruent with the organization's mission statement?

Are the nursing-related structural components of the organization supportive of practice from the perspective of the selected theoretical system?

Choosing a Theoretical Perspective to Structure Practice

Choosing a theoretical perspective for practice involves studying available theoretical systems and determining which are congruent with one's view of nursing; including the patient, the nurse, nursing actions, and nursing outcomes. The processes of nursing and the practice models developed vary with the particular theoretical system chosen. These variations are reflected in the descriptions of patient populations served by nursing, the definition of expected outcomes of nursing, the methods by which the expected outcomes can be achieved and the documentation of data related to patients and nursing action.

The theoretical system chosen to structure nursing practice within a healthcare agency should be consistent with the mission statement of the agency. Organizational components should be designed and developed to support practice from the chosen perspective. Research programs should be designed to further the knowledge base about the phenomena of concern. Within educational settings, the theoretical system chosen as the framework for developing the students' concepts of nursing should reflect faculty beliefs about nursing. Nursing courses should be structured around the specified phenomena of concern. Nonnursing courses foundational to fully understanding those phenomena should be offered. See Box 4-3 for suggested questions for developing practice from a selected theoretical system.

Addressing the Theory-Practice Gap

The theory-practice gap has concerned many nurses for some time. Basic nursing programs strongly influence nursing practice. Policies and procedures of employing institutions and the dominance of the medical model in the healthcare field significantly influence the curricula of nursing programs and the daily practice of the nurse after graduation

(Estabrooks, 1997). One cannot help but wonder if the gap partly originates in the introductory nursing programs in which students learn social and biological theories from the perspectives of those disciplines rather than from the perspective of nursing. In addition, although students may be introduced to nursing theories, too commonly the nursing practice before and after graduation is not embedded in the theories of the nursing discipline. Structuring the clinical component of the nursing curriculum from the perspective of a nursing discipline-specific theoretical system would begin to rectify this situation.

The lag between development of nursing theory and its influence on curriculum development means that basic education programs did not socialize many nurses to the usefulness of theory in structuring of nursing practice. Although some essential nursing knowledge was developed in other disciplines, nonnursing elements have tended to dominate clinical practice. Using the knowledge developed within other disciplines and the theories from which they are derived within the practice of nursing requires viewing them from a nursing perspective. Donaldson and Crowley (1978) cautioned that nursing's survival depends on discipline development that can incorporate the knowledge from disciplines but is designed to answer central nursing concerns, such as the effects of particular educational techniques on self-care. Donaldson and Crowley (1978) noted that nurse researchers tended to take for granted that the nursing perspective is understood. This issue is still considered germane; Kenney reproduced Donaldson and Crowley's original article in 1999. This criticism of nurse researchers can be extended to educators and to many current nursing textbooks as well. Developing a nursing perspective and using knowledge associated with related disciplines is not an innate ability. It must be taught. Backscheider (1974) provides an example of the utility of such research for nursing practice (see Chapters 3 and 5).

Summary

- Praxis requires approaching nursing as a practice discipline with both speculative and practical knowledge developed through research and philosophical inquiry.
- Advancing the discipline of nursing requires that the nursing theoretical system be the primary system. Other disciplines may constitute a part of the domain of nursing if they are interpreted from the perspective of a specific nursing theoretical system.
- Moving to a nursing theory–based research and clinical practice requires answering questions about the personal theoretical bases of practice and research. An overall philosophical and logical congruence between the general theory, the focal concept(s), complementary theory or theories, empirical methods, and practical meaning is essential for successful selection and integration of theory into research and practice.
- The chosen theoretical framework may be associated with underlying beliefs about paradigms of inquiry. In selecting a method of discovery, nurses should consider both the paradigm and the nature of the question.
- Key attributes such as reliability, validity, and their appropriateness for the population of study need to be considered in selecting quantitative research instruments.
- Choice of a theoretical system hinges upon congruency between one's views of nursing and of the patient, the nurse, nursing actions, and outcomes.
- Educational and research programs should be developed from the same theoretical perspective to help close the theory-practice gap.

REFERENCES

Backscheider, J.E. (1974). Self-care requirements, self-care capabilities, and nursing systems in the diabetic nurse management clinic. *American Journal of Public Health, 64*(12), 1138-1146.

Beck, C. (1997). Developing a research program using qualitative and quantitative approaches. *Nursing Outlook, 45*(6), 265-269.

Bekel, G. (1998, February-March). *Statements on the object of science: A discussion paper.* Paper presented at the meeting of the Orem Study Group. Savannah, GA. Published in *IOS Newsletter, 7*(1999): 1-3.

Benoliel, J. (1977). The interaction between theory and research. *Nursing Outlook, 25*(2), 108-113.

Boyle, J. (1994). Styles of ethnography. In J. Morse (Ed.), *Critical issues in qualitative research methods.* Thousand Oaks, CA: Sage.

Chenitz, W.C. & Swanson, J.M. (1986). *From practice to grounded theory: Qualitative research in nursing.* Menlo Park, CA: Addison Wesley.

Chinn, P. & Kramer, M. (1999). *Theory and nursing: Integrated knowledge development.* (5th ed.). St. Louis: Mosby.

Cody, W.K. (1996). Drowning in eclecticism. *Nursing Science Quarterly, 9*(3), 86-88.

Cody, W.K. (1997). Of tombstones, milestones, and gemstones: A retrospective and prospective on nursing theory. *Nursing Science Quarterly, 10*(1), 3-5.

Denyes, M.J., O'Connor, N.A., Oakley, D., & Ferguson, S. (1989). Integrating nursing theory, practice, and research through collaborative research. *Journal of Advanced Nursing 14*(2), 141-145.

Denzin, N.K. & Lincoln, Y.S. (1994). Entering the field of qualitative research. In E.K. Denzin & Y.S. Lincoln (Eds.), *Handbook of qualitative research.* Thousand Oaks, CA: Sage.

Donaldson, S.K. & Crowley, D.M. (1978). The discipline of nursing. *Nursing Outlook, 26*(2), 113-120.

Duffy, M.E. (1987). Methodological triangulation: A vehicle for merging quantitative and qualitative research methods, *Image, 19*(3), 130-133.

Estabrooks, C.A. (1997). *Research utilization in nursing: An examination of formal structure and influencing factors.* Unpublished doctoral dissertation, University of Alberta, Edmonton, Alberta, Canada.

Fawcett, J. (1999a). *The relationship of theory and research.* (3rd ed.). Philadelphia: Davis.

Fawcett, J. (1999b). The state of nursing science: Hallmarks of the 20th and 21st centuries. *Nursing Science Quarterly 12*(4), 311-314.

Glaser, B. & Strauss, A. (1967). *The discovery of grounded theory: Strategies for qualitative research.* Chicago: Aldine.

Gortner, S.R. & Schultz, P.R. (1988). Approaches to nursing science methods. *Image 20*(1), 22-24.

Guba, E.G., & Lincoln, Y.S. (1994). Competing paradigms in qualitative research. In E.K. Denzin & Y.S. Lincoln (Eds.), *Handbook of qualitative research.* Thousand Oaks, CA: Sage.

Haase, J.E. & Myers, S.T. (1988). Reconciling paradigm assumptions of qualitative and quantitative research. *Western Journal of Nursing Research, 10*(2), 128-137.

Harré, R. (1998). *The singular self.* Thousand Oaks, CA: Sage.

Holstein, J.A. & Gubrium J.F. (1994). Phenomenology, ethnomethodology, and interpretive practice. In E.K. Denzin & Y.S. Lincoln (Eds.), *Handbook of qualitative research.* Thousand Oaks, CA: Sage.

Kenney, J.W. (Ed.). (1999). Philosophical and theoretical perspectives for advanced nursing practice (2nd ed.). Boston: Jones and Bartlett.

Kerlinger, F. (1973). *Foundations of behavioral research,* (2nd ed.). New York: Hart, Rinehart, and Winston.

Knafl, K.A. & Breitmayer, B.J. (1991). Triangulation in qualitative research: Issues of conceptual clarity and purpose. In J. Morse (Ed.), *Qualitative nursing research: A contemporary dialogue.* Newbury Park, CA: Sage.

Orem, D. (1995). *Nursing: Concepts of practice.* (5th ed.). St. Louis: Mosby.

Orem, D.E. (1997). Views of human beings specific to nursing. *Nursing Science Quarterly 10*(1), 26-31.

Parse, R.R. (1987). *Nursing science: Major paradigms, theories, and critiques.* Philadelphia: W.B. Saunders.

Peck, M.S. (1995). *In search of stones: A pilgrimage of faith, reason, and discovery.* New York: Hyperion.

Rafferty, A. (1995). Art, science, and social science in nursing: Occupational origins and disciplinary identity. *Nursing Inquiry, 2*(4), 141-148.

Reed, P.G. (1996). Transforming practice knowledge into nursing knowledge: A revisionist analysis of Peplau. *Image, 28*(1), 29-33.

Rolfe, G. (1996). Going to extremes: Action research, grounded practice, and the theory-practice gap in nursing. *Journal of Advanced Nursing, 24*(6), 1315-1320.

Schlotfeldt, R.M. (1999). Structuring nursing knowledge: A priority for creating nursing's future. In J.W. Kenney (Ed.), *Philosophical and theoretical perspectives for advanced nursing practice*. (2nd ed.). Boston: Jones and Bartlett.

Silva, M.C. (1977). Philosophy, science, theory: Interrelationships and implications for nursing research. *Image, 9*(3), 59-63.

Strauss, A. & Corbin, J. (1990). *Basics of qualitative research: Grounded theory procedures and techniques*. Newbury Park, CA: Sage.

Strauss, A. & Corbin, J. (1994). Grounded theory methodology: An overview. In E.K. Denzin & Y.S. Lincoln (Eds.), *Handbook of qualitative research*. Thousand Oaks, CA: Sage.

Ulbrich, S.L. (1999). Nursing practice theory of exercise as self-care. *Image, 31*(1), 65-70.

Watson, J. (1999). *Postmodern nursing and beyond*. Philadelphia: Churchill Livingstone.

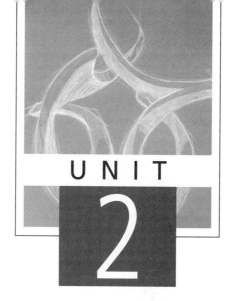

U N I T
2

OVERVIEW of THEORIES, RELATED RESEARCH, and PRACTICE APPLICATIONS

Objectives

- Explore the philosophical underpinnings and central characteristics of selected nursing theoretical systems.
- Examine selected research methods and instruments used for studies guided by nursing theories/models.
- Appraise research conducted with selected nursing theories and models.
- Conceptualize nursing as a program for structuring nursing practice.

Unit 2 presents a selection of specific theoretical systems and middle-range theories. As Chapter 1 stated, a nursing theoretical system consists of a general theory of nursing that can be placed within a philosophical tradition and can structure nursing practice. Within theoretical systems are practical middle-range theories and practice models. Although middle-range theories can be a part of a theoretical system, nursing also has middle-range theories that stand alone. Middle-range theories are limited in range and scope from which hypotheses can be derived and empirically measured. They possess a limited number of concepts related to a specific aspect of a phenomenon.

Included in this unit is work initially developed by Orem, Rogers, Parse, Neuman, King, Roy, Pender, Peplau, and Watson. Each of these theories has evolved to include defined and clarified theoretical elements, descriptions of variations in the elements, research to validate or verify the theoretical components, and described practice modalities. The extent to which each of these is developed varies greatly, as the chapters in this unit demonstrate. In some instances, the connections between research, theory, and subsequent practice applications are well documented. In other instances the associations are less substantial.

Inclusion of a particular theory in this unit depended on a number of factors. First, relevant literature from the Cumulative Index for Nursing and Allied Health Literature (CINAHL) was reviewed. Most studies included were published in the past 10 years. Occasionally, earlier studies were included when they were particularly critical to theory testing or related to practice. Some theorists had a very large number of studies available for inclusion in this book. When this was the case, studies representing continuing programs of research that best supported the theory were selected. For the most part, dissertation research was not included unless it resulted in a subsequent publication. The research sections of the chapters are organized topically by the nature of the research using a given theory.

This unit also explores structuring nursing practice within the various theoretical nursing systems. For some of these systems, extensive work has been undertaken to relate theory to practice. Others are still very much in the speculative stage.

Major topical headings are similar throughout each of the chapters in Unit 2. These headings should facilitate the reading of each chapter and the comparison of different theorists. As with the chapters in Unit 1, each chapter lists key terms at the beginning. These terms are also included in the glossary at the end of the book. Major topical headings in these chapters are ordered as follows:

Theory Title
The Starting Point of the Modeling Process
    Reason for Theory Development (Central Questions)
    Phenomenon of Concern
Description of Theoretical System
    Philosophical Perspecitves
    Description of Model and Theory
Research
    Research Instruments
    Review of Related Research
Praxis and Theory Utilization
    The Variables of Concern for Practice
    Describing a Population for Nursing Purposes
    Expected Outcomes of Nursing
    Process Models
    Practice Models
    Implications for Administration
    Implications for Education
Nexus

Of particular note is the "Nexus" section of each chapter. This section integrates information regarding the status of theory development, empirical support for the theory, and construction of practice based on theory and research application.

Each of the chapters may also include figures, boxes, and tables to highlight information relevant to theory, research, and practice. Figures offer schematic representations of theoretical models, and boxes summarize significant details relevant to theory and practice. Most chapters contain at least two tables: one summarizing research instruments and another summarizing selected research studies. Readers should use these aids in conjunction with text explanations to understand the concepts.

Modeling Nursing from a Realist Point of View

OREM'S SELF-CARE DEFICIT NURSING THEORY

Key Terms

The Self-Care Deficit Nursing Theory (SCDNT) was one of the first models of nursing. Initially developed by Dorothea E. Orem, BSNE, MSNE, RN, FAAN, it was first presented in the 1950s (Orem, 1956) and was formalized and published in 1971. The stated purpose of the theory was to lay out the structure and explicate the domains of nursing knowledge. Further development of the theory by the Nursing Development Conference Group (1973) was described in *Concept Formalization in Nursing*. Since then, Orem and other nursing scholars have worked extensively with the original conceptualizations. The value of this theoretical system has been demonstrated through research and development in practice, education, and administration. This chapter presents a description of the philosophical foundation of the SCDNT, an overview of the theory, and research and practice applications, but a full understanding of the theory can be gained only by reading primary sources and the evolving body of literature, including research reports.

THE STARTING POINT OF THE MODELING PROCESS

Orem began conceptualizing nursing in the 1950s. The logical middle for her was the need to answer the question "What condition exists in a person when that person or a family member or the attending physician or a nurse makes the judgment that a person should be under nursing care?" (1995, p. 433).

Reason for Theory Development

In an oral history interview, Orem said that she needed to include a chapter on hospital nursing services and then a chapter on the art of nursing in the report on her study of nursing administrative positions. "It was in doing that chapter on the art of nursing that I put together a definition of nursing," she explained, "It wasn't the expression of spontaneous, insightful knowing about what nursing is. I actually had to construct it" (Taylor, 1998). Orem's bachelor's and master's degrees in biology gave her some concept of the development of a science. Orem stated, "I knew that it didn't exist in nursing, but to develop nursing science, that wasn't in my mind. I was concerned with expressing what nursing is" (Taylor, 1998). A few years later, Orem had the insight to answer why people need nursing. She reflected:

> From that time onward, the knowledge I had about nursing began to structure itself. It wasn't anything I did deliberately, but the pieces started to come together. Some of the elements of what is now known as Self-Care Deficit Nursing Theory and are recorded in the 1959 *Guides for Developing Curriculum for the Education of Practical Nurses* (Taylor, 1998).

Orem's insight about the nature of nursing stimulated her to construct a definition and description of nursing and led to the formalization of the proper object of nursing. In 1955, Orem defined the essence of nursing care as the "giving of special assistance to the individual in times of illness, during certain periods of natural development and decline, infancy, childhood and old age, as well as in other times of special need such as during pregnancy and childbirth" (p. 95). The following year she wrote that "nursing is an art through which the nurse . . . gives specialized assistance" with the goals of (1) meeting or helping to meet continuous needs for self-care and self-participation in the medical care and (2) helping the patient self-direct personal and medical care (Orem, 1956, p. 85). From this seminal work, Orem identified the proper object, that is, the objective focus that establishes the domain of the discipline. The proper object is congruent with the ontology of the theoretical system and identifies the phenomenon of concern.

Phenomenon of Concern

The primary phenomenon of concern is *nursing and the condition that indicates a person's need for nursing.* The conceptualizations derived from this primary phenomenon or proper object are expressed in the SCDNT. Orem identified the proper object of nursing as persons, specifically those persons who are unable "to provide continuously for themselves the amount and quality of required self-care because of situations of personal health . . . Self-care is the personal care that individuals require each day to regulate their own functioning and development" (Orem, 1995, p. 8). For Orem, the proper object is specifically "persons who are in this state because of the activity-limiting effects of their states of health or because of the nature and complexity of their day-to-day requirements that contribute to regulation of their functioning and development" (Orem, 1995, p. 9). The object also includes children and dependents.

Health and wellbeing are foundational constructs for understanding Orem's conceptualizations of self-care and nursing. Health is described as "a state of a person that is characterized by soundness or wholeness of developed human structures and of bodily and mental functioning" (Orem 1995, p. 101). Well-being is used in the sense of individuals' perceived condition of existence. **Self-care** is conceptualized as the performance of sets of actions that are regulatory of functioning and development for the purpose of maintaining or establishing the state of wholeness or soundness that is called health. Self-care is action or sets of actions that is health promoting. Nursing is action that is focused on the health and wellbeing of persons.

DESCRIPTION OF OREM'S THEORETICAL SYSTEM
Philosophical Perspectives

Moderate Realism and Personalism. The SCDNT developed from the philosophical perspectives of moderate realism (Orem, 1995, 1997) and personalism (Orem, 1995), both of which are associated with Aristotelian Thomism or scholasticism (Wallace, 1983). Realism holds that a world or reality independent of thought exists and that it is possible to acquire knowledge of this world. Moderate realism recognizes that the reality cannot be fully known. Klubertanz (1953) claimed, "we know the existence of a world of sensible beings distinct from ourselves, we know the existence of these beings by our intellect through sense perception; but this evidence cannot be proved. We have a true but incomplete knowledge when we know a singular thing without knowing its singularity" (p. 84.) This view has been described by Wallace (1983) and is supported by philosophers and scholars such as Maritain, Lonergan, and Harré. Banfield (1997) conducted a philosophical inquiry of Orem's theory and placed it within the moderate realist position. She noted:

> Examination and analysis of Orem's work reveals that the SCDNT is based on the view of human beings as unitary beings in the process of becoming, as possessing free-will as well as other qualities. (The) moderate realist position . . . supports reality as existing independent of thought. However, a realist view of reality does not negate the view that human beings are experiencing beings, beings that attribute meaning based on their experiences (p. 79).

"Personalism is a philosophy predicated upon the irreducibility and primacy of personal categories" (Gallagher, 1998). Donohue-White (1997) described personalism as "founded on the fundamental concepts of participation, interpersonal community, and solidarity. Participation takes place on the 'I-Thou' level and entails joining with others. To participate is to be a co-agent of the community's activities and life, including its self-understanding and self-governance" (p. 453). With a foundation of the individual person as person, personalism affirms both the unique, essentially unrepeatable individuality of the person and the essentially social, relational, contextualized character of the person. The person is by essence a radically concrete, particular, embodied subjectivity directed to other persons and the world . . . an essential structure which is living becoming, developing, being actualized. To be a human person is to be essentially embodied . . . subjectivity and body compose an integrated whole in which personal subjectivity informs the body and the body expresses subjectivity. The human person is . . . irreducible and unrepeatable, that is, radically concrete, particular, and irreducible to non-personal being (p. 454).

Ontological Realities. Orem (1995) identified the realities that establish the ontology of SCDNT as "(a) persons in space-time localizations, (b) attributes or properties of these persons, (c) motion or change, and (d) products brought into being" (p. 170). The person is viewed as an essential substantial unity. Wallace states, "The essential unity of man is manifest from the fact that the same concrete being who experiences a bodily presence also recognizes this presence as that of a person who thinks. The mental activity of thinking and the material givenness of the body are both manifestations of one and the same human reality" (1996, p. 161).

Orem's ontological premises focus on the nature of person and the nature of human action (1995). The SCDNT is based on the view of humans as unitary beings in the process of becoming, possessing free will as well as other qualities (Orem, 1997). Self is an essential element in Orem's work. Orem (1997) subscribes to Weiss' description of person, which defines personhood as "being at once a self and a person with a distinctive I and me" (1980, p. 128). The self is embodied and therefore has biological life. In addition, there are psychological, rational, and spiritual dimensions to the self. All require attention if the person is to continue to mature and be healthy. Self-care must include attention to the biological dimension.

Orem and Vardiman (1995) described the psychological dimension of positive mental health as including the "modes of functioning of individuals in life situations that express their uniquely human qualities and personal development as they live and work with other persons in their communities . . . [and] positive mental health also requires understanding of the language, concepts, knowledge, and social customs of the communities" (p. 165). The rational dimension means that the person is able to symbolize, communicate, and interact with others. The rational dimension defines the person as an agent with the capacity to deliberate and choose, make judgments and take action. One can use these actions toward one's own ends by directing them toward the environment. Orem is less explicit about spirituality. Baker (1998) conceptualized spirituality as a sociocultural conditioning factor. Of Orem's work, Baker stated that "it can be inferred that spirituality, or the spiritual dimension of persons, is an integrating force" (p. 7). This inference is based, in part, on the philosophers that Orem cites as foundational to her conceptualizations, namely Lonergan, Maritain, Harré, and Wallace.

Orem identified the premises underlying the SCDNT in 1973. She notes that although "they have been referred to at times as assumptions, they are more properly referred to as premises since they were and are advanced as true and not merely assumed (1995, p. 169).

BOX 5-1

Basic Premises Underlying the SCDNT

- Human beings require continuous deliberate inputs to themselves and their environments in order to remain alive and to function in accord with natural human endowments.
- Human agency—the power to act deliberately—is exercised in the form of care of self and others, in identifying needs for self and others, and in making needed input.
- Mature human beings experience privations in the form of limitations for action in care of self and others involving the making of life-sustaining and function-regulating inputs.
- Human agency is exercised in discovering, developing, and transmitting to others ways and means to identify needs for self and others and make inputs to self and others.
- Groups of human beings with structured relationships cluster tasks and allocate responsibilities for providing care to group members who experience privations for making required deliberate input to self and others.

From: Orem, D.E. (1995). *Nursing: Concepts of practice*. (5th ed.). St. Louis: Mosby.

These premises, which are presented in Box 5-1, directly relate to the proper object and the ontology as previously described.

Knowledge of the human self as agent—that is, as one capable of deliberate action—and of the human self in relation to others provides the base for understanding SCDNT.

Description of Models and Theories

The general theory of nursing, SCDNT, consists of three theories: theory of nursing systems, theory of self-care, and theory of self-care deficits. Orem described the theory of nursing systems as the "unifying theory" within a triad of systems (Parse, 1987, p. 74). The **theory of nursing systems** is shown in the model in Figure 5-1, a hierarchy of interlocking systems (Nursing Development Conference Group, 1979, p. 112). The **theory of self-care** describes the purpose for taking care of self and the capacity for taking such action, and for being able to act on behalf of others. The **theory of self-care deficit** or dependent-care deficit is the "core of the general theory because it expresses the human condition that exists when people need nursing" (Orem, 1987). Understanding the self as imperfect—that is, as subject to limitations in knowledge, judgment and decision, and action—is the basis for understanding the theory of self-care deficit. Understanding the self in relation to others provides the basis for understanding the theory of nursing systems and the concepts of dependent care.

Throughout his or her life, a person faces choices of personally and culturally acceptable actions. Purposeful actions are called deliberate. Deliberate actions of persons are based on their judgments about what is appropriate under certain conditions and circumstances. Orem proposed a model of deliberate action that forms the basis for understanding both self-care and nursing (Orem, 1995, p. 165).

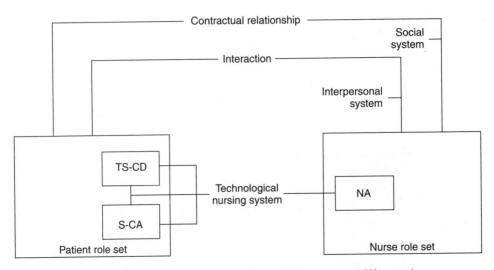

Key: TS-CD = therapeutic self-care demand, S-CA = self-care agency, NA = nursing agency.

FIGURE 5-1   The Hierarchy of Interlocking Systems (From Nursing Development Conference Group. (1979). *Concept formalization in nursing: Process and product.* (2nd ed.). Boston: Little, Brown.) Copyright Dorothea Orem.

Actions that seek a goal are described in phases. Phase I begins with investigation, proceeds to reflective understanding and judgments, and concludes with a decision about the ends sought and the means used. Phase II proceeds from the decision about what will be done and the design for doing it, to actions through which the end is reached and success or failure determined. Phase II also includes actions through which the work is planned and controlled (Orem, 1995).

Orem's conceptualizations about nursing are also related to the concept of care. In the fifth edition of *Nursing: Concepts of Practice*, she presents her thoughts about care and caring and makes critical distinctions between general views of caring and nursing-specific views. These are important distinctions as nurses seek to develop nursing discipline-specific knowledge.

Concepts associated with personalism are a part of the basis for helping and caring for others. Understanding personalism and concepts of person-in-relation is essential to the theoretical conceptualization of dependent-care and of nursing. Both of these are relational concepts. As defined by Orem, the interpersonal dimension is one of the three dimensions of a nursing system. The other two dimensions are the social-cultural system and the technological system. Their relationship is shown in Figure 5-1. Figure 5-2 depicts the relationships of the basic elements of the general theory (Orem, 1995, p. 435).

Orem described the nature of the theoretical elements as follows:

Nurse and patient have concrete referents, namely, the persons who fulfill these roles. The terms nursing, self-care, and dependent care signify behavioral processes. Self-care agency, dependent-care agency, and nursing agency stand for

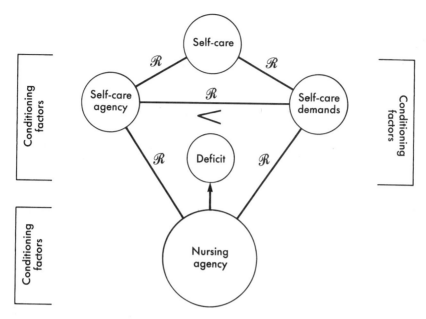

FIGURE 5-2   A conceptual framework for nursing. (From Orem, D. (1995). *Nursing: Concepts of practice.* (5th ed.). St. Louis: Mosby.)

abstractions about the nature of powers and capabilities of persons to engage in these named forms of care. Self-care requisite is a term that signifies a specific need for regulation of human functioning and development. Therapeutic self-care demands signifies all the care measures necessary to meet existent and emerging self-care requisites of individuals at particular times. Self-care deficit or dependent-care deficit signifies that the nature of a therapeutic self-care demand of individuals exceeds the powers and capabilities that constitute individuals' self-care agency or dependent-care agency (1995, p. 12).

Other useful models for further theory development, research, or practice applications are the process model of deliberate action (Figure 5-3) that forms the basis for understanding the concepts of self-care and nursing, the basic psychologic model of action (Figure 5-4) with three sub-models, and the physiologic model of action (Figure 5-5).

Orem's other models (1997) that should be examined are the model of self-care operations and their results, power components, foundational human capabilities and dispositions, models of the categories of elements of TSCD, and a model of constituent elements of a TSCD and their derivation. Other models based in SCDNT include those by Geden and Taylor (1999), who developed a model of collaborative self-care systems; Taylor and Renpenning, who developed models for multiperson situations of family and community (in Orem, 1995); and Taylor and Godfrey (1999), who proposed a model for nursing ethics using Orem's theory. Along with the theory of dependent care, models of dependent-care also have been proposed (Taylor, McLaughlin-Renpenning, Geden, Neuman, & Hart, 2001).

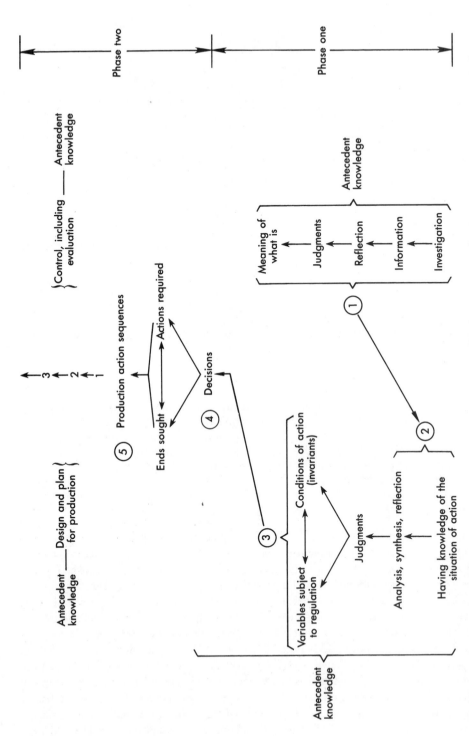

FIGURE 5-3 Process Model of Deliberate Action. (From Orem, D. (1995). *Nursing: Concepts of practice.* (5th ed.). St. Louis: Mosby.)

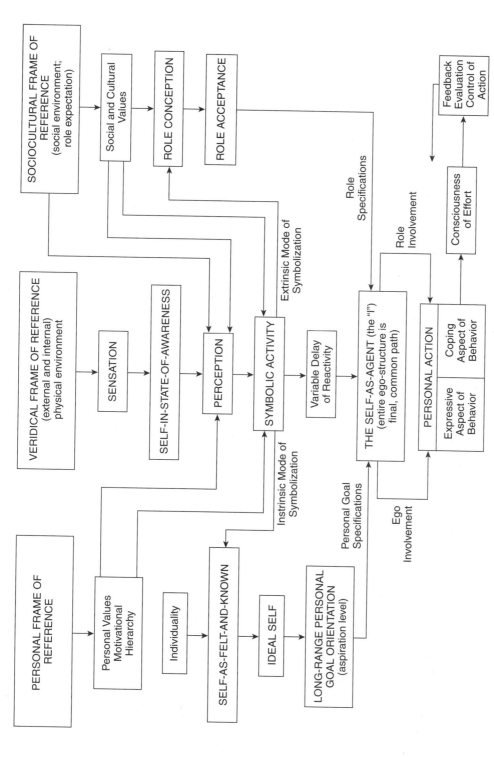

FIGURE 5-4 Basic Psychological Model of Action (From Nursing Development Conference Group. (1979). *Concept formalization in nursing: Process and product.* (2nd ed.). Boston: Little, Brown. Developed by Louise Hartnett.). Copyright Dorothea Orem.

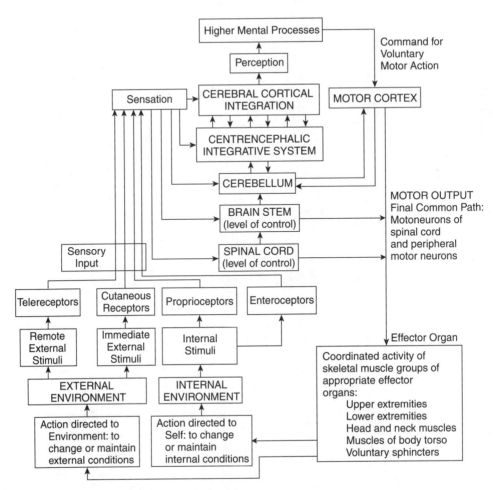

FIGURE 5-5 Basic Physiological Model of Action (From Nursing Development Conference Group. (1979). *Concept formalization in nursing: Process and product.* (2nd ed.). Boston: Little, Brown. Developed by Louise Hartnett.). Copyright Dorothea Orem.

RESEARCH DERIVED FROM SELF-CARE DEFICIT NURSING THEORY

The epistemology of realism supposes that a world of nature exists "independently of the knower's thinking about it, that objects and events are real and can be known through sensory experience, and that the natural light of the intellect is adequate to the task of knowing them as they are" (Wallace, 1996, p. 142). Orem (1988a) described the epistemology congruent with her conceptualizations about nursing and nursing science, which are congruent with those of Maritain. Orem posited that nursing science is practical science with speculative and practical knowledge. To the extent that a practical science engages in causal analysis, it can speculate and use analytical procedures similar to those of the speculative sciences. A practical science actually seeks to produce or construct its object and needs scientific knowledge in order to do so. Consideration of practical science should include concern for the ideas of action science (Orem, 1997). Research from this theoretical perspective should be both speculative and practical. Nursing sciences are grounded in the reality of deliberate human action and are limited by the object of nursing in the society. Practice-oriented sciences seek to know not purely for the sake of knowing but for the sake of making and doing (NDCG, 1979). In a welcome statement to the Sixth International Self-Care Conference, Bangkok, Thailand, 2000, Orem (2000) asked, "Given the accumulating results of theory developments, how should these results be structured toward the formal organization of discrete nursing sciences?" (p. 4). She identified two sets of nursing sciences: the practical sciences and the foundational sciences. The foundational sciences are specific to nursing and include (1) the science of self-care, (2) the science of the development and exercise of self-care agency, and (3) the science of human assistance for persons with health associated self-care deficits. The practical sciences are structured using the concepts of nursing systems—wholly compensatory nursing science, partly compensatory nursing science, and supportive educative nursing science. The preponderance of research relates to the foundational sciences.

Research Instruments Measuring Self-Care

As Orem's Self-Care Deficit Nursing Theory developed, instruments to measure the concept of self-care were lacking. The ability to measure aspects of self-care agency is considered critical because measures of self-care can guide nursing interventions. Over time, several instruments have been developed measuring specific self-care aspects. Comments regarding the reliability and validity of instruments used to measure self-care can be found in Table 5-1. Interpretation of information on the table may be facilitated by referring to the section discussing on evaluating reliability and validity of research instruments.

Exercise of Self-Care Agency. Kearney and Fleischer (1979) developed the Exercise of Self-Care Agency Scale (ESCA) to measure patients' self-appraisal of their self-care behaviors. The ESCA is a 43-item, five-point Likert scale developed around five dimensions of self-care: self-responsibility, motivation to care for oneself, application of knowledge regarding self-care, valuing healthcare priorities, and self-esteem. Likert scale ratings range from items being "very uncharacteristic" to "very characteristic." Items are scored from 0 to 4, to yield a total possible high score of 172, which indicates a high degree of exercise of self-care agency (McBride, 1987). The ESCA is usually completed in 8 to 10 minutes (Riesch & Hauck, 1988).

The ability of the ESCA to measure the concept of self-care was established initially through content validity evaluations by a panel of five experts (Kearney & Fleischer, 1979). Construct validity was established by comparing the ESCA to the Adjective Check List (ACL) and Rotter's Internal-External Locus of Control (I-E Scale) (see Table 5-1). These findings showed promise for the new measure of self-care.

McBride (1987) continued the ESCA validation process by using the instrument with 62 post–basic training nursing students and with 57 diabetic patients. Positing that factors in this instrument were related to Kearney and Fleischer's five indicators, McBride selected Guglielmino's Self-Directed Learning Readiness Scale (SDLRS) as a part of the construct validation process. Split-half reliabilities fell slightly below the correlations that Kearney and Fleischer found (see Table 5-1). Additionally, stability correlation for the patient group

Text continued on p. 86

TABLE 5-1

Selected Research Instruments Used to Measure Self-Care

Instrument	Study/Year	Reliability and Validity
Exercise of Self-care Agency Scale (ESCA) 43-item Likert scale	Kearney and Fleischer, 1979	Five experts established content validity. Stability, internal consistency, and construct validity were tested with 84 nursing students and 153 psychology students. Five-week test/retest reliability for nursing students was $r = 0.77$. All students completed the ESCA, the Adjective Check List, and the Internal-External Locus of Control Scale. Internal consistency, calculated with split-half reliabilities and a Spearman-Brown formula, were $r = 0.80$ on first testing and $r = 0.81$ on second testing with nurses and $r = 0.77$ for testing with psychology students. For construct validity, significant positive correlations were demonstrated between self-care agency and self-confidence ($r = 0.23$, $p \leq 0.05$), achievement ($r = 0.32$, $p \leq 0.01$), and intraception ($r = 0.26$, $p \leq 0.05$). A negative correlation between self-care agency and abasement was found ($r = -0.35$, $p \leq 0.01$). As self-care increased, abasement decreased. Locus of control failed to influence self-care agency.
ESCA	McBride, 1987	Reliability and validity were assessed using 62 post–basic nursing students and 57 adult diabetic patients. Both nursing student and diabetic patients completed a 5-week test/retest reliability assessment ($r = 0.76$ and 0.55 respectively, $p < 0.000$). Internal consistency, which was evaluated with split-half reliabilities, was also significant ($r = 0.78$ and 0.74 respectively, $p < 0.000$). Construct validity was assessed by correlating the eight factors of the Self-Directed Learning Readiness Scale (SDLRS) to the ESCA. Four factors were predicted to be significant: self-concept, initiative, self-understanding, and acceptance of responsibility for learning. ESCA scores correlated significantly with SDLRS scores (nurses $r = 0.5$, diabetic patients $r = 0.3$). Only nurses had significant correlations on the four selected SDLRS factors ($r = 0.27$ to 0.48). Nurses had positive correlations with the SDLRS subscales of love of learning ($r = 0.59$), tolerance of risk ($r = 0.26$), creativity ($r = 0.49$), and view of life long-learning ($r = 0.56$). Patients had significant ESCA correlations with love of learning ($r = 0.34$), creativity ($r = 0.49$), and view of life-long learning ($r = 0.29$).
ESCA	Riesch and Hauck, 1988	A composite sample of 506 pregnant women; labor coaches; adolescents; and university faculty, staff, and students completed the ESCA. Principal components analysis with varimax rotation was used to establish construct validity. Investigators deemed eight items consistently loading at less than 0.4 on the identified factors conceptually incompatible with the intent of the ESCA. Therefore 35 items were used for the final solution. Factor analysis identified four factors supporting the theorized dimensions of self-care agency: self-concept, initiative, knowledge, and information seeking. The four-actor solution accounted for 40% of the variance.

Denyes Self-Care Agency Instrument (DSCAI) 35 items with response format of 0% to 100%	Denyes, 1982	One hundred sixty-one adolescents aged 14 to 18 years were randomly divided into two groups and responded to a DSCAI. Both data sets were subjected to exploratory factor analysis with varimax rotation and compared. Internal consistency reliability ranged from 0.86 to 0.89. Six factors emerged from the factor analysis: (1) ego strength and decision-making capability, (2) relative valuing of health, (3) health knowledge and decision making experience, (4) physical energy levels, (5) feelings, and (6) attention to health.
Perception of Self-Care Agency (PSCA) 48-item, 6-point Likert scale	Hanson and Bickel, 1985	Five experts established content validity, and 456 nonhospitalized adults' responses to the PSCA were used to assess reliability and construct validity. The internal consistency coefficient alpha was 0.93. Principal components factor analysis with orthogonal rotation revealed five factors that accounted for 86% of the variance: (1) cognitive abilities, (2) cognitive limitations, (3) motor abilities, (4) motivation, and (5) repertoire of skills.
Dependent Care Agent Instrument Questionnaire for Mothers (DCA) 39-item, 5-point Likert scale	Moore and Gaffney, 1989	Seven mothers of well children between the ages of 1 and 20 identified content areas for item development. Content validity of items was established by 12 faculty with a background in Orem's theory. A pilot study was completed with 27 mothers in order to test for possible social desirability response bias. The pilot study used the Marlowe-Crowne Social Desirability Scale. Low correlations ($r = 0.14$, $p = 0.25$) indicated that subjects provided authentic answers. When tested with 475 mothers, the internal consistency was established at 0.91. Factor analysis revealed 12 factors. Universal care requisites were identified by the following: (Factor 1) social interaction, activity, and normalcy; (Factor 4) elimination; (Factor 5) water; (Factor 7) air; (Factor 9) rest; and (Factor 10) food. (Factor 2), health and safety focus, combined universal requisite of hazards with health deviation dimension. A developmental dimension was found in (Factor 3) social responsibility and (Factor 6) social interaction. The health deviation dimension was represented by (Factor 8) seeking medical assistance. Factors 11 and 12 were less interpretable.
55-item, 5-point Likert scale	Mosher and Moore, 1998	To make the DCA more relevant for mothers caring for children with cancer, 16 items were added, for a total of 55 items. Internal consistency for revised instrument was 0.93.

Continued

TABLE 5-1

Selected Research Instruments Used to Measure Self-Care—cont'd

Instrument	Study/Year	Reliability and Validity
Self-as-Carer Inventory (SCI) 40-item, 6-point equal interval scale	Geden and Taylor, 1991	Content validity was established by a panel of three experts to assess item clarity and validity. A second content analysis to assess relevancy of items to Orem's 10 power components was completed (CVI = 94%). Fifty-six students completed the SCI. Test/retest reliability was 0.85 for total scores and ranged from 0.54 to 0.83 on subscales. Preliminary factor analysis led to further revision. Five hundred eighty-five respondents completed the revised SCI for a subsequent test of internal consistency and factor analysis. Respondents also judged themselves as healthy or unhealthy and rated their general health and degree of self-care. On final testing Cronbach's alpha was 0.96 for the total SCI. Significant Pearson correlations were found in response to the SCI and questions on general health, current health, and amount of self-care ($r = 0.29$, 0.26, and 0.36, $p \leq 0.0001$, respectively). Principal components factor analysis with oblique rotation identified four factors, accounting for 52% of variance. Factors included: (1) knowledge of self, (2) judgment and decisions affecting production of self-care, (3) attention to and awareness of self and self monitoring, and (4) physical skills and satisfaction with self-care routines.
Appraisal of Self-Care Agency (ASA) 24-item, 5-point Likert scale (English or Dutch) Format A (ASA-A): self-appraisal Format B (ASA-B): appraisal of others	Evers, Isenberg, Philipsen, Senten, and Brouns, 1993	Construct validity was assessed with a randomly selected sample of 40 nursing home patients, 30 residents of a personalized care facility, 30 residents of a service flat, and 40 independent residents in the community. Older adults who depended less on institutionalized care had higher ASA scores. Community elders demonstrated greater self-care agency than those in assisted living ($t = 3.38$, $\underline{df} = 61$, $p < 0.001$). Assisted living residents exhibited greater self-care agency than those in personalized care facilities ($t = 2.75$, $\underline{df} = 57$, $p < 0.008$). Differences in ASA scores for elders in personalized care facilities and nursing home residents were not significant, although ASA scores were higher for those in personalized care facilities.

Child and Adolescent Self-Care Practice Questionnaire 35-item, 5-point Likert scale	Moore, 1995	To create the Child and Adolescent Self-Care Practice Questionnaire, items were developed, assessed for readability, and sent to seven content experts for evaluation. Following content evaluation, 40 items were retained. Four hundred seventy-one students aged 9 to 18 were given the Child and Adolescent Self-Care Practice Questionnaire, the DSCAI, and the ESCA. Following statistical analysis, five items were deleted, yielding a 35-item instrument. Coefficient alpha was 0.83. Concurrent validity between the Child and Adolescent Self-Care Practice Questionnaire and DSCAI and ESCA was $r = 0.54$, $p \leq 0.001$; and $r = 0.58$, $p \leq 0.001$ respectively. Confirmatory factor analysis using LISREL identified underlying dimensions of the questionnaire. The goodness of fit index for a 10 factor model was 0.848, indicating a moderate fit. Factors included: responsibility, food, schoolwork, hazards, activity and social interaction, rest, hand washing, skipping meals, and hygiene. The tenth factor was less interpretable.
The Children's Self-Care Performance Questionnaire 51 items	Mosher and Moore, 1998	A variation of the Child and Adolescent Self-Care Practice Questionnaire was developed for children with cancer. Sixteen items were added to the original instrument to increase relevancy for children with cancer. Internal consistency reliability of revised instrument was 0.83.
Mental Health Self-Care Agency Scale (MH-SCA) 35 item, 5-point Likert scale	West and Isenberg, 1997	Content validity was assessed through an expert panel's review of items for relevance to mental health self-care and for inclusion of Orem's power components. The CVI for 33 of 35 items was 0.83, with an overall scale CVI of 0.94. Power component CVI was 0.88 for 33 items, with an overall CVI of 0.94. Internal consistency reliability was 0.90. Construct validity was established with a known-groups technique administered to depressed and nondepressed women. Participants also completed the ASA-A. Nondepressed women scored significantly higher on MH-SCA than depressed women ($t = -5.86$, $p < 0.000$), thus supporting investigators' proposed prediction for scale performance. Nondepressed women had higher ASA scores ($t = -3.72$, $p < 0.001$), which indicated higher self-care capacity than in depressed women.

was substantially below that of the nurse group. In terms of construct validity, the ESCA scores for both patients and nurses were significant, but the hypothesized relationships between four selected SDLRS factors held true only for the nurse group.

Using a principal components factor analysis, Riesch and Hauck (1988) completed subsequent testing of the ESCA. Four factors emerged from the ESCA: self-concept, initiative and responsibility, knowledge and information seeking, and passivity. Because eight items consistently failed to load onto a factor, Riesch and Hauck completed the analysis using only 35 items and recommended the shorter scale. Feedback from respondents led the researchers to recommend changing the item response choices to phrases ranging from "very like me" to "very unlike me" (p. 254).

Although the ESCA was an important early instrument in the measure of self-care agency, some nursing scholars have criticized Kearney and Fleischer's ambiguous incorporation of dispositional characteristics into their definition of self-care agency (Gast, Denyes, Campbell, Hartweg, Schott-Baer, & Isenberg, 1989). Additionally, McBride's findings (1987) question the stability and theoretical predictability of the ESCA with patient groups. Finally, after factor analysis, Riesch and Hauck (1988) suggested significant changes in the ESCA since some items fail to load on identifiable factors and since feedback indicated confusing item responses. Researchers should consider these issues when selecting this instrument to measure self-care agency.

Denyes Self-Care Agency Instrument. Using an early definition of self-care by the Nursing Development Conference Group and drawing heavily on developmental theories of Piaget, Kohlberg, and Tanner, Denyes (1982) developed a 35-item Likert scale to measure self-care agency in adolescents. The Denyes Self-Care Agency Instrument (DSCAI) indicates the ability of adolescents to make decisions on their own behalf and to manage self-care. Factor analysis revealed six factors, including ego strength and health decision making capability, valuing of health, health knowledge, physical energy levels, feelings, and attention to health (see Table 5-1). Strong levels of internal consistency reliability were found. One strength of the DSCAI is that eight of the ten power components of self-care theorized by the Nursing Development Conference Group are incorporated into Denyes' instrument (Gast, Denyes, Campbell, Hartweg, Schott-Baer, & Isenberg, 1989).

Denyes Self-Care Practice Instrument. To clearly differentiate measurement of self-care agency from practices, Denyes (1988) developed a 17-item self-response instrument measuring general self-care actions (e.g., following through on health decisions) and specific actions (e.g. following a balanced diet). Item responses range from 0% to 100%. She cited evidence of content and construct validity derived from her original instrument development work (Denyes, 1982). In a study of 369 adolescents, which used a 22-item form of the DSCPI, internal consistency reliabilities ranged from 0.84 to 0.92 on the DSCPI (Denyes, 1988). Using a revised 17-item DSCPI, internal consistency was reported to be 0.88 (Frey & Denyes, 1989).

Perceived Self-Care Agency. Hanson and Bickel (1985) developed the Perceived Self-Care Agency Questionnaire (PSCA) to measure the ten power components of self-care agency. It is a 48-item, six-point Likert scale with item responses ranging from "never like me" to "always like me." Although reported internal consistency reliability is strong for the total scale, only five rather than the predicted ten factors emerged from the factor analysis. Hanson and Bickel believed that the five-factor solution accounted for seven of the ten components.

Weaver (1987) criticized the use of orthogonal rotation in Hanson and Bickel's factor analysis. He theorized that because orthogonal rotation does not allow intercorrelations between factors, the interrelationships of some of the power components prevented an accurate structure from being derived from the factor analysis. Using a convenience sample of 467 adults, confirmatory and exploratory factor analyses using linear structural relations analysis (LISREL) failed to find an adequate data fit. Additionally, although the internal consistency reliability was strong for the total scale score (0.94), reliabilities for the factors identified by Hanson and Bickel were low, with the exception of the cognitive factor, which ranged from 0.46 to 0.92. These findings led Weaver to question the usability of the PSCA as a measure of self-care agency. However, Weaver's assertions have been challenged on the basis that factor reliabilities are adequate for heterogeneous uncorrelated factors and that confirmatory factor analysis is inappropriate for early instrument development (Cleveland, 1989).

Bottorff (1988) assessed the usability of the PSCA with a group of 27 nursing home residents who were 60 years or older. Only four of the 27 residents were able to complete all items on the PSCA. Areas of difficulty included language comprehension for item stems, inaccuracies concerning residents' personal circumstances, double negatives in some item stems, and the length of the phrases in the responses. Bottorff concluded that the PSCA was not appropriate for use in older adults.

Dependent Care Agent Questionnaire. When Moore and Gaffney (1989) wanted to study mothers' performances of self-care activities for children, no instruments existed to measure activities of the dependent-care agent as described in Orem's SCDNT. Thus they designed the Dependent Care Agent Questionnaire to assess dependent-care activities of mothers performing self-care for children. Following initial testing, the DCA contained 39 items with a five-point Likert scale format. Possible scores on the DCA range from 39 to 225, with higher scores indicating increased performance of care by the dependent-care agent. Instrumentation testing was completed with an adequate sample size and resulted in an excellent internal consistency reliability. One area of concern is that twelve factors are identified through factor analysis. Interpreting Factors 11 and 12 has proven particularly difficult. However, DCA factors are associated clearly with Orem's SCDNT and account for 63.5% of the variance. Moore and Gaffney (1989) suggest that the wide variance in Orem's requisites for self-care could account for some of the difficulty in developing a more cohesive instrument.

The original DCA was designed for use with mothers of healthy children. In order to make the instrument more useful for studying mothers of children with cancer, 16 items were added, for a total of 55 items. With this revised version, now called the Dependent-Care Agent Performance Questionnaire, potential instrument scores range from 55 to 275. High scores continue to indicate greater performance of dependent-care activities.

Appraisal of Self-Care Agency. The Appraisal of Self-Care Agency (ASA) is a 24-item Likert scale with five response categories developed to measure whether individuals can meet their self-care needs (Evers, Isenberg, Philipsen, Senten, & Brouns, 1993). Individual scores can range from 24 to 120, with higher scores indicating greater self-care agency. Two formats of the instrument are available: one for self-appraisal (Form A) and the other for appraising another person (Form B).

The ASA has been translated into Dutch and tested for construct validity using a known-groups method with a sample of older adults living either in a nursing home, a personalized care facility, a service flat, or in independent homes in the community. Researchers found predicted differences in self-care agency. Respondents with higher scores on the ASA demonstrated lower levels of dependence on others for self-care activities. These findings indicate that Orem's Theory of Self-Care Deficit can be tested within Dutch culture (Evers, Isenberg, Philipsen, Senten, & Brouns, 1993).

Self-As-Carer Inventory. Significantly modifying the PSCA, Geden and Taylor (1991) developed the Self-As-Carer Inventory (SCI) as a measure of self-care agency. The SCI is a 40-item, six-point equal interval scale in which respondents can choose between two anchor points of "very accurate" to "very inaccurate." The maximum score value of 40 indicates a high degree of perceived ability to care for self, whereas the minimum value of 240 indicates a low ability. The scale, which includes four items per component and eight items for two subsections on the first component, is designed to represent each of the 10 power components.

Content validity was established for relevance, clarity, and representation of the 10 power components. Test-retest reliability was strong for the total scale, with slightly lower estimates for the subscales—particularly the subscale of the repertoire of interpersonal skills needed for self-care. Construct validation using factor analysis indicated strong theoretical validity. These findings were supported by correlations of responses regarding general health, current health, and amount of self-care to SCI total scores (see Table 5-1).

Child and Adolescent Self-Care Practice Questionnaire. The Child and Adolescent Self-Care Practice Questionnaire is a 35-item, 5-point Likert scale that can determine children's and adolescents' performances as self-care agents (Moore, 1995). Initial attempts at establishing reliability and validity met with modest success. Internal consistency reliability was adequate, particularly for a new instrument. An existing instrument to measure adolescent self-care practices (DSCAI) and a measure of adult self-care agency (ESCA) established only moderate levels of concurrent validity. Although a 10-factor solution identified factors consistent with Orem's model, there are limitations to the derived solutions (see Table 5-1). The reliability and validity of the Child and Adolescent Self-Practice Questionnaire has been established only with children and adolescents between the ages of 9 to 18. Use with other age-groups requires additional instrument testing.

The Child and Adolescent Self-Care Practice Questionnaire was designed for healthy children. In order to use this instrument with children with cancer, Mosher and Moore (1998) added 16 items pertinent to this population. The added items included taking medications, reporting symptoms, and keeping healthcare appointments. Reliability for this revised instrument was similar to that of the original questionnaire. Mosher and Moore (1998) modified the title of the instrument to the Children's Self-Care Performance Questionnaire.

Mental Health Self-Care Agency Scale. To facilitate description of how individuals were capable of engaging in mental health–related self-care West and Isenberg (1997) developed the Mental Health Self-Care Agency Scale (MH-SCA). This 35-item, 5-point Likert scale is a self-report questionnaire. Scale items incorporate Orem's concepts of self-care agency, including the ability to perform self-care operations, enabling capabilities (power components), and foundational capabilities. To ensure that elements related to mental health were captured, five types of human functioning were incorporated. These included (1) affective (life satisfaction, emotional experience, or management of frustration or anxiety), (2) cognitive (thinking processes and thought content), and (3) perceptual functioning (ability to accurately absorb and interpret sensory information), (4) patterns of activity (behavioral aspects), and (5) valuative processes (acquisition of values and finding direction and purpose).

Content validity was established using a two-step process—one step for item relevance and a second to ensure inclusion of Orem's power components of self-care. Strong content validity was achieved for the scale in terms of relevance and incorporation of power components (see Table 5-1). A pilot study administered the MH-SCA along with the Appraisal of Self-Care Agency (ASA-A) and the Center for Epidemiological Studies Depression Scale (CES-D). Pilot studies indicated strong internal consistency reliability. Construct validity was established using a known-groups technique. Nondepressed women performed more self-care activities than depressed women performed. This matched investigators' predictions for the MH-SCA. Additionally, nondepressed women also had higher ASA scores, thus indicating higher levels of self-care abilities than depressed women. The findings of the pilot study strongly supported the reliability and validity of the MH-SCA.

Summary of Instruments Measuring Self-Care Agency. Instruments measuring self-care continued to evolve and become stronger as concepts related to self-care developed. Commonalties exist between some instruments. McBride (1991) identified knowledge, attention, self-concept, and skill/action as common components of the DCSAI, the ESCA, and PSCA. Although shortcomings have been identified in all instruments, newer instrument revisions such as the SCI demonstrate stronger theoretical underpinnings of self-care agency. Despite shortcomings such as the ESCA's reliability in patient populations and the PSCA's reliability in older adult populations, instruments such as the ASA are being used with other cultural groups and with a variety of ages. The MH-SCA permits a focus on mental health. Although refinement of instruments needs to continue and new instruments related to specific aspects of self-care agency need to be developed, methods are available to operationalize and measure self-care.

Review of Related Research

In order to become clinically useful, self-care theory must be linked to practice through research. Research provides a potential mechanism for testing the tenets of Orem's theory. A particularly good example is Denyes' study (1988) of health promotion in adolescents. In other studies, theory provides a perspective or theoretical point of view for a study (Geden, 1989). Regardless of the nature of a study, researchers must logically tie research questions, assumptions, variable operational definition, and discussion of findings to the theoretical perspective. These linkages help to clarify the nature of the research problem and measurement of variables, and they help investigators to tie their findings back to the theoretical frame of references.

An example in which these linkages are well connected is a study by Jirovec and Kasno (1990), which studied the influences of environmental constraints on the self-care agency of nursing home residents. This study combined self-care agency as defined by Orem with elements of social learning theory and social breakdown theory in an effort to assess limitations that environmental factors imposed on older adults' self-care. The study hypotheses were explicitly congruent with the theoretical frames of reference, leading investigators to propose that constraints within nursing homes would impede elders' self-care. Instruments explicitly measured self-care agency (ASA-A), environmental constraints (Perceived Environmental Constraints Index), and the ability to perform activities of daily living (Katz Index of Activities of Daily Living). Investigators then discussed the findings theoretically and proposed that basic conditioning factors suggested in Orem's theory influence self-care abilities. In this manner, investigators ensured that the problem of study was congruent with the theory, that variable measurement was linked to theory, and that findings tied back to propositions found within the theory. Ideally, these linkages should be the goal of all investigators.

The SCDNT has been used in numerous settings, with groups of all ages, with health considerations ranging from health promotion to management of specific diseases, for multicultural clients, and for curricula and information systems and electronic documentation. Table 5-2 lists selected research studies and identifies their purposes, methods, and findings. These studies and their fit and congruence with the SCDNT are also discussed in the text. Reviewed studies were categorized into the following topical areas: health and illness, pain, self-care and children, older adults, documentation, and education.

Health and Illness. The SCDNT has been used to guide studies in health promotion and in patient management of specific chronic illnesses such as cancer, diabetes mellitus, and cardiovascular disease. Orem (1995) proposes that individuals must perform or have performed activities that maintain regulatory functions, including (1) maintenance of sufficient intake of air, water, and food; (2) provision of care regarding elimination processes; (3) balance of rest and activity and solitude and social interaction; (4) prevention of hazard; and (5) promotion of normalcy. Successful self-care must be learned and deliberately performed. The SCDNT indicates that a lack of maturity or occurrence of illness limits self-care activities to the degree that individuals may be unable to perform self-care, thus creating a self-care deficit. The Theory of Nursing Systems holds that nurses, through the exercise of their nursing agency, can regulate the development and exercise of self-care agency by others. Nurses may partially or totally compensate for self-care deficits when the need exists. Research centered on health promotion or illness care reflects patients' abilities to perform self-care or, when self-care is not feasible, nurses' abilities to intervene to varying degrees. Research related to health and illness includes studies that simply describe self-care activities of particular groups as well as studies that test the effectiveness of nursing interventions.

Denyes (1988) used the theories of self-care and self-care deficit in her study of health promotion in adolescents. One strength of this study was the close alignment of variables with Orem's theoretical concepts in the study of health promotion. Denyes clearly defined aspects of Orem's theory being tested, followed with related hypotheses, and then incorporated the SCDNT in the discussion. In examining the influence of basic conditioning factors on self-care, Denyes found that an absence of health problems was associated with higher levels of self-care. Younger adolescents and males reported more self-care behaviors, but the demonstrated relationship was modest. This finding provides limited support for Orem's contention that a relationship exists between basic conditioning factors and self-care agency and self-care. Denyes discovered a moderate relationship between self-

Text continued on p. 100

TABLE 5-2

Selected Self-Care Research Studies

Study/Year	Purpose	Methods	Findings
HEALTH AND ILLNESS			
Aish and Isenberg, 1996	The study investigated the influence of nursing care on nutritional self-care of myocardial infarction patients. Investigators hypothesized that fostering self-care agency would improve health habits and that self-efficacy would promote healthy eating.	Sixty-two men and 42 women who had experienced a myocardial infarction during the last 5 years kept three 24-hour food diaries, responded to the Food Habits Questionnaire (FHQ), the SCA, and the Eating Habits Confidence Scale (EHCS). Subjects were randomly assigned to a control or treatment group. The treatment group received home visits to review food habits and preparation and to answer be questions about lifestyle modifications. The treatment group also received three follow-up phone calls over a 6-week period to encourage following a healthy lifestyle.	Ninety-eight of subjects had just experienced a first MI while the remaining subjects had a first MI up to 5 years ago. Seven weeks post- discharge, the treatment group exhibited lower total fat and saturated fat intake ($t = -5.10$ and -3.56 respectively, $p < 0.001$) and lower FHQ scores ($t = -1.78$ and -3.56, $p < 0.05$). The treatment group significantly increased self-care agency and self-efficacy over seven weeks, whereas the control group increased only in self-efficacy. Increases in self-efficacy did not impact dietary choices. Investigators concluded that intervention could positively impact self-care agency and subsequently improve nutritional choices of MI patients.
Campbell and Weber, 2000	The study tested a model, based on Orem's SCDNT, of women's responses to battering.	One hundred seventeen women responded to questions on age, education, cultural and socioeconomic group value of wife-mother role, and acceptability of hitting women. Instruments included Conflict Tactics Scale (abuse), Tennessee Self-Concept Scale (esteem), DSCAI, the Symptom Checklist, and Beck Depression Inventory. Simultaneous structural equation modeling ascertained the fit of the proposed model.	The final model had an adequate, mediocre fit ($\chi^2 = 57.9$, $p < 0.094$, with 45 $\underline{df}$ and a ratio of 1:1.28). The goodness of fit index was originally 0.920 and was 0.811 when adjusted. Root mean square was 0.074. The proposed model accounted for 45% of variance in health.

Continued

TABLE 5-2		
Selected Self-Care Research Studies—cont'd		
Study/Year	Purpose	Methods	Findings
Denyes, 1988	The study tested relationships between self-care and self-care deficit. Specific relationships included self-care agency with health problems, conditioning factors and self-care, and self-care agency and self-care.	An aggregate of 369 adolescents from several studies completed questions related to health problems, demography, presence of health problems, the DSCAI; the Denyes Self-Care Practice Instrument (DSCPI), and the Denyes Health Status Instrument (DHSI). Correlations and regressions were used to assess relationships of several factors to self-care.	The presence or absence of health problems weakly correlated to self-care ($r = 0.12$, $p < 0.018$). Younger adolescents ($r = -0.13$, $p < 0.01$) and males ($r = 0.11$, $p < 0.04$) engaged in more self-care. A moderate relationship between self-care agency and self-care existed ($r = 0.38$, $p < 0.000$). The combined effects of self-care, self-care agency, and health problems explained 41% of variance in general health state.
Dodd, 1982	The study identified self-care behaviors used to counteract side effects of chemotherapy for cancer patients.	Forty-eight cancer patients undergoing chemotherapy responded to the Chemotherapy Knowledge Questionnaire and the Self-Care Behavior Questionnaire to determine patterns of self-care behaviors used to respond to chemotherapy side effects.	Patients reported an average of 7.69 side effects, with a severity of 2.85 on a 5-point scale. Patients correctly identified 3.13 side effects attributed to chemotherapy and 4.56 side effects not attributable to chemotherapy. Patients engaged in a limited number of self-care behaviors (0.81) that were modestly effective (3.05). Lack of knowledge was a contributing factor to the initiation of limited self-care activities.
Dodd, 1983	The study was a continuation of Dodd, 1982, and it assessed the effect on self-care of providing information about side effect management techniques (SEMT) to cancer patients receiving chemotherapy.	Forty-eight cancer patients were randomly assigned to four groups. One group received information about drugs, a second information about SEMT, a third a combination of drugs and SEMT, and the fourth was not given any systematic information.	Patients receiving SEMT reported initiating more self-care behaviors to counteract side effects of chemotherapy and more effective actions than patients not receiving SEMT ($F (1,44) = 7.60$, $p < 0.01$). Post-intervention self-care behaviors were similar to pre-intervention behaviors but occurred in greater numbers. The increase in self-care behaviors was attributed to increased knowledge level.

Dodd, 1988a	The study determined the nature and frequency of self-care behaviors of breast cancer patients undergoing chemotherapy. Duration of side effects; perceived effectiveness of self-care behaviors; source of ideas for self-care behaviors; relationship of severity with distress of experience, side effects, and initiation of self-care behaviors; and influence of moderator variables were determined.	Thirty women who had completed surgery and were initiating a chemotherapy regimen completed a Self-Care Behavior Log, the State-Trait Anxiety Inventory, and the Multidimensional Health Locus of Control at initiation and 6 to 8 weeks following the beginning of chemotherapy. The study assessed demographic variables that potentially influence self-care behaviors.	Patients initiated an average of 0.16 self-care behaviors for each chemotherapy side effect. Patients initiated self-care behaviors within one day of experiencing a side effect with behaviors perceived as moderately effective. Patients indicated they were most often the source of ideas for self-care behaviors (60%), followed by the physician (25%), the nurse (7%), and family (7%). Ratings for severity of side effects and distress were moderate and exhibited a moderate correlation ($r = 0.65$, $p > 0.002$). Patients exhibited high internal locus of control, which may have contributed to patients' feelings that they were most significant source of self-care information.
Dodd, 1988b	The study assessed the effect of proactively providing side effect management (SEM) information to cancer patients undergoing chemotherapy.	Sixty chemotherapy patients were randomly assigned to either a treatment or control group. Participants from both groups completed pretreatment interviews, including the Karnofsky Performance Status Scale, the STAI, and the MHLC. Subjects also were given a SCB log. The treatment group was given an explanation of how to use SEM materials to prevent or alleviate side effects from chemotherapy. Six weeks following the initial interview, a post-intervention interview collected information regarding disease and treatment variables, and the Karnofsky, STAI, and MHLC, and SCB logs were collected.	Patients who received SEM information scored significantly higher on all self-care behavior ratios and performed significantly more preventative self-care behaviors ($t = 2.6$, $p < 0.012$). The group receiving SEM delayed intervention initiation for 4 hours, as compared to 7 hours for the control group, but this time difference was not statistically significant. Both groups had average side effect severity and distress ratings. Patients receiving SEM information experienced a significant increase performance status by the end of the study.

Continued

TABLE 5-2

Selected Self-Care Research Studies—cont'd

Study/Year	Purpose	Methods	Findings
Geden and Taylor, 1999	The study described collaborative care systems in which couples shared the work of self-care.	In this descriptive study, 108 couples completed two forms of the SCI, discussing personal self-care agency and that of partners. Also completed were the Couple Form of the Family Adaptability and Cohesion Evaluation Scales (FACES II), the Caregiver Reciprocity Scale, and self-reports of health at the moment and in general.	Individuals indicated that they were capable of caring for themselves, and couples were found to be connected and flexible. Stepwise multiple regression indicated that cohesion, dyad gender, and health explained 27% of variance in the collaborative care system. Two variables—total family scores and health—contributed to 23% of variance. Caregiver reciprocity did not contribute to the model.
Hanucharurnkul, 1989	The study determined whether social support and basic conditioning factors of age, marital status, and socioeconomic status can predict self-care, living arrangements, and stage and site of cancer.	A convenience sample of 112 adults with cervical or head and neck cancer undergoing radiotherapy in Bangkok, Thailand, responded to the Self-Care Behavior Questionnaire (SCQB), the Social Support Questionnaire (SSQ), and sociodemographic questions related to income, education, and Occupational Prestige Scale.	Family members and healthcare providers were found to be the most likely sources of support. Hierarchical multiple regression revealed that the socioeconomic indicator of occupational prestige accounted for the greatest potion of self-care variance (21%). Social support contributed to 17% of the variance, and site of cancer explained 6% of the variance associated with self-care.
Kubricht, 1984	The study identified cancer patients' perceived therapeutic self-care demands while receiving outpatient radiation therapy.	Open-ended interview questions were used to collect data regarding changes in 30 participants' lives since beginning radiotherapy. Data were transcribed and categorized according to Orem's six universal self-care requisites.	The study identified 553 self-care requisites: protection from hazards (20.4%), food and water (19.7%), rest and activity (19.5%), normality (12.8%), solitude and social interaction (5.6%), and air (5%). All subjects had therapeutic self-care demands related to excrements, rest/activity, food/water, protection from hazards, and being normal. Seventy-six percent of subjects expressed changes related to solitude and social interaction, and 50% had changes related to the air category.

Pickens, 1999	The study investigated perceptions of individuals with serious mental illness about their mental illness, their desire for normalcy, and their self-care actions to promote and maintain normalcy.	Nineteen qualitative interviews were reviewed in a secondary analysis of two previous studies to investigate a serendipitous finding regarding normalcy. Content analysis techniques were used to perform thematic analysis of the data.	Participants expressed a desire to "have normal things and experiences, [do] meaningful activities, and [be] well, safe, free, and independent" (p. 235). Self-care actions to maintain normalcy included rejecting labels, working, focusing on symptoms of others, managing emotional pain and distress, and trying to be better through actions such as taking medications.
Walker and Grobe, 1999	The study explored the construct of thriving as integration of self-care in the areas of nutritional, psychosocial, and lifestyle-related concerns of childbearing women.	In secondary analysis, 145 postpartum women were assessed at 3 and 12 months. The three month assessment considered weight, lifestyle components (Food Habits Questionnaire, Aerobic Exercise Scale, Personal Lifestyle Questionnaire), and psychosocial status (Weight Locus of Control Scale, Body Cathexis Scale, Self-Control Schedule). At 12 months, the weight and psychosocial assessments were repeated.	Factor analysis revealed four dimensions associated with postpartum thriving: (1) psychosocial distress, (2) lifestyle patterns, (3) weight, and (4) body image.
PAIN Villarruel, 1995	The ethnographic study considered basic conditioning factors of culture and dependent self-care agency associated with pain in Mexican-Americans.	Twenty-two key and 14 general Mexican-American informants were observed and interviewed about selected theoretical concepts from Orem's theory in order to discover cultural meanings, expressions, self-care, and dependent-care actions related to pain.	Four themes emerged. These included meanings, expressions, care of self, and care of others. Pain and suffering were viewed as synonymous and associated with sense of loss. Pain was to be accepted and was associated with fulfilling one's role. Care by and for others found to be an important cultural expression.

Continued

TABLE 5-2

Selected Self-Care Research Studies—cont'd

Study/Year	Purpose	Methods	Findings
Denyes, Neuman, and Villarruel; 1991¹	Two studies were conducted to determine what nursing actions were used to prevent and alleviate pain in hospitalized children.	Ethnographic interviews were completed with 13 nurses to determine their views in caring for children with pain, actions taken to prevent and alleviate pain, involvement of parents and children, and believed effectiveness of pain-relieving actions. Following the interviews, 87 pediatric nurses were surveyed to determine the frequency of pain-relieving actions and to identify actions that were perceived most effective.	The findings identified six nursing action patterns for pain relief: (1) doing for child (medicating, talking, touching), (2) modifying environment (call physician, room dim, noise down, etc.), (3) engaging child in care (repositioning self, assist with care, pillow to cough, imagery, etc.), (4) engaging parent (read to child, hug, back rub, apply cool cloth), (5) teaching child (relaxation, distraction, pain prevention), and (6) teaching parent (what to watch for, understanding pain). Staff nurses used seven actions for pain relief often. These included the following: (1) talking to child, (2) preparing for procedures, (3) asking the child where it hurts, (4) preparing parents for procedures, (5) gentle handling, (6) rewarding the child, and (7) involving and supporting parents. The most effective actions were administration of medications, physical comfort measures, diversion, tender loving care, involving and supporting parents, preparation for procedures, repositioning, and talking calmly and soothingly.

SELF-CARE AND CHILDREN

Frey and Denyes, 1989

The study measured the impact of basic conditioning factors and universal and health deviation self-care on health and control of pathology.

Thirty-seven diabetic patients aged 11 to 19 responded to DSCPA, DiSCPI, U-SC, DHSI, questions of age, gender, birth order, mother's employment, religious participation. Subjects also completed the Hollingshead Four Factor Index (income measure), the BSI, and GSI. Zero order correlations measured relationships between U-SC basic conditioning factors. Stepwise multiple regression determined the contribution of basic conditioning factors to U-SC. Pearson correlations examined the relationship between the DSCPI and health. Hierarchical multiple regression tested the relationships between basic conditioning factors; U-SC, and health. Pearson correlations examined relationships between basic conditioning factors and HD-SC.

Age and health symptoms were negatively correlated with U-SC ($r = -0.38$, $p = 0.02$, and $r = -0.47$, $p = 0.004$ respectively). Younger youths reported more U-SC. Those with fewer health symptoms reported more U-SC. Age and health symptoms jointly explained 35% of the variance. Youths with higher levels of U-SC had higher levels of health ($r = 0.72$, $p = 0.001$). Health symptoms and U-SC explained 64% of the variation in health. There were no significant correlations between basic conditioning factors and HD-SC. A moderate negative relationship existed between HD-SC and the DiSCPI score that was regressed with the glycosylated hemoglobin levels ($r = -0.46$, $p = 0.009$). Those with higher HD-SC better controlled their IDDM. This explained 21% of the variance of metabolic control.

Gaffney and Moore, 1996

The study tested the theory of self-care in children and examined the relationship between mothers' dependent-care performance and basic conditioning factors.

A convenience sample of 380 mothers aged 23 to 57 years with children aged 1 to 16 years responded to the DCA and the Basic Conditioning Factors Questionnaire. Simultaneous regression analysis identified which of basic conditioning factors accounted for variance in dependent-care activity.

Although the sample was primarily Caucasian, 16% of mothers were immigrants to America. With all of the basic conditioning factors included, 13% of the variance in dependent agent performance was explained ($R = 0.354$, $p = 0.0001$). Significant factors were age and ethnicity. Internal consistency for DCA was 0.88.

Mosher and Moore, 1998

This descriptive study examined relationships between self-concept and self-care, dependent-care, and basic conditioning factors for children with cancer. The self-concepts of children both on and off of therapy were compared.

Subjects consisted of a nonprobability sample of 74 cancer patients aged 9 to 18 and their mothers. Children completed the Children's Self-Care Performance Questionnaire and Piers-Harris Children's Self-Concept Scale. Mothers completed the Dependent Care Agent Performance Questionnaire. Health providers completed Cosmetic and Functional Impairment Ratings Scale. Pearson correlations were used to assess relationships. Stepwise regression assessed the relationship between self-concept and basic conditioning factors.

Researchers discovered a small but significant relationship between self-concept and self-care practices ($r = 0.233$, $p < 0.046$) and dependent-care practices ($r = 0.228$, $p < 0.05$). Age was the only significant basic conditioning factor related to self-concept, explaining 7% of variance. Older children demonstrated lower self-concept ($F = 4.96$, $p = 0.03$). No differences between self-concept of children currently receiving treatment and those who had completed it were found.

Continued

TABLE 5-2

Selected Self-Care Research Studies—cont'd

Study/Year	Purpose	Methods	Findings
OLDER ADULTS			
Jirovec and Kasno, 1990	The study determined the influence of patient characteristics and environmental constraints provision of self-care by nursing home residents.	Eighty-three conveniently selected nursing home residents were assessed for self-care agency using the ASA-A. Environmental constraints were examined using the Perceived Environmental Constraints Index, and the ability to perform activities of daily living (ADL) was assessed using the Katz Index of ADL.	African-Americans demonstrated higher levels of self-care agency than Caucasians ($t = 2.54$, $p < 0.02$). Previously self-employed persons had significantly higher perceptions of their self-care agency than other groups (white collar professionals, blue collar workers, and homemakers) ($F_{(3, 77)} = 4.07$, $p < 0.01$). Lower self-care agency scores occurred in residents who felt that the nursing home environment produced dependency and that the rules were too restrictive.
Jirovec and Kasno, 1993	Basic conditioning factors were operationalized and used to predict nursing home residents' self-care abilities.	Hierarchical multiple regression determined predictors of self-care.	Accounting for a total of 20% of the variance in self-care scores, occupation and race were the only significant predictors for self-care.
Faucett, Ellis, Underwood, Naqvi, and Wilson; 1990	The study determined whether implementating the SCDNT altered nursing home staff members' perspectives on promoting self-care activities. It addressed the nature of nursing assessments and patient-care goals.	Two 50-bed nursing home care units were selected and assigned to serve as experimental and control units. On the experimental unit, two clinical nurse specialists directed the implementation of the SCDNT over a 2½ year period. Care records for last six months of implementation were reviewed to elicit common problem categories and number of interventions elicited. Structured interviews were conducted with staff of both units to elicit descriptive data about nurses' perspectives on care. Interviews were rated for nurse consideration of resident self-care capabilities and the use of concepts related self-care.	Twelve common problems on both units were identified. Falls were mentioned more frequently on the control unit ($p < 0.01$). The number of interventions on each unit was similar except for fall risk. Staff interviews revealed similarities in acquiring information about family, and sociocultural and medical histories and in assessing general physical and mental status, and specific assessments of bowel and bladder continence, skin condition, and orientation. Experimental nurses were more comprehensive and consistent in their assessment approach and organized functional assessment into areas related to universal requisites. SCDNT nurses facilitated resident participation in care to achieve goals.

DOCUMENTATION

Rossow-Sebring, Carrieri, and Seward; 1992

The study evaluated the outcomes of implementing Orem's Self-Care Model on nurse attitudes and charting behaviors.

Twenty nurses with an average age of 46 and an average of 23 years of work experience who worked on one of three medical surgical units in an institution implementing Orem's Self-Care Model completed the Nurse Attitudes Instrument before implementation and one year after. Randomly selected charts were reviewed to evaluate whether they met seven criteria related to assessment, expected outcomes, nursing actions, and patient responses.

Satisfaction with nursing and the value of patient teaching changed significantly following implementation of the Orem model. Baccalaureate nurses were more likely to be satisfied than nurses prepared at the AD or diploma level. Documentation remained approximately the same one year after program implementation A small increase in the number of actions relevant to nursing problems were documented.

EDUCATION

Berbiglia, 1991

A case study assessed use of and satisfaction with the SCDNT as a theoretical framework for a BS nursing program.

Structured interviews were conducted with five administrators, three faculty, and 10 students. Document analysis was completed on the school philosophy, texts, conceptual framework, college bulletin, curriculum guide, most recent self-study, course syllabi, handouts, and transparencies. Curriculum implementation was compared to an ideal implementation, which included the following: understanding the SCDNT, conceptualizing nursing within that framework; Orem's seven areas of nursing knowledge (profession, jurisprudence, history, ethics, economics, social field, and sciences), personal knowledge, and four types of instructional material (printed materials, situations, health-care participants, and audiovisuals).

Faculty, students, and administrators were satisfied that the curriculum elements matched the ideal perspective. All three groups perceived that goals, objectives, content, and evaluation were near agreement with the ideal perspective of use of the SCDNT. The major inconsistency found was variation in interpreting the nursing process.

care agency and self-care behaviors. Forty-one percent of the variance found in the general state of health could be predicted by the variables of self-care agency, self-care behaviors, and health problems. This indicates that health problems, as basic conditioning factors, influence health outcomes.

Geden and Taylor (1999) proposed a collaborative care system (CCS) in which couples functioned as a social unit that shared self-care. Although it was based on the central tenets of Orem's SCDNT, the focus of CCS differs from the traditional focus on individual self-care. Investigators perceived the CCS as a "unique whole formed through the informal negotiation for care by two adults" in which each member made a unique contribution to self-care (p. 330). In this instance the whole is considered greater than the sum of the individual parts, and the parts work integrally within the system to provide a whole. Cohesion within the couple dyad and the couple's appraisal of health accounted for 27% of the CCS. The study provided tentative support for the CCS, but additional variables that could contribute to the explanatory value of the model need to be added. The concept of self-care occurring within the context of a dyad is a new variation of the tenets of self-care. Additional areas for investigation include examining development and maintenance of the self-care dyads and renegotiation of the CCSs in changing health situations.

Walker and Grobe (1999) used the SCDNT to examine the construct of thriving during the postpartum period. The SCDNT's conceptualization of the self-care regulatory functions through which humans maintain life provided a broad context for the study. Thriving was perceived as an extension of the power component of self-care agency and was related to the integration of nutritional, psychosocial, and lifestyle concerns during the childbearing process. Specifically, Walker and Grobe wanted to further elaborate on basic factors influencing self-care requisites and self-care agency. In a secondary data analysis derived from a study of nutritional components, lifestyle components, and psychosocial status, investigators found four factors that influenced postpartum thriving. These included psychosocial distress, lifestyle patterns, weight, and body image. The emotional and psychological effects of weight gain, depressive symptoms, body image dissatisfaction, and lifestyle pattern influenced the balance of self-care demands with self-care agency. This study provided preliminary evidence that the construct of thriving in postpartum women is viable and has connections to the SCDNT.

Hanucharurnkul (1989) found that basic conditioning factors of social support, occupational prestige (measuring socioeconomic status), and cancer site and stage (measuring health state) contributed to differences in self-care characteristics for cancer patients receiving radiotherapy in Bangkok, Thailand. This study supported Orem's proposal that basic conditioning factors influence self-care. However, some of Orem's basic conditioning factors, such as age, marital status, and living arrangements, did not significantly influence self-care. Kubricht (1984) identified self-care demands of cancer patients undergoing radiotherapy as food and water, rest and activity, normality, solitude and social interaction, and air. These concerns are congruent with universal requisites identified by Orem (1985), which include (1) maintenance of sufficient intake of air, water, and food; (2) provision of care associated with elimination; (3) maintenance of a balance between rest and activity; (4) avoidance of hazards to life; (5) functioning and well-being; and (6) promotion of normalcy.

Dodd (1982, 1983, 1988a, 1988b) and Dibble (Dodd & Dibble, 1993) performed a series of investigations examining the frequency with which cancer patients engaged in self-care behaviors to counteract chemotherapy side effects and the influence of knowledge giving on self-care performance. In her initial study Dodd (1982) found that patients experienced an average of eight side effects during chemotherapy, three of which were directly attributable to the therapy. These side effects were moderately severe; however, cancer patients engaged in less than one self-care behavior per side effect. Dodd attributed the limited self-care behaviors to lack of information from physicians and nurses. Her conclusion concurs with Orem's suggestion that patient self-care actions are limited by knowledge of what they can do for themselves. Dodd (1983) then examined the influence of offering information regarding side effect management on self-care. The patient group that was offered knowledge of side effect management engaged in a greater number of behaviors to counteract the side effects and reported a higher degree of effectiveness for those actions, thus supporting Orem's contention that self-care activities need to be learned and deliberate.

In an extension of her work, Dodd (1988a) examined breast cancer patients' self-care management. Thirty women initiating chemotherapy completed a Self-Care Behavior Log (SCB), the State-Trait Anxiety Inventory (STAI), and a Multidimensional Health Locus of Control (MHLC) at the beginning of chemotherapy and 6 to 8 weeks later. As in the previous studies (Dodd, 1982, 1983) patients initiated few self-care behaviors in response to side effects perceived as moderately severe. One difference from the earlier studies was that subjects did not delay initiation of self-care behaviors. Most participants exhibited a strong internal locus of control that led them to feel they had control over their situations. This, in turn, impacted self-reliance in initiating self-care activities. These findings once again demonstrated Orem's contention that knowledge influences self-care activities. State anxiety decreased between initiation of chemotherapy and the second interview, and anxiety levels decreased as side-effect management improved.

To assess whether knowledge of side-effect management would impact self-care, Dodd (1988b) assigned 60 cancer chemotherapy patients to either control or experimental groups. The experimental group received materials about side effect management and instructions for use of the materials. Following 6 weeks of chemotherapy, patients receiving the side effect information management materials performed significantly more preventative self-care behaviors to reduce chemotherapy-related side effects. Once again Orem's contention that knowledge is key to self-care was upheld.

In a study specifically testing Orem's Theory, Dodd and Dibble (1993) examined predictors of self-care in cancer patients. Predictors of self-care included demographic characteristics, performance status (Karnofsky Performance Status Scale), affective state (Profile of Mood State [POMS]), social support (Norbeck Social Support Questionnaire), ability to manage a situation, self-care ability (ESCA score, Self-Care Behavior Checklist), and prior health-promoting activities (Health-Promoting Lifestyle Profile [HPLP]). Basic conditioning factors related to self-care included lower performance status, lower social support, and more formal education. One of Orem's power components, self-care agency, was found to predict self-care. This finding was unexpected. High anxiety increased self-care behaviors and seemed to reflect participants' increased vigilance in maintaining self-care behaviors.

To assess the influence of nursing intervention on the self-care nutritional habits of myocardial infarction patients, Aish and Isenberg (1996) tried to determine prior dietary behavior and offer information about modifying patients' dietary lifestyles. Follow-up visits emphasized healthy self-care behaviors. Participants receiving the dietary support intervention demonstrated significant increases in self-care agency and self-efficacy for eating. Findings from this study were congruent with Orem's suggestion that individuals are capable of self-care and that nursing intervention can foster and support self-care agency.

In a secondary analysis from two previous qualitative studies, Pickens (1999) explored different aspects of the desire for normalcy in seriously mentally ill patients. Orem's SCDNT suggests that normalcy is associated with human functioning and development within social groups that permit achievement of human potential and that satisfy the desire to be normal. Normalcy was defined as having normal things and experiences; doing meaningful activities; and being well, safe, free, and independent. Prevention of actual or potential hazards supported Orem's notion of universal self-care requisites and promoted normalcy. The concept of universal self-care requisites was supported by Pickens' finding that balancing activity and rest and solitude and social interaction promoted normalcy. Thus nurses should practice acceptance and support toward this end.

In a theory-testing study of the SCDNT, Campbell and Weber (2000) proposed that basic conditioning factors of age, education, and culture would influence the relational conflicts of frequency and severity of abuse and sex abuse. They further proposed that relational conflicts would in turn influence self-care agency as measured by the Tennessee Self Concept Scale (self esteem) and the DSCAI (power components of self-care). This in turn would influence health (functional integrity related to presence of injury and physical symptoms) and well-being (as exhibited by depression and measured by the Beck Depression Inventory). Investigators hypothesized that women who experienced abuse would have poorer functional integrity and greater depression. The investigators aimed to extend Orem's SCDNT to include relational conflict. In a sample of women experiencing serious marital problems, Campbell and Weber predicted 45% of the variance in health outcomes in a modified model. Relational problems were demonstrated to have a greater influence on physical and mental health than self-care. Campbell and Weber attributed this finding to women's lack of control in battering. This model supported the idea that the basic conditioning factors of age and education influence relational factors and self-care. Additionally, self-care influences health factors. Campbell and Weber recommended further research with a larger sample size and assessment of more variables to increase the explanatory power of the model.

Findings from studies regarding health and illness provide an incomplete picture of the linkages between basic conditioning factors and self-care. Orem posited that internal and external factors called basic conditioning factors would influence individual ability to engage in self-care or affect the type of self-care required. Basic conditioning factors included age, gender, education, health state, sociocultural orientation, healthcare systems, family systems, patterns of living, environment, and adequacy of resources. Additionally, self-care agency was proposed to affect the ability to meet self-care demands. Basic conditioning factors that were shown to influence self-care activities included health state, knowledge levels (Dodd, 1988a, 1988b; Dodd & Dibble, 1993), age and education (Campbell & Weber, 2000). However, basic conditioning factors of age, marital status, and living conditions were found to inconsistently influence self-care activities (Dodd & Dibble, 1993; Hanucharurnkul, 1989). Self-care agency consistently affected the ability to meet self-care demands (Dodd, 1982, 1983, 1988a, 1988b; Dodd & Dibble, 1993). Further research could determine the roles of basic conditioning factors on self-care, explore effective nursing interventions for patients with self-care deficits, and improve self-care capabilities.

Pain. Villarruel (1995) used an ethnographic approach to discover Mexican-American expressions and meanings of pain and associated self-care activities. Orem's theoretical constructs of self-care agency and dependent-care agency (caring for self and others), self-care requisites, and the relations of self-care requisites to basic conditioning factors were found relevant to the phenomena of study. Four themes were associated with Mexican-American interpretations of pain and self-care perspectives. Pain was perceived as an encompassing life obligation to be borne without inflicting pain on others. Thus it should be hidden and endured stoically. Care for others and helping others is central in the pain experience. Informants used self-care behaviors to promote pain relief. The sense of obligation to care for others reflected Orem's concepts of dependent-care. Villarruel suggested that Mexican-American decisions to forgo self-care in favor of caring for others needs to be considered in Orem's theory. This study provided an important cultural context from which pain can be understood and from which effective culturally competent interventions can be designed. Although Villarruel's study supported concepts found in Orem's theory, a new avenue—forgoing self-care in favor of caring for others—was discovered. Orem's theory does not address this particular phenomenon.

Denyes, Neuman, and Villarruel (1991) conducted a pair of studies to determine the pain relief actions and action patterns expert nurses used in caring for children in pain. The second study examined the frequency with which the general nursing staff used pain-relieving actions. Orem had described five methods of helping or nursing action systems: doing for, guiding, supporting, providing a developmentally supportive environment, and teaching. In ethnographic interviews of expert nurses, Denyes, Neuman, and Villarruel discovered that nurses used 156 pain management actions, which could be grouped into six patterns: (1) doing for the child, (2) modifying the environment, (3) engaging the child in care, (4) engaging parent or family in care, (5) teaching the child, and (6) teaching the parent. Nursing actions such as application of heat, cold, or pain medication were directed toward the pain, whereas distraction or diversion techniques were directed away from the pain. This study's strength was the method in which investigators tied nursing actions for pain relief to Orem's concept of "acting for" or "doing for" and "guiding or directing." Nurses who were "acting for or doing for" actively engaged the child and parents in care or another activity. Nurses using a teaching method for the child and parents exhibited "guiding or directing." Investigators also tied Orem's concept of "creating a developmental environment" to nursing actions of allowing visitors and sharing pain relief measures. Physical environmental behaviors such as dimming the room and providing quiet also created "a developmental environment." None of the action patterns studied reflected Orem's concept of "supporting."

In the second study of general nursing staff, investigators discovered that the top methods for pediatric pain relief were medications, comfort measures, distraction, tender loving care, parental involvement, preparing the child, repositioning, and calmly talking with child. Five of these actions agreed with those previously identified by the expert nurses. Two actions expert nurses viewed as particularly effective—guided imagery and giving the child choices—were not considered effective by staff nurses and were used only occasionally. The study findings can prompt further testing of pain relief protocols for children. Additionally, findings indicate that nursing actions for pain may be either wholly or partially compensatory, depending on child's or parent's needs, and that nursing action systems can effectively intervene.

Self-Care and Children. Frey and Denyes (1989) used the SCDNT to study the influence of basic conditioning factors on universal self-care (U-SC) and health deviation self-care (HD-SC) in adolescents with insulin-dependent diabetes mellitus (IDDM). The impact of self-care was measured in terms of control of illness. Clear connections between the identified study variables and the SCDNT were found. Self-care variables were operationalized with two instruments: (1) the Denyes Self-Care Practice Instrument (DSCPI) to measure general care actions and specific care actions, and (2) the Diabetic Self-Care Practice Instrument (DiSCPI) to measure self-care when health deviations occurred. Health was measured using the combined score of the Self-Perception Profile for Children (SPPC) and the Denyes Health Status Instrument (DHSI). Basic conditioning factors were measured via interview questions, the Hollingshead Four Factor Index (reflecting socioeconomic status), the Brief Symptom Inventory (BSI) (reflecting health state), and the General Severity Index (GSI) (reflecting health state). Each of these instruments was congruent with the SCDNT. Frey and Denyes concluded that findings provided insight about U-SC and HD-SC in that relationships were demonstrated between universal and health deviation self-care. However, Frey and Denyes questioned whether U-SC and HD-SC were different, since the basic conditioning factors of age and health state correlated only with U-SC and not with HD-SC. None of the other basic conditioning factors (age, income, illness severity) correlated with health deviation in self-care, which suggests that basic conditioning factors do not directly influence this type of self-care. In summary, the Frey and Denyes study provides empirical support for a selected concept of the SCDNT but fails to support a direct relationship between condition factors and HD-SC.

Gaffney and Moore (1996) tested Orem's Theory of Self-Care Deficit by examining the relationship between dependent-care agent performance and selected conditioning factors. Gaffney and Moore examined Orem's SCDNT and specifically the ideas that dependent-care performance is related to capabilities of the dependent and that dependent care is related to age and other basic conditioning factors. Mothers were perceived as the dependent care agents who performed self-care activities unable to be performed by the child. The Dependent Care Agent Questionnaire (DCA)—a measure of caregivers' performance of self-care activities for children—and the Basic Conditioning Factors Questionnaire—short answer questions—were completed. Only two basic conditioning factors, child age and ethnicity, predicted dependent-care agent performance. Increasing age reduced performance of self-care activities for dependents. Although this study upholds Orem's SCDNT, it does not measure the basic conditioning variables. Work needs to be completed on measurement of basic conditioning factors before further research is undertaken.

Gaffney and Moore's study (1996) focused on dependent-care agency for healthy children. In a follow-up study, Mosher and Moore (1998) focused on self-concept, children's self-care, and dependent agent self-care of children with cancer. The study centered on Orem's proposition (1995) that self-care and dependent care must meet universal self-care requisites such as those for air, food, water, rest, activity, elimination, social interaction, solitude, hazards, and normalcy. Feelings of normalcy included development and maintenance of a realistic self-concept. Researchers also were guided by Orem's proposition that conditioning factors such as age, gender, and sociocultural orientation influence self-care. Illness was perceived to influence the ability to manage self-care requisites. Mosher and Moore's study supported Orem's propositions and revealed relationships between self-concept and self-care and between self-concept and dependent-care practices. Children with higher self-concepts performed more self-care and received more support in performing self-care from their mothers. This study was the first time the relationship between self-care and self-concept had been documented for seriously ill children. Only age correlated with self-concept. This finding provided only partial support for Orem's proposition regarding the role of basic conditioning factors. The demonstrated relationship between self-concept and self-care necessitates further research to address strategies that could promote positive self-concept in children. Likewise, the connection between self-concept and dependent agent care calls for investigation of strategies that would promote greater dependent agent care. Because older children with cancer had lower self-concepts, additional interventions may be needed to improve self-concept in older children with serious illness.

Older Adults. Self-care for older adults has become a particular concern. Allowing nursing home residents to maintain control of self-care is believed to benefit both physical and psychological health. Orem posited that self-care agency was a product of day-to-day living and was influenced by knowledge, environment, and ability to perform effective care actions. The studies discussed in the following paragraphs address older adults' self-care in residential environments.

Jirovec and Kasno (1990) examined the impact of patient characteristics and environmental constraints on self-care provision by nursing home residents. This study linked clearly to Orem's SCDNT in theoretical frame of reference and variable conceptualization, with each of the basic conditioning factors listed and specific indicators delineated. For example, sociocultural orientation was measured by years of education, race, and previous occupation, and health state was measured using an Activities of Daily Living index and a morale scale. Self-care agency was related to the basic conditioning factors of race and nature of previous occupation. These two variables accounted for 20% of the variance found in self-care scores (Jirovec & Kasno, 1993). African-Americans and individuals previously self-employed had higher perceptions of self-care agency. Residents who felt that the nursing home environment prevented them from completing things they wanted to do exhibited lower self-care agency. Although conditioning factors of patterns of living (the perception that nursing home living fostered dependence) and morale correlated with self-care, these variables failed to account for any additional variance in self-care. Findings support Orem's suggestion that basic conditioning factors of sociocultural orientation and life experience influence self-care. However, other basic conditioning factors suggested by Orem, such as age, sex, and family system, failed to influence self-care participation.

Faucett, Ellis, Underwood, Naqvi, and Wilson (1990) examined the impact of Orem's SCDNT as a practice framework on nursing assessment and goal planning for nursing home residents. Orem's concepts of satisfying universal care requisites to maintain life and promote health and well-being and basic conditioning factors guided study planning. Nursing roles focused on instances of actual or potential patient failure to provide self-care. Two and a half years following implementation of Orem's SCDNT, investigators found that nurses on the SCDNT unit were more comprehensive and organized in their assessment approach, organizing functional assessment in the areas related to universal care requisites. For example, a functional assessment might question the resident's ability to manage food and fluid or regulate elimination patterns. Both are areas suggested in Orem's universal self-requisites. SCDNT nurses facilitated resident participation in care. For example, the nurses' goals might focus on a resident learning wound care or maintaining social interaction skills. This study emphasized the need for theory-guided practice and provided a basis for further study to determine the effectiveness of theory-based practice. In this study, application of Orem's theory to a practice setting clarified the philosophy of practice and the role of nursing. Using Orem's SCDNT provided a common language for communicating needs and promoted consistency in care delivery.

Documentation. Documentation is a critical step in providing nursing care. However, this aspect of care had been neglected in SCDNT nursing studies. Rossow-Sebring, Carrieri, and Seward (1992) evaluated the effects of the implementation of the SCDNT on nursing attitudes and charting behaviors following implementation of Orem's model. Although they found that overall nursing satisfaction increased following implementation of nursing based on Orem's theory, the influence on charting was somewhat mixed. Investigators proposed that increased satisfaction could be attributed to the dynamic created by bringing the nursing staff together to work on the documentation project. However, 1 year after program implementation, investigators found that nurses charted with about the same frequency. Documentation of nursing actions relevant to identified problems increased slightly. Documentation of family responses to educational interventions increased as did the number of appropriate client referrals. This study demonstrates that, although the generated changes may not be as widespread as desired, Orem's SCDNT can usefully guide documentation.

Education. Berbiglia (1991) evaluated the use of the SCDNT in curriculum implementation for a baccalaureate nursing program. Data were gathered by interviewing administrators, faculty, and students, and by examining curriculum-associated materials. The descriptive study revealed student and faculty commitment to the SCDNT. Although the curriculum was closely congruent with an ideal conception of an SCDNT-based curriculum, Berbiglia discovered differences in the way the nursing process was interpreted among administrators, faculty, and students. On the whole, the SCDNT proved to be a useful organizing framework for a nursing education program. The study suggested that the SCDNT could give direction to education and, potentially, to nursing as a discipline. Further research should be conducted in other educational programs where the SCDNT is used as a basis for the curriculum.

Usefulness of Theory to Research. Work completed by Aish and Isenberg (1996), Denyes (1988), Frey and Denyes (1989), Jirovec and Kasno (1990), and Campbell and Weber (2000) most strongly reflects Silva's theory-testing priorities (1986). These studies clearly used Orem's SCDNT as a conceptual frame of reference to identify study questions, used the theoretical perspective when planning for variable measurement, and discussed findings in light of their contribution to the theoretical frame. Each of these studies clearly cited Orem's theory as the basis for research. Dodd's (1983, 1988a, 1988b, 1997; Dodd & Dibble, 1993) studies consistently identify Orem as a theoretical frame of reference and address her theory in the discussion. However, variable conceptualization linking to Orem is not as clear. Of all the study series, Dodd and Dibble's study (1993), which deals specifically with Orem's power components, comes closest to fulfilling Silva's criteria for adequate theory use.

Dodd's study (1983) of the influence of education on self-care activities represents one of the earlier intervention studies. Aish and Isenberg's study (1996) of nutritional self-care of myocardial patients demonstrated that nursing care could influence self-care agency. Research findings have offered mixed support for the SCDNT. The connection between self-care agency and self-care has been established consistently. However, the influence of basic conditioning factors is less convincing because research findings have been mixed. Race has been found to be a basic conditioning factor affecting self-care, but it has not been examined in many studies. Factors such as age, marital status, and socioeconomic status have inconsistently correlated to self-care. In some instances, direct support of health deviation self-care failed to materialize despite the connection between selected basic conditioning factors and universal self-care. Suggestions for future studies include the following:

- Specific theory-testing studies
- Multicultural studies
- Studies regarding self-care needs and activities associated with different acute and chronic illnesses and health promotion
- Intervention studies to assess the effectiveness of nursing interventions, patient-initiated self-care, and family-associated self-care.

PRAXIS AND THEORY UTILIZATION: DESIGNING NURSING PRACTICE PROGRAMS WITHIN THE THEORETICAL SYSTEM OF SELF-CARE DEFICIT NURSING THEORY

Individuals and healthcare organizations widely use the SCDNT to design nursing practice programs. Clarifying the proper object of nursing and implementing composite theories of self-care, self-care deficit, and nursing systems provides direction for specifying the boundaries of nursing practice within a multidisciplinary environment, identifying the goal of nursing, and developing process and practice models. As previously described, the inability to perform the required quantity and quality of self-care creates the proper object of nursing. The focus of nursing is not health, disease, or care—it is the person(s) with health-derived or health-associated self-care deficits. Although the early applications to practice focused on the individual, the literature also has described extensions to family and community (Taylor, 1989; Taylor & McLaughlin, 1990; Taylor & McLaughlin-Renpenning, 2001).

Self-care is a recurring theme in the healthcare literature. Much of that literature views self-care as a derivation of a philosophical base of independence. Practicing nursing from the perspective of the SCDNT requires that nurses conceptualize self-care in a manner consistent with the theory. Self-care within this theory stems not from independence but from the condition of being human. It is care that individuals must perform on their own behalf to promote development and to maintain life, health, and integrated functioning (Orem, 1995). The necessity of self-care exists regardless of whether the individual can perform such care. A person's inability to perform health-related self- or dependent-care creates a need for nursing. Nursing is an action system, and nurses produce the **nursing system,** composed of the patient(s), the nurse, and the actions and interactions between nurse and patient(s).

BOX 5-2

Nursing System Variables by Unit of Service

1. When the unit of service is an individual:
   a. The patient variables of self-care, therapeutic self-care demand, and self-care agency and the relational variable of self-care deficit
   b. The nurse variable of nursing agency
   c. Basic conditioning factors, foundational capabilities, and dispositions condition the patient variables and the nurse variable
2. In a dependent-care situation:
   a. The patient and nurse variables as identified above
   b. The capabilities of the care provider namely the dependent care agency and the relational variable of dependent care deficit
3. When the unit of service is the family:
   a. The self-care systems of persons making up the family unit, the therapeutic self-care demand and self-care agency of those persons, and the interactions among the foregoing variables in relation to meeting the functions of the family associated with self-care
   b. Nursing agency
4. When the unit of service is a multiperson unit of service such as a community:
   a. The self-care systems and therapeutic self-care demand and agency of persons making up the multiperson unit of service
   b. The conditioning factors modifying the self-care systems, therapeutic self-care demand, development, operability, and adequacy of self-care agency of persons making up the unit of service
   c. Nursing agency
   d. Community systems in operation
   e. Therapeutic systems in operation

The Variables of Concern for Practice

The variables of concern for practice are those that make up the nursing system in relation to the variations in unit of service (Box 5-2). These have been identified and described by Orem (2001), the Nursing Development Conference Group (1979), Taylor (1989), Taylor and McLaughlin (1990), and Taylor, McLaughlin-Renpenning, Geden, Hart, and Neuman (2001). Case study and research are clarifying the underlying structure of each for practice purposes. The primary sources in the reference section of this chapter provide more extensive description and explanation.

Therapeutic self-care demand is foundational to practicing nursing from the perspective of the SCDNT. The therapeutic self-care demand summarizes all of the actions required over time to meet known self-care requisites. A self-care requisite expresses the goals of actions necessary for regulating an aspect(s) of human functioning and development (Orem, 1995). There are three categories of self-care requisites or goals of self-care: *universal*, which are common to all persons; *developmental*, which are particular to the person's developmental stage; and *health deviation*, which address particular health states. Each self-care requisite consists of the factor to be controlled or managed and the action to be taken. A sampling of self-care requisites is reproduced in Box 5-3.

> ## BOX 5-3
>
> ### Sample of Self-Care Requisites
>
> **UNIVERSAL SELF-CARE REQUISITES**
> - The maintenance of a suffient intake of air
> - The maintenance of a sufficient intake of water
> - The maintenance of a sufficient intake of food
> - The provision of care associated with elimination processes and excrements
> - The maintenance of a balance between activity and rest
>
> **DEVELOPMENTAL SELF-CARE REQUISITES**
> Provision of conditions that promote development
> - Provide and maintain an adequacy of materials and conditions for development of the human body.
> - Provide and maintain physical, environmental, and social conditions that ensure feelings of comfort and safety, the sense of being close to another, and the sense of being cared for.
> Engagement in self-development
> - Seek to understand and form habits of introspection and reflection to develop insights about self, one's perception of others, relationships to others, and attitudes toward them.
> - Seek to accept feeling and emotions as leading, after reflection on them, to insights about self and about relationships to others, to objects, or to life situations.
> Interference with development
> - Provide conditions and promote behaviors that will prevent the occurrence of deleterious effects on development.
> - Provide conditions and experiences to mitigate or overcome existent deleterious effects on development.
>
> **HEALTH DEVIATION SELF-CARE REQUISITES**
> - Seeking and securing appropriate medical assistance.
> - Being aware of and attending to the effects and results of pathological conditions and states, including effects on development.

From Orem, D.E. (1995). *Nursing: Concepts of practice.* (5th ed.). St. Louis: Mosby.

Orem (2001) offers a complete listing of the self-care requisites and required general sets of actions.

Self-care agency is persons' ability to know and meet their continuing requirements for self-care in order to regulate their own human functioning and development (Orem, 1995). It is a theoretical construct. The NDCG (1979), comprised primarily of nursing practitioners, specified real world referents for self-care agency through case analysis and research studies. Self-care agency is conceptualized as a threefold construct (Figure 5-6). These include the following:

- Self-care operations of knowing, decision making, and acting with the abilities associated with each operation. These operations are derived from action theory.
- The ten power components, which are abilities specific to self-care (Box 5-4) capabilities and dispositions identified as being foundational to deliberate action (Table 5-3).

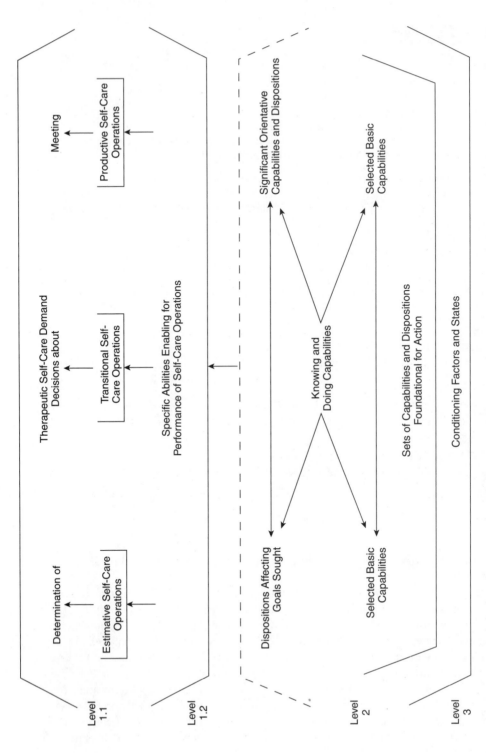

FIGURE 5-6 Three structural levels for diagnostic processes directed to the patient variable self-care agency. (From Nursing Development Conference Group. (1979). *Concept formalization in nursing: Process and product.* (2nd ed.). Boston: Little, Brown) Copyright Dorothea Orem.

TABLE 5-3

Capabilities and Dispositions: A Survey List of Human Capabilities and Dispositions Foundational to Self-Care Agency, with a List of Factors and States that Condition the Capabilities and Dispositions

Conditioning Factors and States	Selected Basic Capabilities I	Selected Basic Capabilities II	Knowing and Doing Capabilities	Dispositions Affecting Goals Sought	Significant Orientative Capabilities and Dispositions
Genetic and Constitutional Factors	Sensation Proprioception Exteroception	Attention	Rational Agency	Self-under-standing Self-awareness	Orientations to: Time Health Other Persons Events Objects
Arousal State	Learning	Perception	Operational Knowing	Self-image Self-value	Priority System or Value Hierarchy Moral Economic Aesthetic Material Social
Social Organization	Exercise or Work	Memory	Learned Skills Reading Counting Writing Verbal Perceptual Manual Reasoning	Self-acceptance Self-concern	Interest and Concerns Habits
				Acceptance of Bodily Functions	Ability to Work with the Body and its Parts
Culture				Willingness to Meet Needs of Self	Ability to Manage Self and Personal Affairs
Experience	Regulation of the Position and Movement of the Body and its Parts	Central Regulation of Motivational Emotional Processes	Self-consistency in knowing and doing	Future Directions	

From Nursing Development Conference Group. (1979). *Concept formalization in nursing: Process and product.* (2nd ed.). Boston: Little Brown. Copyright Dorothea Orem.

Basic conditioning factors influence therapeutic self-care demand. For example, culture influences how a person maintains sufficient intake of food. The scope of these factors and the relationship of these factors to therapeutic self-care demand and self-care agency are illustrated in Figure 5-7.

Self-care deficit is a relational construct, not a value statement. It expresses the disparity between therapeutic self-care demand and self-care agency when the self-care agency is inadequate.

Self-care systems are the sequences of action performed by individuals to meet their self-care requisites.

Nursing agency refers to nurses' empowerment to act and know. It also refers to nurses' abilities to help patients to accomplish self-care and to regulate patients' self-care agency through legitimate interpersonal relationships (Orem, 1995).

Dependent-care agency is the "capabilities of persons to know and meet the therapeutic self-care demands of persons socially dependent on them or to regulate the development or exercise of these persons' self-care agency" (Orem 1995, p. 457).

Dependent-care deficit is also a relational statement. It describes the relationship between the self-care deficit of the dependent (the required assistance) and dependent-care agency (the capabilities of the care provider). Identification of a dependent-care deficit indicates a need for further assistance.

Describing a Population for Nursing Purposes

Describing a population through the SCDNT in order to develop a nursing practice program begins with organizing the most commonly recurring and valuable variable(s) for nursing. These variables may be one or more of the components of the therapeutic self-care demand, basic conditioning factors, components of self-care agency, and so on (Taylor, 1987). Allison and McLaughlin-Renpenning (1998) and Taylor and McLaughlin-Renpenning (2001) have developed a schema based in the SCDNT for analyzing a nursing population in an organized fashion. Population descriptions of this sort have been useful in developing client assessment standards (Vancouver Health Department [VHD], 1988), computerized information systems (Bliss-Holtz, McLaughlin, & Taylor,

Pattern of living
of
THIS INDIVIDUAL
MAN, WOMAN, CHILD
of this

Age   Gender
in this

Development state   Health state
affected by
Health care systems factors

Family system factors   Socio-cultural factors
Availablility of resources
and
Environmental factors

FIGURE 5-7 Basic Conditioning Factors (From Orem, D. (1995). *Nursing: Concepts of practice.* (5th ed.). St. Louis: Mosby.)

1990), patient classification systems (Allison & McLaughlin-Renpenning, 1998) and similar patient-centered tools of practice. Allison (1985) illustrated the use of the theory in the development of a nursing production design model and development of a nursing practice program for persons with spinal cord injuries. The Vancouver Health Department and the Mississippi Methodist Rehabilitation Hospital later used this model in developing assessment guidelines for a variety of classifications of populations (Allison & McLaughlin-Renpenning, 1998).

Expected Outcomes of Nursing

The expected outcomes of nursing are related to the variables of concern. Box 5-5 includes a sample of expected outcome categories derived from the SCDNT.

Process Models

The process models described by Orem (2001) make explicit three separate functions: design, planning, and production. The process models address nursing and self-care as deliberate action, the regulatory functions required to maintain life and health, and the operations required to accomplish those functions. *Operations* refers to the series of acts involved in a particular form of work, an instance or a method of efficient, productive activity. Regulation refers to control of or adjustment to a particular requirement, such as the self-care requisites express.

Orem has identified seven essential operations of nursing practice through which nurses come to know what is required in a nursing situation and how to perform accordingly. These operations are outlined in Box 5-6. These operations are broader than those traditionally referred to as *the nursing process*, which Orem calls the professional-technological component of the nursing systems. It includes diagnosis and prescription, design and planning, and production and control (Orem, 1995) and is shown in Table 5-4.

BOX 5-5

Sample of Expected Outcome Categories Derived from SCDNT

1. Self-care/self-management system
   1.1 Adequate or taking action to modify
   1.2 Integrated into broader system of living
2. Therapeutic self-care demand
   2.1 Calculates:
      2.1.1 What needs to be done
      2.1.2 Best method(s) to use
      2.1.3 Time sequence
      2.1.4 Equipment
3. Self-care agency
   3.2 Self-care operations performed
      3.2.1 Knowing
      3.2.2 Decision making
      3.2.3 Acting

From Allison, S.E. & McLaughlin-Renpenning, K.E. (1999). Nursing administration in the 21st century: A self-care theory approach. Walnut Creek, CA: Sage.

BOX 5-6

Nursing Practice Operations

- Securing demographical data about persons in the role of nurse's patient and information about the nature and boundaries of each patient's healthcare situation and nursing's jurisdiction within these boundaries.
- The taking of a nursing history to obtain information about persons' perceptions of therapeutic self-care demands, their development and exercise of self-care agency, and about their conditions and patterns of living.
- Establishing and maintaining a legitimate and functional unity of persons for the production of nursing.
- Determining the current values and probable foreseen changes in basic conditioning factors that are affecting or may positively or negatively affect patients' therapeutic self-care demands or their self-care agency.
- Performing the professional-technologic operations of nursing diagnosis, nursing prescription, nursing regulation, or treatment with associated evaluation and control operations and case management.
- Development of designs for the production of regulatory nursing care with attention to continuing nursing diagnosis and prescription.
- Maintaining an overview of the social, interpersonal, and professional-technological features of each nursing practice situation in the interests of situational management.

From Orem, D.E. (1995). *Nursing: Concepts of practice*. (5th ed.). St. Louis: Mosby.

Practice Models

Several practice models are reported in the literature. Integrating knowledge and direction from physiology, learning theory, systems theory, and nursing theory, Backscheider (1974) describes a practice model for assessing patient self-care abilities and designing nursing systems for a diabetic population. This model emphasizes the interrelationship of therapeutic self-care demand and self-care capabilities with nursing as a mediating system that complements self-care incapacities. Linking the data to Piaget's learning theory specified the knowledge, skills, and abilities required to manage diabetes. The necessary motivational and orientational capabilities were also identified and used to structure the nursing system. This model exemplifies structuring nursing knowledge around descriptions of self-care capabilities and limitations for self-care. It also models deriving the therapeutic self-care demand for specific patient populations and structuring nursing knowledge around that demand.

Horn and Swain (1977) and the Nursing Development Conference Group (NDCG) (1979) performed early work in the development of practice models. Horn and Swain studied criterion measures of nursing care. This is an example of work underlying the development of practice models. The NDCG related self-care actions to the demand to regulate a therapy in developing an "Ideal General Set of Actions." (see Box 3-1). This model, along with the diagnostic considerations of self-care agency, is the basis for the development of assessment guidelines and documentation tools in practice settings (Allison & McLaughlin-Renpenning, 1998).

TABLE 5-4

The Professional-Technological Process of Nursing

Variable of Concern	Diagnosis	Prescription	Design	Planning	Production
Therapeutic self-care demand, calculated by relating basic conditioning factors and self-care requisites.	Determine conditioning effect of basic conditioning factors on self-care requisites of concern. Evaluate adequacy of self-care practices in relation to known components of the therapeutic self-care demand.	Specify actions to be taken to meet therapeutic self-care demand. Determine organization of required actions. Specify roles of nurses, patient, others in meeting therapeutic self-care demand.	Describe amount, timing and reasons for nurse-patient contact. Describe contributions of persons involved in meeting or making adjustments to the therapeutic self-care demand.	Specify time, place, environmental conditions, equipment, and supplies required for the regulatory operations.	Nursing system: An action system with goal of meeting the therapeutic self-care demand.
Self-care agency: Adequacy of self-care operations (knowing, decision making, acting). Adequacy of power components. Conditioning effect of foundational capabilities and dispositions.	Evaluate adequacy of self-care agency for meeting components of therapeutic self-care demand and willingness to do so. Determine potential for development and exercise of self-care agency.	Specify roles of nurses, patient, in relation to development and or regulation of the exercise of self-care agency.	Describe contributions of persons involved in regulating the exercise and or development of self-care agency.	Specify time, place, environmental conditions, equipment, and supplies required for the regulatory operations.	Nursing system: An action system with goal of regulating the exercise and development of capabilities for self-care.

Continued

TABLE 5-4

The Professional-Technological Process of Nursing—cont'd

Variable of Concern	Diagnosis	Prescription	Design	Planning	Production
Dependent-care agency.	Determine adequacy of dependent-care agency for calculating and meeting therapeutic self-care demand of dependent and willingness to do so.	Specify and organize actions to be taken to meet therapeutic self-care demand of dependent.	Describe the amount, timing, and reasons for nurse-patient contact; describe contributions of persons involved in regulating the exercise and/or development of dependent-care agency.	Specify time, place, environmental conditions, equipment, and supplies required for the regulatory operations.	Dependent-care system: An action system to meet therapeutic self-care demand of the dependent and for regulating development and exercise of self- and dependent care capabilities.
Adequacy of dependent-care operations (knowing, decision making, acting).					
Adequacy of capabilities for dependent-care.	Determine potential for development and exercise of dependent-care agency.	Specify roles of nurses, patient, and dependent-care agent in meeting therapeutic self-care demand and dependent-care demand.			
Disposition for dependent-care.					

The NDCG (1979) also developed a model of the variance between therapeutic self-care demand and self-care agency in stroke patients and a corresponding model of the range over which nursing agency should vary. These models help nurses to think from a population perspective in relation to nursing variables. They stimulate and pattern the development of a categorization of variables for describing patient populations (Allison & McLaughlin-Renpenning, 1998). This work also was foundational to the initial conceptualization of the relational databases integral to the nursing component of a computerized patient record (Bliss-Holtz, 1996).

Dodd (1997) has developed systematic guidelines for examining the balance between needs, capabilities, and limitations in the exercise of self-care agency to enhance personal health. These guidelines are the result of a series of descriptive studies extending from 1978 to 2000. Publication of these studies has contributed to the understanding of the therapeutic self-care demand and health deviation self-care requisites of persons undergoing chemotherapy and radiation therapy. These studies have provided additional information about the links between conditioning factors and self-care and self-care agency.

Several partial practice models have been developed for persons with particular health issues. Jaarsma, Halfens, Senten, Huijer Abu Saad, and Dracup (1998) developed a model for persons with advanced heart failure. Aish and Isenberg (1996) addressed self-care in relation to nutrition for myocardial infarction patients. Hagopian (1996) developed a partial design model for persons undergoing radiation therapy. Hart and Foster (1998) contributed to the literature in relation to a practice model for pregnant women. The work of Fawdry, Berry, and Rajacich (1996) and Baker (1998) contributed to the development of practice models for dependent-care situations.

Implications for Administration

This nursing theory can assist in decision making related to designing, delivering, and managing the production of nursing within an organization. The SCDNT provides a structure for analyzing cases, developing population descriptions, developing practice models and rules of practice within an organization, and designing programs of nursing that reflect the concerns of nursing, medicine, and other disciplines. By laying out the operations of nursing practice and introducing the concepts of design units, control functions, and management, Orem provides administrators with an understanding of the scope of nursing. The design units provide a basis for establishing the cost of nursing (Orem, 1995). The development of the variables associated with the SCDNT and the descriptions of the relationships among those variables clearly illustrates the complexity of nursing. The SCDNT also provides nursing administrators with a language for discussing the concerns of nursing within the interdisciplinary healthcare world. For example, many healthcare organizations expect nurses with vocational/technical preparation to function beyond their capabilities. Explaining this to persons other than nurses has been problematic, as nursing so commonly is considered a collection of tasks.

The SCDNT provides the means for developing a clinical information system that can provide data about the outcomes of nursing (Allison, 2000). Furthermore, the available data about the development and exercise of self-care agency provide a concise and meaningful basis for referral from one service to another, such as moving from critical care to a step-down unit. Healthcare agencies can also provide one another with information on a patient's self-care management ability, for example, upon his or her discharge from an acute care facility to community care. This information might also indicate that a patient no longer requires nursing service (VHD, 1988).

The diagnostic structure of self-care agency as developed by Orem and her colleagues can be used as a framework for analyzing cases and structuring nursing knowledge in the practice arena. This would be a significant contribution to the discipline.

Implications for Education

Some nursing education programs, both basic or and continuing/in-service, use the SCDNT (Berbiglia, 1991). An SCDNT-based curriculum addresses the variables of therapeutic self-care demand as conditioned by the basic conditioning factors and self-care agency required to meet that demand. For example, an in-service education program for persons undergoing cardiac surgery would include the following:

- Information about the surgery and associated therapeutic plan
- The common components of the therapeutic self-care demand for this population at particular points in time
- The process for determining the therapeutic self-care demand for specific patients
- The characteristics of self-care agency required to meet the therapeutic self-care demand
- The diagnostic considerations about self-care agency in relation to therapeutic self-care demand
- The characteristics of an appropriate nursing system

STATUS OF THEORY DEVELOPMENT

The development of the SCDNT is described in relation to the stages of theory development described in Unit 1 (see also Orem, 1995).

- Stage I: *Description with Descriptive Explanation of Properties of Persons*. This work is reasonably well developed, despite ongoing need to amplify and extend understanding of the elements and properties.
- Stage II: *Variations of Nursing Elements and Relationships*. Work is in progress in this area. The development of family and community nursing situations by Taylor (1989) and Taylor and McLaughlin (1990) are examples of Stage II work. Another example is the theory of dependent care with the related terms of dependent-care agency, dependent-care demand, and dependent-care deficit being developed by the Orem Study Group.
- Stage III: *Nursing Cases and Their Natural History*. Some case studies have been published (Orem & Taylor, 1986; Taylor, 1988). A model of nursing systems design structures insightful analysis of patient or case material (Orem, 1995). Case studies articulate the work done in Stages I and II by providing the material for researchers and theorists to learn variations of nursing elements and relationships.
- Stage IV: *Models and Rules for Nursing Practice*. Models for practice can be found in the literature. Work by Horn and Swain (1977) on development of criterion measures of nursing care is an excellent example of Stage IV work. Jaarsma, Halfens, Senten, Huijer Abu Saad, and Dracup (1998) developed a model for patients with advanced heart failure.
- Stage V: *Models and Rules for Provision of Nursing for Populations*. Allison and McLaughlin-Renpenning (1998) present examples of Stage V work.

NEXUS

The SCDNT is a theoretical system worthy of further study for nurses who believe that the human person is a substantial unity with the capacity for deliberate action (agency) and that nursing is an interpersonal, interactive action system within a sociocultural context. Orem's SCDNT is one of the more fully developed models of nursing. Orem continues to work on refinements of the SCDNT. She has authored several articles (Orem, 1996, 1997; Orem & Vardiman, 1995) since the fifth edition of her text (1995). A sixth edition was published in 2001 and includes many new or expanded conceptualizations about nursing and nursing science. She has worked with a group of scholars who have published or presented the results of that work (Taylor, McLaughlin-Renpenning, Geden, Hart, & Neuman, 2001; Orem, Bekel, & Denyes, 2001).

The model of nursing includes dependent-care and individual, family, and community nursing situations. Orem's conceptualizations of health and well-being allow for both objective and subjective considerations. She is clear in her views of the nature of nursing as practice discipline and practical science. The moderate realism perspective supports speculative and practical knowledge. Research conducted from that perspective can be either qualitative or quantitative. Research using the SCDNT is growing, and the theory has proven to be a useful guide for research. Although much work that remains to be done, research also has supported the theory. Orem began and continues her work from the perspective of practice. The theory itself is limited, but the explanations and conceptualizations that flesh out the theory identify the complexities of nursing practice.

REFERENCES

Aish, A.E. & Isenberg, M. (1996). Effects of Orem-based nursing intervention on nutritional self-care of myocardial infarction patients. *International Journal of Nursing Studies, 33*(3), 259-270.

Allison, S.E. (1985). Structuring nursing practice based on Orem's theory of nursing: A nurse administrator's perspective. In J. Riehl-Sisca (Ed) *The science and art of self-care*. Norwalk, CT: Appleton-Century-Crofts.

Allison, S.E. (2000, February). Self-Care Deficit Nursing Theory: A framework for specifying nursing outcomes. Paper presented at the Sixth International Self-Care Deficit Nursing Theory Conference. Bangkok, Thailand.

Allison, S.E. & McLaughlin-Renpenning, K. (1999). *Nursing administration in the 21st century: A nursing theory approach*. Walnut Creek, CA: Sage.

Backscheider, J. (1974). Self-care requirements, self-care capabilities and nursing systems in the diabetic nurse managed clinic. *American Journal of Public Health, 64*(12), 1138-1146.

Baker, S. (1998). The relationships of self-care agency and self-care to caregiver strain as perceived by female family caregivers of elderly parents. *Journal of the New York State Nurses Association, 28*(1), 7-11.

Banfield, B.E. (1997). A philosophical inquiry of Orem's self-care deficit nursing theory. (Doctoral dissertation, Wayne State University, 1997), *Dissertation Abstracts International, 58*, B5885.

Berbiglia, V.A. (1991). A case study: Perspectives on a self-care deficit nursing theory-based curriculum. *Journal of Advanced Nursing, 16*(10), 1158-1163.

Bliss-Holtz, J. (1996). Using Orem's theory to generate nursing diagnoses for electronic documentation. *Nursing Science Quarterly, 9*(3), 121-125.

Bliss-Holtz, J., McLaughlin, K. & Taylor, S.G. (1990). Validating nursing theory for use within a computerized nursing information system. *Advances in Nursing Science, 13*(2), 46-52.

Bottorff, J. (1988). Assessing an instrument in a pilot project: The self-care agency questionnaire. *Canadian Journal of Nursing Research, 20*(1), 7-16.

Campbell, J. & Weber, N. (2000). An empirical test of a self-care model of women's responses to battering. *Nursing Science Quarterly, 13*(1), 45-53.

Cleveland, S. (1989). Re: Perceived self-care agency: A LISREL factor analysis of Bickel and Hanson's Questionnaire. *Nursing Research, 38*(1), 59.

Denyes, M.J. (1982). Measurement of self-care agency in adolescents. *Nursing Research, 31*(1), 63.

Denyes, M.J. (1988). Orem's model used for health promotion: Directions from research. *Advances in Nursing Science, 11*(1), 13-21.

Denyes, M.J., Neuman, B.M., Villarruel, A.M. (1991). Nursing actions to prevent and alleviate pain in hospitalized children. *Issues in Comprehensive Pediatric Nursing. 14*(1), 31-38.

Dodd, M.J: (1982). Assessing patient self-care for side effects of cancer chemotherapy—part I. *Cancer Nursing, 5*(12), 447-451.

Dodd, M.J. (1983). Self-care for side effects in cancer chemotherapy: an assessment of nursing interventions—part II. *Cancer Nursing, 6*(1), 63-67.

Dodd, M.J. (1988a). Patterns of self-care in patients with breast cancer. *Western Journal of Nursing Research, 10*(1), 7-24.

Dodd, M.J. (1988b). Efficacy of proactive information on self-care in chemotherapy patients. *Patient Education & Counseling, 11*(3), 215-225.

Dodd, M.J. (1997). Self-care: Ready or not. *Oncology Nursing Forum, 24*(6), 983-990.

Dodd, M.J. & Dibble, S.L. (1993). Predictors of self-care: A test of Orem's model. *Oncology Nursing Forum, 20*(6), 895-901.

Donohue-White, P. (1997). Understanding equality and difference: A personalist proposal. *International Philosophical Quarterly, 37*(4), 441-456.

Evers, G., Isenberg, M., Philipsen, H., Senten, M., & Brouns, G. (1993). Validity testing of the Dutch translation of the appraisal of self-care agency scale. *International Journal of Nursing Research, 30*(4), 331-342.

Faucett, J., Ellis, V., Underwood, P., Naqvi, A., & Wilson, D. (1990). The effect of Orem's self-care model on nursing care in a nursing home setting. *Journal of Advanced Nursing, 15*(6), 659-666.

Fawdry, M.K., Berry M.L., & Rajacich, D. (1996). The articulation of nursing systems with dependent care systems of intergenerational caregivers. *Nursing Science Quarterly, 9*(1), 22-26.

Frey, M. & Denyes, M. (1989). Health and illness self-care in adolescents with IDDM: A test of Orem's theory. *Advances in Nursing Science, 12*(1), 67-75.

Gallagher, S. (1998). *Personalism: A brief account.* URL http://www.canisius.edu/~gallaghr/pers.html.

Gaffney, K. & Moore, J. (1996). Testing Orem's theory of self-care deficit: Dependent care agent performance for children. *Nursing Science Quarterly, 9*(4), 160-164.

Gast, H., Denyes, M., Campbell, J., Hartweg, D., Schott-Baer, D., & Isenberg, M. (1989). Self-care agency: Conceptualizations and operationalizations. *Advances in Nursing Science, 12*(1), 26-38.

Geden, E. (1989). The relationship between self-care theory and empirical research. In J.P. Riehl-Sisca (Ed.). *Conceptual Models for Nursing Practice* (3rd ed.) Norwalk, CT: Appleton & Lange.

Geden, E. & Taylor, S. (1991). Construct and empirical validity of the self-as-carer inventory. *Nursing Research, 40*(1), 47-50.

Geden, E. & Taylor, S. (1999). Theoretical and empirical description of adult couples' collaborative self-care systems. *Nursing Science Quarterly, 12*(4), 329-334.

Hagopian, G.A. (1996). The effects of informational audiotapes on knowledge and self-care behaviors of patients undergoing radiation therapy. *Oncology Nursing Forum, 23*(4), 697-700.

Hanson, B. & Bickel, L. (1985). Development and testing of the questionnaire on perception of self-care agency. In J. Riehl-Sisca (Ed.), *The science and art of self-care*. Norwalk, CT: Appleton-Century-Crofts.

Hanucharurnkul, S. (1989). Predictors of self-care in cancer patients receiving radiotherapy. *Cancer Nursing, 12*(1), 21-27.

Hart, M.A. & Foster, S.N. (1998). Self-care agency in two groups of pregnant women. *Nursing Science Quarterly, 11*(4), 167-171.

Horn, B.J. & Swain, M.A. (1977). *Development of criterion measures of nursing care*. Ann Arbor, MI: University of Michigan Department of Hospital Administration.

Jaarsma, T., Halfens, R., Senten, M., Huijer Abu Saad, H., & Dracup, K. (1998). Developing a supportive-educative program for patients with advanced failure within Orem's general theory of nursing. *Nursing Science Quarterly, 11*(2), 79-85.

Jirovec, M. & Kasno, J. (1990). Self-care agency as a function of patient-environmental factors among nursing home residents. *Research in Nursing & Health, 13*(5), 303-309.

Jirovec, M. & Kasno, J. (1993). Predictors of self-care abilities among the institutionalized elderly. *Western Journal of Nursing Research, 15*(3), 314-326.

Kearney, B. & Fleischer, B. (1979). Development of an instrument to measure self-care agency. *Research in Nursing and Health, 2*(1), 25-34.

Klubertanz, G. P. (1953). *The philosophy of human nature*. New York: Appleton-Century-Crofts.

Kubricht, D.W. (1984). Therapeutic self-care demands expressed by outpatients receiving external radiation therapy. *Cancer Nursing, 7*(2), 43-52.

McBride, S. (1987). Validation of an instrument to measure exercise of self-care agency. *Research in Nursing and in Health, 10*, 311-316.

McBride, S. (1991). Comparative analysis of three instruments designed to measure self-care agency. *Nursing Research, 40*(1), 12-16.

Moore, J. & Gaffney, K. (1989). Development of an instrument to measure mothers' performance of self-care activities for children. *Advances in Nursing Science, 12*(1), 76-84.

Moore, J. (1995). Measuring the self-care practice of children and adolescents: Instrument development. *Maternal-Child Nursing Journal, 23*(3), 101-108.

Mosher, R. & Moore, J. (1998). The relationship of self-concept and self-care in children with cancer. *Nursing Science Quarterly, 11*(3), 116-122.

Nursing Development Conference Group. (1973). *Concept formalization in nursing: process and product*. Boston: Little, Brown.

Nursing Development Conference Group. (1979). *Concept formalization in nursing: process and product*. (2nd ed.). Boston: Little, Brown.

Orem, D.E. (1955). *Indiana hospitals: A report*. Indiana State Board of Health.

Orem, D.E. (1956). Hospital nursing service, an analysis. Indianapolis, 1956. Division of Hospital and Institutional Services, Indiana State Board of Health.

Orem, D.E. (1985). Nursing: Concepts of practice. (3rd ed.). New York: McGraw-Hill.

Orem, D.E. & Taylor, S. (1986). Orem's general theory of nursing. In P. Winstead-Fry (Ed.), *Case Studies in Nursing Theory* New York: National League for Nursing.

Orem, D.E. (1987). Orem's general theory of nursing. In Parse, R.R. *Nursing science: Major paradigms, theories, and critiques*. Philadelphia: W.B. Saunders.

Orem, D.E. (1988a). The form of nursing science, *Nursing Science Quarterly, 1*(2), 75-79.

Orem, D.E. (1988b, November). A perspective on theory based nursing. Paper presented at 7th Annual Self-Care Deficit Nursing Theory Conference, St. Louis, MO.

Orem, D.E. (1995). *Nursing: Concepts of practice*. (5th ed.). St. Louis: Mosby.

Orem, D.E. (1996). The world of the nurse. *International Orem Society Newsletter, 4*(1), 2-7.

Orem, D.E. (1997). Views of human beings specific to nursing. *Nursing Science Quarterly 10*(1), 26-31.

Orem, D.E. (2000, February). A message from Dorothea Orem, Savannah, Georgia, USA. Presented at the Sixth Annual International Self-Care Deficit Nursing Theory Conference. Bangkok, Thailand.

Orem, D.E. (2001) *Nursing: Concepts of practice*. (6th ed.). St. Louis: Mosby.

Orem, D.E., Bekel, G. & Denyes, M.J. (2001). Self-care, a foundational nursing science. *Nursing Science Quarterly*.

Orem, D.E. & Vardiman, E. (1995). Orem's nursing theory and positive mental health: practical considerations. *Nursing Science Quarterly 8*(4), 165-173.

Parse, R.R. (1987). *Nursing science: Major paradigms, theories, & critiques*. Philadelphia: W.B. Saunders.

Pickens, J. (1999). Living with serious mental illness: The desire for normalcy. *Nursing Science Quarterly, 12*(3), 233-239.

Riesch, S. & Hauck, M. (1988). The exercise of self-care agency: An analysis of construct and discriminant validity. *Research in Nursing and in Health, 11*(4), 245-255.

Rossow-Sebring, J., Carrieri, V., & Seward, H. (1992). Effect of Orem's model on nurse attitudes and charting behavior. *Journal of Nursing Staff Development 8*(5), 207-212.

Silva, M.C. (1986). Research testing nursing theory: State of the art. *Advances in Nursing Science, 9*(1), 1-11.

Taylor, S.G. (1987). Defining clinical populations from Self-Care Deficit Theory perspective. Theory-based nursing process and product: Using Orem's Self-Care Deficit Nursing Theory in practice, education, and research. Presented at the Fifth Annual Self-Care Deficit Theory conference. St. Louis, MO.

Taylor, S.G. (1988). Nursing theory and nursing process: Orem's theory in practice. *Nursing Science Quarterly 1*(3), 111-119.

Taylor, S. (1989). An interpretation of family within Orem's general theory of nursing. *Nursing Science Quarterly*, *2*(3), 153-160.

Taylor, S.G. (1998). The development of Self-Care Deficit Nursing Theory: An historical analysis. *International Orem Society Newsletter, 4*(2), 7-11.

Taylor, S.G. & Godfrey, N.S. (1999). The ethics of Orem's theory. *Nursing Science Quarterly, 12*(3), 202-207.

Taylor, S. & McLaughlin, K. (1990). Orem's theory of nursing and community nursing. *Nursing Science Quarterly*, *3*(4), 153-160.

Taylor, S. & McLaughlin-Renpenning, K. (2001). The practice of nursing in multiperson situations, family, and community. In D.E. Orem, *Nursing: Concepts of practice.* (6th ed.). St. Louis: Mosby.

Taylor, S., McLaughlin-Renpenning, K., Geden, E., Hart, M.A., & Neuman, B. (2001). A theory of dependent-care. *Nursing Science Quarterly, 14*(1), 39-47.

Vancouver Health Department. (1988). *Assessment Standards.* Vancouver, Canada. Author.

Villarruel, A.M. (1995). Mexican-American cultural meanings, expressions, self-care, and dependent care actions associated with experiences of pain. *Research in Nursing and Health, 18*(5), 427-436.

Walker, L. & Grobe, S. (1999). The construct of thriving in pregnancy and postpartum. *Nursing Science Quarterly, 12*(2), 151-157.

Wallace, W.A. (1983). Essay VIII: Being in a scientific practice discipline. In W.A. Wallace (Ed.), *From a realist point of view, essay on philosophy of science.* (2nd ed.). Lanham, MD: University Press of America.

Wallace, W.A. (1996). *The modeling of nature: Philosophy of science and philosophy of nature in synthesis.* Washington, DC: Catholic University of America.

Weaver, M. (1987). Perceived self-care agency: A LISREL factor analysis of Bickel and Hanson's questionnaire. *Nursing Research, 36*(6), 381-387.

West, P. & Isenberg, M. (1997). Instrument development: The Mental Health-Related Self-Care Agency Scale. *Archives of Psychiatric Nursing, 11*(3), 126-132.

CHAPTER 6

Modeling Nursing From an Energy Field Perspective

ROGERS' SCIENCE of UNITARY HUMAN BEINGS

Key Terms

energy field, p. 125
helicy, p. 126
integrality, p. 126
pandimensional, p. 125
pattern, p. 125
resonancy, p. 126
unitary human being, p. 125

The Science of Unitary Human Beings (SUHB) focuses on the wholeness of reality and of human beings as a part of that reality. First developed by Rogers in 1961 in response to the need for conceptual structures in nursing education, it developed into a major theoretical system. The first description of Rogers' model was published in 1970. Her generalizations founded continued development of knowledge about the unity and wholeness that she considers the theoretical basis for nursing.

Rogers refined her model after its publication in 1970. She wrote a number of articles but never revised the original work. She postulated a theory of accelerating evolution, revised and refined the principles of homeodynamics (Box 6-1), and introduced the concept of pandimensionality. Other scholars focused on issues including pattern, time, and perception of human time and health. Barrett, Malinski, and others operationalized the theoretical elements to be used empirically. Others, most notably Parse and Newman, developed qualitative methodologies for research and practice. Both Parse's Theory of Human

---

BOX 6-1

Principles of Homeodynamics

- Principle of resonancy: Continuous change from lower to higher frequency wave patterns in human and environmental fields
- Principle of helicy: Continuous innovative, unpredictable, increasing diversity of human and environmental fields.
- Principle of integrality: The continuous mutual human field and environmental field process.

From Rogers, M.E. (1990). Nursing: Science of unitary, irreducible human beings: Update 1990. In E.A.M. Barrett (Ed.), *Visions of Rogers' science-based nursing*. New York: National League for Nursing Press.

Becoming, and Newman's work continue in the tradition of Rogerian science. Parse's work is presented in Chapter 7.

Coinciding with Rogers' death in 1994, F.A. Davis Co. published *Martha E. Rogers: Her Life and Her Work*, a compilation that included commentary from noted Rogerian scholars Malinski, Phillips, and Barrett (1994), who provide much information on Rogers' life and the context within which her work developed. In the same book, proponents of the SUHB describe the significance of her work.

THE STARTING POINT OF THE MODELING PROCESS

Rogers started by looking for the way in which human beings could be conceptualized as the object of nursing. She was concerned that development encompass science from a traditional perspective but be based in a concept of the human being who is integral with the environment. Rogers focused on science, which she defined as "an organized abstract body of knowledge arrived at from scientific research and logical analysis" (1988, p. 100). She wanted a philosophy, based in science, of the nature of human beings and the universe. Sarter (1988) proposed that "Rogers' outlook is based on the most recent theories in the biological sciences, and on the attempts of some contemporary philosophers to include these insights into a coherent worldview" (p. 60).

Reason for Theory Development

Rogers' impetus for theory development appears in her early book *Educational Revolution in Nursing*, published in 1961. She considered this volume groundwork for her philosophy and for theoretical concepts in nursing. Rogers (1961) proposed significant nursing concepts and a theory development process that would lead to a rational framework for professional education. In a later work, Rogers (1970) noted that she was motivated by a strong conviction that nursing practice needed to be underwritten by substantive knowledge.

Rogers' initial work (1961) identified a foundation for nursing professional education based in a "substantial organized body of theoretical knowledge fundamental to nursing" (p. 23). Rogers felt strongly that the development of nursing theory was crucial to further progress in the profession. For Rogers, nursing theories are never static; they provide the operational basis for knowledgeable practice. Nursing theory is "rooted in the broad founda-

TABLE 6-1	
Key Definitions Specific to the Science of Nursing	
Key Words	**Definition**
Energy Field	The fundamental unit of the living and the non-living. Field is a unifying concept. Energy signifies the dynamic nature of the field. A field is in continuous motion and is infinite.
Pattern	The distinguishing characteristic of an energy field perceived as a single wave.
Pandimensional	A nonlinear domain without spatial or temporal attributes.
Unitary Human Being Human field	An irreducible, indivisible, pandimensional energy field identified by pattern and manifesting characteristics specific to the whole and which cannot be predicted from knowledge of the parts.
Environment Environmental field	An irreducible, pandimensional energy field identified by pattern and integral with the human field.

From Barrett, E.A.M. (Ed.), (1990). *Visions of Rogers' science-based nursing.* New York: National League for Nursing.

tion of knowledge that characterized the liberally educated man" (p. 24). She wanted nursing science to recognize the unitary nature of the person integral with the environment. Rogers continued refining the language in order to emphasize general knowledge of the universe and specific knowledge about nursing. Her work incorporated ideas from both philosophy and science. Rogers cites such sources as Lewin, Barzun, Asimov, Bertalanffy, Burr and Northrop, Arendt, Polanyi, deChardin, Bohm, and Gleick.

Rogers posited a number of questions related to the nature of human beings and the universe in her early work and noted their relevance to nursing. In 1961, Rogers asked questions that form the basis for our understanding nursing: "What is man? Where does he fit into the universe? Is he subject to the same laws that govern the physical world? What is life? How can man be conceptualized, consistent with the world as we know it?" (1961, p. 16). She introduced the idea of life as a manifestation of energy and humans as integral parts of an expanding universe that moves on through time and space. The theoretical content of nursing, for Rogers, focuses on the life process of human beings and thus is nursing's focus.

Phenomenon of Concern

Rogers consistently referred to the structure of her work as the Science of Unitary Human Beings from which theories will be derived. Structural elements of the SUHB are called *building blocks* and include energy fields, a universe of open systems, pattern, and four-dimensionality, now conceptualized as pandimensionality (1992a). Rogers has iterated this focus on nursing science as an organized abstract system of unitary, irreducible, and indivisible energy fields in many of her writings (1988, 1990, 1992a, 1994). The specific definitions of relevant terms are provided in Table 6-1.

DESCRIPTION OF ROGERS' THEORETICAL SYSTEM
Philosophical Perspectives

A New Worldview. Rogers posited her work as evolving from a new worldview, the basis of which is science, defined as "an organized body of abstract knowledge arrived at from scientific research and logical analysis" (1988, p. 100) and "identified by the phenomenon central to its concern" (p. 99). Rogers "acknowledges the ultimate unity, or wholeness, of the universe" (Sarter, 1988, p. 74). Rogers holds that the "energy field is integral with the environment," while at the same time "every energy field is identified by a unique pattern, which implies that it has a personal, ontological reality" (Sarter, 1988, p. 74). Rogers refers to man as "a unified phenomenon subject to natural laws . . . man's consciousness and creativity are integral dimensions of man's wholeness" (1970, p. 34). The ontology of wholeness provides the basis for Rogers' work.

The phenomenon of concern to nursing, according to Rogers, is people and their environments, whereas the purpose of nurses is to promote health and well-being for all persons. In 1970, she identified the model of the "life process in man" as nursing's conceptual model. She deemed nursing a humanitarian science with a focus on the irreducible nature of individuals—unitary human beings—and environment. The fundamental ontological unit is the human energy field (Sarter, 1988). Rogers described the continuous mutual process between the human being and his or her environment in terms of **resonancy, helicy,** and **integrality,** all of which are homeodynamic principles (see Box 6-1). The human being is an energy field in constant interaction with the environment. Postulates underlying the system include energy field open system, pattern and patterning, pandimensionality, and the theory of accelerating evolution. The theory of accelerating evolution holds that "[t]he reality of evolutionary change is explicit. Man's development through time reflects growing complexity of pattern and organization" (Rogers, 1970, p. 27). Manifestations of relative diversity in field patterning describe the continuous change in human-environment process.

Language of Rogers' Theoretical System. Rogers' theoretical system prefers the term *practice modalities* over *interventions* because of the linear and causal connotation of the latter. Terms that connote linearity and causality, such as *prediction, probability, intervention, interaction,* and *stasis* are not appropriate. Descriptions in the literature of the nurse as human energy field in continuous mutual process with patient are sparse. Malinski (1994) synthesized the evolution of the SUHB and identified the contemporary vocabulary of the work, notably *patterning* and *pandimensionality.* Patterning replaces the metaphor of repatterning, and pandimensionality replaces four-dimensionality or multidimensionality. Malinski's work points out language's limitations in conveying Rogers' intentions. Rogers initially used the vocabulary of old paradigms to express her new worldview. Although Rogers conceptualized the universe as nonlinear, temporal, and nonspatial, she relied nevertheless on linear, temporal, and spatial referents to describe human patterns. Until the language and metaphors of the new view are identified and accepted, this natural limitation remains. As with any system, specific terms with specific meanings are essential for the development of nursing science.

Supporting Sciences. Sciences that support Rogers' work include quantum physics, systems, chaos, and complexity. Quantum physics presents the principles of unpredictability, energy, and waves (Gribbin, 1998). Quantum physics applies the principles to subatomic particles; however, the relationships between and among the various particles and waves have been used metaphorically at other levels, as in Zohar and Marshall's *The Quantum Society* (1994). The application of quantum physics at the human and social level is a matter of metaphor and analogy.

Rogers used concepts of systems theory in her work. She depicted a pandimensional universe of open systems (1981, 1988, 1992a) and used the concept of negentropy to explain increasing diversity and complexity of pattern. Complexity theory, according to Ray, is a "scientific theory of dynamical systems" (1994, p. 91). Chaos theory, a subset of complexity, "deals essentially with the concept of order within disorder" (p. 91). Ray credits Rogers with being the first to introduce complexity to nursing. Vicenz (1994) clearly links chaos and complexity theory to Rogers' work.

Description of Rogers' Model and Theories

Model of Unitary Human Beings. Structural elements of Rogers' model of unitary human beings include definitions of terms, postulates accepted as assumptions, principles of homeodynamics, and correlates of human patterning (Sarter, 1988). These are presented in Box 6-1 (principles), and Table 6-1 (definitions). No sketches or schematics are found in the available literature. Rogers recognized the difficulty of efforts to schematize four-dimensionality; she did not develop a symbolic model but used the "Slinky" toy in her early work to illustrate nonrepeating, unidirectional rhythmicities. The complexity of Rogers' model, especially as it relates to pandimensionality, makes it difficult to present schematically. Sarter (1988) proposed that Rogers' model is evolutionary in that it is "a process of change toward higher frequency wave patterns and increasing diversity of patterns in the human and environmental fields" (p. 64).

Theories and Models Associated with Rogerian Science. In 1981, Rogers presented her work as a paradigm for nursing as an organized conceptual system based on unitary man and environment as irreducible wholes. Many theories are or can be derived from one paradigm. Rogers identified two theories from her paradigm—accelerating evolution (or change) and the paranormal (1992a). The theory of accelerating evolution proposes that the rate of evolution increases at a continually accelerating pace and that change occurs increasingly rapidly. The paranormal is based in the energy field concept and attributes so-called paranormal events to varying manifestations in field pattern.

The unit of analysis for Rogers is the human energy field, manifested in pattern and recognized by another energy field through pattern recognition in the relative presence. Subatomic wave and particle theory may or may not have meaning in understanding the person. Until the science develops more fully, scholars are limited to metaphors and analogies to explain their hypotheses. *Energy field*, as Rogers (1992a) defines it, consists of energy—the "dynamic nature of the field" (p. 29) and field, which is infinite, unifying, and continually mobile. Rogers does not address issues related to matter or particles. Another energy field's perception of a pattern is not yet addressed from a science perspective. The types of patterns and patterning are described but not explained. It is not known, for example, how an energy field perceives.

Rogers handled the use of energy field theory in a study of family and group pattern manifestations (1992a). As with knowledge development from any paradigm, all extensions or extrapolations must be consistent with the basic phenomenon of concern or ontology. Family is an energy field, and a group is an energy field; each has pattern and exists integrally with the environment energy field.

Barrett conceptualized power as "the capacity to participate knowingly in the process of change characterizing the continuous patterning of human and environmental fields" (1990a, p. 106). She derived this conceptual model from Rogers' principle of helicy. Barrett's model is one of only a few that represent the unitary human perspective. Phillips (1990) suggested that the perspective of human field image is one manifestation of the human energy field in continuous mutual process within the pandimensional universe. Phillips (1990) differentiates human field image (HFI) from body image, noting that HFI synthesizes all the "changes that have occurred in the past and all projected future HFI into what is known as the relative present HFI" (p.14). He describes a concept of health consistent with the HFI perspective as a "eudaemonistic model of health concerned with general well-being and self-realization" (p. 16). Barrett (1990a) developed the methodology of pattern manifestation appraisal and deliberative mutual patterning called practice modalities. Thomas (1990) introduced the Human Environment Encounter Model to clarify the nurse-patient process. Cowling (1990) constructed a template for unitary pattern-based nursing practice as an extension of Barrett's 1988 study and identified nine constituents of pattern-based practice.

RESEARCH DERIVED FROM THE SCIENCE OF UNITARY HUMAN BEINGS

Rogers believed that knowledge development was an open-ended, evolving process. Concepts of pandimensionality and integrality collapse the space-time experience and lead researchers to consider change acausal. This kind of knowing is more congruent with a constructivist than a positivist or postpositivist worldview of science, despite the fact that Rogers began her work when positivism was a commonly accepted worldview.

Consequently, measurement of phenomena within a Rogerian worldview presents challenges. The SUHB is unique because, unlike other science fields, the unitary humans theory is a synergistic phenomenon, the behaviors of which cannot be predicted by the sum of the parts (Cowling, 1986a) and because it transcends accepted notions of time and space (Rawnsley, 1990). This uniqueness creates difficulty because traditional positivist models of quantification are linear and reductionistic, whereas the unitary world is conceptualized as wholistic and nonlinear. Critical problematic elements of the research process include hypothesis formation, variable identification, operationalization and measurement of variables, and research design selection (Cowling, 1986a). Hypotheses accommodating the irreducibility of humans to parts, the premise of noncausality, and continual change are difficult to develop. Sherman (1997) recommended using acausal language in hypotheses and selecting either descriptive or explanatory designs for studies. Barrett (1990a) indicated that quasi-experimental designs also might aid in testing unitary human field practice modalities.

Carboni (1992) suggested that Rogerian research constructs must address the entire system. Additionally, the research process must be considered a changing and mutually processing relationship between the researcher and the research focus. These two aspects are difficult to achieve in a science that relies primarily on quantification. Although qualitative research methods support a more wholistic approach to the study of phenomena, Barrett (1990a) indicated that neither quantitative nor qualitative methods capture the whole.

Unfortunately, it is difficult to divorce theory-based studies from prevalent research methods. Barrett (1990a) suggested that the incongruence between research methods and

Rogerian wholism should be acknowledged but not rejected. Barrett, Cowling, Carboni, and Butcher (1997) indicated that scientific methods are not paradigm-specific but should fit the objectives of the investigation. Barrett (1990a) emphasized that methods of science are tools and should not be confused with the phenomenon of interest. She recommended that the phenomenon of study, the question asked, and the congruence of methods with Rogerian science should determine method selection. To overcome the incongruence between philosophy and science, researchers should focus on manifestations of irreducible wholes—framing research questions in four-dimensional wholism rather than in a three-dimensional context.

Research Instruments

Throughout the history of development of instruments for Rogerian studies, the measurement techniques have been controversial. Whereas early instruments tended to be quantitative, new qualitative Rogerian methods recently have emerged. In 1978, Ference developed one of the first instruments to measure field motion (1986a). Other quantitative measures followed. In 1983 Barrett developed a measure of power that has undergone subsequent refinement (Barrett & Caroselli, 1998). As measures developed, semantic differentials have proven useful, and qualitative investigative techniques have also begun to emerge. Carboni's suggestion (1992) for investigating mutual exploration of the healing human field–environmental field relationship used an experiential approach. Barrett, Cowling, Carboni, and Butcher (1997) suggested that pattern appreciation can be examined through case study. Bultemeier (1997) developed a system of photo-disclosure, which was based on phenomenology and visual research as for data collection and analysis. Efforts exploring new ways to investigate Rogerian phenomena are ongoing. The following is a description of instruments and methods used to measure manifestations of patterning. Table 6-2 presents a summary of instruments developed with the SUHB and offers helpful information on the nature of the instruments and their validity and reliability.

Human Field Motion Test. Developed in 1978, the Human Field Motion Test (HFMT) was the first instrument specifically designed to measure human resonancy. The HFMT consists of two concepts: "my motor running" and "my field expansion," which are measured by a total of 20 semantic differential scales. Ference (1986a) investigated the relationship between human field motion and synergistic development, which included aspects of time experience, creativity, and differentiation. Two dimensions were found to account for the relationship between synergistic development and human field motion. The complexity-diversity dimension reflects a slow-changing pattern and organization. The human field motion dimension was considered a development characteristic that contributed to pattern and organization and accounted for a space-time coordinate. It also has served as a standard of comparison for other human field motion measures that were developed later. Unfortunately, published information on development of the HFMT is limited.

Power as Knowing Participation in Change Tool. The Power as Knowing Participation in Change Tool (PKPCT) was derived from Barrett's power theory, which is based on Rogers' SUHB. Believing that people participate knowingly in change, Barrett (as described in Barrett & Caroselli, 1998) first began work on the PKPCT in 1983. Barrett designed the PKPCT as a series of semantic differential scales that could be used to measure four human field pattern manifestations characterizing power: (1) awareness, (2) choices,

Text continued on p. 134

TABLE 6-2

Research Instruments Using Rogers' Science of Unitary Human Beings

Instrument/Description	Study/Year	Reliability and Validity
Human Field Motion Test (HFMT) 20 semantic scales measure two concepts	Ference, 1986a	Five experts established content validity for initial items. Pilot testing with 43 subjects detected retest reliability of 0.77. Two concepts and 20 scales were retained. The HMFT tested 213 subjects and assessed for retest reliability and construct validity with factor analysis. Retest reliability was 0.70. Correlations of each scale ranged from 0.51 to 0.77; the correlation of the score for each concept ("my motor running" and "my field expansion") to the total test score was 0.87. Three factors emerged, and each scale loaded onto at least one factor. Scale wave frequencies were congruent with judges' predictions. Canonical correlation was used to assess the relationship between the HFMT and synergism, as measured by the Time Metaphor Test, the Adjective Check List, and the Group Embedded Figures Test. Two significant covariants emerged: complexity-diversity pattern, which accounted for 41% of the variance, and human field motion, which accounted for 37% of the variance.
Power as Knowing-Participation in Change (PKPCT) PKPCT VII or Version II 48 items plus four test-retest items using 7-point semantic differential format	Barrett, 1986, 1990b	Two judges' studies were used to establish content validity: (1) rating adjectives to describe power and then rating 43 bipolar adjective pairs; (2) experts rated four contexts of power and 38 items on a semantic differential. Items received mean ratings from 4.0 to 6.75. A pilot study of 267 adults was followed by a study of 625 adults aged 21 to 60. The reliability of the initial PKPCT ranged from 0.63 to 0.99 for the four subscales. Test-retest reliability with a 3-week interval of 25 undergraduate college students ranged from 0.71 to 0.82 for the initial PKPCT and 0.61 to 0.78 for Version II. Factor analysis revealed four factors with loadings ranging from 0.56 to 0.70. Canonical correlations with HFMT accounted for 40% of the variance. In other studies using the PKPCT, internal consistency estimations ranged from 0.81 to 0.93 for the subscales and from 0.94 to 0.97 for the total scale.
Temporal Experience Scale (TES) 24-item, 5-point Likert scale containing three subscales with eight items each	Paletta, 1990	Content validity for metaphors was established by experts. Items were rated according to wave pattern by judges and then classified into patterns using the judges' mean score. Item classification was validated by Rogers. The remaining items were classified by a sample of 305 subjects. Subjected to principal factor analysis with oblique rotation, three factors emerged. Time dragging accounted for 50% variance, time racing for 29%, and timelessness for 21%. Reliabilities were: for time dragging, 0.821; time racing, 0.736; and timelessness, 0.791. The study with 120 subjects found reliabilities of: Dragging = 0.38, Racing = 0.7161, and timelessness, 0.7836. Variables of sex, language, and education influenced one or more of the TES scales and accounted for 2 to 3% of the variance.

Instrument	Citation	Findings
Perceived Field Motion (PFM) 11-item semantic differential with 7-point scale	Yarcheski and Mahon, 1991	Literature review was used to extract 12 adjective pairs describing human field motion. Content validity was established by three experts. During content validation, one pair of adjectives was deleted, for a total of 11 remaining pairs. Principal components factor analysis assessed construct validity. Two factors emerged, with seven items strongly loading on the first factor of motion and potency. Because only two items loaded on the second factor, the factor was not used. Internal consistency reliability was assessed for 116 early adolescents, 116 middle adolescents, and 116 late adolescents (alpha = 0.77, 0.79, and 0.83 for the respective adolescent groups). Reliability for the combined adolescent groups was 0.12.
	Yarcheski and Mahon, 1995	Internal consistency reliability was assessed with 106 early, 111 middle, and 113 late adolescents. Coefficient alpha levels were 0.80, 0.80, and 0.83, respectively.
Human Field Rhythms 1-item, 100 mm visual analog scale (VAS)	Yarcheski and Mahon, 1991	Content validity was derived from Rogers' manifestations of frequencies of human field rhythms. One-day test-retest reliability was reported for 10 early, 10 middle, and 10 late adolescents (r = 0.93, 0.96, and 0.86 respectively). Verbal end descriptors of VAS were congruent with Rogers' theoretical statements.
Mutual Exploration of the Healing Human Field–Environmental Field Relationship	Carboni, 1992	The instrument was designed for experiential research. Configurations of patterns within a field determined the existence of healing nurse-patient relationship. Suggestions were made for mechanisms to establish reliability and validity, but no information was offered for actual use.
Diversity of Human Field Pattern Scale (DHFPS) 16 item, 5-point Likert scale	Hastings-Tolsma, 1992 (as cited in Watson, Barrett, Hastings-Tolsma, Johnston, & Gueldner, 1997); Hastings-Tolsma, 1996	Face (content) validity was established by two experts. In a pilot study with 320 adults, one factor was extracted by principal components analysis. Validity coefficients ranged from 0.36 to 0.62. Correlation of the DHFPS and the HMFT was modest but significant at p = 0.001 (value not stated). Reliability was 0.83. The revised DHFPS was tested with 173 volunteers. Factor analysis demonstrated a unitary factor with validity coefficients ranging from 0.22 to 0.68. Coefficient alpha was 0.81.

Continued

TABLE 6-2

Research Instruments Using Rogers' Science of Unitary Human Beings—cont'd

Instrument/Description	Study/Year	Reliability and Validity
Human Field Image Metaphor Scale (HFIMS) 25 metaphors rated with 5-point Likert scale	Johnston, 1994	Metaphors were generated and validated from literature and expert consultation. The initial metaphor list was expanded, refined, and reduced following consultation with Rogerian scholars. A 32 item HFIMS was pilot-tested with 50 healthy subjects who completed the HFIMS, the IFE, and a demographic data sheet. Principal components analysis revealed six factors, which were reduced to four by deleting two single-item factors. Correlation with IFE = 0.5928 ($p < 0.01$). In the major study of 358 healthy adults, principal component analysis revealed five factors that were reduced to three because two factors had insignificant loadings. Three remaining factors (expressions of clear human field image, expressions of blurred field image, and integrality) accounted for 54.8% of item variance. The remaining 25 items had a Cronbach's alpha of 0.9131. Correlation with IFE was 0.7056.
Index of Field Energy (IFE) 18 pairs drawings with 7-point scale	Gueldner, Bramlett, Johnston, and Guillory 1996	Psychometric testing was completed with two samples of 278 and 357 older adults. Composite internal consistency reliability was reported as 0.9464, and item total correlations ranged from 0.5023 to 0.8038. The IFE has a correlation with the HFMT of 0.6679, with the HFIMS of 0.6647, and the PKPCT of 0.7841. Factor analysis indicates the presence of two factors (nature not specified).
Person-Environment Participation Scale (PEPS) 15-item semantic differential with seven gradations	Leddy, 1995	Psychometric testing was completed with three overlapping samples initially containing 239 ambulatory adults; six months later with 125 adults, of which 104 had previously responded; and one year following initial testing with 136, of which 72 had been previously tested. Internal consistency reliability ranged from 0.90 to 0.94. Test-retest reliability with a 2-to-6-week interval was $r = 0.74$. Stability at 6 months was $r = 0.52$ and at one year was $r = 0.60$. Construct validity, established through principal components factor analysis, revealed two components: expansiveness of participation, accounting for 46.5% of variance, and ease of participation, accounting for 10% of variance. The PEPS inversely correlated to the Fatigue Experience scale ($r = -0.40$) and the Symptom Experience Scale ($r = -0.42$). Discriminant analysis revealed that the PEPS correctly discriminated between persons reporting one or more health problems and those reporting none. Concurrent validity revealed a relationship between sense of coherence and the PEPS scale ($r = 0.70$) and the PKPCT scale ($r = 0.69$).

	Leddy, 1999	Data were analyzed from 53 subjects who had completed all prior PEPS testings in order to assess the stability of the construct of mutual process. Low stability coefficients, ranging from 0.246 to 0.698, indicated the concept of participation as fleeting.
Leddy Healthiness Scale (LHS) 26-item, 6-point Likert scale	Leddy, 1996	Fifteen to 20 items were generated for each of nine theoretical dimensions and yielded 72 items. Following expert review, 24 items were reworded and 13 replaced. CVI for revised scale items ranged from 0.97 to 0.99. The number of items was then reduced to 36, based on corrected item total correlations. A subsample of 125 were used to assess construct factor analysis and convergent and divergent validity as well as internal consistency and stability. Factor analysis reduced the item total to 26. These items were composed of three factors (purpose, power, and connections), which accounted for 51% of total variance. Convergent validity was obtained by comparing: LHS to one item on well-being ($r = 0.62$); LHS to Sense of Coherence Scale ($r = 0.70$); LHS to PKPCT Scale ($r = 0.62$); LHS to Physical Well-Being Scale ($r = 0.74$); LHS to Personal Meaning Index Scale ($r = 0.62$). Divergent validity was tested after 1 year by comparing the LHS to the Fatigue Experience Scale. As fatigue increased, LHS scores decreased ($r = -0.41$). Internal consistency reliability for subscales ranged from 0.66 to 0.87, and total scale reliability ranged from 0.90 to 0.92 over measures made at baseline, 6 months and 1 year. Test-retest reliability for 2 to 6 weeks was $r = 0.86$, 0.58 for 6 months, and 0.61 for 1 year.
	Leddy, 1997	In a follow-up study of 53 women with cancer and 89 healthy subjects, internal consistency of the LHS was 0.93 and test/retest reliability over 2 to 6 weeks was 0.83.
Assessment of Dream Experience (ADE) 20-item, 4-point Likert scale	Watson, 1999	Content validity was assessed by 10 experts. Factor analysis of 100 participants revealed two factors that accounted for 36.8% of the variance: high diversity dream experience and low diversity dream experience. Reliabilities for the two factors were 0.823 and 0.740, respectively. Alpha coefficient for the total scale was 0.84. In the subsequent main study the two factors accounted for 46.3% of the variance, and the alpha coefficient was 0.87.

(3) freedom to act intentionally, and (4) involvement in creating change. Over the years, the PKPCT VI—or Version I—and the PKPCT VII—or Version II—were developed. Version II, now the accepted version, deleted modifications by self, family, or occupation, which were present in the first version, because no statistically significant differences were found (Barrett, Caroselli, Smith, & Smith, 1997).

The PKPCT Version II is a 48-item scale containing four sets of 12 pairs of bipolar adjectives and four retest items, one for each dimension of power. Two types of scoring can be used with the PKPCT. Factor scores are recommended for hypothesis testing (Barrett, 1990b). Alternatively, each power scale can be summed for a score ranging from 12 to 84, or the total scale can be summed for a score ranging from 48 to 336. Higher scores represent greater manifestations of power.

To date, the PKPCT has been used in nearly 40 power studies (Caroselli & Barrett, 1998). Power has been commonly studied with other variables, such as reminiscence, creativity, feminism, life purpose, job diversity and satisfaction, anxiety, empathy, trust, and well-being. Version II has been translated into Japanese, Korean, Swedish, and Finnish (Watson, Barrett, Hastings-Tolsma, Johnston, & Gueldner, 1997); however, the difficulty of reading the PKPCT has led Barrett to recommend that the instrument be used only with subjects who have at least a high school education (Barrett & Caroselli, 1998). The clarity of the PKPCT's instructions has also been questioned. Many have recommended further studies to test the PKPCT's sensitivity in detecting group differences and to establish norms for various populations (Barrett & Caroselli, 1998). Another issue of concern is that PKPCT scores tend to be biased upward, which could be a product of social desirability in responses (Barrett & Caroselli, 1998; Watson, Barrett, Hastings-Tolsma, Johnston, & Gueldner, 1997).

Temporal Experience Scales. The Temporal Experience Scales (TES) collectively consist of three scales: the Time Dragging Scale, the Time Racing Scale, and the Timelessness Scale. Each scale contains eight metaphors rated on a five-point Likert scale. Adequate levels of content and construct validity were established, but the exact process for establishing content validity was not clearly described. For a new instrument, adequate levels of reliability for each of the three scales were demonstrated. Findings during instrument development indicate the TES is useful for measuring sexual, lingual, educational, and occupational biases in adults aged 20 to 50 years (Paletta, 1990). Based on her 1990 study of temporal experience Paletta called for additional development of the TES instrument item configuration and determination of the groups for which the TES is considered an adequate test of temporal experience.

Perceived Field Motion. To measure human field motion in adolescents Yarcheski and Mahon (1991) developed a test of Peceived Field Motion (PFM). The PFM consists of seven adjective pairs, and scores range from a low of seven (perceived slow motion) to a high of 49 (perceived fast motion) (Yarcheski & Mahon, 1995). Internal consistency levels for early, middle, and late adolescents in two studies (Yarcheski & Mahon, 1991, 1995) were adequate for the stage of instrument development. Unfortunately, the internal consistency estimation for combined adolescent groups in the 1991 study was extremely low.

Human Field Rhythms. Human Field Rhythms (HFR) represent the dynamic between the unified whole person and environment. Yarcheski and Mahon (1991) developed a visual analog scale to measure human field rhythms to accompany use of the PFM scale.

This 100-mm visual analog scale contains verbal descriptors of low frequency and high frequency at the two poles of the scale. Subjects respond by placing a mark along the analog scale at the point that best represents their field rhythm. Scoring is accomplished by measuring the mark location from the zero endpoint of the scale. Higher scores represent faster human field rhythms. Content validity is derived only from theoretical frame of reference. Test-retest scores indicate strong stability, but the time span between retesting was short. However, a short retest time span might be appropriate in light of the fluidity of field rhythms.

Mutual Exploration of the Healing Human Field–Environmental Relationship. Carboni (1992) developed the Mutual Exploration of the Healing Human Field– Environmental Relationship to measure changing configurations of energy field patterns that help determine the existence of a healing human field–environmental field relationship. Based on the premise that the healing human field–environmental relationship is a wholistic reflection of a nurse-patient interaction, the Mutual Exploration of the Human Field–Environmental Field Relationship structures joint exploration and description of the healing relationship. Changing configurations reflect affirmations of wholeness and promotion of healing through cooperative relationships between nurses and patients within their environments.

The instrument is designed for experiential research in which participants contribute not only content but also "creative thinking that generates, manages, and draws conclusions from the research" (Carboni, 1992; p. 139). Additionally, the researcher participates in the activity being researched. Although mutual exploration is a joint process, the nurse should facilitate mutual completion. Acknowledgment of mutuality requires validation by both the nurse and patient. The outcome of mutual exploration is a creative understanding of the healing human field–environmental field relationship. Verification of a healing relationship must be evidenced by wholeness and harmony.

Diversity of Human Field Pattern Scale. SUHB field pattern diversity reflects individual capacities to participate in change through involvement in creating transitions and influencing human–environmental field connections (Hastings-Tolsma, 1996). Greater diversity of the human field is thought to promote increasingly varied and innovative field design. To measure field potential, Hastings-Tolsma (1996) created the Diversity of Human Field Pattern Scale (DHFPS), a 16-item, five-point Likert scale. Potential scores range from 80 to 16, with lower scores indicating greater diversity of human field pattern (Watson, Barrett, Hastings-Tolsma, Johnston, & Gueldner, 1997). The DHFPS might elucidate how individuals create change. It shows promise as a new instrument in measuring human field potential. Additional work is needed to further refine the measure of field pattern diversity.

Human Field Image Metaphor Scale. According to Johnston (1994), human field image encompasses the awareness of the infinite wholeness of the human field. Two domains within the human field image—perceived potential and integrality—are measured by the Human Field Image Metaphor Scale (HFIMS). The HFIMS rates 25 metaphors on a five-point Likert scale. Six of the metaphors express a strong sense of potentiality; 12 express a positive perception of integrality; five express restricted potential; and two express a sense of isolation. The scale begins with the stem "I feel," which is followed by presentation of the 25 metaphors. The five-point responses extend from "do not identify" to "totally identify," and scores range from 25 to 125. The HFIMS can shed light on individual health perceptions and health behaviors and might be useful for self-assessment (Watson, Barrett, Hastings-Tolsma, Johnston, & Gueldner., 1997; Johnston, personal communication, April 28, 1999). It is based on the premise that individuals with diverse human field patterns have a sharper, clearer perception of human field image, enabling knowing participation in life choices and changes. Less diverse human field patterns yield a blurred image and a more passive acceptance of life experiences. Initial work on reliability and validity is strong. The HFIMS is available in German and Spanish and has been used to measure field image with a variety of groups, including schizophrenics (Johnston, personal communication, April 28, 1999).

Index of Field Energy. The Index of Field Energy (IFE) measures human field dynamics of older adults or adults who cannot read at a high school level (Gueldner, Bramlett, Johnston, & Guillory, 1996). It consists of 18 pairs of black and white line drawings. Sketches represent low or high frequency. Each sketch pair is connected with a seven-point scale that allows participants to indicate the point that "best describes how you feel right now." Two versions of the IFE are available—a pencil and paper test and a board game (Watson, Barrett, Hastings-Tolsma, Johnston, & Gueldner, 1997). Ongoing work on the IFE will add to the limited information regarding the psychometric testing of the IFE.

Person-Environment Participation Scale. Leddy (1995) developed the Person-Environment Participation Scale (PEPS) to measure mutual process, a manifestation within the SUHB. *Mutual process* describes the integral nature of human and environmental fields. The PEPS is perceived as an extension of available measures that describe the field pattern of motion and is directed specifically toward measuring "experienced expansiveness and ease of mutual process" (Leddy, 1995, p. 23). The PEPS is a semantic differential with a seven-point gradation containing 15 bipolar adjective pairs. Adjectives represent continuity (integrated/fragmented), ease (smooth/turbulent), comfort (calm/ agitated), influence (powerful/powerless), and energy (energetic/lethargic). Scoring is accomplished by reverse scoring selected items and summing the responses for a total instrument score. Scores range from 15 to 105, with higher scores representing higher participation.

Strong internal consistency reliability has been demonstrated psychometrically (Leddy, 1995). Stability scores indicate that participation is a temporary, fleeting, and changing construct (Leddy, 1999). A solid basis exists for initial construct validity. Leddy (1995, 1999) indicates that the PEPS is useful in measuring expansiveness and ease of participation—a phenomenon that could be facilitated through nursing interventions that pattern the environmental field. Examples include noninvasive modalities of therapeutic touch, such as reiki, music, light, or aromatherapy.

Leddy Healthiness Scale. The Leddy Healthiness Scale (LHS) (Leddy, 1996, 1997) measures the perceived purpose, connections, and power that are components of a dynamic process of healthiness. The LHS has 26 items on a six-point Likert scale, and scores can range from a low of 26 to a high of 156. Higher scores indicate healthiness. As a new instrument the LHS demonstrates promise. Content and construct techniques suggest validity, and coefficient alphas for the total scale ranging from 0.90 to 0.93 in three samples from two studies suggest strong internal consistency reliability (Leddy, 1996, 1997). The three factor subscales have lower levels of reliability, but alphas remain sufficient for a new instrument. The instrument's stable measurements even after 6 months to a year are an important strength.

Watson's Assessment of Dream Experience. Watson's Assessment of Dream Experience (ADE) (1999) attempts to measure dreaming in a way consistent with Rogers' conceptualization. Dreaming was a "beyond waking" experience as described by Rogers' longer sleeping/longer waking/beyond waking manifestation. On the 20-item scale, 11 items characterize high diversity dream experience, and nine indicate low diversity dream experience indicators. Participants indicate the extent to which the words on the ADE describe their dreams from the previous two weeks. Adequate internal consistency reliabilities were found for the pilot and main study. Adequate content validity was established, and a beginning basis for construct validity was demonstrated. Watson (1999) indicated that reconsideration of the scoring mechanism may include reporting a high diversity score and a low diversity score. Watson (1999) recommended that the instrument be used with larger and more diverse samples, because women in the instrument development study tended to rate themselves as healthier, more active, and better educated than national norms. Watson plans further refinement of the ADE and seeks greater exploration of the nature and meaning of "beyond waking" experiences.

Photo-Disclosure. Seeking an innovative method to appraise field patterns from a wholistic perspective, Bultemeier (1997) created photo-disclosure. Photo-disclosure is based on a combination of phenomenological and photographic research techniques. Phenomenology approaches research from a wholistic perspective, focusing on the lived reality of research participants. Native photography uses photographs taken by subjects, and photo-elicitation involves participant response to photographs of themselves, their environment, or other photographs. In photo-disclosure, simultaneous native photography and written narrative captures the phenomenon of interest. Rather than the photo serving as a probe, it becomes a data source for capturing lived experience. In Bultemeier's study of women with premenstrual syndrome, women responded to the stems "The title I would give this photo is . . . ;" "I took this photo to show . . . ;" "When I took this photo I felt . . . ;" and "Right now I wish I could . . ." Phenomenological research techniques guided thematic analysis of the data. Gathering data in a wholistic manner without preset limitations on phenomenon description is one advantage of this approach.

Pattern Appreciation. Believing that patterns were a distinguishing characteristic of energy fields, Cowling (1997) proposed pattern appreciation as a "process, an orientation, and an approach for research and practice" (p. 133). Cowling perceives, consistently with the SUHB, that human field patterns are unique. Appreciation permits sensitivity in noticing, perceiving, and recognizing patterns and provides a "grounding context for mutual sharing" (1997, p. 131). Pattern appreciation involves the following (Cowling, 1997):

- Engagement with another for exploration of unitary human field patterns
- Explicit intentions made to participants in mutually derived consent process
- Cocreation for form and structure of engagement
- Documentation of experience, perceptions, and expressions
- Journaling that includes theoretical, methodological, peer review, and general reflective notes
- Development of pattern appreciation profile through synopsis

- Verification of pattern appreciation profile with participant
- Conceptual/theoretical synthesis of pattern information
- Peer review to ensure logical consistency of process
- Audit procedures to review documentation if needed to increase scientific credibility
- Developing a case study report that includes pattern appreciation profile and synthesis

Pattern appreciation can be synoptic, participatory, or transformative. Synopsis seeks the clearest picture of unitary pattern found in data. The process is participatory in that scientist/practitioner and respondent have equal but different shared responsibility. Pattern appreciation is transformative in that it creates new consciousness and awareness that can generate a context for change (Cowling, 1997).

Summary of Research Instruments. Research instruments based on the SUHB reflect both quantitative and qualitative research methodologies. The challenges of measurement within a Rogerian perspective have led to creative efforts such as the Mutual Exploration of the Healing Human Field–Environmental Relationship (Carboni, 1992), Pattern Appreciation (Cowling, 1997), and photo-disclosure (Bultemeier, 1997). Instruments such as the PKPCT have commonly been used in studies based on the SUHB. Other instruments such as Carboni's (1992) Mutual Exploration of the Healing Human Field–Environmental Field Relationship have yet to be used substantively. Although the SUHB's measurement issues have not been solved, instrumentation and research method development have evolved consistently.

Review of Related Research

Research using Rogers' SUHB has encompassed a range of studies describing or testing concepts associated with the three principles of homeodynamics—helicy, resonancy, and integrality. Studies dealing with these concepts can be categorized by power, time passing, creativity, field motion, interactive rhythms, health, and therapeutic touch. Research studies are briefly summarized in Table 6-3, which offers the studies' purposes, measurement methods, and findings.

An overview of Rogerian research follows. Because extensive research has been conducted using the SUHB, the specific studies discussed are intended to be representative. Priority was given to recent, published studies. This limitation is not to negate the importance of early or unpublished work but simply confines discussion to a manageable length. Many studies specifically described the SUHB and its linkage to study variables. In several instances, studies explicitly described propositions that were tested. On the whole, studies tended to be descriptive and/or correlational, which is congruent with thinking about appropriate research strategies for wholistic study. However, more recent studies employing interventional techniques used quasiexperimental, repeated measures or, in two cases, experimental design (Meehan, 1993; Samarel, Fawcett, Davis, & Ryan, 1998). Almost all of the studies used convenience or purposive samples. Support for the SUHB was mixed.

Power Studies. Power is one of the most significantly researched areas of helicy. It has been investigated as the only variable or in conjunction with other areas such resonancy, integrality, feminism, temporal experience, spirituality, health perceptions, life satisfaction, and reminiscence. Over time, Barrett's PKPCT has provided a strong mechanism for assessing power and change.

Text continued on p. 148

TABLE 6-3		
Selected Studies Based on Rogers' Science of Unitary Human Beings		
Study/Year	**Methods**	**Findings**
POWER		
Barrett, 1986	The sample consisted of 625 adults of diverse age, location, and ethnicity. Subjects responded to the HFMT and PKPCT.	Canonical correlation revealed two statistically significant relationships that accounted for 40% of the shared variance between power and field motion.
Bramlett and Gueldner, 1993	Eighty-one healthy adults aged 60 to 86 years were divided into experimental and control groups. The experimental group participated in a process of recollecting past events three times over a 1-week period. Potential subjects were screened using the Short Portable Mental Status Questionnaire. All participants responded the PKPCT (presented as a flip chart). The PKPCT was repeated following experimental intervention and 5 weeks later.	No significant differences were found between experimental and control groups at any of the tests. All subject PKPCT scores dropped between the first and second testing and increased by the third testing.
Caroselli, 1995	Eighty-nine nurse executives from acute care institutions responded to the PKPCT and the Index of Sex Role Orientation (ISRO). Pearson Correlation coefficients of the PKPCT total and subscale scores with the ISRO were used to test hypothesis.	A weak, positive correlation was found between the freedom subscale of the PKPCT and the ISRO ($r = 0.244$, $p < 0.01$). Greater identification with feminism was associated with greater freedom to act intentionally on choices.
Malinski, 1997a	Two hundred depressed and 200 nondepressed women aged 25 to 44 years responded to the PKPCT, TES, Beck's Depression Inventory, and demographic data sheet. Data were analyzed with canonical correlation using the four power concepts (awareness, choices, freedom, and involvement) as dependent variables.	Depressed women demonstrated lower diversity and lower frequency power and temporal experience than nondepressed women.

Continued

Purpose

Barrett, 1986 — This descriptive study examined the relationship between human field motion and power.

Bramlett and Gueldner, 1993 — The study investigated the usefulness of reminiscence and a therapeutic modality to enhance power in healthy older adults. Investigators hypothesized that participation in reminiscent storytelling would increase power and that the increase would be sustained at least 5 weeks.

Caroselli, 1995 — This descriptive correlational study assessed the relationship between power and feminism as perceived by female nurse executives.

Malinski, 1997a — The study determined the relationship of temporal experience and power in depressed and nondepressed women.

TABLE 6-3

Selected Studies Based on Rogers' Science of Unitary Human Beings—cont'd

Study/Year	Purpose	Methods	Findings
POWER—cont'd			
McNiff, 1997	The study investigated the relationship between power, perceived health, and life satisfaction of adults with and without long-term care needs.	Sixty-eight adults with and 68 adults without long-term care needs responded to the PKPCT, Cantril Ladder for Health, and Index of Well-Being. Pearson correlations were used to assess relationship of the three variables for both long-term care group and non–long-term care group. One tailed t compared group differences on variables.	In the long-term care group, power and life satisfaction were associated, and life satisfaction and perceived health were associated ($r = 0.60$; $r = 0.41$, $p < 0.001$, respectively). Power and health were not related. For adults without long-term care needs, power and perceived health, and life satisfaction, and power and life satisfaction were associated ($r = 0.42$; $r = 0.52$, $r = 0.63$, $p < 0.001$ respectively). No differences between groups for the three variables were found.
Smith, 1995	The study aimed to identify relationship between power and spirituality and to compare manifestations of power and spirituality in polio survivors and persons not experiencing a life-threatening event.	One hundred seventy-two polio survivors and 80 persons who had not had polio completed the PKPCT and Spiritual Orientation Inventory (SOI).	A positive relationship between power and spirituality was established ($r = 0.34$, $p < 0.005$). Polio survivors did not exhibit greater power than participants who had not experienced a life-threatening event. Survivors exhibited greater spirituality ($t = 3.79$, $df = 250$, $p = 0.001$).
TIME			
Rawnsley, 1986	The study tested the relationship between perception of speed of time and the dying process.	A purposive sample 41 men and 67 women ($N = 108$) was composed of four groups: (1) Older, Dying; (2) Older, Not Dying; (3) Younger, Dying; and (4) Younger, Not Dying. Subjects completed the Time Metaphor Test (TMT), Time Opinion Survey, and two verbal estimates of time elapsed.	Data were analyzed using one-way ANOVA and Pearson correlations of TMT scores and responses on verbal estimates of time. Dying subjects perceived time as passing faster as evidenced by underestimation of the 50-second time lapse. Younger subjects were more future-oriented. Dying persons exhibited greater unhappiness and boredom.

Paletta, 1990	The descriptive correlational study tested the relationship of the magnitude of temporal experience to human time.	One hundred twenty graduate female nursing students aged 20 to 40 years completed the TES and the Human Time Scale (HTS).	Correlations of the HTS with the three TES indicated relationships in the predicted direction. The relationship between timelessness and HTS was significant ($r = 0.266$, $p < 0.01$). In a stepwise regression the three TES significantly predicted HTS.

CREATIVITY

Cowling, 1986b	The study investigated the principle of helicy, proposing that mystical experience, differentiation, and creativity were related.	One hundred sixty college students were assessed for mystical experience (Hood's Mysticism Scale, Factor I), differentiation (Witken's Group Embedded Figures Test), and Creativity (Creativity Scale from Heilbrun's Adjective Checklist).	As mystical experience increased, creativity increased ($r = 0.333$, $p < 0.01$). Increases in differentiation were associated with increases in creativity ($r = 0.167$, $p < 0.05$. Multiple regression revealed that 14.5% of variance in creativity was attributable to the combination of mysticism and differentiation.
Alligood, 1986	The study described relationships of creativity and actualization with empathy.	Two hundred thirty-six volunteers aged 18 to 60 completed measures of actualization (Personal Orientation Inventory [POI]), creativity (Similes Preference Inventory), and empathy (Hogan Scale).	As actualization increased, empathy increased ($r = 0.269$, $p < 0.001$). Increases in creativity were associated with increased empathy ($r = 0.391$, $p < 0.001$. Multiple regression indicated combined variables of actualization, and creativity explained 21% of variance in empathy.
Alligood, 1991	This study continued the Alligood, 1986 study.	Forty-seven additional volunteers aged 61 to 92 completed the measures of actualization, creativity, and empathy.	With the older sample, as creativity decreased, empathy increased ($r = -0.32$, $p < 0.01$), and actualization and empathy were positively related ($r = 0.68$, $p < 0.01$). Creativity and actualization combined accounted for 48% of the variance in empathy.

Continued

TABLE 6-3

Selected Studies Based on Rogers' Science of Unitary Human Beings—cont'd

Study/Year	Purpose	Methods	Findings
FIELD MOTION (RESONANCY)			
Gueldner, 1986	The study investigated relationship between imposed motion (rocking) and human field motion.	The quasiexperimental design consisted of three groups: (1) rocking at preferred rate (n = 10); (2) rocking at imposed rate of 34 to 36 rocking cycles per minute (n = 13); and (3) control (n = 8). Following a 5-day control regimen, the three groups participated in 5-day treatment regimen, consisting of 10 minutes of rocking at the prescribed rate or not rocking. Field motion was measured with a modified HMFT, and fatigue was assessed by Smith's Restedness-Tiredness Scale (RTS).	Repeated ANOVA measures did not reveal any association between rocking and field motion. A Pearson's correlation between HFMT and RTS scores indicated a positive relationship between field motion and restedness (time 1: r = 0.48, p < 0.01; time 2: r = 0.58, p < 0.01, and time 3: r = 0.48, p < 0.01). Subjects reporting high field motion were more rested.
Matas, 1997	This descriptive study explored the nature of chronic pain as a human-environmental patterning process.	Of the 226 participants, 113 were placed in the chronic pain group and 113 in the comparison group. Subjects were matched for age, race, and sex. Groups were compared on the HFMT and PKPCT using a MANCOVA to control for the covariate of pain medication use. Differences in HFM and PKPCT were analyzed using MANOVA, and questions exploring pattern manifestation within each group were analyzed with Pearson Correlations.	MANCOVA revealed that groups were significantly different when adjusting for opioid use. MANOVA revealed that persons with chronic pain experienced lower frequency patterns and lower power levels. Field motion and power were highly correlated in both the pain and comparison groups (r = 0.71, p < 0.0001 and r = 0.78, p < 0.0001), but no differences in the direction or strength of relationship between the two groups were found.

Yarcheski and Mahon, 1991	The study examined Rogers' original and revised theories of correlates, consisting of perceived field motion, human field rhythms, imaginative pattern, diversity of sensory phenomena (sentience), perception of time moving fast, and waking periods in adolescents.	Three groups of 116 adolescents (early, middle, and late) completed the PFM, HFR, Creativity Scale of the Adjective Check List, Personality Research Form-E, the Fast Tempo subscale from the Time Experience Scale, and the Verran/Snyder-Halpern Sleep Scale. The original theory's prediction was that as adolescents became older, their scores on each measure of correlates would increase. To test the revised theory, investigators predicted early adolescents could manifest correlates of the same relative frequency as late adolescents, and have similar frequency levels of creativity and sentience.	Findings failed to support either the original or revised theory of correlates. No differences in correlates among the adolescent groups were found. A correlation between human field motion and sentience in middle adolescents existed. When examined in distinct adolescent groups, correlations were found between PFM, HFR, creativity, and sentience. Human development as indexed by chronological age was perceived to play a role in emergence of manifestations of human field patterning. Investigators suggested that deletion of terms implying linearity from Rogers' original theory should occur only when clear evidence supporting a revised theory of correlates emerges.
Yarcheski and Mahon, 1995	The study examined four manifestations of human environmental field patterning (field motion, field rhythms, creativity, and sentience) in relation to perceived health status of adolescents.	Three groups of early ($n = 106$), middle ($n = 111$), and late ($n = 113$) adolescents responded to PFM, HFR, the Creativity Scale, the Sentience Scale, the General Health Rating Index, and a demographic questionnaire. Pearson correlations assessed relationships among field patterns and health status.	PFM was related to health status in all three adolescent groups ($r = 0.24$, $p < 0.05$; $r = 0.26$, and 0.44, $p < 0.01$, respectively). HFR and creativity were related to health status only in late adolescents ($r = 0.23$ and 0.20, $p < 0.05$). PMF, HFR, creativity and sentience explained 9% of variance in health status of middle adolescents; whereas in late adolescents, these accounted for 22% of variance.
Watson, 1997	The study explored a different approach for explaining sleep-wake cycles of older adults. It also investigated whether diversity of sleep rhythm and dream experience was related to field motion.	Sixty-six women aged 60 to 83 kept a sleep chart for two weeks and responded to the ADE, HFMT, and TMT.	Most respondents slept between 6 to 8 hours per day. Fourteen percent slept less and 9% slept more. Most woke during the night. As sleep-wake patterns became more diverse, diversity in dream patterns increased ($r = 0.2945$, $p < 0.05$). No associations between sleep-wake patterns or dream experience with either the HFMT and TMT were found.

Continued

TABLE 6-3

Selected Studies Based on Rogers' Science of Unitary Human Beings—cont'd

Study/Year	Purpose	Methods	Findings
INTERACTIVE RHYTHMS (INTEGRALITY)			
Boyd, 1990	The study assessed the intercorrelation of daughters' attachment to mothers, mother-daughter conflict, and dyadic identity. Mother-daughter dyads were felt to represent integrality.	An ex post facto correlational design was used to study 81 mother-daughter dyads with the Attachment Semantic Differential Scale, the Attachment Scale, the Mother Daughter Conflict Scale, and the Tennessee Self-Concept Scale. LISREL analysis examined the fit between the model and the data.	Empirical support was provided for the proposed model. Mother-daughter identification incorporates mutual influence and shared identities, but daughter identity was more influential in overall dyadic identity. Mother-daughter conflict over separation and perceived differences also mediated the relationship, but daughter conflict was a more powerful endogenous variable.
HEALTH			
Leddy, 1997	The study tested relationships among healthiness, fatigue, and symptom experience in women with and without breast cancer.	Eighty-nine healthy subjects were compared to 53 women with breast cancer that had been treated within the past 10 years. Subjects completed the Leddy Healthiness Scale, the Fatigue Experience Scale, and the Symptom Experience Scale (SES).	Women with breast cancer did not differ from healthy women in terms of healthiness or fatigue or the relationships of healthiness, fatigue, and symptom experience. Breast cancer subjects experienced more symptoms than the healthy group ($t = 2.62$, $df = 140$, $p = 0.01$).
Leddy and Fawcett, 1997	The study tested an explanatory theory of healthiness based on Rogers' SUHB.	One hundred twenty-three ambulatory volunteers completed the Person-Environment Participation Scale, Perceived Stress Scale, Energy/Fatigue Scale, Leddy Healthiness Scale, Mental Health Index, Satisfaction with Life Scale, Current Health Status, and Inventory of Symptom Distress.	Path analyses were conducted to assess the theoretical structure. Theorized relationships between participation, change, energy, and healthiness were statistically supported. Paths from participation to other proposed variables of mental health, satisfaction with life, current health status, and symptom distress were deleted.

HEALTH-RELATED

Andersen and Hockman, 1997	The correlational study determined whether change in well-being and change in high-risk drug-related behaviors related to AIDS risk. Effects of a standard treatment protocol and a Rogerian based protocol were compared.	Three hundred seventy-five drug users being tested for HIV received a standard care protocol—consisting of education, counseling, and, if needed, referral. In addition to standard care, another 369 drug users received the LIGHT protocol incorporating bonding, assessment of well-being, and teaching. Initial and 6-month follow-up were completed by 454 subjects. Data were collected through the Risk Behavior Assessment, Global Well-Being Index, and Addiction Severity Index.	All subjects decreased risk behaviors. The LIGHT group also significantly improved well-being, which was associated with a reduction of addiction and risk behaviors. The standard care group did not improve sense of well-being and experienced greater concerns about employment, legal problems, and medical concerns.
Bush, 1997	The study tested the relationship of parental health perceptions and locus of control to healthcare follow-up for children with identified health problems.	A convenience sample of 50 parents or guardians responsible for their child's healthcare completed health perceptions questionnaire, Health Locus of Control Scale, and socioeconomic questionnaire. Twenty-five were parents of children who received follow-up care, and 25 were not.	Locus of control, health beliefs, and socioeconomic factors did not relate to healthcare follow-up for students receiving referrals for healthcare problems.

THERAPEUTIC TOUCH

Meehan, 1993	The single trial, single blinded, three-group design assessed the influence of therapeutic touch on postoperative pain.	One hundred eight postoperative patients were randomly assigned to receive therapeutic touch, a placebo control intervention, or narcotic analgesic for pain. A Visual Analog Scale (VAS) was used before and 1 hour after intervention.	Subjects receiving pain medication experienced significantly greater pain relief than therapeutic touch subjects ($p = 0.001$). Therapeutic touch subjects experienced greater relief than the placebo control subjects, but the difference was not significant. Placebo group patients requested pain medication sooner following treatment than did therapeutic touch subjects ($\chi^2 = 4.69, p < 0.05$).

Continued

TABLE 6-3

Selected Studies Based on Rogers' Science of Unitary Human Beings—cont'd

Study/Year	Purpose	Methods	Findings
THERAPEUTIC TOUCH—cont'd			
Peck, 1998	The study determined whether therapeutic touch (TT) improved functional ability in older adults with arthritis.	A two-group, longitudinal design with repeated treatments assessed the efficacy of TT. Baseline data were collected over 4 weeks, while usual care was given. Forty-five subjects then received TT, while 37 received progressive muscle relaxation (PMR) six times at 1-week intervals. Subjects completed the Arthritis Impact Measurement Scale (AIMS 2) twice during baseline period and following the first, third, and sixth treatments.	TT group baseline AIMS 2 scores were compared to postintervention scores using paired t-tests. The TT group significantly improved hand function, pain, tension, mood, and satisfaction between mean baseline scores and scores following their sixth visit. Significant improvements were found in the PMR group for walking and bending, pain, tension, mood, and satisfaction. Repeated ANOVA measures indicated that TT groups experienced greater mobility and greater hand function.
Samarel, 1992	The phenomenological study described meaning and patient experiences of receiving therapeutic touch.	Twenty participants describing lived experience of receiving therapeutic touch treatments. An initial open-ended interview and a second interview directed toward clarification were used for data gathering.	Experiences prior to treatment were characterized by unmet physiological, mental/emotional, and spiritual needs. The experience of treatment incorporated self-awareness related to physiological relief and emotional nurture. The therapist's roles were important, particularly in relation to trust. Posttreatment positive changes included improved physiological capabilities, renewed emotional outlook, and growing spiritual sense.

| Samarel, Fawcett, Davis, and Ryan, 1998 | The pilot study tested efficacy of dialogue and therapeutic touch on preoperative and postoperative anxiety and mood and postoperative pain. | Thirty-one women undergoing surgery for breast cancer were randomly assigned to experimental or control groups. The State-Trait Anxiety Scale, Affects Balance Scale and Visual Analog Scale—Pain were completed following the pre- and postoperative treatment episodes. Experimental treatment was 10 minutes of therapeutic touch followed by 20-minute dialogue with nurse. Controls listened quietly to music for 10 minutes followed by 20-minute dialogue. | MANCOVA using trait anxiety scores as the covariate revealed that preoperative women in the therapeutic touch group experienced less state anxiety than the control group (Wilks 1 [2,27] = 3.94, p = 0.03; Univariate F [1,28] = 8.15, p = 0.008). There were no preoperative differences in terms of pain or mood and no postoperative differences in anxiety, mood, or pain. |
| Turner, Clark, Gauthier, and Williams, 1998 | The single-blinded randomized clinical trial determined whether therapeutic touch (TT) could produce greater pain relief than sham touch. | Ninety-nine adult burn patients were randomly assigned to TT (n = 62) or sham TT (n = 37) groups. Subjects in each group received TT or sham TT treatments for five days. Baseline questionnaires included the McGill Pain Questionnaire and the Credibility of Therapy Form (CTF). On Day 3, the Visual Analog Scale for Pain (VASP) was administered before and after treatment. On Day 6, the VASP, Visual Analog Scale for Anxiety (VASA), Visual Analog Scale for Satisfaction with Therapy (VASS), and Effectiveness with Therapy Form (ETF) were administered. Eleven subjects donated blood sample drawings for CD4+, CD8+T-lymphocytes on Days 1 and 6. | Mean scores were adjusted, using baseline scores as covariates. Long-term pain control that was assessed with the McGill Pain Questionnaire revealed that TT subjects had significantly less pain than the sham TT group did (Pain rating index: t = 2.76; p = 0.004; Number of words chosen: t = 2.75; p = 0.005). TT subjects had lower anxiety levels (t = 1.90; p = 0.031). There were no differences in satisfaction with therapy or medication usage. The sample was too small to statistically compare blood samples, but CD8+ cell concentrations decreased 13% for TT patients and increased 46% for sham TT subjects. Total CD4+ concentrations increased 15.2% for TT subjects and increased 48.3% for the sham group. Lymphocyte counts increased 1.1% for TT subjects and 38.6% for sham subjects. |

Conceptualizing power as the "capacity to participate knowingly in the nature of change" (p. 174), Barrett (1986) studied power in relationship to field motion concepts of "motor running" and "field expansion." In this process she extended work on field motion by demonstrating that motor running and field expansion were two separate constructs. Following a pilot study ($\underline{N} = 267$), Barrett's main study ($\underline{N} = 625$) used the HFMT and PKPCT. She found that as human field motion increases, so does the ability to participate knowingly. Her study supported conceptual links of the SUHB.

Caroselli (1995) examined the relationship between power and feminism in female nurse executives. This study demonstrated a weak but significant relationship between feminism and one power subscale, the freedom to act intentionally. Although this finding is congruent with Rogerian theory, interpreting the relationship of feminism and power requires consideration of additional factors.

In an intervention study Bramlett and Gueldner (1993) assessed the effectiveness of reminiscent storytelling as a method of maintaining power in the elderly. The study intervention stemmed from Barrett's assertion, derived from the SUHB, that power comes from an individual's ability to gain information, make informed choices, and act on those choices. Bramlett and Gueldner proposed that reminiscent storytelling, as a therapeutic modality, would enhance elders' perceptions of power. Three measures of power were assessed for both the experimental and control groups: at initiation, at 1 week following initiating of storytelling, and 5 weeks later. To make the PKPCT more manageable for elders, a flip chart format presented the metaphors. Both experimental and control groups experienced a small decline in power between the pretesting and first posttesting. Both groups then experienced increased power between the one-week and five-week measures. The value of reminiscence therapy in maintaining power remains unclear.

Several power studies centered on women with illness or significant disability. Malinski (1997a) compared temporal experience and power in depressed and nondepressed women and supported Rogers' homeodynamic principles. Depressed women had lower diversity and lower power and temporal experience. However, the findings did not support the concept of timelessness.

McNiff's (1997) study of adults with long-term care needs examined the relationship of power, perceived health, and life satisfaction. McNiff proposed that power, perceived health, and life satisfaction were pattern manifestations emerging from the diverse continuous mutual human–environmental energy field process proposed by Rogers. She hypothesized that these variables would be associated positively in adults with and without long-term care needs. Findings led her to suggest that perceived health and life satisfaction may complement well-being. Adults with long-term care needs participated knowingly in change, leading McNiff to propose that transcendence may be a key step for individuals with disability as they evolve toward greater diversity. These findings supported Roger's contention that life can transcend difficult circumstances and evolve to a greater diversity.

Smith (1995) investigated the relationship of power and spirituality of polio survivors and compared survivor levels of power and spirituality to levels of persons who had not experienced a life-threatening illness. Her findings of a relationship between power and spirituality supported Barrett's theory of power and Rogers' framework. Smith suggested spirituality grows through continual mutual process and that polio survivors make more choices associated with spirituality. Smith attributed the fact that hypothesized differences in power between survivors and the non-ill failed to materialize to pattern changes over time.

Time Studies. The concept of time passing has been the focus of several studies. In a descriptive study, Rawnsley (1986) proposed that chronological age would influence perceptions of time passing and that time would pass more swiftly for the dying than the healthy. Although she could not support her hypothesis regarding chronological age, she found that the dying perceived time as passing more quickly. Although its methodology was criticized (Fitzpatrick, 1986), Rawnsley's study was the first to empirically test the SUHB. Subsequent changes to the SUHB provided greater clarification of terms (Ference, 1986b).

In a theory-testing study, Paletta (1990) investigated the relationship of temporal experience as measured by the TES to human time as measured by the Human Time Scale (HTS). This study was based on Rogers' postulation that human time is a manifestation of a wholistic developmental process in which time dragging was the least complex of the temporal patterns and timelessness was a more complex field pattern. The time dragging, time racing, and timelessness scales were found to explain 15% of the variance in human time. This study is provided early support for Rogers' construct of temporal experience.

Creativity. Creativity is an aspect of unitary development described in the SUHB. Testing helicy, Cowling (1986b) conducted a descriptive, correlational study of 160 college-age students on mysticism, differentiation, and creativity. One strength of this study was the clear relationship of variables to the SUHB. Cowling's study was based on three conceptualizations of the SUHB, which included: (1) human field patterns represent a wave, in that they move dynamically and continuously toward diversity and innovation; (2) diversity is an identifiable characteristic of a field pattern and can be found in mystical experience and differentiation; and (c) innovation is a characteristic of a human field pattern and is found in creativity. Positive associations between mystical experience and creativity together accounted for a small portion of the variance in creativity. The combination of mystical experience and creativity also accounted for a small portion of variance in creativity. Mystical experience accounted for a greater portion of creativity than differentiation did. As levels of mystical experience increased, so did creativity. As differentiation increased, so did creativity. These findings provide support for the principle of helicy and some tentative support for the concept of a diverse human field pattern.

In a test of helicy, Alligood (1986) hypothesized that creativity, actualization, and empathy were related, and she initially tested the relationships with a group aged 18 to 60 years. Using Rogers' proposal that nature and direction of helicy is innovative, increasingly diverse, and emergent from the continuous mutual process of humans and the environment, Alligood (1986) proposed that empathy is a human field pattern of helicy; creativity exemplifies innovation; and actualization embodies increasing diversity. Positive relationships were found between empathy and creativity and empathy and actualization. Creativity and actualization combined accounted for 21% of the variance in empathy. The presence of a relationship between these variables supported the idea that humans and the environment change together, which is consistent with the SUHB. Alligood (1991) followed her initial study with a second using sample subjects aged 61 to 92 years. An inverse relationship between empathy and creativity weakened support for accelerating change. Clarifying the relationship in older age groups will require further research.

Field Motion Studies. Several studies considered the concept of human field motion. Gueldner (1986) hypothesized a positive relationship between rocking and human field motion. He also speculated that preferred rocking rates would relate more strongly to field motion and that perceived field motion and restedness would relate positively. This study was based on the principle of resonancy, which contends that wave patterns emanating from the human and environmental fields manifest continuous change from lower to higher frequencies. Rocking was an imposed motion. Although no association was found between rocking and field motion, a relationship between field motion and tiredness in the elderly was found. This study did not directly support the principle of resonancy. Gueldner reported difficulty in using the HFMT with less educated subjects. Also, small sample size may have impeded discerning field motion and rocking relationships.

In a study of elderly women, Watson (1997) investigated the sleep-wake patterns of older adults and the association of dreaming, field motion, and time. Although the shared variance of dream experience and sleep-wake cycle was only 8.75%, this study tentatively supports the Rogerian sleeping/longer waking/beyond waking construct. Watson reported difficulties in scoring and interpretation of the TMT and in use of the HFMT with older adults.

Yarcheski and Mahon (1991, 1995) moved the investigation of human field motion to adolescents. A comparison of Rogers' original theory containing developmental language to the revised theory, in which developmental language was removed, did not yield support. Investigators suggested that rhythms and health should be anticipated to emerge developmentally. Other human field manifestations related to health perceptions need to be identified in order to account for more variance associated with health status.

To explore the nature of chronic pain from a Rogerian perspective, Matas (1997) compared subjects experiencing chronic pain to a matched group without pain. Chronic pain sufferers experienced lower field motion and lower power levels than their comparison group. Because field motion was highly correlated to power in both groups, Matas' findings reflected Rogers' concept of a single wave in an energy field. Matas further indicated that chronic pain can be conceptualized as a pattern manifestation and that field pattern appraisal may be useful in describing chronic conditions and promoting intervention.

Therapeutic Touch. Several studies have used the SUHB as a framework for studying therapeutic touch. Samarel (1992) postulated that the homeodynamic principles of helicy, integrality, and resonancy were congruent with the lived experience of individuals receiving therapeutic touch in her phenomenological study. Integrality was expressed through awareness of relationships with others. Pattern changes occurred before, during, and after treatment. They began with low frequency, and later moved to higher frequency. In these senses, the pattern changes were akin to aspects of resonancy and helicy. However, participants expressed change in linear terms, which is potentially problematic for the SUHB since the ideal of a unitary whole is pandimensional and therefore nonlinear and without spatial or temporal attributes.

In an intervention study, Samarel, Fawcett, Davis, and Ryan (1998) used the SUHB to assert that deliberative mutual patterning through therapeutic touch and dialogue would result in lower anxiety, positive moods, and lower pain intensity and distress in pre- and postoperative breast cancer patients. Although women receiving therapeutic touch and dialogue preoperatively experienced less anxiety, quiet time and dialogue were equally effective in improving postoperative anxiety, mood, and pain levels. Nonetheless, this study supports Rogers' assertion that pattern manifestation appraisal and deliberative mutual patterning are associated with human energy field manifestations. In this instance each of the noninvasive modalities of therapeutic touch and dialogue and dialogue and quiet time modified the energy manifestations of anxiety, mood, pain intensity, and distress. Contrary to investigators' predictions, however, therapeutic touch did not correlate more strongly with pattern manifestations than quiet time. Whether quiet time or music followed by dialogue also could be considered a process of patterning remains to be determined.

Proposing that patterning could change a symptom or its meaning, Peck (1998) also envisioned therapeutic touch as a health-patterning modality. Her study investigated the therapeutic touch in comparison to progressive muscle relaxation for treating older adults' arthritis symptoms. Both the therapeutic touch group and progressive muscle relaxation group demonstrated improvement. Both therapeutic touch and progressive muscle relaxation could be considered patterning. This study supports the homeodynamic principles of resonancy and helicy. Resonancy is represented by the fluctuations in energy fields between treatments and corresponding changes in pain. Helicy is characterized by changes in pain.

Meehan (1993) applied the SUHB to therapeutic touch in a slightly different manner. She focused on pandimensionality, which suggests that no linear time or separation of human and environmental fields exists. Meehan explained actions that occur at a distance, such as therapeutic touch, pandimensionally. Her study determined that although therapeutic touch did not reduce pain level, it diminished the need for pain medication. Meehan called for more research to directly test the relationship between therapeutic touch process and propositions derived from the SUHB.

Suggesting that therapeutic touch is a technique can rebalance or replenish depleted, blocked, or unbalanced energy fields affected by illness, Turner, Clark, Gauthier, and Williams (1998) examined the effects of therapeutic touch on burn patients. In a rigorously designed randomized trial, subjects were assigned to a therapeutic touch or sham therapeutic touch group. Researchers measured pain, anxiety, satisfaction with treatment, medication usage, and lymphocyte counts. Therapeutic touch effectively reduced pain and anxiety. However, it did not affect medication use or satisfaction with care. Total lymphocyte concentration decreased in the therapeutic touch group, but the portion of the sample completing physiological measures was very small. This study supports Rogers' contention nurses can intervene to balance and enhance energy fields for ill patients.

Research Summary. Despite some mixed findings, research using a Rogerian framework or a model derived from a Rogerian perspective has supported the SUHB. Rogerian investigators have been commended for their consistent application of the SUHB. Most studies identified strong connections between the dimensions of the SUHB and their variables of study. Perhaps most importantly, the SUHB has provided a theoretical basis for study. Additionally, many studies have been well planned and executed. Measuring instruments and methods, while not problem free, have provided adequate mechanisms for Rogerian discovery. Unfortunately, some SUHB studies offer limited generalizability. Despite sufficiently large sample sizes in many studies, participants often have been selected too conveniently. Moreover, many studies of the SUHB are unpublished dissertations, and what research is available does not tend to move beyond a descriptive level. Although description provides a useful foundation, Rogerian research efforts need to focus on interventional studies that address the methodological issues associated with linear measurement. Examples of such studies include Bramlett and Gueldner (1993); Samarel, (1992); Samarel, Fawcett, Davis, and Ryan (1998); Meehan (1993); and Turner, Clark, Gauthier, and Williams (1998).

In some areas, such as power studies and therapeutic touch, strong foundations for additional research exist. Instrumentation and study methodologies need further study, especially with regard to wholistic measurement. Although research needs to continue in populations of current concern, such as older adults and persons with disabilities, other populations and health concerns need to be added. Children, healthy adults, and health maintenance or illness care interventions, for example, require more research.

PRAXIS AND THEORY UTILIZATION: DESIGNING NURSING PRACTICE PROGRAMS WITHIN THE THEORETICAL SYSTEM OF THE SCIENCE OF UNITARY HUMAN BEINGS

> The unitary nurse considers: Why is the problem occurring in this person at this time? What can the patient do to help eliminate the problem or keep it from happening again? How are the patient's family and co-workers involved and how are they affected? How does the patient feel about what is happening to him or her? Does the patient understand what is happening? *(Manahan & Manahan 1992, in Barrett, 1994.)*

Rogers' perspective defines nursing not only as eradicating symptoms but also as supporting the integral wholeness of human beings (Malinski, 1997b). This perspective allows nurses to extend their focus beyond physical disabilities and body image to the promotion of human field change and human field image (Smith, 1995).

The SUHB is predicated on "a new worldview" (Rogers, 1992a, 1992b). At present, Rogerian practitioners are usually nurses prepared at advanced practice levels—that is, at the master's or doctorate level—who sufficiently understand the new worldview that Rogers proposes to structure practice philosophically. Chapter 3 describes the necessary development that precedes nursing theory and provides direction for practice: (1) making the language explicit, (2) specifying the focus of nursing and associated variables of concern, and (3) developing those variables for practice purposes. The language to describe the "new worldview" has not yet been developed fully nor have the variables been specified for practice purposes. For Phillips (1997), for example, nursing practice flows from theories, which flow from the SUHB, which in turn flows from its underlying philosophy. Rogerian scholars believe SUHB underlies the art—that is, the imaginative and creative application of this foundation—of nursing (Rogers, 1992a). Phillips (1997) challenges Rogerian scholars to

> further elucidate the philosophy of the Science of Unitary Human Beings. The first step might be to look at the words unitary human beings . . . The elucidation and articulation of a Rogerian philosophy requires Rogerian scholars to analyze Rogers' writings within the context of the universe of philosophy and knowledge to elicit the defining attributes of the concept of unitary human beings and its philosophical base (p.16).

This step is a precursor to a Rogerian nursing practice.

The Variables of Concern for Practice

The same limitation in operationalizing variables for study discussed in the previous section hinders development of nursing practice programs within a theoretical system. Although some studies have informed specific practice situations, more variables need to be defined for practice. This cannot occur, however, until the underlying SUHB is developed more fully.

Process Models

Alligood (1994) suggests that the traditional view of nursing as a problem-solving process is not useful for practice within a Rogerian perspective. Rather, nurses provide a decision-making framework. She argues that "theory and practice are not different entities; rather, they are different aspects of the same phenomenon" (1994, p. 228). Because practice from a Rogerian perspective requires knowledge gained in professional nursing education, Alligood considers the SUHB a poor fit for task-oriented vocational nursing. Malinski (1997b) concurs. She describes Rogerian practice as a mutual caring partnership rather than an outcome-focused nursing process (1997b).

Barrett (1988) proposed and updated (1998) *health patterning*, a practice methodology that facilitates patients' well-being through their knowing participation in change. Health patterning is a creative caring partnership of mutual involvement and choices between a patient and a nurse. Knowing participation in change is power, the dimensions of which are awareness, choices, freedom to act intentionally, and involvement in creating change. The processes of health patterning are the following: (1) pattern manifestation knowing—or, "the continuous process of apprehending the human and environmental field" (p. 136), and (2) voluntary mutual patterning—"the continuous process whereby the nurse assists clients to freely choose with awareness ways to participate in their well-being" (p. 136).

Health-patterning modalities include movement/dance/imposed motion, rest/activity, music, imagery, meditation, humor, relaxation, nutrition, affirmations, therapeutic touch, bibliotherapy, and journaling (Barrett, 1992). The Power as Knowing Participation in Change Tool (PKPCT) offers patients a glimpse of their power profiles. The nurse's role is to help patients make informed decisions with knowledge of their options. Health patterning requires knowledge of the SUHB. Meaningful dialogue, centering, genuineness, trustworthiness, acceptance, and knowledgeable caring facilitate patients' knowing participation and thus actualization of their potential well-being.

The PKPCT has been used for 15 years. Caroselli and Barrett (1998) suggest that this tool now could be used to design wellness programs that would enhance feelings of power for older adults in long-term care. Programs also could be designed to strengthen the power of administrators and staff nurses.

Nursing concerns itself with the interaction between humans and their environments, both of which are irreducible energy fields. Patterning-healing modalities allow well-being to emerge. People participate in patterning their own fields. Phillips (1997) has identified some modalities of patterning-healing, including meditation, visualization, imagery, therapeutic touch, music/sound, prayer, art, poetry, storytelling, color, humor, and motion/ dance. Phillips also has listed some characteristics of unitary well-being: awareness of infinite wholeness, unconditional loving, forgiving, freedom of choosing, participating in change, compassion, realizing potentials, peace, joy, integrality with the universe, fulfillment, purpose and meaning in living, recognizing the infinite significance of everything, listening to the flow of energy, and giving-receiving.

Andersen and Smereck (1994) have used Barrett's methodology to develop what they call a personalized nursing process model. The goal of this model is to assist patients in attaining an improved sense of well-being. Pattern manifestation examines well-being, being, not being, and talents. Nurses and caregivers manifest deliberative mutual patterning through loving the patient, intending to help, giving care gently, helping the patient improve well-being, and teaching the process. In turn, the patient should love him or herself, identify concerns, set a goal, be confident and self-motivated, and take positive action. Proponents of this model have demonstrated its utility for practice with populations of substance abusers. They correctly hypothesized that improving well-being would reduce directly the high risk behaviors associated indirectly with AIDS.

Practice Models

The development of practice models derived from this theoretical system is in the beginning stages. Further development of the variables for practice purposes and of practice theories will facilitate continuing development of the models.

Carboni (1995a) has derived a theory of Rogerian nursing practice entitled "Enfolding Health-as-Wholeness-and-Harmony." By integrating theory and practice, she attempts a conceptual understanding required to identify and test theoretical statements. The process of inquiry becomes an integral part of the practice. She proposes a theoretical perspective to guide nursing practice and a research methodology integral to that practice (Carboni, 1995b).

Cowling's description (1993) of the nurse-patient relationship in the unitary model supports Carboni's approach. He contrasts systems thinking, which has been such a dominant force in nursing, with a unitary perspective, in which the focus of nursing is on "aspects of the situation and not on the relationship of parts as in systems thinking" (p. 202). A nurse-patient encounter involves mutual simultaneous shaping. Interrelating is a construction process during which both the nurse and patient interact with the human variables or phenomena. Cowling further suggests that these variables are more constructs than fundamental aspects of reality. Observations are "the momentary manifestations of pattern" (p. 204).

Cowling (1997) integrates scientist and practitioner roles as he describes a scientist/practitioner model of nursing facilitating knowledge development through case studies. He suggests that in working with individuals "the surface display of information be considered in the context of unitary patterning and that pattern be given attention as the referent for practice and for creating a knowledge base of science for the practice of nursing" (p. 53). He describes a process of pattern appreciation that involves being open to the experience, perception, and expressions of another as representative of pattern manifestations. A pattern profile is developed by examining data from experience, perception, and expressions. The pattern profile is context-based and is verified by the participant. The pattern profile suggests possible strategies for accomplishing the patient's intent. This activity leads to practical or theoretical knowledge development.

Defining pain as "an emergent expression of human–environmental field patterning—experienced as a hurt" (1997, p. 90), Matas offered a rudimentary practice model that considers unitary human field patterning manifestations by using the HFMT and the PKPCT. Although the limited sample precludes generalization of the findings, they nonetheless indicate that field pattern appraisal is useful for describing chronic pain. With further research, this finding could provide a new direction for the treatment of such pain. Nursing strategies developed within this framework would facilitate human growth toward higher frequency patterning. Using music, sound and motion, meditation, dream journaling, nature explorations, imagery hypnosis, and therapeutic touch also are consistent with this perspective. Matas identifies the following specific areas of study that have implications for changing nursing practice (1997):

- Clinical trials using blue light to support field pattern transformation
- Exploring the use of the PKPCT and HFMT as outcome measures in studying chronic pain
- Designing and testing interventions for chronic pain based on Barrett's power theory
- Designing and testing strategies for chronic pain which enhance the unfolding of human-environmental patterning process in the direction of higher frequency patterning

Smith's study (1995) of power and spirituality in polio survivors also could lead to a practice model. This study extends the exploration of spirituality within Rogers' framework to a theory of spirituality. Spirituality is defined from a humanistic perspective, incorporating both religious and nonreligious expressions. The findings support Barrett's theory "that people who have the capacity to participate knowingly in change . . . also have the ability to change the nature of their participation" (Smith, 1995, p. 137). This study suggests nurses should expand their scope of activity to the promotion of power and spirituality.

Implications for Administration

In keeping with the perspective that there should be congruence between ontology, epistemology and methodology, the worlds of Rogerian nurses are quite different from the worlds of nurses practicing in most healthcare agencies today. Rogerian practice requires a major shift in thinking about the role of nursing in an organization and the organizational structure required to support that practice.

Caroselli (1994) describes an organizational structure that emanates from a philosophy congruent with SUHB and that would support nursing practice from this perspective, but she does not provide a detailed description of that nursing practice. The organization she envisions would emphasize participatory management, from which knowing participation in change stems. The statement of philosophy would reflect this value. The chief nursing executive would function as "leader-as-teacher." A model of shared governance is most congruent with Rogerian nursing practice since it supports the value of knowing participation. A relatively "flat" organizational structure would comprise specialists in Rogerian science, change theory, and nursing administration as well as research advisors responsible for developing research programs that include all nurses. The research advisor would work closely with the financial advisor and details of the finances would be available to all nurses to allow their knowing participation. Staff development would proceed from a competency perspective with modalities consistent with the Rogerian perspective.

Implications for Education

Basic and continuing education programs require major changes in order to practice nursing within this theoretical framework. However, before the changes can be designed, the SUHB must be developed more fully.

NEXUS

The development of the SUHB has taken several tracks. Research studies and methods are developing into a substantive body of knowledge that offers potential for nursing practice. While traditional science methodologies are manifested in the work described above, creative measurement strategies continue to evolve. Other nursing scholars, focusing on the further development of the conceptual expressions, moved to develop other models or theories. Newman's work (1994) on health as expanding consciousness and Parse's Theory of Human Becoming are notable, but it is not yet clear how these fit into Rogers' SUHB. A sign of the legacy of Rogers and the SUHB is the Society of Rogerian Scholars. This group fosters further theoretical development through exchange of ideas, elaboration of unitary knowing perspectives, and dissemination of information. These efforts should continue to develop a definitive perspective of viewing human beings and nursing.

REFERENCES

Alligood, M.R. (1986). The relationship of creativity, actualization, and empathy in unitary human development. In V.M. Malinski (Ed.), *Explorations on Martha Rogers' Science of Unitary Human Beings*, Norwalk, CT: Appleton, Century, & Crofts.

Alligood, M.R. (1991). Testing Rogers' theory of accelerating change: The relationships among creativity, actualization, and empathy in persons 18 to 92 years of age. *Western Journal of Nursing Research, 13*(1), 84-96.

Alligood, M.A. (1994). Toward a unitary view of nursing practice. In M. Madrid and E.A.M. Barrett (Eds.), *Rogers' scientific art of nursing practice*. New York: National League for Nursing Press.

Andersen, M. & Hockman, E.M. (1997). Wellbeing and high-risk drug use among active drug users. In M. Madrid (Ed.), *Patterns of Rogerian knowing*. New York: National League for Nursing Press.

Andersen, M.D. & Smereck, G.A.D. (1994). Personalized nursing: A science-based model of the art of nursing. In M. Madrid and E.A.M. Barrett (Eds.), *Rogers' scientific art of nursing practice*. New York: National League for Nursing Press.

Barrett, E.A.M. (1986). Investigation of the principle of helicy: The relationship of human field motion and power. In V.M. Malinski (Ed.). *Explorations on Martha Rogers' Science of Unitary Human Beings*. Norwalk, CT: Appleton, Century, & Crofts.

Barrett, E.A.M. (1988). Using Rogers' Science of Unitary Human Beings in nursing practice. *Nursing Science Quarterly, 1*(2), 50-51.

Barrett, E.A.M. (1990a). Rogerian patterns of scientific inquiry. In E.A.M. Barrett (Ed.), *Visions of Rogers' science-based nursing*. New York: National League for Nursing Press.

Barrett, E.A.M. (1990b). A measure of power as knowing participation in change. In O. Strickland & C. Waltz (Eds.), *The measurement of nursing outcomes: Measuring client self-care and coping skills, Volume 4*. New York: Springer.

Barrett, E.A.M. (1992). Innovative imagery: A health patterning modality for nursing practice. *Journal of Holistic Nursing 10*(2), 154-166.

Barrett, E.A.M. (1994). Rogerian scientists, artists, revolutionaries. In M. Madrid and E.A.M. Barrett (Eds.). *Rogers scientific art of nursing practice*. New York: National League for Nursing Press.

Barrett, E.A.M. (1998). A Rogerian practice methodology for health patterning. *Nursing Science Quarterly, 11*(4), 136-138.

Barrett, E.A.M., Caroselli, C., Smith, A.S., & Smith, D.W. (1997). Power as knowing participation in change: Theoretical, practice, and methodological issues, insights, and ideas. In M. Madrid (Ed.), *Patterns of Rogerian knowing*. New York: National League for Nursing Press.

Barrett, E.A.M. & Caroselli, C. (1998). Methodological ponderings related to the Power as Knowing Participation in Change Tool. *Nursing Science Quarterly, 11*(1), 17-22.

Barrett, E.A.M., Cowling, W.R., Carboni, J.T., & Butcher, H.K. (1997). Unitary perspectives on methodological practices. In M. Madrid (Ed.), *Patterns of Rogerian knowing*. New York: National League for Nursing Press.

Boyd, C. (1990). Testing a model of mother-daughter identification. *Western Journal of Nursing Research, 12*(4), 448-468.

Bramlett, M.H. & Gueldner, S.H. (1993). Reminiscence: A viable option to enhance power in elders. *Clinical Nurse Specialist, 7*(2), 68-74.

Bultemeier, K. (1997). Photo-disclosure: A research methodology for investigating unitary human beings. In M. Madrid (Ed.), *Patterns of Rogerian knowing.* New York: National League for Nursing Press.

Bush, M. (1997). Influence of health locus of control and parental health perceptions on follow-through with school nurse referral. *Issues in Comprehensive Pediatric Nursing, 20*(3), 175-182.

Carboni, J.T. (1992). Instrument development and the measurement of unitary constructs. *Nursing Science Quarterly, 5*(3), 134-142.

Carboni, J.T. (1995a). Enfolding health-as-wholeness-and-harmony: A theory of Rogerian nursing practice. *Nursing Science Quarterly,* 8(2), 71-78.

Carboni, J.T. (1995b). A Rogerian process of inquiry. *Nursing Science Quarterly,* 8(2), 22-37.

Caroselli C. (1994). Opportunities for knowing participation: A new design for the nursing service organization. In M. Madrid and E.A.M. Barrett (Eds.), *Rogers' scientific art of nursing practice.* New York: National League for Nursing Press.

Caroselli, C. (1995). Power and feminism: A nursing science perspective. *Nursing Science Quarterly,* 8(3), 115-119.

Caroselli, C. & Barrett, E.A.M. (1998). A review of the power as knowing participation in change literature. *Nursing Science Quarterly, 11*(1), 9-16.

Cowling, W.R. (1986a). The Science of Unitary Human Beings: Theoretical issues, methodological challenges, and research realities. In V.M. Malinski (Ed.), *Explorations on Martha Rogers' Science of Unitary Human Beings.* Norwalk, CT: Appleton, Century, & Crofts.

Cowling, W.R. (1986b). The Relationship of mystical experience, differentiation, and creativity in college students. In V.M. Malinski (Ed.), *Explorations on Martha Rogers' Science of Unitary Human Beings.* Norwalk, CT: Appleton, Century, & Crofts.

Cowling, W.R. (1990). A template for unitary pattern-based nursing practice. In E.A.M. Barrett (Ed.), *Visions of Rogers' science-based nursing.* New York: National League for Nursing.

Cowling W.R. (1993). Unitary knowing in nursing practice. *Nursing Science Quarterly, 6*(4), 201-207.

Cowling W.R. (1997). Case study: A pattern appreciation method. In M. Madrid (Ed.), *Patterns of Rogerian Knowing.* New York: National League for Nursing Press.

Ference, H.M. (1986a). The relationship of time experience, creativity traits, differentiation, and human field motion. In V.M. Malinski (Ed.), *Explorations on Martha Rogers' Science of Unitary Human Beings.* Norwalk, CT: Appleton, Century, & Crofts.

Ference, H.M. (1986b). Critique of Rawnsley's study. In V.M. Malinski (Ed.), *Explorations on Martha Rogers' Science of Unitary Human Beings.* Norwalk, CT: Appleton, Century, & Crofts.

Fitzpatrick, J. (1986). Critique of Rawnsley's study. In V.M. Malinski (Ed.), *Explorations on Martha Rogers' Science of Unitary Human Beings.* Norwalk, CT: Appleton, Century, & Crofts.

Gribbin, J. (1998). *The search for superstrings, symmetry, and the theory of everything.* Boston: Little, Brown & Co.

Gueldner, S.H. (1986). The relationship between imposed motion and human field motion in elderly individuals living in nursing homes. In V.M. Malinski (Ed.), *Explorations on Martha Rogers' Science of Unitary Human Beings.* Norwalk, CT: Appleton, Century, & Crofts.

Gueldner, S.H., Bramlett, M.H., Johnston, L., & Guillory, J.A. (1996). Index of Field Energy. *Rogerian Nursing Science News,* 8(4), 6.

Hastings-Tolsma, M. (1996). Diversity of Human Field Pattern Scale. *Rogerian Nursing Science News,* 8(4), 6-7.

Johnston, L.W. (1994). Psychometric analysis of Johnston's Human Field Image Metaphor Scale. *Visions, 2*(1), 7-11.

Johnston, L. Personal Communication. April 28, 1999.

Leddy, S.K. (1995). Measuring mutual process: Development and psychometric testing of the Person-Environment Participation Scale. *Visions, 3*(1), 20-31.

Leddy, S.K. (1996). Development and psychometric testing of the Leddy Healthiness Scale. *Research in Nursing and Health, 19*(5), 431-440.

Leddy, S.K. (1997). Healthiness, fatigue, and symptom experience in breast cancer. *Holistic Nursing Practice, 12*(1), 48-53.

Leddy, S.K. & Fawcett, J. (1997). Testing the theory of healthiness: Conceptual and methodological issues. In M. Madrid (Ed.), *Patterns of Rogerian Knowing*. New York: National League for Nursing.

Leddy, S.K. (1999). Further exploration of the psychometric properties of the Person-Environment Participation Scale: Differentiating instrument reliability and construct stability. *Visions, 7*(1), 55-57.

Malinski, V.M. (1994). Emergence of the Science of Unitary Human Beings. In *Martha E. Rogers: Her life and her work*. Philadelphia: F.A. Davis.

Malinski, V.M. (1997a). The relationship of temporal experience and power as knowing participation in change in depressed and nondepressed women. In M. Madrid (Ed.), *Patterns of Rogerian Knowing*. New York: National League for Nursing.

Malinski, V.M. (1997b). Rogerian health patterning: Evolving into the 21st century. *Nursing Science Quarterly, 10*(3), 115-116.

Malinski, V.M., Phillips, J.R., & Barrett, E.A.M., (1994). *Martha E. Rogers: Her life and her work*. Philadelphia: F.A. Davis.

Matas, K.E. (1997). Human patterning and chronic pain. *Nursing Science Quarterly, 10*(2), 88-96.

McNiff, M. (1997). Power, perceived health, and life satisfaction in adults with long-term care needs. In M. Madrid (Ed.), *Patterns of Rogerian Knowing* New York: National League for Nursing.

Meehan, T.C. (1993). Therapeutic touch and postoperative pain: A Rogerian research study. *Nursing Science Quarterly, 6*(2), 69-78.

Newman, M.A. (1994). *Health as expanding consciousness*. (2nd ed.). New York: National League for Nursing.

Paletta, J.L. (1990). The relationship of temporal experience to human time. In E.A.M Barrett (Ed.), *Visions of Rogers' science-based nursing*. New York: National League for Nursing Press.

Peck, S. (1998). The efficacy of therapeutic touch for improving functional ability in elders with degenerative arthritis. *Nursing Science Quarterly, 11*(3), 123-132.

Phillips, J.R. (1990). Changing Human Potentials and Future Visions of Nursing: A Human Field Image Perspective. In E.A.M. Barrett (Ed.). *Visions of Rogers' science-based nursing*. New York: National League for Nursing Press.

Phillips J.R. (1997). Evolution of the science of unitary human beings. In M. Madrid (Ed.), *Patterns of Rogerian Knowing*. New York: National League for Nursing Press.

Rawnsley, M.M. (1986). The relationship between the perception of the speed of time and the process of dying. In V.M. Malinski (Ed.), *Explorations on Martha Rogers' Science of Unitary Human Beings*. Norwalk, CT: Appleton, Century, & Crofts.

Rawnsley, M.M. (1990). Structuring the gap from conceptual system to research design within a Rogerian worldview. In E.A.M. Barrett (Ed.), *Visions of Rogers' science-based nursing*. New York: National League for Nursing.

Ray, M.A. (1994). Theoretical considerations: Complexity and nursing science. *Nursing Science Quarterly 11*(3), 91-93.

Rogers, M.E. (1961). *Educational revolution in nursing*. New York: Macmillan.

Rogers, M.E. (1970). *An introduction to the theoretical basis of nursing*. Philadelphia: F.A. Davis Co.

Rogers, M.E. (1981). Science of unitary man: a paradigm for nursing. In G.E. Lasker (Ed.), *Applied systems and cybernetics: Systems research in healthcare, biocybernetics, and ecology*. New York: Pergamon Press.

Rogers, M.E. (1988). Nursing science and art: A prospective. *Nursing Science Quarterly, 1*(3), 99-102.

Rogers, M.E. (1990). Nursing: Science of unitary, irreducible, human beings: Update 1990. In E.A.M. Barrett (Ed.), *Visions of Rogers' science-based nursing*. New York: National League for Nursing Press.

Rogers, M.E. (1992a). Nursing science and the space age. *Nursing Science Quarterly, 5*(1), 27-34.

Rogers, M.E. (1992b). Space-age paradigm for new frontiers in nursing. In M.E. Parker (Ed.), *Nursing Theories in Practice*. New York: National League for Nursing Press.

Rogers, M.E. (1994). The Science of Unitary Human Beings: Current perspectives. *Nursing Science Quarterly, 7*(1), 33-35.

Samarel, N. (1992). The experience of receiving therapeutic touch. *Journal of Advanced Nursing, 17*(6), 651-657.

Samarel, N., Fawcett, J., Davis, M., & Ryan, F. (1998). Effects of dialogue and therapeutic touch on preoperative and postoperative experiences of breast cancer surgery: An exploratory study. *Oncology Nursing Forum, 25*(8), 1369-1376.

Sarter, B. (1988). *The stream of becoming: A study of Martha Rogers' theory*. New York: National League for Nursing Press.

Sherman, D.W. (1997). Rogerian science: Opening new frontiers of nursing knowledge through its application in quantitative research. *Nursing Science Quarterly, 10*(3), 131-135.

Smith, D.W. (1995). Power and spirituality in polio survivors: A study based on Rogers' science. *Nursing Science Quarterly, 8*(3), 133-139.

Thomas, S.D. Intentionality in the human-environment encounter in an ambulatory care environment. In E.A.M. Barrett (Ed.), *Visions of Rogers' science-based nursing.* New York: National League for Nursing Press.

Turner, J., Clark, A., Gauthier, D., & Williams, M. (1998). The effect of therapeutic touch on pain and anxiety in burn patients. *Journal of Advanced Nursing, 28*(1), 10-20.

Vicenz, A.E. (1994). Chaos theory and some nursing considerations. *Nursing Science Quarterly 7*(2), 36-42.

Watson, J. (1997). Using Rogers' model to study sleep-wake pattern changes in older women. In M. Madrid (Ed.), *Patterns of Rogerian knowing.* New York: National League for Nursing.

Watson, J. (1999). Measuring dreaming as a beyond waking experience in Rogers' conceptual model. *Nursing Science Quarterly, 12*(3), 245-250.

Watson, J., Barrett, E.A., Hastings-Tolsma, M., Johnston, L., & Gueldner, S. (1997). Measurement in Rogerian science: A review of selected instruments. In M. Madrid, (Ed.), *Patterns of Rogerian knowing.* New York: National League for Nursing Press.

Yarcheski, A. & Mahon, N.E. (1991). An empirical test of Rogers' original and revised theory of correlates in adolescents. *Research in Nursing and Health, 14*(6), 447-455.

Yarcheski, A. & Mahon, N.E. (1995). Rogers' pattern manifestations and health in adolescents. *Western Journal of Nursing Research, 17*(4), 383-397.

Zohar, D. & Marshall, I. (1994). *The quantum society.* New York: Morrow.

Modeling Nursing From Unitary and Existential Perspectives

PARSE'S THEORY of HUMAN BECOMING

*Key Terms*_____

coconstituting, p. 164
cocreating, p. 164
cotranscending, p. 164
human becoming, p. 162
meaning, p. 164
originating, p. 166

powering, p. 166
rhythmicity, p. 164
transcendence, p. 164
transforming, p. 166

Rosemarie Rizzo Parse first introduced her theoretical conceptualization of nursing under the title *Man-Living-Health* (1981), later known as the Theory of Human Becoming. Parse's work proceeds from Rogers' Science of Unitary Human Beings. In her first exposition of the theory, Parse created assumptions about man and health, and she stated principles, concepts, theoretical structures, and an overall schema of the theory (1981) Parse refined the theory in 1992 and 1997 and she renamed her conceptualizations and changed the language of the assumptions to reflect the more inclusive term *human* rather than *man* (Parse, 1997a). In 1992, she developed the Institute of Human Becoming to assist persons in learning and living her theory. Ongoing scholarly work has established and refined the research and practice methodologies. Parse founded and edits the journal *Nursing Science Quarterly*.

THE STARTING POINT OF THE MODELING PROCESS

Parse is a second-generation nursing theorist in that her work clearly extends from Rogers'. It uses the same level of abstraction yet is a theoretical system in its own right. Parse (1997a) called her early work a synthesis of Rogers' principles and concepts with existential-phenomenological tenets and concepts. Parse's early work focuses on health and defines it as "the process of becoming as experienced by a person" (1981, p. 14). The redefined focus is on **Human Becoming,** a "unitary construct referring to the human being's living health" (1997, p. 32). In 1992 and again in 1997, Parse updated the philosophical assumptions and later synthesized them in terms of Human Becoming.

Reason for Theory Development

Parse's theory surfaced over years of her lived experiences and interrelationships. She offered her work as a contribution toward a unique body of nursing knowledge. The Theory of Human Becoming attempts to answer Rogers' questions (see Chapter 6). Noting the limitations of existing perspectives, Parse wanted to "focus on moving with other possibilities for nursing" (1997a, p. 32). She sought a science approach for nursing grounded in the human sciences and "rooted in the belief that humans participate with the universe in the cocreation of health" (Parse, 1992, p. 32).

The Theory of Human Becoming was created as an alternative to traditional natural science nursing in response to the limitations inherent in the totality perspective (Parse, 1981). The totality perspective, Parse contends, includes "viewing human beings as bio-psycho-social-spiritual organisms that interact linearly with the environment. Health is physical, mental, social, and spiritual well-being that human beings strive for through manipulation of the environment" (Fawcett, 1993). In the preface to *Illuminations*, Parse elaborates:

> These limitations were most visible in four major ways:
>
> - The value priorities of the person were subordinated to a set of norms defined by medical science.
> - The nurse, rather than the patient, was considered the expert on health.
> - The meaning of lived experiences was not the focus of nursing; a human science approach had not yet been conceptualized.
> - The potential contributions of nursing as a unique discipline were obfuscated by the natural science approach to research and practice.
>
> As an alternative to traditional, the Human Becoming Theory focuses on the experience of humans as freely choosing beings who cocreate health in mutual process with the universe. The person is respected as the expert on his or her own health, and the meaning of lived experiences is honored. This theory, then, rooted in the human sciences, clearly requires a different approach to research and practice (1997b).

Phenomenon of Concern

The object of Human Becoming Theory is universal human health experiences that surface in the human-universe process and reflect being-becoming, value priorities, and quality of life (Parse, 1992). The central focus of practice is the meaning of lived experiences in enhancing quality of life for unitary human beings. These lived experiences include paradoxical unities—such as certainty-uncertainty, revealing-concealing, enabling-limiting, and connecting-separating—regarded as natural rhythms of life. Nursing's goal is improved quality of life. The primary mode of practice is "true presence," described under Practice in this chapter. The specific concepts of human being and health are defined in the Theory section.

DESCRIPTION OF PARSE'S THEORETICAL SYSTEM

The Theory of Human Becoming includes philosophical and theoretical levels and research and practice methodologies. These elements constitute the theoretical system.

Philosophical Perspectives

Parse describes and categorizes her worldview with the simultaneity paradigm, which is characterized by beliefs that (1) human beings "are synergistic; more than and different from the sum of their parts" and in "mutual rhythmical interchange with the environment, and (2) "[health] is a process of becoming; living a set of value priorities" (Fawcett, 1993, p. 57).

Cody (1995c) identified the goals of nursing within the simultaneity paradigm as "oriented toward quality of life and evolving patterns of living for the person and family" (p. 145). Parse identified the basic themes of the philosophical assumptions of her theory as "meaning, rhythmicity, and transcendence" (1997a, p. 32). Although Parse does not emphasize the Rogerian ideas of nonspatial, nontemporal human and environment energy fields, she does not reject them. Parse is most concerned with the human unity and the meaning humans assign to human-universe-health situations. She describes persons' properties through assumptions and principles. The descriptive properties of persons are expressed through lived experience. The properties described refer to all persons—the nurse as well as the patient.

Existential Phenomenology. In the first published edition of the theory (1981), Parse identified the existential-phenomenological tenets of intentionality and human subjectivity along with concepts of coconstitution, coexistence, and situated freedom. Existential philosophy stresses individual existence, subjectivity, individual freedom, and choice. Phenomenology is concerned with describing human experiences or the objects of experience. Phenomenological methodology is described under the Research section of this chapter. Anyone using Parse's theoretical system to guide research and practice needs to be grounded in this philosophy.

Parse (1981) identified a number of philosophers and theorists in addition to Rogers whose work helped her shape the theory: Heidegger, Sartre, Husserl, and Merleau-Ponty are her predominant influences. The synthesis of their existential concepts with Rogerian principles of helicy, complementarity, and resonancy in addition to concepts of energy field, openness, pattern and organization, and four-dimensionality (now referred to as pandimensionality) resulted in nine philosophical assumptions. Three principles are posited from these assumptions, which in turn give rise to theoretical structures. The essence of Parse's theory is found in the principles, concepts, and theoretical structures (Figure 7-1) and the evolution of the ontology of human becoming (Figure 7-2).

The Language of Human Becoming. The language used within a theoretical system, especially one that proposes a new worldview, must be specific to that theoretical system. Because of the complexity of the language used in Parse's theory, readers should refer to Parse's original writings for clarification. Parse (1997a) noted that the Theory of Human Becoming has created new language for the discipline. The use of the gerund in "Becoming"

Relationship of Principles, Concepts, and Theoretical Structures of Man-Living-Health

Principle 1: Structuring meaning multidimensionally is cocreating reality through the languaging of valuing and imaging.

Principle 2: Cocreating rhythmical patterns of relating is living the paradoxical unity of revealing-concealing and enabling-limiting while connecting-separating.

Principle 3: Cotranscending with the possibles is powering unique ways of originating in the process of transforming.

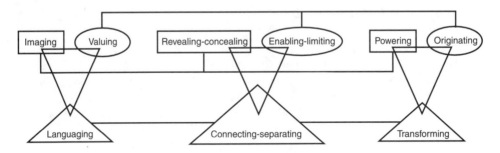

Concepts in the *squares:*
Concepts in the *ovals:*
Concepts in the *triangles:*

Powering emerges with the *revealing-concealing of imaging.*
Originating emerges with the *enabling-limiting of valuing.*
Transforming emerges with the *languaging of connecting-separating.*

FIGURE 7-1   Principles, concepts, and theoretical structure of human becoming. (From Parse, R.R. (1998). *The Human Becoming school of thought.* Thousand Oaks, CA: Sage.)

focuses action in the present. The prefix "co" refers to the mutuality of human life processes. **Cocreating, coconstituting,** and **cotranscending,** like existential phenomenology, describe the experience of the person in the here and now. Existentialists' primary concern is with human existence as distinct from its essence. They examine the reality of being, the nature of the individual. Figure 7-2 depicts the relationship between the Science of Unitary Human Beings and existential phenomenology in the evolution of the theory and science.

Philosophical Level of Parse's Model. Parse synthesized Rogerian and existential-phenomenological concepts and tenets into nine assumptions. The major themes of meaning, rhythmicity, and transcendence are reflected in the assumptions. **Meaning,** according to Parse, refers to the linguistic and imagined content and the interpretation one gives to some thing or event. **Rhythmicity** refers to the "patterning of human-universe mutual process" (Parse, 1998, p. 29). **Transcendence** refers to reaching beyond ordinary limits. Four of these concepts relate to the nature of the human, and five relate to health as a process of becoming. Figure 7-1 includes the philosophical assumptions of the Human Becoming Theory, written at the philosophical level of discourse (Parse, 1997a). These philosophical assumptions were synthesized into three assumptions about human becoming (Parse, 1997a, p. 33):

- Human becoming is freely choosing personal meaning in situation in the intersubjective process of relating value priorities.

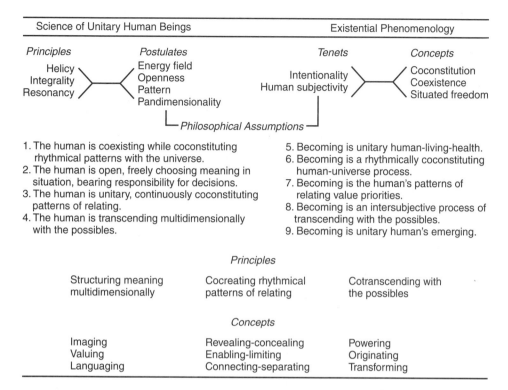

Science of Unitary Human Beings		Existential Phenomenology	
Principles	*Postulates*	*Tenets*	*Concepts*
Helicy Integrality Resonancy	Energy field Openness Pattern Pandimensionality	Intentionality Human subjectivity	Coconstitution Coexistence Situated freedom

Philosophical Assumptions

1. The human is coexisting while coconstituting rhythmical patterns with the universe.
2. The human is open, freely choosing meaning in situation, bearing responsibility for decisions.
3. The human is unitary, continuously coconstituting patterns of relating.
4. The human is transcending multidimensionally with the possibles.

5. Becoming is unitary human-living-health.
6. Becoming is a rhythmically coconstituting human-universe process.
7. Becoming is the human's patterns of relating value priorities.
8. Becoming is an intersubjective process of transcending with the possibles.
9. Becoming is unitary human's emerging.

Principles

Structuring meaning multidimensionally	Cocreating rhythmical patterns of relating	Cotranscending with the possibles

Concepts

Imaging Valuing Languaging	Revealing-concealing Enabling-limiting Connecting-separating	Powering Originating Transforming

FIGURE 7-2 Evolution of the ontology of human becoming. (From Parse, R.R. (1998). *The Human Becoming school of thought.* Thousand Oaks, CA: Sage.)

- Human becoming is cocreating rhythmical patterns of relating in mutual process with the universe.
- Human becoming is cotranscending multidimensionally with the emerging possibles.

Description of Models and Theories

Theoretical Principles. The principles of the theory follow directly from the philosophical assumptions and are written at a theoretical level of discourse. These are (Parse, 1981, p. 69):

- Principle 1. Structuring meaning multidimensionally is cocreating reality through the languaging of valuing and imaging.
- Principle 2. Cocreating rhythmical patterns of relating is living the paradoxical unity of revealing-concealing and enabling-limiting while connecting-separating.
- Principle 3. Cotranscending with the possibles is powering unique ways of originating in the process of transforming

The relationship of these principles to concepts and theoretical structures is shown in Figure 7-1.

Theoretical Structures. Parse's first book (1981) presented schemata that model her conceptualizations. She offered three relationships of concepts that are "nondirectional propositions . . . non-causal in nature . . . and consistent with the assumptions and principles of the theory" (1992, p. 39). These propositions are called theoretical structures. Parse (1992) put these forth to guide research and practice and noted that additional theoretical structures need to be written at lower levels of discourse. These structures—**powering, originating,** and **transforming**—are presented in Figure 7-1. Powering is the "pushing-resisting process" present in all change (Parse, 1998, p. 47). Originating is inventing or creating new ways of living with the paradoxes of daily living. Transforming involves the human-universe process as the human coparticipates in changing in a deliberate way.

RESEARCH DERIVED FROM THE THEORY OF HUMAN BECOMING

Initial investigational techniques for developing Parse's Theory of Human Becoming were qualitative—primarily phenomenological and ethnographic. Support for Parse's theory was bolstered by these qualitative techniques and in 1987 led to a research method directly tied to the theoretical constructs. Parse (1996a, 1997a) now describes her method as a phenomenological and hermeneutic one that values the research participants for sharing their experiences. This approach relies on interpretation to understand lived phenomena. Attention to participant language is important because the researchers translate the participants' responses into the language of science. Parse synthesized the works of Kaplan (1964) with the artistic qualities of "order, design, composition, balance, and harmony" into the following (Parse, 1987, p. 173):

- The methodology is constructed to be in harmony with and evolve from the ontological beliefs of the research tradition.
- The methodology is an overall design of precise processes that adhere to methodological rigor.
- The methodology specifies the order within the processes appropriate for inquiry within the research tradition.
- The methodology is an aesthetic composition with balance in form.

Parse (1997a) considers her research method a mechanism for enhancing the knowledge base for the discipline of nursing. This method provides a different worldview from the traditional natural science perspective and is most congruent with constructivism. The following are additional assumptions that underlie Parse's research method. These assumptions, which regard human beings and their relationship to the human universe, are the following (Parse, 1992, p. 41):

- Humans are open beings in mutual process with the universe. The construct *human being* refers to the human-universe-health process.
- Human becoming is uniquely lived by individuals. People make reflective and prereflective choices in connection with others and the universe, which incarnate their health.
- Descriptions of lived experiences enhance knowledge of human becoming. Individuals and families can describe their own experiences in ways that shed light on the meaning of health.
- Researcher-participant dialogical engagement uncovers the meaning of phenomena as humanly lived. The researcher in true presence with the participant can elicit authentic information about lived experiences.

- The researcher, through inventing, abiding with logic, and adhering to semantic consistency during the extraction-synthesis and heuristic interpretation processes, creates structures of lived experiences and weaves the structure with the theory in ways that enhance the knowledge base of nursing.

These assumptions must be congruent with the research method to result in good science.

The purpose of the Parse method is to uncover "universal lived experiences of health" (Parse, 1994, p. 57). Parse (1997a) suggested that researchers must commit to understanding lived experiences. Phenomena for study are universal health experiences that surface in the human-universe process. Parse (1996a) believes that universal experiences are those that all humans experience and would describe if given an opportunity. These experiences reflect being-becoming, value priorities, and quality of life (Parse, 1997a). Examples Parse (1996a) cites include "hope, joy-sorrow, restriction, freedom, considering tomorrow, persevering through difficulty, grieving, and persisting while wanting to change" (p. 59). The emerging phenomena's structures simultaneously encompass the remembered, the now moment, and the not-yet.

Parse's method of study includes identification of entities for study, scientific processes of investigation, and details of processes appropriate for inquiry (Parse, 1987). Box 7-1 outlines Parse's research method. Specific processes of the method include participant selection, in which persons who live the experience are invited to participate in the study. Invitees give authentic accounts and engage in dialogue. Dialogical engagement follows participant selection. This involves researcher-participant discussion in which the researcher is "truly present" with the participant (Parse, 1987). Dialogues are unstructured; the direction emerges from the nature and structure of the participant's lived experience. Many types of media describing the phenomenon of study—including words, drawings, metaphors, photographs, music, and movement—can be incorporated into dialogues (Parse, 1997a). Dialogical engagement is a unique method of eliciting descriptions from participants.

BOX 7-1

Processes of Parse's Research Method

- Participant selection
- Dialogical engagement
- Extraction synthesis
  - Extracted from participant's language
  - Written in researcher's language
  - Propositions formulated from participant's essences
  - Core concepts extracted and synthesized
  - Structure of experience synthesized
- Heuristic interpretation
  - Structural integration
  - Conceptual interpretation

From Parse, R.R. (1987). *Nursing science: Major paradigms, theories, and critiques*. Philadelphia: W.B. Saunders.

Extraction-synthesis permits the researcher to move from participant description to a conceptualization of phenomena in scientific language. Dialogues are tape-recorded and transcribed, permitting the researcher to dwell on the experience. Dwelling is the process of reflecting on the information participants shared. It allows the investigator to become thoroughly familiar with the information shared. Five steps occur in extraction-synthesis process:

1. Essences or expressions of a core idea stated in the participant's language are extracted from the transcriptions.
2. The researcher synthesizes the essences, trying to capture the basic nature of the participant-described phenomenon, and then puts the description in scientific language that allows other professionals to easily understand it.
3. For each participant's description, a joining nondirectional statement or proposition is formulated
4. Concepts from the formulated propositions are extracted in order to capture the central meaning of the propositions.
5. Researchers synthesize the structure of the lived experience by developing a statement that conceptualizes the core concepts and answers the research question.

Heuristic interpretation is a structural and conceptual integration of propositions connected to the structure of the theory. Heuristic interpretation is an analytical process that involves careful examination and abstraction in which the structure of the lived experience is interpreted in light of Human Becoming Theory. This interpretative process "weaves the ideas of the structure as lived into the theory and propels it to posit ideas for research studies and possible practice activities" (Parse, 1987, p. 177).

An excellent example of the explicit steps of a research study using Parse's research method is her study of laughing and health (Parse, 1994). Essences were extracted from each individual discussion. For example, one participant said, "Well, I feel usually if I laugh, I'm happy. Even if it is just for a while, you know. Joy. And I think whatever my ache or pain is, it goes away." (Parse, 1994, p. 59). Parse's extracted statement read, "the participant laughs a lot and finds it a joy to laugh since it makes her feel good; it takes away her aches and pains and gives her a lift when she's down" (Parse, 1994, p. 59). From this extracted essence Parse drew a synthesized essence, which stated that "frequent mirthful episodes with personal delight foster contentment deflecting suffering while lightening burdens" (p. 59). The formulation of the composite is: "The lived experience of laughing and health is delightful contentment arising through frequent mirthful engagements deflecting suffering while lightening burdens" (p. 59). Once propositions were formulated for all participant essences, Parse extracted core concepts for the study.

In this study, three core concepts associated with laughing and health included "a buoyant vitality," "mirthful engagements prompting an unburdening delight deflecting disheartenments," and "emerging in blissful contentment" (p. 61). In the heuristic interpretation, for the structured concept "a buoyant vitality," Parse identified the structural integration as "exuberant exhilaration" and the conceptual interpretation as "languaging the enabling-limiting of powering" (p. 61). Structural and conceptual integrations were completed for each structural concept. The final structural statement regarding the interconnectedness of laughing and health was "laughing and health is a potent buoyant vitality sparked through mirthful engagements, prompting an unburdening delight deflecting disheartenments while emerging with blissful contentment" (p. 59).

Review of Related Research

Research using the Human Becoming Theory is predominately qualitative. Most recent studies specifically use Parse's research method. Research studies engage diverse age-groups, but older adults have been the focus of many studies. Research topics center around what Parse would describe as universal human experiences: laughter, joy, grieving, quality of life and suffering, aging, living with illness, homelessness, and workplace issues. Table 7-1 summarizes selected research studies using Parse's Theory of Human Becoming.

Laughter/Joy-Sorrow. Parse conducted several studies of laughter and health. The first was a phenomenological study that used van Kaam's method to study descriptions of laughter by 30 people over age 65. Parse (1993) found many similarities in descriptions of laughing and discovered that participants related laughing and health. The structural definition of laughing that emerged from this study was a "buoyant immersion in the presence of unanticipated glimpsings promoting harmonious integrity, which surfaces anew through contemplative visioning (Parse, 1993, p. 41). In a subsequent study, Parse (1994) used her research method to further the understanding of the interconnectedness between laughing and health for individuals age 65 and over, and she connected her findings to the Human Becoming Theory. Language used to describe laughter included "potent buoyant vitality" that reflected joy and exhilaration (p. 59). "Mirthful engagements prompting an unburdening delight deflecting disheartenments" resonated with Parse's concept of connecting-separating in transforming imaging (p. 60). The process was perceived as rhythmical, "being with," and paradoxical in that it involves both delight and disheartenment. The concept "emerging with blissful contentment" was identified as a product of laughter associated with health (p. 61). In these two studies, health was not conceived as a process of disease or its absence but rather as a process of becoming in which values emerge and change. Laughing provided a way of becoming in the moment and in that way is relevant to health. Parse (1994) suggested that "buoyant vitality" is the energy of health and that contentment is a "plenitude of health" that arises through mirth (p. 62). This concept supports the Human Becoming Theory. Further investigation into concepts of "buoyant vitality" or "blissful contentment" could be promising. New dimensions of understanding could offer unique insights about nurse-patient engagement.

Examining a different but related phenomenon, Parse (1997c) investigated the paradoxical structure of joy/sorrow in women over age 65. Core concepts of "pleasure amid adversity" represent patterns of transforming imaging (p. 84). "Cherished contentment" reflects treasuring or valuing, which reflects a sense of satisfaction with accomplishments (p. 85). "Benevolent engagement" represents connecting-separating with family, friends, and strangers. Experiences of joy-sorrow consist of the ups and downs of everyday living. In this study, joy and sorrow were found to be a pattern of health with a paradoxical rhythm of ups and downs cocreated in the process of the human-universe. This supports Human Becoming Theory's concept of paradoxical processes. Identified core concepts warrant further investigation to increase insights into these universal lived experiences.

Text continued on p. 176

TABLE 7-1

Selected Studies Based on Parse's Theory of Human Becoming

Study/Year	Purpose	Methods	Findings
LAUGHTER Parse, 1993	The study uncovered structural definition of laughing in persons over age 65.	Thirty men and women over age 65 wrote descriptions of laughing and all of their thoughts and feelings associated with the experience. Their descriptions were analyzed with van Kaam's phenomenological method.	Four common elements emerged: buoyant immersion, harmonious integrity, contemplative visioning, and unanticipated glimpsings. Synthesis of the final definition of laughing was "buoyant immersion in the presence of unanticipated glimpsings, prompting harmonious integrity which surfaces anew in contemplative visioning" (p. 41).
Parse, 1994	The study uncovered the structure of lived experience of laughing and health.	Twenty men and women over age 65 participated in a dialogical engagement about the experience of laughing and health.	"The lived experience of laughing and health was a potent buoyant vitality sparked through mirthful engagements, prompting an unburdening delight deflecting disheartenments while emerging with blissful contentment" (p. 58).
JOY-SORROW Parse, 1997c	The study uncovered the structure of joy-sorrow in women over age 65.	Eleven women over 65 years of age engaged in audiotaped and videotaped dialogues about joy-sorrow.	Joy-sorrow is "pleasure amid adversity emerging in the cherished contentment of benevolent engagements" (p. 84).
GRIEVING Cody, 1991	The study generated a structure of the lived experience of grieving a personal loss.	Using the process of dialogical engagement, four participants described experiences with personal losses.	Grieving a personal loss is "intense struggling in the flux of change, while a shifting view fosters moving beyond the now, as different possibilities surface in dwelling with and apart from the absent presence and others in light of what is cherished" (p. 64).

Cody, 1995a, 1995b	The study specifically investigated the structure of grieving for families living with AIDS.	Ten families participated in dialogical engagement to describe their experiences of grieving. The families were diverse and included gay male couples, a husband and wife, and a male and female partner, and daughters, companions, sisters, and brothers.	Four concepts were explicated: easing-intensifying with the flux of change, bearing witness to aloneness with togetherness, possibilities emerging with ambiguity, and confirming realms of endearment.
SERENITY			
Kruse, 1999	The study investigated the meaning of serenity for survivors of life-threatening illness.	Ten cancer survivors described the meaning of serenity in their lives. Parse's research method and photos were used to facilitate description of serenity.	The four extracted concepts included steering-yielding with the flow, savoring remembered visions of engaging surroundings, abiding with aloneness-togetherness, and attesting to a loving presence.
QUALITY OF LIFE/SUFFERING			
Allchin-Petardi, 1998	The study described perservering through ovarian cancer.	Parse's research method was used with eight women with ovarian cancer who described the concept of perserving.	The three core concepts included deliberately persisting, propelling fortitude, and powering valuing.
Carson and Mitchell, 1998	The study investigated the experience of living with persistent pain.	Seventeen participants offered narratives regarding their experiences.	Three themes emerged: forbearance surfaces with the drain of persistent anguish; isolating retreats coexist with comforting engagements; and hope for relief clarifies priorities for daily living.
Daly, 1995	The study explored the experience of suffering.	Nine participants participated in dialogical engagement to describe their experience of suffering.	Suffering is "paralyzing" anguish with glimpses of precious possibilities emerging with entanglements of engaging-disengaging while struggling in pursuit of fortification" (p. 253).

Continued

TABLE 7-1

Selected Studies Based on Parse's Theory of Human Becoming—cont'd

Study/Year	Purpose	Methods	Findings
QUALITY OF LIFE/SUFFERING—cont'd			
Fisher and Mitchell, 1998	This qualitative study examined the quality of life of inpatients receiving psychiatric care.	Twenty-four psychiatric inpatients participated in semistructured interviews. Interviews were analyzed by tape review, thematic identification, and consideration of theoretical framework and literature.	Three major themes emerged: reflective moments illuminate shifting priorities (remembering how things used to be); upset and calm change patterns of being with and apart from others (sense of discomfort in relationships); and distant hopes fuel the relentless struggle to carry on (reflects relentless struggle to carry on).
Parse, 1996a	The study explored the meaning of quality of life for person's living with Alzheimer's disease.	Five men and 20 women with beginning or moderate Alzheimer's disease shared the meanings of their quality of life.	Quality of life for Alzheimer's patients was found to be a "contentment with the remembered and now affiliations that arises amidst the tedium of the commonplace, as an easy-uneasy flow of transfiguring surfaces with liberating possibilities and confining constraints, while desiring cherished intimacies yields with inevitable distancing in the vicissitudes of life, as contemplating the ambiguity of the possible emerges with yearning for successes in the moment" (p. 130).
Baumann, 1994	The study explored the experiences of mothers and children who were homeless.	An exploratory, descriptive design guided discussions of 13 mothers and 25 children living in two shelters. Open-ended questions were used to explore the meaning of not having a place of their own, the unfolding of relationships, and changing views of possibility.	Meaning of not having a place of one's own was "a sense of gratitude for protection, mingling with the discomfort of restriction and exposure, giving rise to fears and reassurances as detachment from cherished others surfaces discordance with unfamiliar patterns, while novel engagements bring pleasure as insights and struggles surface new possibles as well as disillusionment" (p. 165).

Continued

Baumann, 1996	The study explored the concept of "feeling uncomfortable" as experienced by children with no place of their own.	Parse's research methodology was used to explore experiences of 16 homeless children 4 to 16 years of age. Dialogical engagement provided a format for unstructured sessions.	The central finding was feeling that being uncomfortable was "a disturbing uneasiness with the unsureness of aloneness with togetherness amidst longing for personal joyful moments" (p. 153).
AGING Mitchell, 1995	The study generated a description of the meaning of restriction-freedom in older persons.	Twelve persons 75 to 92 years of age participated in dialogical engagement to describe their experiences of restriction-freedom.	"The lived experience of restriction-freedom in later life is anticipating limitations amidst unencumbered self-direction as yielding to change fortifies resolve for moving beyond" (p. 171).
Futrell, Wondolowski, and Mitchell, 1993	The study elicited a structural definition of aging from the oldest older adults living in Scotland.	One hundred elders living in Scotland participated in interviews regarding the meaning of aging. Data collection and analysis were guided by van Kaam's steps of phenomenological analysis.	The meaning of aging was "intensifying engagements as transfigurations signify maturity tempering the unavoidable with buoyant serenity" (p. 191).
Gates, 2000	The study uncovered the meaning of caring for an elderly relative.	Nine middle-aged and older individuals were interviewed regarding their experiencing of caring for a loved one. Interviews were analyzed using van Kaam's method of phenomenological analysis.	Five common themes were discovered: poignant remembering (offered a historical context), dogged continuing (effort and endurance of situation), nurturant giving and confirmatory receiving (caring for others contributes to quality of life), swells of enjoyment and tides of sorrow (moments that break routine as opposed to day-to-day routine), and uplifting togetherness and valleys of aloneness (connectedness to cared for loved one or to others despite sense of isolation from desired activities).
Mitchell, 1994a	The study uncovered the meaning of being an elder.	Six hundred narrative stories written by Canadians on personal experiences in later life were analyzed using van Kaam's phenomenological method. Analysis was completed from the 5000 descriptive expressions.	A structural definition being a senior was "engaging the now while rolling with the vicissitudes of life as refined astuteness surfaces a buoyant unburdening. It is as though shifting rhythms propel discovery through grateful abiding in wondering awareness as anticipation of new possibles enlivens connectedness and altruistic commitments affirm self amidst the retrospective pondering of everyday" (p. 74).

TABLE 7-1

Selected Studies Based on Parse's Theory of Human Becoming—cont'd

Study/Year	Purpose	Methods	Findings
AGING—cont'd			
Rendon, Sales, Leal, Piqué, 1995	The study explored the experience of aging of community-dwelling elders living in Valencia, Spain.	van Kaam's phenomenological method was used to study nine community-dwelling elders regarding their lived experience of aging.	Aging for community dwelling elders was "confirming triumphs through the forceful enlivening of bridled potency" (p. 154).
Jonas, 1992	The study explored the meaning of being an elder in Nepal.	Twenty-five individuals were interviewed about the meaning of being an older adult in Nepal.	The meaning of being and older adult in Nepal is "cherishing necessities for survival intermingles with the rapture of celebration with important others, as diminishing familiar patterns expand moments of respite, while regard from others affirms self and changing customs create comfort-discomfort as what-was unfolds into new possibles" (p. 174).
Davis and Cannava, 1995	The study explored the meaning of retirement for older persons who were performing artists and now living in Italy.	A descriptive, exploratory method was used to interview eight artists regarding their experiences following retirement from the performing arts.	Retirement of performing artists was the "emerging of an unburdening lightness as esthetic interconnections surface the was and will-be in the now moment as the diversity of everydayness enlivens through communion-solitude while anticipating the transposing vistas of the inevitable prompts treasuring the now in confirming a perpetual artistic legacy" (p. 13).

WORKPLACE

Mitchell and Heidt, 1994	The study generated the structure of the experience of wanting to help another.	Eight nurses who incorporated nontraditional modalities (therapeutic touch) participated in dialogical engagement about their desire to help.	The experience of wanting to help another was "directing intentions to nurture amidst uplifting affirmations with others while dissonant constraints unfold new possibilities" (p. 123).
Janes and Wells, 1997	The study described experiences of caring by nurses using Human Becoming Theory as a basis for practice.	A phenomenological approach guided 10 interviews with persons age 65 years or older who were hospitalized for medical problems. Colaizzi's method for protocol analysis was used to analyze data.	Emerging themes included coming together around instrumental tasks, nurses being there for patients, and nurse's pleasing way. Experience of relating to nurses invoked "feelings of being both cared for and looked after: One will not be neglected or abandoned, or will one be treated with anything less that human kindness and respect" (p. 217).
Northrup and Cody, 1998	The study described changes following implementation of Parse's Theory of Human Becoming in a psychiatric setting.	A descriptive, qualitative method was used to discover changes on three acute-care psychiatric units that adopted Human Becoming Theory as a basis for practice. Interviews with nurses, patients, unit managers, and hospital supervisors were conducted preimplementation, midimplementation, and postimplementation. Written questionnaires were also completed by nurses, unit managers, and supervisors. Chart audits were completed at each of the three data collection points.	Preimplementation nurse interviews focused on techniques of care and functional status of clients. Therapeutic intervention was aimed at control and shaping more desirable behavior. Themes changed by midinterview and postinterview. Care became more person-focused rather than problem-focused. Listening habits changed as nurses became more comfortable with permitting patients to set the tone. Topics for discussion shifted to those the patient selected. Job satisfaction improved as nurses became more committed to applying the theory.

Grieving. Using Parse's research method, Cody (1991) described another universal phenomenon—grieving. Cody found that the structure of personal grieving was characterized by four core concepts. "Intense struggling in the flux of change" incorporated confrontation of personal mortality, struggling toward possibility, affirming self, and easing and intensifying of immobilizing agony (p. 64). The "shifting view that fosters moving beyond now" reflected transformation and the rise of a new view or sense of self (p. 65). "Dwelling with and apart from the absent presence and others" represented connecting-separating where there was simultaneous involvement and noninvolvement with the absent presence and others (p. 64). "Different possibilities surfacing in light of what is cherished" demonstrated valuing of choices and possibilities. The structure of grieving Cody described is congruent with Parse's principle of cotranscendence, in which power can provide unique mechanisms for transforming. Findings indicate that grief is an ongoing process of being and becoming in which individuals, while living among others and cherishing involvements, move forward toward a new perspective. Further study on the grief of the dying or on grief unrelated to death could be explored with Parse's theory.

Broadening his study of personal grieving, Cody (1995a, 1995b) examined grieving in families living with Autoimmune Deficiency Syndrome (AIDS). "Easing and intensifying with the flux of change" represented a multidimensional process in which families handled both welcome and unwelcome change (p. 108). "Bearing witness to aloneness with to-getherness" reflected the connections within grieving families and the options of living with and apart from one another (p. 108). "Possibilities emerging without ambiguity" exemplified the paths chosen in grieving from multiple possibilities in light of complex relationships (p. 108). Finally, "confirming realms of endearment" embodied the concept of valuing what mattered in terms of grief and the meaning of the loss itself (p. 108).

This was the first study to use Parse's research method for families rather than individuals. Structuring meaning through mutual reflection of cherished images, an aspect of Parse's concept of cocreating reality, lends credence to Human Becoming Theory. Moreover, HIV families, who live in the presence of others' grief while experiencing personal loss, demonstrated cocreated rhythmical patterns of living in paradoxical unity. The struggles and joys of these families led to transformations. All of these factors provide support for Parse's theory. Areas of suggested study include examining experiences of being with and apart from loved ones, doing the best in an impossible situation, and bearing witness to suffering.

Serenity. Kruse (1999) documented ovarian cancer survivors' descriptions of serenity. Photographs were used to enhance the descriptions of serenity. The resulting structural statement was "steering-yielding with the flow arising with savoring remembered visions of engaging surroundings, as abiding with aloneness-togetherness attests to a loving presence" (p. 147). The concept of serenity incorporates powering, a fundamental process in which self-affirmation allows cancer patients to let go and move with the flow while still focusing on important life aspects. Serenity for these cancer patients also reflected connecting-separating, in which patients spoke of being alone and together with others. Kruse suggested that this concept of serenity can guide practitioners in the nurse-to-person process for patients experiencing a life-threatening illness.

Quality of Life and Suffering. Quality of life was another phenomenon investigated with Parse's research method (Parse, 1996b). In a study of Alzheimer's patients, four themes supported Parse's concept of paradoxical rhythms. "Contentment with the remembered and now affiliations arises amidst the tedium of the commonplace" encompassed Alzheimer's patients' lives now as compared to their lives in the past (p. 130). The "easy-uneasy flow of transfiguring surfaces with liberating possibilities and confining constraints" represented the sometimes smooth, sometimes difficult changing patterns of living (p. 108). "Desiring cherished intimacies yields with inevitable distancing in the vicissitudes of life" recognized the wish for family closeness but acceptance of being apart (p. 108). Finally, "contemplating the ambiguity of the possibles emerges with yearning for successes in the moment" reflected participants' consideration of their futures (p. 108).

In a different setting, Fisher and Mitchell (1998) conducted a qualitative study focusing on the quality of life of psychiatric inpatients. This study supported Parse's suggestion that humans have unique realities. Mental inpatients expressed these realities through their shifting priorities with day-to-day life changes. Reflecting on the past and present with changing relationships offered both comfort and discomfort. Struggles in relationships could be both upsetting and calming and thus exhibited a paradoxical rhythm. Parse's concepts of transforming, originating, and powering were supported in patient descriptions of perservering in hopes of improving their situations. Fisher and Mitchell suggest that nurses can facilitate patient exploration of meaning, relationships, and hopes through a participatory practice in which nurses are truly present with patients.

Suffering is closely connected to the concept of quality of life. Daly (1995) identified three core concepts associated with suffering: (1) "paralyzing anguish with glimpses of possibility," (2) "entanglements of engaging-disengaging," and (3) "struggling in pursuit of fortification" (p. 253). These concepts discern the anguish of suffering from the positive aspects of individuals' lives. Possibilities remained even in the face of suffering. These concepts reflected the valuing, connecting-separating, and powering posited in Human Becoming Theory.

Allchin-Petardi (1998) examined a concept related to suffering—women's perseverance during ovarian cancer. Persevering through a difficult time was described as "deliberately persisting with significant engagements while shifting life patterns" (p. 174). In the conceptual integration, persevering was described as "powering valuing in the connecting-separating of originating" (p. 174). Powering was reflected in participants' forging ahead in spite of diagnosis and treatment and in reflecting and acting on values. Parse's connecting-separating was evidenced by moving toward support systems found in significant relationships and away from relationships or engagements perceived to be unsupportive. Shifting life patterns reflected Parse's "will-be with the now" concept, in which participants choose to live in new ways. This research expanded insights about the concept of perseverance, a concept that needs further description. Perseverance is not merely persisting but involves significant human engagements.

Carson and Mitchell (1998) studied patients who live with persistent pain. The persistent anguish of pain was generated by physical symptoms and reflected the individual lived realities of the sufferers. The concept of isolating retreats while also participating in comforting engagements reflects Parse's paradoxical rhythm of connecting and separating as well as revealing and concealing their pain from others. Hope for relief exemplifies Parse's suggestion of transcendence, in which participants thought about and remembered being pain-free. Parse's concept of powering is found in the personal strategies used to obtain relief. This study provided insight into lives of people experiencing chronic pain. Further research could examine the ways in which these individuals conduct themselves in terms of disclosure and obtaining pain relief.

Homelessness. Two studies by Baumann (1994, 1996) explored homelessness. In the 1994 study of mothers and children, displacement and moving to a shelter was agonizing but was preferred over being on the streets. Participants were relieved at being in a shelter but frustrated with not getting out. Residential displacement, relocation, and shelter policies were found to disconnect family members from themselves and others. Families expressed possibilities through dreams for the future. However, some felt that dreams were squelched by Social Services. Learning about self generated other possibilities. Powering as described by Human Becoming Theory occurred as mothers attempted to maintain control. Originating, another focus of Parse's theory, was evidenced as new shelter relationships developed. Transforming was exhibited as familiar ways of being were influenced by new insights and awareness. This study uncovered important aspects of living without a place of one's own. These aspects, including experiencing and creating freedom, dignity, and privacy, and mothers' desires not to burden others, should be further investigated.

Baumann's 1996 study focused on homeless children and their sense of feeling uncomfortable. A unique characteristic of the dialogical engagement was the use of drawings to explain the concept of feeling uncomfortable. Three core concepts included "disturbing uneasiness" which reflected an explicit tacit knowing of being uncomfortable (pp. 154-155). The "unsureness of aloneness" exemplified the ambiguity experienced with destructive caring and uncaring engagements and losses (p. 156). "Longing for personal joyful moments" mirrored yearning and also reflected ways children could affirm themselves. Feeling uncomfortable was found to be paradoxical and powerful. These concepts support Parse's Theory of Human Becoming with unsureness of aloneness reflecting connecting-separating, and longing for personal joyful moments exemplifying yearning for lightness that is a part of powering. This research could be expanded by further exploring identified core concepts.

Aging. In addition to Parse's laughter studies with persons age 65 and over, several other studies investigated aging. Some used phenomenological methods, and some used Parse's research method. In a study on the restriction of freedom in older adults, Mitchell (1995) identified core concepts related to anticipating limitations, having unencumbered self-direction, and yielding to change as a fortification of resolve to move beyond. These concepts and description provided a sense of how older adults learned to live with change by adjusting. They felt restricted by loss of activities but enabled by the choice to change. This study generated concepts related to languaging, valuing, and imaging; the paradoxical nature of the human-universe relationship; and powering, originating, and transforming as posited by the Theory of Human Becoming. Suggested research directions include exploring turbulent times, seeing things in a new light, feeling free to pursue dreams, looking to the future, getting involved in something new, feeling good about helping others, and recalling special memories.

Some aging studies have provided a crosscultural perspectives. Futrell, Wondolowski, and Mitchell (1993) studied 100 of the oldest residents of Scotland and found that the meaning of aging was best described as "intensifying engagements as transfigurations signify maturity tempering the unavoidable with buoyant serenity" (p. 191). Mitchell's study (1994a) of 600 narratives written by Canadians revealed some common elements, including the intensifying engagements which were propelled by an energy and enthusiasm found in later life. The concept of buoyancy found in the Futrell, Wondolowski, and Mitchell study (1993) is similar to Mitchell's findings. Courage, understanding, and strength are important characteristics. Anticipation of possibles was important in accounting of both studies. Future research should be directed toward how attitudes shape experience in later life and how those attitudes are chosen. Exploration of how transfigurations influence health would also provide valuable information in working with elders.

Rendon, Sales, Leal, and Piqué (1995) studied older adults living in Valencia, Spain and found that elders described triumphs in living but also experienced the paradox of being limited while remaining vital and alive. A sustaining resolve to move forward reflected elements of strength and courage congruent with other studies. In this study, confirming triumphs is linked to Parse's principle of valuing; bridled potency reflects rhythmicity; and the paradox of revealing and concealing while connecting/separating and forceful enlivening reflects powering.

Nepalese older adults also described the paradox of aging (Jonas, 1992). For these elders, paradoxes emerged in terms of possibility and limitation, changing customs but having a sense of cultural loss, and rejoicing in celebrations while struggling with day-to-day life.

Davis and Cannava (1995) studied a special segment of older adulthood—retired performing artists living in a retirement community. Once again paradoxical themes emerged with concern over losses but the presence of new possibilities. The retired performers feared losing themselves as they gave up performing but discovered new interests in passing on an artistic legacy. Compared to descriptions of other older adult groups, this was a unique manifestation of the paradoxes of aging.

Gates (2000) explored the experience of caring for an elderly loved one. Thematic findings provided insight into the experience of caregiving and support for Parse's Theory of Human Becoming. Memories were a way of providing history and constructing individual meaning for caregiving. The endurance required for providing long-term caregiving reflects the concept of powering. Cotranscending was exemplified in the nurturant giving, and cocreating was reflected in the paradoxical rhythm of the joy and sorrows embedded in care giving and in the sense of togetherness and isolation of missed activities. This study helps to provide a view of caregiving embedded within the concept of human becoming.

Workplace. Parse's theory has provided a frame of reference for practice issues. Mitchell and Heidt (1994) explored the phenomenon of wanting to help another with eight nurses who used therapeutic touch. The first concept, "directing intentions to nurture," represented choosing ways of being in the helping process and shepherding others (p. 123). Participants had longstanding desires to help. "Uplifting affirmations with others" depicted the learning, changing, and connecting that occurred in the helping process (p. 124). This aspect was cherished or valued by participants. "Dissonant constraints unfold into new possibilities" reflected the constraint of wanting to help but not being able to. However, new possibilities emerged even amidst limitations. These findings support Parse's principles regarding meaning, rhythmicity, and transcendence. Findings provide insight into the nature of nurse-person relationships and the outcomes of living in true presence with others.

Janes and Wells (1997) examined older adult experiences of receiving care from nurses who used the Theory of Human Becoming. Nurses on a medical unit that had adopted Parse's theory as a guide for practice 3 years before the patient interviews. Patients felt cared for and treated with kindness and respect. Although time with nurses was driven by the completion of instrumental tasks, extra attention enhanced the hospital experience. Patients appreciated the accessibility of the nurses and believed nurses were committed to meeting their needs. The value of Human Becoming Theory was confirmed in that patients felt their values as human beings were confirmed in their relationships with nurses.

Northrup and Cody (1998) evaluated the influence of using Human Becoming Theory on three acute-care psychiatric units. Their qualitative interviews, questionnaires, and chart audits began before implementation of Human Becoming Theory as a basis for practice and continued at the midpoint and after implementation. On some units, investigators found dramatic shifts in perspectives from nurses who adopted the theory's tenets. Patients were viewed as people rather than problems, and nurses valued patient perspectives in planning care. Patients found nurses to be more available and respectful of their views. Managers reported that job satisfaction and personal transformations were enhanced. Investigators recommended that successful implementation of Human Becoming Theory in practice include an on-site facilitator familiar with the theory, allocation of sufficient resources for learning, management endorsement of the theory, and administrative support for continued education.

Research Summary. Studies demonstrate support for the Human Becoming Theory. Concepts related to Parse's principles have been demonstrated in several studies. It should be noted that at this time, the number of studies remains relatively small. A strength of Parse's research method is that data analysis is systematically guided, since a critical feature of any qualitative research is evidence of systematic analysis. Each of the study reports using Parse's research method presents data from each step of analysis and conclusions in the form of extracted essences and then propositions for each participant. Core concepts and then heuristic analysis is presented. Evidence supporting findings is consistently and clearly delineated. The descriptive nature of the study findings can generate further research and provide insight into the nature of universal lived experiences.

Whenever a theorist conducts research to support his or her theory, potential bias presents a difficulty. Having the theory's preconceptions tied so closely to the processes of data collection and analysis may sway interpretation of findings. Chinn (1995) pointed out that theory potentially serves as a barrier to discovery when it obscures an investigator's ability to recognize new possibilities. Although the concept of dialogical-engagement encourages participants to reveal their experiences, the lenses through which findings are interpreted are invested heavily in the perspectives derived from the Theory of Human Becoming. From this perspective, discovery may be limited. Finally, while description is illuminating and can offer valuable insight for practice, it does not provide a basis for demonstrating outcomes of interventions beyond a descriptive level. This is a potentially limiting factor in testing interventions based on Human Becoming Theory.

PRAXIS AND THEORY UTILIZATION: DESIGNING NURSING PRACTICE PROGRAMS WITHIN THE HUMAN BECOMING SCHOOL OF THOUGHT

Parse (1998) described the linking between theory, research, practice, and education as a sequence including philosophical assumption, conceptual system, theory development, and scholarly research. The findings of the research are linked back to the conceptual system and frame of reference with implications for theory development, further research, and practice. This in turn leads to an expansion of the body of nursing knowledge. Thus theory, research, practice and education are interrelated, which is essential to the development of nursing science and nursing knowledge.

The Variables of Concern for Practice

The variables of concern for practice within the Human Becoming school of thought are process variables as reflected in the language of the theory: *cocreating, coconstituting, cotranscending*. Parse's writings provide a complete description of the meaning of the variables.

Describing a Population for Nursing Purposes

Describing a population for nursing purposes precedes designing nursing for groups of people. No patient population descriptions within the perspective of the Human Becoming school of thought were found in the literature that was reviewed.

Expected Outcomes

The term *expected outcomes* does not fit well with the Human Becoming Theory (Mitchell, 1998). The goal of the discipline of nursing is quality of life, and the goal of the nurse is "to be truly present with people as they enhance their quality of life" (Parse, 1998, p. 68). Nurse-patient interaction should achieve the plans, goals, and priorities for change in personal patterns of knowing. Only the person living the life can describe quality of life. Therefore there is no standard against which to measure quality of life, and such measurement is not consistent with this theory.

Process Models

Parse refers to a practice methodology rather than to the nursing process. The methodology includes illuminating, synchronizing rhythms, and mobilizing transcendence (Box 7-2). Note that Parse does not refer to a nursing diagnosis or patient problems. The knowledge and capabilities beneath these processes need to be specified, and education programs for practicing nurses need to be developed. At present, the richest sources of information are case studies, reports of research in the literature, and Parse's own writings.

   Within the Human Becoming school of thought, the goal of nursing is being "truly present with people as they enhance their quality of life" (Parse, 1998, p. 69). Parse describes

---

BOX 7-2

Practice Methodology Proposed by Parse

1. Illuminating meaning is explicating what was, is, and will be. Explicating is making clear what is appearing now through languaging.
2. Synchronizing rhythms is dwelling with the pitch, yaw, and roll of the human-universe process. Dwelling with is immersing with the flow of connecting-separating.
3. Mobilizing transcendence is moving beyond the meaning moment with what is not yet. Moving beyond is propelling with envisioned possibles of transforming.

From Parse, R.R. (1998). *The Human Becoming school of thought*. Thousand Oaks, CA: Sage.

the processes related to true presence and ways of changing health in true presence as being achieved through the following actions:

- Preparation
- Focused attention on the moment at hand
- Face-to-face discussion
- Silent immersion
- Lingering presence

Changing health occurs through the following:

- Creative imagining of particular changes to a situation
- Affirming personal becoming
- Recognizing the paradoxical

Mitchell (1998) describes the process, developed by the nurses at Sunnybrook Hospital in Toronto, Canada, for guiding practice from the perspective of the Theory of Human Becoming (Box 7-3). Dialogue is the essence of this process. As with the traditional nursing process, consideration of the person's lived experiences as problems to be solved has no place in this methodology (Mitchell, 1991). Rather, determining a nursing diagnosis creates an ethical dilemma for nurses practicing from this perspective as "the process of labeling is the exercise of power over another which sets the stage for human suffering" (Mitchell, 1991, p. 100). In Box 7-3, note the strong emphasis on listening, clarifying, addressing the patient's/family's concerns, discussing options, and being nonjudgmental. Mitchell, Bernardo, and Bournes (1997) relate patient views about encounters with nurses practicing from the perspective of Human Becoming, in which the healing nurse-person relationship is the essence of practice. The goal of nursing is enhancing quality of life for the patient. This is manifested in nurses' accommodating patients' wishes for variations in treatment regimens and schedules. Nurses helped patients make decisions, and patients felt they were treated as human beings. Nurses listened to and respected patients and did not judge them.

BOX 7-3

Dialogue as the Essence of Nursing Practice

1. Initiate discussions to clarify issues, concern, and wishes as expressed by patient/families. Seek depth about the person's particular wishes for care and information. Focus on the individual's/family's personal meaning and views of life.
2. Clarify the meanings, concerns, and priorities individuals want to discuss or change.
3. Discuss options, alternatives, and anticipated consequences as seen by the person. Create open, honest, nonjudgmental engagements.
4. Record descriptions of changing life situations as described by persons and groups. Record staff activities that support the person's wishes for change and care. Record how individuals evaluate healthcare and how they view progression toward their desired health and quality of life.

From Mitchell, G.J. (1998). Standards of nursing and the winds of change. *Nursing Science Quarterly, 11*(3), 97-98.

Descriptions of practice situations in the literature focus on "being with" the individual/ family. In addition to the dialogue process described, nurses practicing from this perspective seek the patient's and family's views of the situation while performing the technical procedures. They are also conscious of and attend to their own attitudes, approaches, and interactions with the patient and the family. Nurses working from this perspective do not attempt to judge another nor to direct their choices or actions. Rather, through processes such as those described in Boxes 7-2 and 7-3, they support individuals and groups of persons as they clarify their own intentions, fears, and hopes.

Practice Models

Because each situation is perceived as unique, practice models and rules of practice have not been developed from this perspective. It is possible that some guidelines for practice that are consistent with Human Becoming Theory will result from research studies such as Carson and Mitchell's study (1998) of persistent pain. Within the descriptions of the unique experience of living with persistent pain, the researchers found themes shared by all study participants. These included "forbearance surfaces with the drain of persistent anguish," "isolating retreats coexist with comforting engagement," and "hope for relief clarifies priorities of daily living" (p. 1246). The researchers suggest that these themes could be investigated further to help nurses better understand people's choices about disclosing their personal realities. This type of work might lead to related practice models.

Since there are no practice models, reading Human Becoming research studies is essential for nurses who wish to practice from this perspective. Such research has been identified as the source of development of nursing knowledge (Parse 1997d, 1998). The focus of research reported in the literature includes the lived experiences of persons with varying health states and in varying stages of development.

Implications for Administration

The organizational structure and the systems and procedures developed by an organization to ensure service delivery have a major impact on the nature of nursing practice in a health care agency (Allison & McLaughlin-Renpenning, 1998; Mitchell, 1998). Administrators must clearly think through the direction for provision of care mandated by mission statements, policy statements, patient/nursing standards, and similar tools of organizations. A major task for administration is ensuring consistency between the values espoused by nurses practicing from a particular theory base and the systems, procedures and evaluation standards developed by the service delivery organization. For example, evaluating the effectiveness of nursing practiced from the perspective of the Human Becoming Theory requires differentiating evidence relating to skill, outcomes associated with procedures, and service delivery from knowledge that informs the nurse-person process. Evidence that indicates the benefit of nursing comes from the descriptions by patients and families of changes in health and quality of life that result from nursing care (Mitchell, 1999).

Studies of nurses practicing within the Human Becoming Theory indicate that nurses see patients as unique persons in relationship with others rather than as problems. Emphasis is on the person rather than on procedures and treatments (Mitchell, 1994b). The focus of nurse-patient discussions appears to shift from procedures to relationship issues. This changed focus is accompanied by an increase in job satisfaction (Northrup and Cody, 1998). Moreover, some nurses expressed an increased understanding of nursing as a scientific discipline. However, nurses commonly express this feeling when practice based in specific nursing theory is introduced; this response does not appear to be unique to any one theoretical perspective (Fitch, Rogers, Ross, Shea, Smith, & Tucker, 1991; Frederickson & Williams, 1997; Walker, 1993).

In reference to a community group of persons diagnosed with genital herpes, Kelly (1995) describes the contrast between traditional nursing and practice guided by the Theory of Human Becoming. Over the period of 10 weeks in which seven 75-minute discussion sessions were held, the nurse developed an understanding of the experience of living with herpes. Kelly went on to further analyze this experience and to formulate what she called a "loose agenda for community-based practice" (p. 130). This included the following (Kelly, 1995, p. 130-131):

- Knowing the cycle of irresponsibility stops here brings priorities forward in action, whereas keeping facades in relationships both protects and causes worries
- Wanting to be "moving real" with intentions to turn your world around, yet saying the time is not right for either reaching out or risking vulnerability because it is not easy
- Seeing the center of the universe as being true to the purpose of self, yet separating from the center to find "a love relationship between two persons which creates a vacuum" in regard to the future

Kelly went on to identify certain characteristics of a "Parse nurse." These included being respectful and nonjudgmental, honoring the importance of "facades," and respecting that each person knows his or her own way and that it is always evolving, and exploring joy and spontaneity in the presence of suffering.

Northrup and Cody (1998) recommend that organizations implementing nursing practice from the Human Becoming perspective include a facilitator knowledgeable in the theory at the master's or doctorate level. Adequate resources need to be allocated for staff education. Organizations should also ensure that management endorses practice from this perspective and provides administrative support for appropriate continuing education. An ongoing program of research related to the health concerns of the population being served is essential as research generates the knowledge base for nursing practice. Research programs based in other schools of thought will have little relevance (Mitchell, 1999).

Implications for Education

Nursing practice within the human becoming school of thought involves a specific worldview. This worldview, at present, is not generally the basis of nursing education programs or nursing textbooks. Although Parse (1981) described a curriculum based in Human Becoming Theory that directs development of basic and continuing education programs, this worldview, at present, generally is not the basis of nursing education programs or textbooks. An understanding of existential phenomenology is probably necessary to practicing from the perspective of the Theory of Human Becoming. This presupposes at least a baccalaureate degree that includes courses in philosophy as a requirement for entry to practice. Research literature is not a common source of information for practicing nurses (Estabrooks, 1998). Disseminating the body of knowledge generated by this school of thought to practicing nurses should include publication in what Estabrooks calls the "trade" journals—*The American Journal of Nursing, The Canadian Nurse,* and state and provincial nursing journals and newsletters—as well as the nursing science and nursing research journals. In addition, continuing education programs and/or in-service education programs need to be designed and delivered to disseminate this view and to develop the knowledge base to support practice from this perspective.

NEXUS

With some background in philosophy, one will find that Parse's work is simple to grasp conceptually; the difficulty is in the level of knowledge necessary to use this approach in research and practice. The basic concepts and assumptions are philosophically congruent and logically consistent. It is important to recognize the depth underlying the ideas presented. Without a background in philosophy, the language and the ideas may appear difficult and confusing. It is important to understand that Parse believes that one does not simply use or apply her theory. One lives it (1997a).

REFERENCES

Allchin-Petardi, L. (1998). Weathering the storm: Persevering through a difficult time. *Nursing Science Quarterly, 11*(4), 172-177.

Allison, S.E. & McLaughlin-Renpenning, K.E. (1998). *Nursing Administration in the 21st century: A self-care theory approach.* Thousand Oaks, CA: Sage.

Baumann S.L. (1994). No place of their own. *Nursing Science Quarterly, 7*(4), 162-169.

Baumann S.L. (1996). Feeling uncomfortable: Children in families with no place of their own. *Nursing Science Quarterly, 9*(4), 152-159.

Carson, M.G. & Mitchell, G.J. (1998). The experience of living with persistent pain. *Journal of Advanced Nursing, 28*(6), 1242-1248.

Chinn, P.L. & Kramer, M. (1995). *Theory and nursing: A systematic approach.* (4th ed.). St. Louis: Mosby.

Cody, W. (1991). Grieving a personal loss. *Nursing Science Quarterly, 4*(2), 61-68.

Cody, W. (1995a). The lived experience of grieving, for families living with AIDS. In R. Parse (Ed.), *Illuminations: The human becoming theory in practice and research.* New York: National League for Nursing Press.

Cody, W. (1995b). The meaning of grieving for families living with AIDS. *Nursing Science Quarterly, 8*(3), 104-114.

Cody, W. (1995c). About all those paradigms: Many in the universe, two in nursing. *Nursing Science Quarterly, 8*(4), 144-146.

Daly, J. (1995). The lived experience of suffering. In R. Parse (Ed.), *Illuminations: The human becoming theory in practice and research.* New York: National League for Nursing Press.

Davis, D.K. & Cannava, E. (1995). The meaning of retirement for communally-living retired performing artists. *Nursing Science Quarterly, 8*(1), 8-16.

Estabrooks, C.A. (1998). Will evidence-based nursing practice make practice perfect? *Canadian Journal of Nursing Research 30*(1), 15-36.

Fawcett, J. (1993). From a plethora of paradigms to parsimony in worldviews. *Nursing Science Quarterly, 6*(2), 56-58.

Fitch, M., Rogers, M., Ross, E., Shea, H., Smith, I., & Tucker, D. (1991). Developing a plan to evaluate the use of nursing conceptual frameworks. *Canadian Journal of Nursing Administration, 4*(1), 22-28.

Fisher, M. & Mitchell, G. (1998). Patients' views of quality of life: Transforming the nursing knowledge base. *Clinical Nurse Specialist, 12*(3), 99-105.

Frederickson, K., & Williams, J.K. (1997). Nursing theory-guided practice: The Roy adaptation model and patient/family experiences. *Nursing Science Quarterly, 10*(1), 53-54.

Futrell, M., Wondolowski, C., & Mitchell, G. (1993). Aging in the oldest old living in Scotland: A phenomenological study. *Nursing Science Quarterly, 6*(4), 189-194.

Gates, K. (2000). The experience of caring for a loved one: A phenomenological study. *Nursing Science Quarterly, 13*(1), 54-59.

Janes, N.M. & Wells, D.L. (1997). Elderly patients' experiences with nurses guided by Parse's theory of human becoming. *Clinical Nursing Research, 6*(3), 205-224.

Jonas, C.M. (1992). The meaning of being an elder in Nepal. *Nursing Science Quarterly, 5*(4), 171-175.

Kaplan, A. (1964). *The conduct of inquiry.* Scranton, PA: Chandler Publishing Company.

Kelly, L.S. (1995). Parse's theory in practice with a group in the community. *Nursing Science Quarterly, 8*(3), 127-132.

Kruse, B. (1999). The lived experience of serenity: Using Parse's research method. *Nursing Science Quarterly, 12*(2), 143-150.

Mitchell, G.J. (1991). Nursing Diagnosis: An ethical analysis. *Image, 23*(2), 99-103.

Mitchell, G.J. (1994a). The meaning of being a senior: Phenomenological research and interpretation with Parse's nursing theory. *Nursing Science Quarterly, 7*(2), 70-79.

Mitchell, G.J. (1994b). Parse's theory based practice and research. *Nursing Science Quarterly, 7*(3), 107-109.

Mitchell, G.J. (1995). The lived experience of restriction-freedom in later life. In R. Parse (Ed.), *Illuminations: The Human Becoming Theory in practice and research.* New York: National League for Nursing Press.

Mitchell, G.J. (1998). Standards of nursing and the winds of change. *Nursing Science Quarterly, 11*(3), 97-98.

Mitchell, G.J. (1999). Evidence-based practice: critique and alternative view. *Nursing Science Quarterly, 12*(1), 30-35.

Mitchell, G.J., Bernardo, A., & Bournes, D. (1997). Nursing guided by Parse's theory: Patient views at Sunnybrook. *Nursing Science Quarterly, 10*(1), 55-56.

Mitchell, G.J. & Heidt, P. (1994). The lived experience of wanting to help another: Research with Parse's method. *Nursing Science Quarterly, 7*(3), 119-127.

Northrup, D.T. & Cody, W.K. (1998). Evaluation of the Human Becoming Theory in practice in an acute-care psychiatric setting. *Nursing Science Quarterly, 11*(1), 23-30.

Parse, R.R. (1981). *Man-living-health.* New York: Wiley Medical Publication.

Parse, R.R. (1987). *Nursing science: Major paradigms, theories, and critiques.* Philadelphia: W.B. Saunders.

Parse, R.R. (1992). Human becoming: Parse's theory of nursing. *Nursing Science Quarterly, 5*(1), 35-42.

Parse, R.R. (1993). The experience of laughter: A phenomenological study. *Nursing Science Quarterly, 6*(1), 39-43.

Parse, R.R. (1994). Laughing and health: A study using Parse's research method. *Nursing Science Quarterly, 7*(2), 55-64.

Parse, R.R. (1996a). The Human Becoming Theory: Challenges in practice and research. *Nursing Science Quarterly, 9*(2), 55-60.

Parse, R.R. (1996b). Quality of life for persons living with Alzheimer's disease: The Human Becoming perspective. *Nursing Science Quarterly, 9*(3), 126-133.

Parse, R.R. (1997a). The Human Becoming Theory: The was, is, and will be. *Nursing Science Quarterly, 10*(1), 32-38.

Parse, R.R. (1997b). *Illuminations: The Human Becoming Theory in practice and research.* New York: National League for Nursing.

Parse, R.R. (1997c). Joy-sorrow: A study using the Parse research method. *Nursing Science Quarterly, 10*(2), 80-87.

Parse, R.R. (1997d). Transforming research and practice with the Human Becoming Theory. *Nursing Science Quarterly, 10*(4), 171-174.

Parse, R.R. (1998). *The Human Becoming school of thought.* Thousand Oaks, CA: Sage.

Rendon, D.C., Sales, R., Leal, I. & Piqué, J. (1995). The lived experience of aging in community-dwelling elders in Valencia, Spain: A phenomenological study. *Nursing Science Quarterly, 8*(4), 152-157.

Walker, D. (1993). A nursing administrator's perspective of use of Orem's Self-Care Deficit Nursing Theory. In M. Parker (Ed.), *Patterns of nursing theories in practice.* New York: National League for Nursing Press.

CHAPTER 8

Modeling Nursing From a Systems Perspective

THE NEUMAN SYSTEMS MODEL

Key Terms

client/client system, p. 188
flexible line of defense, p. 191
lines of resistance, p. 191
normal line of defense, p. 191
primary prevention, p. 191
secondary prevention, p. 191

stressor, p. 191
tertiary prevention, p. 191
wholism, p. 190

The Neuman Systems Model (NSM) was first presented in 1972. A conceptual model for nursing was considered a unifying factor for a course for graduate students in nursing. The model was subtitled "a total person approach to viewing client problems" (Neuman & Young, 1972, p. 265). It extended beyond the illness model and "[provided] a frame of reference for the practice of nursing" (p. 265). This work was the basis for a chapter and later a book (Neuman, 1974, 1982, 1989, 1995). In 1989 Neuman added spirituality as a variable to the model. She expanded the concept of environment to include "created environment" (Neuman, 1990) and developed the "Neuman Nursing Process and Prevention as Intervention Formats" for implementation of the model (1995, p. 18-20). Extensive use of the model in research, education, and practice can be found in the literature. In 1988 Neuman founded the Neuman Systems Model Trustees Group, Inc. to "preserve, protect, and perpetuate the integrity of the Model for the future of nursing" (1995, p. 700). The trustees are a group of nursing scholars who support the testing and application of the model and its adaptation to clinical practice.

THE STARTING POINT OF THE MODELING PROCESS

Neuman started by developing a model that integrated many variables known through practice and nursing literature. It is a general model—it is not specific to any one nursing specialty. The development of the model is toward research and practice. The systems view is considered a philosophy in itself. Therefore development of the philosophical foundations is unnecessary. Explication of the philosophy, however, is necessary.

Reason for Theory Development

Neuman and Young (1972) noted that graduate students in nursing wanted exposure to a breadth of nursing problems before limiting themselves to the study of a specific problem area. They developed the NSM to unify concepts important in nursing and to provide a focal point for student learning. A systems model organized the many variables into a whole. The model was designed for use in nursing, but Neuman posited its appropriateness for other health disciplines as well (1995). She viewed the adoption of the NSM as a "two-edged sword" in that it can foster a common perspective but in so doing may mask the distinctive contributions of nursing (1989, p. 87).

Phenomenon of Concern

All of the phenomena of nursing, or nursing variables, form a domain organized into a system. A system is defined as "a family of relationships among the members acting as a whole" (International Society for System Science [ISSS], 1999), and system theory is a "theory of organized complexity" (Hazzard, 1971, p. 383). Purpose, process, interaction, integration and emergence are characteristics of systems and have become the central phenomena for any system designer. Neuman justified the use of the systems approach to nursing because the "nursing system will benefit . . . through better organization, specificity, and cohesion of its increasingly complex components" (1989, p. 3). Focusing on the expansiveness of a system, Neuman believes that the "complex nursing phenomena can be placed within a logical and empirically valid open systems perspective; as the number of parts and subparts increases, the whole expands" (p. 5). Neuman's model is shown in Figure 8-1. The NSM is presented as a wellness model (Neuman, 1990) that "extends beyond the illness and includes the concepts of problem-finding and prevention, and the newer behavioral science concepts and environmental approaches to wellness" (Neuman & Young, 1972, p. 265). The specific phenomena of concern to Neuman are the relationships among all stressors, the reactions to these stressors, and reconstitution factors within a general systems structure. The object of nursing is the **client/client system,** which may be an individual family, group, or even a "social issue" that is described as an "open system in interaction and total interface with the environment" (Neuman, 1989, pp. 22-23).

DESCRIPTION OF NEUMAN'S THEORETICAL SYSTEM
Philosophical Perspectives

General System Theory. The NSM provides a comprehensive, flexible, wholistic, and system-based perspective for nursing (Neuman, 1996). The model focuses on the response of the client system to actual or potential environmental stressors. Neuman's worldview is congruent with tenets of general system theory as put forth by von Bertalanffy (1968). Systems philosophy reorganizes ways of thinking and knowing perceived reality. The cosmology and ontology are constituted by the processes and relationships of the system itself (ISSS, 1999). Banathy (1999) described the development of system models in two stages: (1) creating a general system model,

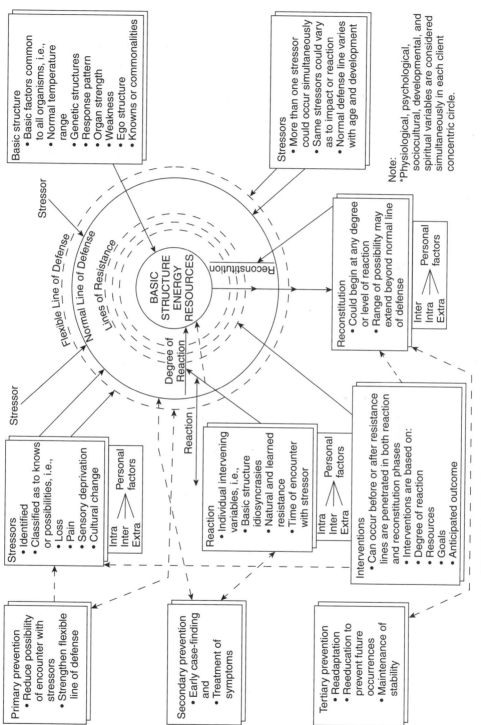

FIGURE 8-1   The Neuman Systems Model. (Copyright © 1970 Betty Neuman.)

and (2) transforming the general model into specific content. In the first stage, many types of system models can be constructed, including systems-environment models, functions/structure models, and process models. The second stage is concerned with the integration of the models and elements of the models into one's thinking and the application in real-life contexts; this stage is called internalization and application. The NSM is primarily a functions/structure model. The work of Neuman and other scholars is primarily second stage work. In 1995, Neuman presented a process "format" to describe how to use the model. The model structures the development of theory relevant to understanding the characteristics of the system and its implementation, but it is not in itself a theory. The works of Gestalt, Teilhard deChardin, Bernard Marx, and Selye were foundational to NSM (Freese, Beckman, Boxley-Harges, Bruick, Harris, Hermiz, Meininger, & Steinkeler, 1998). Others whose views are compatible with the NSM include systems theorists/scientists Ashby (1972), Emery (1969), Klir (1972), Lazarus (1981), Lazlo (1972), and Putt (1978).

System theory (and hence the NSM) is concerned with wholeness, dynamic interaction, and organization. System terms, notably "wholeness, order, differentiation, goal directedness, stressors, stability, and feedback, are homologous (analogous or similar) to nursing concepts" (Neuman, 1995, p. 9). **Wholism** is seen as both a philosophical and biological concept. The NSM is developed as an open system and reflects the structure and elements of General System Theory. Lowry, Walker, and Mirenda (Neuman, 1995) consider the model a way of viewing clients both wholistically and multidimensionally, within a systems perspective. Furthermore, they believe that the model "clearly reflects continuous interaction occurring between clients and their environment, dynamic and reciprocal in nature, leading to growth and congruence with an organismic worldview" (p. 70). Descriptions of the elements, the relationships among the elements, the purpose, process, interaction, integration and emergence of the system provides ontological structure. The specific language of NSM is based in the concepts of stress and reaction to stress as well as in the systems language.

Description of Model and Theories

The diagram of the NSM has remained unchanged since its original development, although some of the model concepts were refined (Reed, 1993) (see Figure 8-1). The model is described through four additional models depicting the subsystems of client, health, environment, and nursing.

In 1990, *spirituality, created environment,* and *energy* were defined in addition to the original conceptualizations, and new relationships were posited. The created-environment profoundly affects client functioning with the energy used for personal development and system maintenance. These concepts led to a theory of optimal client system stability to describe the wellness focus of the model and the purpose of the system.

Neuman conceptualized health as the state of system balance and described it on a wellness-illness continuum. NSM is considered a wellness model (1995, p. 25). Neuman identified ten assumptions inherent within the NSM that may also be viewed as propositions (Box 8-1). The components of the model are listed in Box 8-2. The work by Neuman and others is not set out as theory, with the exception of Koertvelyessy's work (Neuman and Koertvelyessy, 1986) on a theory of client stability associated with the assumptions and theory elements that equate client stability with wellness (Neuman, 1989).

BOX 8-1

Assumptions/Propositions of the Neuman Systems Model

1. Though each individual client or group as a client system is unique, each system is a composite of common known factors or innate characteristics within a normal, given range of response contained within a basic structure
2. Many known, unknown, and universal environmental **stressors** exist. Each differs in its potential for disturbing a client's usual stability level, or normal line of defense. The particular interrelationships of client variables—physiological, psychological, sociocultural, developmental, and spiritual—at any point in time can affect the degree to which a client is protected by the flexible line of defense against possible reaction to a single stressor or a combination of stressors.
3. Each individual client/client system has evolved a normal range of response to the environment that is referred to as a **normal line of defense,** or usual wellness/stability state. The normal line of defense can be used as a standard from which to measure health deviation.
4. When the cushioning, accordion-like effect of the **flexible line of defense** is no longer capable of protecting the client/client system against an environmental stressor, the stressor breaks through the normal line of defense. The interrelationships of variables—physiological, psychological, sociocultural, developmental, and spiritual—determine the nature and degree of system reaction or possible reaction to the stressor.
5. The client, whether in a state of wellness or illness, is a dynamic composite of the interrelationships of variables—physiological, psychological, sociocultural, developmental, and spiritual. Wellness is on a continuum of available energy to support the system in an optimal state of system stability.
6. Implicit within each client system are internal resistance factors known as **lines of resistance,** which function to stabilize and return the client to the usual wellness state (normal line of defense) or possibly to a higher level of stability following an environmental stressor reaction.
7. **Primary prevention** relates to general knowledge that is applied in client assessment and intervention in identification and reduction or mitigation of possible or actual risk factors associated with environmental stressors to prevent possible reaction. The goal of health promotion is included in primary prevention.
8. **Secondary prevention** relates to symptomatology following a reaction to stressors, appropriate ranking of intervention priorities, and treatment to reduce their noxious effects.
9. **Tertiary prevention** relates to the adjustive processes taking place as reconstitution begins and maintenance factors move the client back in a circular manner toward primary prevention.
10. The client as a system is in dynamic, constant energy exchange with the environment.

From Neuman, B.M. (1995). *The Neuman Systems Model.* (3rd ed.). Norwalk, CT: Appleton & Lange.

BOX 8-2

The Components of the Neuman Systems Model

The Client/Client System	Internal environment
Flexible line of defense	External environment
Variables	Created environment
Physiological	Health
Psychological	Wellness-illness continuum
Sociocultural	Client system stability
Developmental	Nursing
Spiritual	Prevention as intervention
Lines of resistance	Primary
The normal line of defense	Secondary
Environment	Tertiary

RESEARCH DERIVED FROM THE NEUMAN SYSTEMS MODEL

The NSM is a wholistic framework that reflects human complexity and the broad context of healthcare interactions. This complexity makes it difficult to study problems representing the global range of concepts. To facilitate research, Fawcett (1995) proposed a structure to enable use of the NSM in studying specific nursing problems. Fawcett (1995) suggested that conceptual models such as the NSM guide middle-range theory development and research model selection. Because conceptual models are not directly observable in the world, middle-range theory can be useful in clarifying more specific concepts and propositions. It can be the vehicle for observation and empirical testing. Empirical indicators are the actual instruments, study conditions, and research procedures used to examine a particular concept derived from middle-range theory. They represent the most concrete components or concepts of middle-range theory. Using Fawcett's schema, theory can be generated by moving from the NSM to the empirical indicators, analyzing data from empirical indicators, and, finally, applying it to an emerging middle-range theory.

An example of the conceptual-theoretical-empirical structure can be found in Lowry and Anderson's study (1993) of ventilator dependency. This study used several concepts from the NSM within a created environment, including several theoretical variables specified in the middle-range theory, and then identified empirical indicators. For example, the NSM concept of extrapersonal stressor was delineated by the theoretical research variable of mechanical ventilation, which was measured by the empirical indicator of multiple failed weaning attempts. Interpersonal factors were a concept from the model; the research variable was social support; and the empirical indicator was perceived social support. This approach delineated several empirical indicators of the ventilator study.

Fawcett (1995) proposed six rules for the conduct of all theory-driven nursing research and then specifically applied them to the NSM (Box 8-3).

According to the first rule, phenomena permissible for study include the following (Fawcett, 1995, p. 463):

- physiological, psychological, sociocultural, developmental, and spiritual variables
- properties of the central core of the client system

> ## BOX 8-3
>
> ### Rules for Conceptual Model–Based Research
>
> Fawcett's rules for using conceptual models in research identify the following:
> - Phenomena to be studied
> - Distinctive nature of the problems to be studied and the purpose to be fulfilled by the research
> - Subjects who are to provide the data and the settings in which data are to be gathered
> - Research designs, instruments, and procedures to be employed
> - Methods for reducing and analyzing data
> - Nature of contributions that the research will make to the advancement of knowledge

Modified from Fawcett, J. (1995). Constructing conceptual-theoretical-empirical structures for research: Future implications for use of the Neuman systems model. In B. Neuman (Ed.), *The Neuman Systems Model*. (3rd ed.). Norwalk, CT: Appleton & Lange.

- properties of the flexible and normal lines of defense as well as lines of resistance
- characteristics of the internal, external, and created environments
- characteristics of intrapersonal, interpersonal, and extrapersonal stressors
- elements of primary, secondary, and tertiary prevention interventions

The second rule specifies that clinical problems of study should be those dealing with the impact of stressors on client system stability in terms of physiological, psychological, sociocultural, developmental, and spiritual variables. These studies should examine lines of defense and resistance. According to Fawcett, a function of Neuman Systems research is predicting the effects of interventions at the primary, secondary, or tertiary levels.

According to the third rule, subjects can include client systems of "individuals, families, groups, communities, organizations or collaborative relationships between two or more individuals" (Fawcett, 1995, p. 463). Data may be collected in multiple settings, including inpatient, ambulatory, home, and community. It should include client systems, investigator perceptions, and strategies of negotiated goal setting. The fourth rule specifies that inductive or deductive research, using either quantitative or qualitative designs, is acceptable. The fifth rule indicates analytical techniques associated with either quantitative or qualitative designs are permissible. Finally, the sixth rule indicates that research should advance understanding of the influence of preventive interventions on stressors and client system stability (Fawcett, 1995).

Fawcett (1995) followed her rules with a set of guidelines for constructing NSM-based studies. The guidelines state that investigators must acknowledge the model as the underlying study guide. Acknowledgement must be followed by a discussion of the model sufficient to clarify the relationship between the model and study purpose. Relevant linkages between model and study variables must be stated. In addition, propositions of the model and the study aims or hypotheses must be established. Study methods must reflect the model in terms of selection of appropriate subjects, instruments that adequately measure concepts, and appropriate data analysis methods. In the discussion of study findings, conclusions should reflect the adequacy of the theory and the credibility of the model.

Louis (1995) applied Fawcett's guidelines for use of a conceptual model in research as criteria for evaluating Neuman-based studies. The specific criteria she addressed required that studies do the following (Louis, 1995, pp. 476-478):

- Provide an outline of the phenomena to be investigated
- Direct the method to be used in the investigation
- Guide data collection and analysis
- Guide the interpretation of the findings
- Direct the use of findings for future studies and nursing practice

These guidelines proved useful for study evaluation.

Research Instruments

Instrumentation derived from the research rules should enable measurement of specific empirical indicators. A broad array of instruments that use the NSM as a conceptual framework have measured a variety of research variables. The instruments selected usually reflect the stressors or responses to the stressors under investigation. Consequently, readers will see many different measuring instruments in Neuman-based studies. For example, Lowry and Anderson's study (1993) on ventilator dependency measured the stressor of mechanical ventilation by counting the multiple failed weaning attempts. Another example is Gigliotti's study (1999), which used the Norbeck Social Support Questionnaire to measure interpersonal relationships as a test of the flexible line of defense in women with multiple role stress. Two instruments—the Spiritual Care Scale and the Levels of Cognitive Functioning Assessment Scale—are derived more specifically from the NSM (Table 8-1).

Spiritual Care Scale. The Spiritual Care Scale (SCS) was developed by Carrigg and Weber (1997) and was specifically derived from the NSM. It measures the spiritual aspect of Neuman's client system. Carrigg and Weber developed the SCS to differentiate between spiritual and psychosocial aspects of nursing care. The SCS is a 27-item, 4-point Likert scale that was refined using expert nurses' written definitions of spiritual and psychosocial care. Internal consistency reliability for the SCS is strong, and the content validity is acceptable. Construct validity as established by factor analysis identified a spiritual and a psychosocial component that accounted for a total of 60% of the variance. The instrument clearly identifies a spiritual component. This relatively new instrument shows promise as a measurement of a spiritual component of care.

Levels of Cognitive Functioning Assessment Scale. Adapted from the Rancho Los Amigos Levels of Cognitive Functioning instrument, the Levels of Cognitive Functioning Assessment Scale (LOCFAS) was developed by Flannery (1995) to assess cognitive functioning in clients with traumatic brain injuries. The assessment aimed to enhance rehabilitative efforts through appropriate planning. Agreement for experts using the LOCFAS was very high, but inexperienced raters had lower agreement. This indicates a need for education regarding instrument use. Criterion-related validity was very strong. However, this finding is unsurprising, since the Rancho Los Amigos Levels of Cognitive Functioning Scale, from which the LOCFAS was adapted, was the selected criterion. Chiverton and Flannery (1995) reported the LOCFAS a useful measure of the degrees of reaction of cognitively impaired clients. This information is then used to propose primary, secondary, or tertiary interventions.

TABLE 8-1		
Research and Assessment Instruments Based on the Neuman Systems Model		
Instrument/Description	**Study/Year**	**Reliability and Validity**
Spiritual Care Scale (SCS) 27-item, 4-point Likert scale	Carrigg and Weber, 1997	The Content Validity Index for the original 30-item SCS was 0.83. Content analysis revealed three dimensions of faith, empowerment, and meaningfulness. Psychometric testing with two groups of registered nurses ($N = 144$) revealed internal consistency of 0.94 for the total scale, 0.95 for the spiritual subscale, and 0.92 for psychosocial subscale. Construct validity was established via a principal components factor analysis with a two-factor solution. The spiritual component— consisting of faith, empowerment, and meaningfulness— accounted for 42% of the variance, and the psychosocial component accounted for an additional 18% of variance.
Levels of Cognitive Functioning Assessment Scale (LOCFAS) Five assessment levels	Flannery, 1995	Content validity was established by an expert panel. Interrater reliability of five written vignettes established high agreement among experts (level of cognitive kappa $= 1.00$ and individual items kappa $= 0.997$) and modest agreement among inexperienced raters (M agreement $= 0.839$; $SD = 0.006$; and individual items M agreement $= 0.83$; $SD = 0.052$). Intrarater reliability with a 2-week interval was $M = 0.86$ ($SD = 0.88$). Criterion-related validity, which was assessed with the Rancho Los Amigos Levels of Cognitive Functioning Scale, was high ($r = 0.929$).

Review of Related Research

Research conducted using the NSM has been diverse. Studies of physiological, psychological, sociocultural, developmental, and spiritual categories identified by the NSM have been conducted. Intrapersonal, interpersonal, and extrapersonal stressors have been explored through research, as have concepts of primary, secondary, and tertiary prevention. One strength of some the published research is their clear theoretical ties to the model. For example, Gigliotti (1999) clearly ties Neuman's concept of stressors to a middle-range theory that examines role conditions. This is linked subsequently to maternal and student roles occupied by women who are suspected of experiencing multiple role stress. Flexible lines of defense are conceptualized as personality characteristics measured by Maternal Role and Student Role Questionnaires and as interpersonal relationships that are measured by Norbeck's Social Support Questionnaire.

A difficulty with research using the NSM is that some studies need to isolate aspects of the model to facilitate measurement. Although this approach may facilitate measurement and control of variables, it diminishes the wholism that is central to the theory. The NSM suggests that five person variables (physiological, psychological, sociocultural, developmental, and spiritual) enable the flexible line of defense to ward off environmental stressors. To create a study with a realistic scope, Gigliotti (1999) selected two of these variables— psychological and sociocultural—to investigate the impact of multiple role stress on mothers who are also students. The developmental variable of age, not originally considered as part of the study focus, was discovered to influence multiple role stress.

As the following discussion indicates, a positive aspect of NSM-based research is the variety of age-groups and settings that have been studied. Because many studies encompass more than one aspect of Neuman's model in terms of variables of study, stressors, and lines of defense, research in this review is organized around the areas of inpatient settings, community settings, academic applications, and workplace concerns. Table 8-2 summarizes selected studies using the NSM.

Research about Inpatient Issues. Inpatient practice sites have been the setting for testing many NSM-based nursing interventions. Nursing practice research using the NSM includes interventions for a variety of problems and descriptive research. Intervention research focuses on primary, secondary, and tertiary prevention measures. Descriptive research concentrates on depicting stressors that clients experience. The concepts of . prevention and intrapersonal, interpersonal, and extrapersonal stressors are key to descriptive research using the NSM. Intervention studies tested nursing measures that could be used alone or in conjunction with other therapies to promote client wellbeing and prevent complications.

Leja (1989) investigated the effectiveness of guided imagery on postsurgical depression in older adults. Guided imagery was conceived as a primary prevention measure to counteract the stressors of hospitalization and surgery that could lead to depression. The NSM was supported in that depression scores for the guided imagery group were lower 1 week after discharge. However, no significant differences were found between the group receiving routine discharge teaching and those receiving guided imagery teaching. The small sample size could have influenced study outcomes.

Sabo and Michael (1996) also investigated a stress reduction strategy that used personal messages with music to reduce anxiety and minimize the side effects of cancer chemotherapy. Nurse-prescribed interventions aimed to minimize stressor reaction and strengthen the flexible lines of defense. During their chemotherapy, clients who listened to taped music with a message from their physicians experienced lower anxiety levels. However, the interventions did not decrease the chemotherapy side effects. The experimental and control groups experienced equally severe side effects. The anxiety reduction supports NSM concepts of minimization of stressor reactions.

Gavigan, Kline-O'Sullivan, and Klumpp-Lybrand (1990) investigated regular turning—a primary prevention technique for coronary artery bypass graft clients—and its influence on pulmonary postoperative complications and length of stay. Although turning did not impact incidence of atelectasis or length of stay, the control group experienced a greater frequency of increases in temperature. Unfortunately, the outcome of postoperative turning on the incidence of atelectasis did not support the NSM.

Waddell and Demi (1993) examined the effectiveness of an intensive partial hospitalization program (IPHP) for the treatment of anxiety disorders. The NSM guided individualized therapy that encompassed the biological (pharmacotherapeutical), cognitive, and behavioral techniques for treating anxiety disorders. Investigators found that using a wholistic approach to decrease stressors, as the NSM suggests, was an effective intervention with agoraphobic clients. It significantly reduced fear, avoidance behaviors, panic attacks,

Text continued on p. 211

TABLE 8-2

Selected Studies Based on the Neuman System Model

Study/Year	Purpose	Methods	Findings
INPATIENT			
Ali and Khalil, 1989	The study examined the influence of preoperative educational intervention on anxiety levels of Egyptian bladder cancer clients.	Pretest/posttest control design was used for control ($n = 15$) and intervention ($n = 15$) groups. Intervention was a semistructured teaching program about the nature of surgery and allowed time for clients to express anxieties. The State-Trait Anxiety Inventory was administered preoperatively, on the third postoperative day, and before discharge. Data were analyzed using MANOVA followed by univariate F tests.	Preoperative educational clients had significantly lower anxiety levels than the control group on postoperative day 3 (F (1, 28) 94.58, $p < 0.00$) and at discharge (F (1, 28) 301.47, $p < 0.00$). Qualitative themes included fear of cancer, body mutilation and distortion, and impact of surgery on social and marital relationship.
Bass, 1991	The study identified the support needs of parents of neonatal intensive care clients.	The study included semistructured interviews with 18 parents from two hospitals. Data were analyzed with content analysis and subsequent quantification.	Six hundred thirty-four need statements were categorized into broad content areas. Parents most needed information, person-related support, attachment/parenting, physical support, spiritual support, and staff support.
Bowman, 1997	This descriptive study investigated the contextual variable of planned versus unplanned hip surgery on pain, sleep, and delirium.	Forty-three consecutively admitted subjects participated—26 with planned surgery and 17 with unplanned hip surgery. Data were collected with Mini Mental Status examination (MMS), a visual analog scale for pain, and a 7-point Likert assessment of sleep quality.	The unplanned surgery group experienced greater delirium (47% versus 27%). Unplanned surgery subjects reported greater pain on some days. Subjects who experienced delirium reported the highest levels of pain. Unplanned surgery participants expressed fear about future mobility and lifestyle changes and placed trust in God. Planned surgery subjects feared unexpected complications but expected improvements in lifestyle and placed faith in doctors and caregivers.

Continued

TABLE 8-2

Selected Studies Based on the Neuman System Model—cont'd

Study/Year	Purpose	Methods	Findings
INPATIENT—cont'd			
Breckenridge, 1997a	This qualitative study was designed to elicit client perceptions of decision making about dialysis as a treatment modality.	A grounded theory method guided by the NSM. A Degner and Beatons Life-Death Decisions framework was used to interview and analyze data from 13 males and nine female end-stage renal disease clients. Six open-ended interview questions used to elicit information.	A theory of Patient's Choice of a Treatment Modality versus Selection of a Client's Treatment Modality emerged. Two patterns and 11 themes were identified. Dialysis modality was selected by either clients, significant others, or health providers. Decision themes included: self, access-rationing, significant other, living, physiological demands, experts, receiving care, independence versus dependence, lack of client choice, and client preference.
Breckenridge, 1997b	A secondary analysis identified factors that influenced clients' dialysis decisions.	Data were examined for themes related to the system variables identified by the NSM.	NSM system variables of physiological, psychological, sociocultural, developmental, and spiritual factors found to influence dialysis modality decisions.
Clark, Cross, Deane, and Lowry, 1991	This was a descriptive study of the spiritual needs of hospitalized clients.	A convenience sample of 15 hospitalized adults participated in structured interviews regarding hospitalization experience.	The most significant factors were trust, meaningful support systems, and respect for personal beliefs.
Gavigan, Kline-O'Sullivan, and Klumpp-Lybrand, 1990	This interventional study investigated the effects of regular turning on pulmonary complications and on length of stay for coronary artery bypass clients.	Fifty clients were randomly assigned to experimental ($n = 18$) and control groups ($n = 32$). Experimental group turned every two hours between supine and left or right lateral position. Control clients remained flat the first 24 hours postoperatively. Portable chest radiographs for first three days compared.	Both groups exhibited left-sided atelectasis, but the control group had a greater frequency of fever during first 24 hours ($p = 0.015$). There were no significant differences in length of stay.

Heffline, 1991	The study compared the effectiveness of radiant heat, radiant heat and meperidine combined, and radiant heat and fentanyl combined in treating postanesthesia shivering.	Twenty-nine subjects were randomly assigned to three groups. All received radiant heat and blankets for shivering. Additionally, the first group received normal saline, the second meperidine, and the third fentanyl. Data were gathered using electromyography, mean arterial pressure (MAP), heart rate (HR), rate pressure product (RPP), and oxygen saturation. Comparisons between shivering subjects and one hundred forty-nine nonshivering subjects also were made.	Data showed no significant differences among the three groups with regard to treatment. At the end of shivering cycles, statistically significant differences were found in MAP, HR, and RPP. Younger subjects and those receiving anesthesia for longer periods tended to shiver. Those receiving larger amounts of IV fluid administration tended to shiver.
Hinds, 1990	The study explored personal and contextual factors that influence quality of life for lung cancer clients.	A retrospective cross-sectional study of 87 lung cancer clients identified the relationship of information needs, family functioning, and learned resourcefulness to quality of life.	Thirty percent of the variance in quality of life was explained by prognosis, surgery, current radiotherapy, performance status, self-control skills, preference for information, and age-group.
Leja, 1989	This pilot study investigated the effectiveness of guided imagery on postsurgical depression in older adults.	Ten adults were randomly assigned to a control group receiving routine discharge teaching (RDT) or an experimental group receiving guided imagery teaching (GIDT). The Beck Depression Inventory (BDI) was completed before discharge and 1 week after discharge.	Beck Depression Inventory scores were significantly lower for the GIDT group 1 week after discharge (t = 3.588, p = 0.025). Although mean BDI postdischarge scores were lower for the GIDT group, no significant differences in BDI post scores between the RDT and GIDT groups were noted.

Continued

TABLE 8-2		
Selected Studies Based on the Neuman System Model—cont'd		
Study/Year	Purpose	Methods	Findings
INPATIENT—cont'd			
Loescher, Clark, Atwood, Leigh, and Lamb, 1990	The study explored the impact of cancer experience on survivors.	Seventeen cancer survivors responded to 22 open-ended questions on the Cancer Survivor Questionnaire. Content analysis was used to analyze responses using NSM as guide.	Treatment-related physiological stressors included decreased lung capacity, hearing loss, or mobility. Needs included access and health protection. Psychological concerns included fear of recurrence and feeling of hypochondria. Needs comprised wanting to hear other survivor stories and need for reassurance and control. Socioeconomic stressors included overprotective family members, discrimination, decreased social activities, and employment concerns. Needs for support and talking about experience were present. Life patterns were permanently changed.
Lowry and Anderson, 1993	This pilot study explored NSM client system variables that influenced weaning from mechanical ventilator.	Ten ventilator-dependent clients with a history of weaning failure responded to Multidimensional Health Locus of Control Scales (MHLC), a 1-item hope scale, the Norbeck Social Support Questionnaire, and the Anderson-Lowry Ventilation Scale. Only four subjects completed both data collection interviews.	MHLC scores were similar to normed scores for chronic clients. Hope levels increased when successful weaning occurred. Social support was important for all subjects. Subjects maintained fear of mechanical ventilation.

Maligalig, 1994	This qualitative study investigated parents' perceptions of stressors associated with pediatric ambulatory surgery.	Six pairs of parents with children aged 1 to 3 years responded to six open-ended questions in a semistructured interview. Content analysis was completed on the transcribed interviews.	Intrapersonal stressors included anxiety about child's feelings, laboratory tests and procedures, fear of surgery risk, fear of unknown, and apprehension about and desire for positive outcome. Interpersonal stressors comprised separation anxiety of parents and anxiety waiting to hear from surgeon. Extrapersonal stressors were availability of resources to use at home, and financial security.
Radwanski, 1992	This descriptive study examined practices of pain control for clients with spinal cord injuries who were experiencing chronic pain.	Sixteen subjects completed a pain analog scale, the Drug Use Inventory (DUI), McGill Comprehensive Pain Questionnaire (MCPG), the Drug Use for Chronic Pain Management Survey and the Chronic Pain Modifier Questionnaire.	Reports of pain perceptions varied: above, at, or below the injury. Severity of pain was low during the interview; clients reported medication use when pain was only slightly higher than the average pain score. Alcohol was used for pain relief alone or in conjunction with other drugs, but alcohol use declined after the injury. Use of over-the-counter medications increased after the injury.
Rodrigues-Fisher, Bourguignon, and Good, 1993	The study investigated the effect of increasing dietary fiber and fluid on laxative use in nursing home residents.	A convenience sample of 15 laxative-dependent residents was followed for a baseline period and for 6 months following intervention. Intervention consisted of slow reduction of laxatives accompanied by program of fiber and fluid intake. Repeated measures MANOVA were used for analysis.	Significant MANOVA (Wilks lambda = 0.444, $p = 0.001$) was followed by repeated measures ANOVA. The number of bowel movements increased significantly by month 3 but returned to baseline by month 6 ($F_{(6,84)} = 2.83$, $p = 0.015$). Laxative and stool softener use decreased ($F_{(6,84)} = 4.30$, $p = 0.001$) over 5 months but increased at month 6.

Continued

TABLE 8-2

Selected Studies Based on the Neuman System Model—cont'd

Study/Year	Purpose	Methods	Findings
INPATIENT—cont'd			
Sabo and Michael, 1996	The study evaluated the benefits of listening to taped music with a message during chemotherapy for reducing anxiety and severity of side effects.	Fifty subjects in a control group and 50 in an experimental group responded to the Spielberger State Anxiety Inventory (SSAI) and Cancer Chemotherapy and Side Effects Inventory. Experimental subjects listened to taped music and messages from the physician while receiving chemotherapy.	The anxiety scores of the experimental group decreased between the pretest and posttest ($t = 3.32$; $p < 0.001$). Anxiety gain score reductions between control and experimental group were significantly different ($t = 2.19$; $p < 0.015$). The experimental group was less anxious following treatment than the control group. No differences were found in severity of side effects.
Waddell and Demi, 1993	The study evaluated the effectiveness of an intensive partial hospitalization program (IPHP) for treatment of anxiety disorders.	A comparative design was used to contrast pretreatment and posttreatment data for 32 clients completing a 2- to 5-week partial hospitalization program. Measures included Agoraphobic Cognitions Questionnaire (ACQ), Body Sensations Questionnaire (BSQ), Mobility Inventory for Agoraphobia (MI), and Symptom Checklist 90-Revised (SCL90-R).	Scores of ACQ and BSQ were lower posttreatment ($t = 4.48$, $p < 0.001$, and $t = 4.67$, $p < 0.001$). This indicated decreased fear levels. The severity of impaired functioning significantly decreased, as was indicated by lower scores on each MI subscale. Somatization, phobic anxiety, general anxiety, obsessive-compulsive behaviors, interpersonal sensitivity, and depression were significantly reduced following treatment as measured by the HSCL-90-R subscales.
Ziemer, 1983	This intervention study investigated the effects of the type of information given on postsurgical coping.	One hundred eleven clients were randomly assigned to three groups. Group 1 received procedural information; Group 2 received procedure and sensation information; and Group 3 received procedure, sensation, and coping information. Data were collected using Physical Coping Behavior Scale, Psychophysiological Coping Behavior Scale, a list of client symptoms, a 5-point Pain Intensity scale, and a 4-point Distress scale.	No differences were found in Physical Coping Behaviors, Psychophysiological Coping Behaviors, number of symptoms, pain intensity, or distress. Although subjects in Group 3 remembered receiving coping information, simply having the information did not motivate them to use specific coping behaviors.

COMMUNITY

Barker, Robinson, and Brautigan, 1999	This prospective study investigated the effectiveness of psychiatric nurse visitation on readmission rate of clients with depression.	Sixty-nine male and female adults discharged from a mental health unit were followed for readmission during a 60 day period. Clients ($n = 12$) who received follow-up were visited by a psychiatric nurse for the purpose of mental health interventions. Remaining clients ($n = 57$) were followed for readmission rates.	Significant differences between the visitation and nonvisitation groups ($df = 1$, $\chi 2 = 6.698$, $p = 0.008$) were found. The twelve clients receiving follow-up had no readmission, whereas the nonvisited group had a 39% readmission rate ($n = 22$).
Beynon and Laschinger, 1993	The study examined attitudes toward theory-based practice before and after educational sessions.	Nineteen community health nursing managers responded to the Adjective Rating Scale (ARS) and Nursing Theories Opinionnaire (NTO) before education, after the second session, and 6 months later. Managers participated in three educational sessions on the NSM.	Managers had positive attitudes toward theory-based practice that were increased and sustained for a 6 month period. Recommendations for implementing theory-based practice were made.
Blank, Longman, and Atwood, 1989	This descriptive study identified anticipated home care needs for cancer outpatients and their caregivers.	Eight cancer clients and eight caregivers responded to the Neuman-based interview guides, which were used to assess stressors. Content analysis was used to analyze transcribed data.	Client needs from intrapersonal stressors included treatment uncertainty, physical restriction/role change, anger/depression, and isolation. Lack of support was an interpersonal stressor. Extrapersonal stressors were transportation and finances. The needs that caregivers and clients identified were deemed congruent.

Continued

TABLE 8-2

Selected Studies Based on the Neuman System Model—cont'd

Study/Year	Purpose	Methods	Findings
COMMUNITY—cont'd			
Bowdler and Barrell, 1987	This descriptive study assessed multidimensional health needs of homeless persons.	Investigators used an indicator approach (chart audits at a free clinic), a key informant approach (telephone survey of key providers), and survey approach (health shelter interviews of 295 residents) to identify health needs.	A chart audit revealed 9% of clinic visitors had been released from jail within past month, 33% were day laborers, and 11% had previous psychiatric inpatient stays. Physical problems included hypertension, respiratory problems, and infectious parasitic diseases. Key informants indicated lack of money was major barrier to health. Substance abuse and mental illness were common problems, and physical problems were related to nutritional disorders, weather related injuries, seizure disorders, heart disease, and high blood pressure. Provider interviews confirmed financial barriers to care, mental disorders, substance abuse, loneliness, and heavy alcohol consumption. Limb disorders and hypertension were the most commonly reported physical health problems.
Bueno, Redeker, and Norman, 1992	This epidemiological study analyzed motor vehicle crash data in an urban trauma center.	Medical records of 864 motor vehicle crash victims were reviewed to ascertain gender, age, restraint use, intoxication, and mortality.	Safety restraints were not used in 84% of the accidents. Thirty-six percent of drivers or pedestrians were intoxicated at the time of the accident. Survival was significantly associated with restraint use. Females were more likely to use restraints, and males were more likely to be intoxicated. Alcohol use and lack of restraint use were associated.

Decker and Young, 1991	The study assessed self-perceived care needs of primary caregivers of home-hospice clients.	Nineteen primary caregivers participated in a needs assessment interview regarding intrapersonal, interpersonal, and extrapersonal stressors with regard to physiological, psychological, sociocultural, developmental, and spiritual aspects of the caregivers' situations. Qualitative and quantitative items were incorporated.	Caregivers perceived their overall health status as good although most were able to leave the home for only limited time periods. Coping was good, but some were overwhelmed by situational demands. Interpersonal stressors included lack of support, lack of information, and lack of service coordination. Extrapersonal stressors involved finances and legal concerns.
Grant and Bean, 1992	The study described the needs of informal caregivers of adults with head injuries.	Eighty-four informal caregivers were randomly selected from the mailing lists of two head injury foundations and responded to a questionnaire on needs. Needs were categorized by the investigators and by three content experts in the NSM.	Individuals identified a mean of 4.6 needs each. One hundred ten different needs were identified with 37 intrapersonal stressors, 24 interpersonal stressors, and 49 extrapersonal stressors. Physiological variables comprised 29 needs—58 psychosocial, and 16 spiritual.
Hanson, 1999	The study identified beliefs that differentiated smokers and nonsmokers in African-American, Puerto Rican, and non-Hispanic white adolescent females.	Four hundred thirty adolescent female clients at family planning clinics completed questionnaires on smoking behavior and the Fishbein-Ajzen-Hanson Questionnaire (FAHQ) on belief-based measures of attitude, norms, and perceived behavioral control. Logistic regression was used for analysis.	The attitude beliefs model correctly predicted smoking status in 94% of African-American subjects, 90% of Puerto Rican subjects, and 96% of non-Hispanic white subjects. Belief norms correctly predicted smoking status in 86% of African-American subjects and 71% of Puerto Rican and non-Hispanic white subjects. Perceived behavioral controls correctly predicted smoking status in 84% of African-American subjects, 81% of Puerto Rican subjects, and 85% of non-Hispanic white subjects.

Continued

TABLE 8-2

Selected Studies Based on the Neuman System Model—cont'd

Study/Year	Purpose	Methods	Findings
COMMUNITY—cont'd			
Mackenzie and Laschinger, 1995	The study evaluated NSM theory-based nursing (TBN) diagnoses generated by public health nurses.	Thirty-seven public health nurses—22 in a NSM theory-based practice and 15 in agency without specific theory—generated nursing diagnoses for a fictitious case. The Ziegler Characteristics of Diagnosis Tool (ZCDT) was used to score quantity and quality of diagnostic judgments.	One hundred forty-one diagnostic judgments were generated. Sixteen were determined to be medical diagnoses; 41 were incomplete nursing diagnoses; and 84 met criteria for nursing diagnoses. Of the 84 diagnoses, 55 were derived from nursing database and 29 from medical database. Use of nursing database generated more nursing diagnoses, but use of this database rather than a medical database did not improve the quality of the diagnoses. Non-TBN practice nurses generated more nursing diagnoses per nurse. TBN failed to influence quality of diagnosis.
Mannina, 1997	The study evaluated the effectiveness of combined pure tone threshold audiometry and tympanometry as opposed to audiometry alone.	Forty-one elementary students were evaluated with audiometry with tympanometry ($\underline{N} = 84$ ears).	Twenty-eight ears passed pure tone and tympanometry. Ten failed pure tone but passed tympanometry. Twenty-eight passed pure tone but failed tympanometry. Sixteen failed both pure tone and tympanometry.
Montgomery and Craig, 1990	This descriptive correlational study investigated stress levels and health practices of wives of alcoholics.	A convenience sample of 33 women was selected from 3 alcohol treatment centers. Interviews were conducted using Perceived Stress Level visual analog scale and FANTASTIC Lifestyle Checklist.	Two thirds perceived stress levels as high. The greatest interpersonal stressor was poor relationships with husbands; extrapersonal stressors centered on occupational and financial concerns. Wives reported minimal alcohol consumption, and only 40% reported smoking. Better health habits and improved mental health were associated with lower stress levels ($\underline{r} = -0.393$, $\underline{p} < 0.03$; $\underline{tau} = -0.412$, $\underline{p} < 0.003$).

Continued

ACADEMIC

Carroll, 1989	The study considered role deprivation of students in a traditional curriculum versus those enrolled in new curriculum based on the NSM.	One hundred ninety-four students enrolled in a Neuman-based curriculum were compared to 174 students in a medical model–based curriculum. The Role Conception-Role Deprivation Scale by Corwin was used to measure role deprivation.	Role deprivation was found to be significantly greater for students in the NSM-based curriculum ($t = -2.56$, $\underline{df} = 367$, $p < 0.05$).
Gigliotti, 1999	The study investigated multiple role stress as a moderator of the flexible line of defense of mothers who are also students.	One hundred eighty-eight women responded to the Perceived Multiple Role Stress scale (PMRS), the Maternal Role Involvement Questionnaire (MRIQ), the Student Role Involvement Questionnaire (SRIQ), and the Norbeck Social Support Questionnaire (NSSQ).	Maternal and student role involvement and social support did not influence PMRS for the total group. However, a maternal age of 37 or greater influenced role stress. Regression analysis revealed maternal and student involvement contributed 11% to PMRS, and social support added an additional 5% to the explanation of variance. In a subsequent regression, maternal and student involvement with low social support accounted for 8% of PMRS. In the total regression model, 24% of variance explained in PMRS by age, maternal and student role involvement, and social support.
Hainsworth, 1996	This experimental study investigated the influence of a death education program on nurse attitudes toward care of the dying.	Twenty-eight nurses were randomly assigned to control or experimental groups. Participants responded to Attitudes, Subjective Norms, and Behavioral Intentions of Nurses Toward Care of the Dying Persons and Their Families (ASBID). Experimental group nurses participated in three 2-hour classes about personal death awareness, communication with the dying, and care for the caregiver. The ASBID was administered before classes, 1 week following classes, and—for the experimental group—1 year after the class.	Significant differences were found only on the subjective subscale of the ASBID. In that instance, experimental group nurses had higher scores ($\underline{F} = 7.795$, $p < 0.010$).

TABLE 8-2

Selected Studies Based on the Neuman System Model—cont'd

Study/Year	Purpose	Methods	Findings
ACADEMIC—cont'd			
Speck, 1990	The study examined the effect of guided imagery on the anxiety level of baccalaureate (BS) nursing students performing their first injections.	Anxiety about performing injections was evaluated using a quasiexperimental posttest design that compared an experimental and control group. Twenty-six nursing students were randomly selected, with 16 assigned to the experimental group and 10 to the control. In addition to injection techniques, the experimental group received guided imagery instruction. Anxiety was measured using the chemical dot (Biodot) system, the State-Trait Anxiety Inventory (STAI), performance time, and performance score.	ANCOVA using the baseline STAI scores as the covariate revealed significant differences between the two groups. The guided imagery group has less anxiety, as measured by the STAI ($F = 8.514$, $df = 1, 24$, $p = 0.008$). No differences were noted in performance time, performance scores, or Biodot readings.
WORKPLACE			
Brown, Sirles, Hilyer, and Thomas, 1992	The study investigated the effect of a back school rehabilitation program for injured workers.	Seventy employees with back injuries who participated in 6-week back school were compared to 70 injured employees not participating. Dependent variables included lost work time, lost time cost, medical cost, and number of injuries.	The back school group experienced fewer subsequent injuries 6 months after intervention ($p = 0.001$). Although not it was not statistically significant, the back school group experienced a cost savings of $9,743 after intervention. Back school subjects lost fewer work days after treatment than before treatment.

Sirles, Brown, and Hilyer, 1991	The study evaluated back strength, flexibility, psychological well-being, and pain for back school rehabilitation program participants.	Seventy-four back school participants were evaluated before and after treatment. Subjects completed the Acuflex I Sit and Reach test, a 20-point pain rating scale, the Nottingham Health profile, the Psychological Wellbeing Scale, the Spielberger Anxiety Scales, and the Beck Depression Inventory.	Back strength increased ($t = 5.29$, $p < 0.01$), as did back flexibility ($t = 6.27$, $p < 0.01$). Pain decreased ($t = 3.73$, $p < 0.01$). Psychological well being improved in terms of sleep ($z = 2.24$, $p < 0.05$), pain ($z = 3.75$, $p < 0.01$), and physical mobility ($z = 3.13$, $p < 0.01$). Subjects had greater overall wellbeing ($t = 3.75$, $p < 0.05$), less anxiety ($t = 3.42$, $p < 0.05$), less depression ($t = 2.44$, $p < 0.01$), more positive well being ($t = 3.03$, $p < 0.05$), improved general health ($t = 2.65$, $p < 0.05$), and improved vitality ($t = 2.91$, $p < 0.05$).
Koku, 1992	The study evaluated the influence of counseling on back pain severity.	Forty back school participants who were randomly selected to receive individual counseling were compared to a group that did not receive counseling. The McGill Pain Questionnaire was completed at the beginning and end of the program.	No significant differences in severity of back pain between participants receiving counseling and those who did not were found.
Collins, 1996	This descriptive study examined the relationship of work stress, hardiness, and burnout of hospital staff nurses.	One hundred thirteen full-time staff nurses responded to the Personal Views Survey (hardiness), the Tedium Burnout Scale, and the Nursing Stress Scale. Correlations were used for data analysis.	Nurses with higher levels of hardiness experiences less stress ($r = -0.22$, $p < 0.01$) and lower levels of burnout ($r = -0.56$, $p < 0.01$). Higher levels of stress were associated with more burnout ($r = 0.39$, $p < 0.01$).
Courchene, Patalski, and Martin, 1991	The study examined the health status of pediatric nurses who routinely administered Cyclosporine A (CyA).	Twenty-two pediatric nurses administering CyA and 31 medical surgical nurses with no CyA exposure completed the Health Status Questionnaire. Data were analyzed for homogeneity of proportions using a chi square.	Of the CyA-exposed nurses, 72% handled the substance daily. Symptoms that were more likely to be reported by CyA-exposed group were constipation ($\chi^2 = 9.34$, $p < 0.01$), tinnitus ($\chi^2 = 7.78$, $p < 0.02$), and headache ($\chi^2 = 6.12$, $p < 0.05$).

Continued

TABLE 8-2

Selected Studies Based on the Neuman System Model—cont'd

Study/Year	Purpose	Methods	Findings
WORKPLACE—cont'd			
Gellner, Landers, O'Rourke, and Schlegel, 1994	This survey assessed real and perceived safety risks of community health nurses (CHN).	Thirty-five CHNs were surveyed about the person, safety, risk, environment, nursing intervention, and prevention.	Nurses worked at all times of day or night. Most perceived themselves as cautious and expressed concern for personal safety. Safety measures were recognizable clothing, escorts, and safety rules. Risks in the home environment included violence, crime, guns, and drug abuse.
Marsh, Beard, Adams, 1999	This study tested a theoretical model based on Selye's stress theory and NSM to confirm the mediational effect of spiritual well-being and hardiness on job stress and burnout among nurses.	Two hundred eight RNs completed the Stress Diagnostic Survey, JAREL Spiritual Well-Being Scale, Personal Views Survey, and Maslach Burnout Inventory. Structural equation modeling was used for model testing.	The proposed model achieved a good fit with observed findings. Job stress had a direct, positive effect of burnout (0.55). Spiritual well-being directly and negatively affected burnout (−0.36). Spiritual well-being had a moderate direct, positive effect on hardiness (0.40). Hardiness had a small negative, indirect effect on burnout (−0.27). Spiritual wellbeing operating through hardiness had a small, indirect negative effect on burnout among nurses (−0.107).
Vaughn, Cheatwood, Sirles, and Brown, 1989	The study investigated the effect of progressive muscle relaxation (PMR) on stress among clerical workers.	The Stress Response Index (SRI) was used to assess stress level of eight experimental subjects who were taught PMR and 10 control subjects. Subjects were pretested with SRI and posttested 4 weeks after intervention.	ANCOVA using the pretest scores as covariates revealed significant difference between experimental and control group SRI scores ($E = 11.01$, $p = 0.005$). The PMR group experienced lower stress.

somatization, phobic anxiety, general anxiety, obsessive-compulsive behaviors, interpersonal sensitivity, and depression. This study supports Neuman's concept of wholistic interventions for decreasing stressors.

Heffline (1991) compared the use of radiant heat versus pharmacological agents such as meperidine and fentanyl for their usefulness in treating postanesthesia shivering. The nursing intervention of radiant heat was aimed at reestablishing physiological stability and reducing the degree of reaction to a stressor breaking through the flexible line of defense. Heffline found that radiant heat alone worked as well in reducing postanesthesia shivering as combinations of radiant heat and meperidine or fentanyl did. This lends support to using radiant heat as a primary intervention to prevent postanesthesia shivering and substantiates the NSM concepts of degrees of reaction to stressors and primary prevention.

Rodrigues-Fisher, Bourguignon, and Good (1993) used a tertiary prevention program of fiber and fluid intake to maintain bowel elimination in older adult nursing home residents. The number of bowel movements increased by the third month but had returned to baseline by the sixth month. Laxative and stool softener use decreased to their lowest points at 4 and 5 months, respectively, but had increased by the sixth month. Frequency of use, however, was approximately half that of the baseline period. The finding that some participants were able to discontinue laxatives and stool softeners was clinically significant.

Ziemer (1983) completed one of the early intervention projects in the area of education, investigating the effects of providing clients with information before surgery. Unfortunately, her findings failed to support the concept that coping was improved by providing information. Subjects given procedure information, those given procedure and sensation information, and those receiving procedure, sensation, and coping information all exhibited similar degrees of coping skills and reported the same intensity of pain and distress. These similarities led Ziemer to question the sufficiency of the intervention. This study did not support Neuman's concept that primary prevention increases resistance to stressors.

Ali and Khalil (1989) examined the effects of a psychoeducational intervention completed 1 to 2 days preoperatively on anxiety levels of Egyptian bladder cancer clients. Clients receiving this primary prevention measure postoperatively demonstrated lower levels of anxiety. This study supported the idea that nursing interventions can strengthen resistance to stressors and the flexible line of defense.

Several descriptive studies (Bowdler & Barrell, 1987; Lowry & Anderson, 1993; Breckinridge,1997a, 1997b) used the NSM to explore contextual variables that might influence phenomena experienced by clients. The wholistic focus of the NSM proposes that context provides important indicators of response to stressors. Ultimately, this information can be useful in planning interventions.

Bowdler and Barrell (1987) used the NSM as a conceptual framework to identify health needs of homeless persons. Investigators considered this study the assessment phase of the nursing process. The composite profile was a single male in his mid-to-late thirties with financial limitations. Mental problems, including substance abuse, were prevalent. Many physical problems existed, with limb disorders and hypertension being the most common. Healthcare tended to be episodic and usually was received at a local teaching hospital. Investigators recommended a wholistic approach—similar to Neuman's suggestion—to address full range of stressors that homeless clients encounter.

Hinds (1990) studied contextual factors that predict quality of life for lung cancer clients. Significant factors influencing quality of life included prognosis, surgery, current radiotherapy, performance status, self-control skills, preference for information, and age-group. Hinds completed a systematic review of the NSM and established congruence of these personal and contextual factors within the model. This study considers clients with lung cancer whose flexible lines of defense, normal lines of defense, and lines of resistance were penetrated. Life-threatening core penetration had occurred. In the environment, interpersonal stress factors reflected age, performance status, informational styles, resourcefulness, prior surgeries, and prognosis. Interpersonal and extrapersonal stress factors were related to involvement with healthcare personnel, clinic staff, and institutional policies. Health was conceived as variance from wellness and reflected in quality of life. Nursing protected the client by strengthening lines of resistance and maintaining the highest possible level of functioning. Secondary interventions aimed to reduce symptoms, tension, and fear. Tertiary interventions were directed toward maintaining client stability.

Bowman (1997) studied sleep satisfaction, pain perception, and psychological concerns of older adults undergoing planned and unplanned hip replacement. Delirium occurred more commonly in clients who had unplanned hip surgery. Both groups of clients had unsatisfactory postoperative sleep levels, but the unplanned hip surgery group experienced more days with unsatisfactory sleep levels. Pain levels were also greater on some days for the unplanned hip surgery group, particularly for those who experienced delirium. The NSM was valuable in considering multiple contextual variables that influence client response and well-being; however, investigators only loosely identified the linkages between the findings and the model.

In an effort to further describe spirituality—one of Neuman's five interdynamic variables—Clark, Cross, Deane, and Lowry (1991) interviewed 15 adults about their hospitalization. Investigators suggested that illness and loss depleted energy, leading to spiritual needs and concerns. The presence of nurses and their caregiving contributed to the sense of client well-being. Important common patterns described by clients included trust, meaningful support systems, and respect for personal beliefs. A shortcoming of this study is its failure to tie its findings to the NSM. However, trusting relationships, supportive environments, sensitivity to the client's belief system, integration of spiritual concerns into the plan of care, and ownership of the nursing role in healthcare systems were key interventions.

Examining the stressor of chronic pain, Radwanski (1992) described postinjury methods of treating chronic pain from spinal cord injuries. Radwanski proposed that stressors such as addiction and pain altered family and social relationships. Over-the-counter drugs alone or in combination with alcohol were used for pain relief. The NSM was loosely associated with the study. Radwanski suggested that client stressors must be managed through teaching clients new behaviors for response to pain.

In a study strongly connected to the theoretical tenets of the NSM, Lowry and Anderson (1993) studied Neuman client system variables to determine which might influence weaning from mechanical ventilation. Study variables were tightly linked to concepts of stressors, with mechanical ventilation as the research variable and failed weaning attempts as the empirical indicator. Physiological, developmental, psychological, and spiritual intrapersonal variables were assessed. Unfortunately, only four clients were able to complete the study protocol, which involved two interviews using several instruments. Investigators found that internal locus of control increased with likelihood of discharge and level of hope increased when clients completed ventilation. However, fear continued to be a factor during the entire period of mechanical ventilation. Investigators suggested that shorter instruments and use of the concept of mastery rather than locus of control would facilitate future study.

Breckenridge (1997a, 1997b) used a grounded theory approach to develop a model of decision making regarding dialysis modalities. Decisions were split between those made by clients, significant others, and healthcare providers. Financial resources, independence, and physiological issues influenced decision making. In a secondary analysis, Breckenridge (1997b) used the qualitative findings to describe a middle-range model of wholistic nursing practice for clients with end-stage renal disease. The model was developed within the context of the NSM. Physiological factors were related to dialysis as necessary for life and accessibility to dialysis sites. Psychological factors reflected power to make treatment decisions, whereas sociocultural issues related to financial issues and support from significant others. Developmental issues were related to level of independence, and spiritual issues centered around "counting blessings" (p. 59). Breckenridge's initial study and secondary analysis, which led to a model of wholistic nursing practice for end-stage renal disease clients, supports Fawcett's proposal (1995) of developing middle range theory derived from a conceptual model. Breckenridge's model specifically ties to the NSM and focuses in a very manageable way on nursing interventions for end-stage renal disease clients.

Several descriptive studies using the NSM focused on clients' significant others. Bass (1991) studied the needs of parents of infants in neonatal intensive care (NICU). The wholistic nature of the NSM guided the process of identifying needs and examining individual adaptation to stressors. Bass found parents most needed information, followed by person-related support, time for attachment/parenting, physical support for new mothers, spiritual support, and staff support. With these findings Bass was able to propose primary prevention measures such as ongoing nursing assessment of client and family needs, secondary prevention, and tertiary measures of information giving and personal support.

In another study of parents, Maligalig (1994) assessed perceptions of stressors in pediatric ambulatory surgery. Using the NSM as a guide for the qualitative methodology, Maligalig found that parents identified intrapersonal, interpersonal, and extrapersonal stressors experienced by children and their parents. Coping strategies identified as part of the normal lines of defense included seeking information, identifying resources, discussing concerns, using social support mechanisms, and rationalizing decisions about the child's surgery. Other strategies included acting calm, keeping occupied, keeping silent, crying, turning to faith or philosophy, and denying the situation. Findings suggested useful strategies congruent with the NSM concepts of primary, secondary, and tertiary prevention for decreasing the impact of stressors.

Loescher, Clark, Atwood, Leigh, and Lamb (1990) used the NSM to analyze the impact of the cancer experience on long-term survivors. Physiological, psychological, and socioeconomic stressors were identified. Investigators found that the cancer experience disrupted and permanently impacted life patterns. Adapting to personal and interpersonal changes and getting on with living were the two predominant themes. Stressors continued beyond diagnosis and treatment, and reconstitution was found to be an ongoing process. Relationships were renegotiated as intrapersonal and interpersonal levels of intimacy were disrupted. Survivors used four methods of reconstitution: personal counseling, counseling for family members, support or peer discussion groups, and talking to family and friends.

In summary, an intriguing aspect of the inpatient studies is the number that were intervention-oriented. Nursing studies tend to be description-oriented, but the NSM readily suggests a basis for intervention, as was indicated by the research from inpatient settings. There has been a wide array of interventions studies. Leja (1989) used guided imagery to decrease anxiety; Sabo and Michael (1996) used music and taped messages from the physician to decrease anxiety in cancer chemotherapy clients; Gavigan, Kline-O'Sullivan, and Klumpp-Lybrand (1990) explored the effect of turning on the occurrence of atelectasis in coronary artery bypass clients; Waddell and Demi (1993) investigated the effectiveness of individualized therapy for clients in a intensive partial hospitalization program for clients with anxiety disorders; Heffline (1991) compared radiant heat to the use of pharmacological agents in treating postanesthesia shivering; Rodrigues-Fisher, Bourguignon, and Good (1993) examined the outcome of a program of fiber and fluid intake on elimination in older nursing home residents; and Ziemer (1983) and Ali and Khalil (1989) explored the effectiveness of educational interventions.

These intervention studies tend to aim toward primary, secondary, or tertiary prevention as proposed by the NSM. Although a small number of the studies failed to demonstrate support for the NSM, many provided substantial support for the concepts of stressor reduction and prevention. Sabo and Michael (1996) found reduced anxiety but no fewer chemotherapy side effects for clients listening to music tapes. Using a wholistic individualized intervention, Waddell and Demi (1993) reduced fear and panic attacks for clients with anxiety disorders. Heffline (1991) found radiant heat prevented postanesthesia shivering. Ali and Khalil (1989) demonstrated that education decreased postoperative anxiety. For studies failing to exhibit significant differences postintervention (Leja, 1989; Gavigan, Kline-O'Sullivan, & Klumpp-Lybrand, 1990; Rodrigues-Fisher, Bourguignon, & Good, 1993; Ziemer, 1983) the sufficiency of the intervention or sample size rather than the NSM tended to be in question. Although some of these studies did not demonstrate statistical significance, they nonetheless hold clinical significance. For example, in the Rodrigues-Fischer, Bourguignon, and Good study (1993), some participants were able to discontinue laxative use.

Use of a theory in clinical practice also affects validation of that theory. Several descriptive inpatient studies were linked to the NSM and resulted in proposed clinical interventions. Bowdler and Barrell (1987) used their findings from their study describing health needs of homeless persons to propose a wholistic intervention approach as suggested by the NSM. Hinds' study (1990) of contextual factors predicting quality of life in lung cancer clients used the NSM to organize findings and suggest secondary and tertiary interventions. Bowman (1997) found the NSM useful in a multiplicity of contextual variables influencing outcomes for clients undergoing hip replacement surgery. Breckenridge (1997a, 1997b) developed a middle-range model from the NSM for intervention with clients with end-stage renal disease. Maligalig (1994) delineated coping patterns congruent with the NSM and identified strategies for reducing stressors. Unfortunately, descriptive studies such as those by Clark, Cross, Deane, and Lowry (1991) and Radwanski (1992) failed to adequately tie findings back to the NSM in their interpretations.

Additional research in inpatient settings can be directed toward interventions that can reduce potential and actual stressors. Several interventions studies have been completed, but numerous opportunities for continuing this line of research remain. In addition, many opportunities for descriptive research guided by the NSM exist. Such research can be directed toward stressor identification, contextual factors, and correlational studies of the relationship between selected stressors or contextual factors and client outcomes.

Research in Community Settings. A number of NSM studies were conducted in community settings. One topic of particular note was assessment of stressors for family members or caregivers. Montgomery and Craig (1990) investigated the stress levels and health practices of the wives of alcoholics. The NSM provided a view of wives as a composite of physiological, psychological, sociocultural, developmental, and spiritual variables. The nature of stressors was linked to the NSM. However, instrument reliability and validity was weak. Investigators found stress level to be inversely related to health status. Researchers suggested stressor assessment for wives of alcoholics.

Decker and Young (1991) investigated the self-perceived care needs of primary caregivers of home-hospice clients. NSM concepts related to intrapersonal, interpersonal, and extrapersonal stressors guided data analysis. The identification of stressors in each area led to five community nursing diagnoses supported with the data collected. The population was at risk for the following (Decker & Young, 1991, pp. 151-153):

- Health problems related to the physical demands of caring for the patient and insufficient rest and sleep
- Role constriction/role fatigue related to large number of caregivers living alone with the patient, few "breaks" from role a manifested by requests for increased respite relief, complaints about being homebound
- Insufficient support related to little assistance from friends and neighbors, variable levels of assistance from other family members, and feelings of being overwhelmed by demands of the situation
- Lack of information related to requests for information, particularly concerning the death experience
- Lack of service coordination related to care being provided by several different agencies as manifested by caregiver complaints of too many people being involved in care and not knowing [whom] to call for what

This qualitative study supported Neuman's concept of stressors, and the model directly guided the data analysis process.

Grant and Bean (1992) used the NSM in a descriptive study to identify and classify needs of informal caregivers for adults with head injuries. Investigators found unmet care needs in all categories of stressors that encompassed physiological, psychosocial, and spiritual needs. Intrapersonal stressors included time for self, time for social activities, assurance of care, physical rest, emotional rest, and meeting needs of head injured adults. Intrapersonal needs encompassed need for support groups, friends to assist with housekeeping, supportive family and friends, and supportive health professionals. Extrapersonal stressors resulted from need for respite care, day care programs, alternative housing, transportation, information, individuals to care for the client, financial support for sociocultural care, and information about psychosociocultural resources. The NSM was found to be useful in categorizing needs and represents a wholistic client view, in which stressors and variables are interrelated.

Blank, Longman, and Atwood (1989) interviewed outpatients with cancer and their caregivers and established that intrapersonal, interpersonal, and extrapersonal stressors were present. Moreover, cancer outpatients and their caregivers had the same perception of stressors. These findings provided a basis for needs assessment of cancer outpatients and their caregivers based on stressors identified in the NSM.

Barker, Robinson, and Brautigan (1999) examined the effectiveness of follow-up care by psychiatric home nurses on the readmission rates of clients with depression. Using the NSM as a guide, researchers proposed that mental health nurse home visits would eliminate environmental forces that might act as stressors and affect system stability. For clients receiving home visits, psychiatric nurses completed assessment of stressors and coping skills, teaching about the therapeutic regimen, and reinforcing compliance. None of the clients who received home visits was readmitted, despite histories of many previous readmissions. This study convincingly supported Neuman's concept that primary prevention (reduced possibility of stressor encounter), secondary prevention (early case finding and treatment), and tertiary prevention (readaptation, further education, and maintenance of stability) strengthens the flexible line of defense. In this instance these interventions were attributed to preventing psychiatric readmission.

In a slightly different study, implementation of theory-based practice that used the NSM in community settings was evaluated. Beynon and Laschinger (1993) studied public health nurse managers before and after and educational programs on theory-based practice. Managers who had moderately positive attitudes toward theory-based practice at the beginning increased and maintained those attitudes for six months following the educational intervention. Recommendations were made regarding a process for implementing theory-based practice in community settings.

Mackenzie and Laschinger (1995) undertook evaluation of the use of the NSM in a community-based practice by investigating the number and quality of theory-based nursing diagnoses. Unfortunately, use of theory-based nursing practice failed to generate any difference in quality of nursing diagnosis. One positive finding was that more nursing diagnoses were generated with a nursing database than with a medical one.

Hanson (1999) examined crosscultural beliefs about smoking among adolescent females. In a comparison of African-American, Puerto Rican, and non-Hispanic white females, Hanson developed logistic regression models regarding beliefs about smoking in order to determine whether differences existed within the ethnic groups. Using a dual theoretical framework of the NSM and Ajzen's Theory of Planned Behavior, Hanson proposed that stressors were beliefs about smoking, and lines of defense that smoking represented. Hanson's goal was to identify noxious and beneficial stressors that could generate health promotion interventions to discourage cigarette smoking.

African-American smokers believed more often than Puerto Ricans and non-Hispanic whites that smoking was enjoyable, would make them feel good, would not affect breathing despite the increased chance for heart disease, and was worth the financial expense of cigarettes. Puerto Rican smokers felt more often than African-Americans and non-Hispanic whites that smoking was enjoyable, made them feel good, was not bad for their health, and made it harder to breathe. Non-Hispanic white smokers felt smoking was enjoyable, helped them relax, and was bad for their health. In terms of subjective norm beliefs, African-American mothers and best friends were most likely to influence behavior, whereas Puerto Ricans were most influenced by mothers and a broader group of friends. Non-Hispanic whites were most influenced by boyfriends in shaping their smoking behaviors. For perceived behavioral control beliefs, smokers in all the groups were most influenced by stress and being around others who smoked. The study's finding that specific factors, including ethnicity, may influence smoking contributes significantly to practice guided by the NSM. Use of this information as primary prevention should permit targeted interventions to reduce stressors.

Unlike inpatient-based studies, most studies in community settings were descriptive. Barker, Robinson, and Brautigan (1999) provided support for the NSM concept that primary, secondary, and tertiary interventions can strengthen the lines of defense. Hanson (1999) was able to identify relevant information that would permit targeted smoking intervention as proposed by the NSM. Two studies on caregivers (Montgomery & Craig, 1990; Decker & Young, 1991) provided support for the NSM concept of stressors. Grant and Bean (1992) and Blank, Longman, and Atwood (1989) found that the NSM provided a wholistic framework in which to view caregivers' stressors. Beynon and Laschinger (1993) and Mackenzie and Laschinger (1995), in community-based studies, investigated the attitudes toward and the impact of theory-based practice. Their findings were not specifically related to the NSM.

Research in Academic Settings. Although the NSM has been a commonly used theoretical framework in education, research in academic settings focuses primarily on student intervention and use of the NSM within the curriculum. Speck (1990) studied the influence of guided imagery on the anxiety levels of baccalaureate nursing students giving their first injections. She tied study variables to Neuman's concept of stressors and their potential to disturb the normal lines of defense. Study findings partially supported the NSM, leading Speck to suggest that guided imagery could be a valuable tool for anxiety reduction in nursing students.

Hainsworth (1996) tried an educational intervention to positively influence nurse attitudes toward care of the dying. Such care was perceived to be a stressor for nurses as they tried to work with clients and families to manage their reactions to stressors. The research partially supported the contention that education could influence attitudes because the area of subjective norms differed significantly. However, no other differences were found. The study's limitations were a small sample size and the use of an instrument with limited reliability.

Carroll (1989) studied the influence of curriculum revision on the role deprivation of baccalaureate nursing students. In the new curriculum implementation, the NSM was used as a guiding framework as opposed to the medical model in the old curriculum. Students in the NSM conceptually based curriculum experienced greater role deprivation than students in a curriculum based on a traditional medical model. Carroll attributed both these differences to a substantial decrease in the number of program and clinical hours and to the focus of early courses on primary prevention. Additionally, hospital clinical experiences tended to be in institutions still based on the medical model.

Gigliotti (1999) was concerned about multiple role stress potentially experienced by women who were both mothers and students. She conceptualized both maternal and student roles as interpersonal and extrapersonal stressors as identified in the NSM. The psychological involvement in these roles was considered a psychological variable in the flexible line of defense, and interpersonal relationships were considered a sociocultural variable in the flexible line of defense. Perceived multiple role stress was considered an invasion of the normal line of defense. Maternal age moderated role stress. For older women, age influenced maternal and student role involvement, which in turn increased the multiple role stress. Social support exerted negative pressure on the flexible line of defense because women 37 years of age and older had slightly larger social networks. Gigliotti suggested that these findings reflected a variable in the NSM flexible line of defense in which women experienced anxiety when relationships failed to accommodate the changing self and thus generated anxiety. A surprising finding of the study was that the developmental variable of age intervened in the psychological and sociocultural variables under study. Gigliotti did not initially include age as a study factor influencing the flexible line of defense. Gigliotti also suggested that traditional statistical analyses such as analysis of variance might fail to identify potential interactions in complex relationships.

Interventional studies indicated that guided imagery could reduce stressors as suggested by the NSM (Speck, 1990) or education to decrease anxiety regarding death (Hainsworth, 1996). Carroll (1989) discovered students felt role deprivation in a curriculum based on the NSM. Gigliotti (1999) discovered multiple role stress in women over the age of 37 who were both students and mothers. Greater research on the use of the NSM in educational programs needs to occur. The Gigliotti study underscores some of the difficulties in studying the complex wholistic variables suggested by the NSM.

Workplace Studies. Both in healthcare and in the general sector, the workplace has served as a setting for a number of studies using the NSM. One intervention study dealt with the concept of intervention with back injury. Brown, Sirles, Hilyer, and Thomas (1992) studied the effects of a back school program on lost work time, lost time cost, medical cost, and number of injuries in municipal employees. Using the NSM, investigators proposed that lines of resistance could be strengthened through exercise and education—the intervention initiated in back school. All employees improved, but back school employees experienced significantly fewer subsequent injuries and saved more than $9,000. Although this study supports the NSM concept of strengthening lines of resistance, investigators failed to tie findings back to the NSM.

In an associated study, Sirles, Brown, and Hilyer (1991) found that participants in a 6-week back school program exhibited greater back strength and flexibility. Additionally, participants exhibited improvements in psychological well-being, depression, anxiety, and perceptions of pain. Investigators suggested that interventions were methods of enhancing lines of defense. Once again, these interventions strengthened the lines of defense, reconstituting the individual at a higher level of wellness.

As a third aspect of the back school study, Koku (1992) evaluated the influence of a tertiary prevention measure in the form of a counseling program on severity of low back pain of municipal city employees. Short, individual counseling sessions for clients demonstrated no influence on pain severity in comparison to clients who did not receive counseling. Koku recommended exploring other avenues to reduce client stressors.

In another workplace study, Vaughn, Cheatwood, Sirles, and Brown (1989) assessed a primary prevention strategy of progressive muscle relaxation (PMR) aimed to reduce stress levels of female clerical workers. The resulting stress reduction supported Neuman's theory that primary prevention can strengthen lines of defense.

In a hospital study Courchene, Patalski, and Martin (1991) examined the self-reported health status of pediatric nurses who administered Cyclosporine A (CyA). CyA represented an environmental stressor capable of penetrating lines of defense or resistance. Nurses handling CyA on a frequent basis were compared to a control group of nurses. Those handling CyA reported symptoms such as constipation, tinnitus, and headache more often than did those in the control group. Although the sample size was small, some tentative evidence supporting CyA's penetration of lines of defense was found. An implication of this study is that nurses need to apply NSM principles of primary prevention to themselves.

Collins (1996) examined the relationship of work stress, hardiness, and burnout of hospital staff nurses. The NSM provided a basis for assessing the degree of response stress and mediating stressors through education. Hardiness was associated with low levels of stress and burnout, and stress and burnout were found to be associated. Nurses experiencing greater stress were more likely to experience burnout. Correlations in this study were small but significant and offered tentative support for the impact of stressors on the lines of defense. Collins failed to directly tie findings from this study back to the NSM.

Using a theoretical model based on Selye's stress theory (1974) and the NSM, Marsh, Beard, and Adams (1999) investigated the mediational effect of spiritual well-being and hardiness on job stress and burnout among nurses. Investigators proposed that job stress would be mediated by NSM variables that were spiritual (spiritual well-being, life satisfaction, life responsibility, and self-actualization), psychological (hardiness, commitment, challenge, and control), sociocultural (social support), developmental (age), and physiological (increased blood pressure, pulse, blood flow to muscles, respiration, metabolic rate, glucose level, and gastric movement). If the flexible line of defense prevented penetration of the normal line of defense, investigators proposed an absence of burnout (emotional exhaustion, depersonalization, and presence of personal accomplishment). Variables actually measured in this study were spiritual well-being, hardiness, social support, age, and burnout. Other model variables were considered latent variables. The proposed model was found to fit the observed data and led to the conclusion that spiritual well-being functioned indirectly through hardiness to influence levels of burnout. Several specific findings indicated this linkage. Higher levels of job stress were associated with greater burnout. Nurses with greater spiritual well-being evidenced higher levels of hardiness and exhibited lower levels of burn out. This study supported the NSM view of the total person as a composite of mind, body, and spirit. The spiritual aspect consciously or unconsciously can control the mind and influence well-being. The aspect of spiritual well-being was shown to affect the psychological variable of hardiness. A strength of this study is the care that investigators used in tying variables of research to the proposed model based on the NSM. Additionally, their discussion directly linked their findings back to the model.

Gellner, Landers, O'Rouke, and Schlegel (1994) investigated environmental stressors that influence the safety of the community health nursing workplace. Using the NSM as a guide, community health nurses were perceived as persons functioning within a complex environment with health and safety concerns. Nurses made visits at all hours and were concerned about their personal safety. Urban areas were perceived as high risk, and nurses felt a safety education program was needed. Behaviors that decreased fears included wearing recognizable identification, carrying a nursing bag and portable phone, and using an escort service for evening visits. Findings from this study were used to develop a Community Risk-Reduction Plan, which is an example of a primary prevention modality.

In a school-based study, Mannina (1997) compared the combined use of pure tone audiometry and tympanometry with pure tone audiometry alone. The NSM emphasis of wellness was used to frame the study. Hearing testing was considered to be either primary, secondary, or tertiary prevention for school children, depending on their level of hearing. More middle-ear disease was discovered with the combination assessment mechanisms than would have been found with either system alone. Findings were not tied to the NSM, but secondary and tertiary measures were recommended for discovering hearing loss.

The NSM was used a guide for an epidemiological study of motor vehicle crash data from an urban trauma center. Motor vehicle crashes were perceived as stressors that threaten wellness. Bueno, Redeker, and Norman (1992) found the following:

- More than 80% of motor vehicle crash victims were not wearing safety restraints at the time of the crash.
- One third of drivers was intoxicated.
- Women were more likely to wear restraints than men.
- Men were more likely to be intoxicated than women.
- Intoxicated crash victims were less likely to use restraint devices.

Using the NSM and these epidemiological findings as a basis for intervention, investigators indicated lines of defense must be strengthened to prevent additional stressors such as automobile accidents and to strengthen lines of defense through prevention.

To summarize workplace research, the back studies (Brown, Sirles, Hilyer, & Thomas, 1992; Sirles, Brown, & Hilyer, 1991; Koku, 1992; Vaughn, 1989) were the only intervention studies, all of which were related aspects of one large intervention program. Descriptive information on stressors of hospital and community nurses was obtained by Courchene, Patalski, and Martin (1991); Collins (1996); and Gellner, Landers, O'Rourke, and Schlegel (1994), and primary prevention measures congruent with strengthening lines of defense were derived. Perhaps the strongest study of this group is the model testing study by Marsh, Beard, and Adams (1999), which examined the effect of spiritual well-being and hardiness on job burnout of nurses. Further descriptive research of stressors, the influence of stressors on lines of defense, and effectiveness of interventions is needed.

Research Summary. The NSM has provided a framework for diverse nursing research studies, and investigators find the NSM helpful in conceptualizing research variables. An important point is that many studies provided support for selected concepts in the NSM. Some studies reflected only minimal use of the NSM according to the criteria classified by Silva (1986), other studies demonstrated strong theoretical ties. A number of studies have used the NSM for descriptive purposes. Some studies, however, are conceptualized within the NSM framework, identifying variables of interest from the NSM and driving research methods and analysis by model concepts (Blank, Longman, & Atwood, 1989; Clark, Cross, Deane, & Lowry, 1991; Courchene, Patalski, & Martin, 1991; Gavigan, Kline-O'Sullivan, & Klumpp-Lybrand, 1990; Gigliotti, 1999; Hinds, 1990; Lowry & Anderson, 1993; Rodrigues-Fisher, Bourguignon, & Good, 1993; Ziemer, 1983). A particular strength of each of the listed studies is that they tie their recommendations for intervention back to NSM concepts. All studies need to have these linkages and tie findings and proposals for new research back to the theoretical basis of the study.

The NSM has guided many theses and dissertations and has resulted in numerous research publications. Programs of research using the NSM need to be established to link additional connecting theory to phenomena of interest. To date, individual studies have limited generalizability to a variety of practice settings. Studies tend to be isolated and unconnected and fail to build uniformly strong support. More theory-testing studies similar to that of Marsh, Beard, and Adams (1999) need to be completed. Smith and Edgil (1995) have proposed that the future of NSM use lies in middle-range theory testing within the NSM. The Institute for the Study of the Neuman Systems Model has been established to assist in accomplishing the goal of middle-range theory testing. Goals of the Institute are to facilitate collaborative and multisite research efforts. This structure should be instrumental in unifying research efforts and facilitating development of middle-range theory.

Future research studies can be directed toward the following:

- Stressor identification
- Identification of the impact of contextual variables
- The impact of primary, secondary, and tertiary prevention on the flexible line of defense, the normal line for defense, and lines of resistance in clients, caregivers, and students

The potential for the NSM has only begun to be explored. Nurses have the opportunity to examine many variables identified within the wholistic context of the NSM. Greater effort in tying findings of future studies back to the tenets of the NSM is necessary.

PRAXIS AND THEORY UTILIZATION: DESIGNING NURSING PRACTICE PROGRAMS WITHIN NEUMAN'S THEORETICAL SYSTEM

Neuman has indicated that her model relates to practice, research, and education; however, she has not described the relationship as explicitly as Parse and Roy have described their own theories. The NSM has been particularly well received in community health settings. It is interdisciplinary, but it also is a systems model that uses the terms *primary, secondary,* and *tertiary prevention,* which are common in public health. Neuman describes the focus of nursing as keeping the client system stable through accuracy both in assessing the actual and possible effects of environmental stressors and in assisting client adjustments required for an optimal wellness level (Neuman, 1995). Neuman does not describe how the concern of other disciplines using the model might vary from those of nursing.

The Variables of Concern for Practice

The components of the NSM are listed in Box 8-2. The definitions of concepts associated with the model tend to be broad (Neuman, 1995). Development of the substantive structure of the concepts still requires work. For example, nursing is defined as "a unique profession concerned with all variables affecting clients in their environments" (p. 46). The characteristics of the uniqueness need to be specified to elucidate the domain and boundaries of nursing. To illustrate the variation in definitions of some NSM concepts, Table 8-3 lists definitions extracted from selected publications.

Describing a Population for Nursing Purposes

A literature review found no examples in which the NSM was used to describe populations. Additional specification of the components of the NSM is required before the model should be used for describing a population for nursing purposes.

Text continued on p. 226

TABLE 8-3

Definition of Terms

Author	Lines of Defense and Resistance	Variables	Stressors	Environment
Rodriguez, 1995	Flexible line of defense—health and mental status of resident Normal line of defense—body's defenses	Physiological—deterioration of body systems Psychological—cognitive changes Sociocultural—retirement, family/friend separation, death of spouse Developmental—experiencing last developmental stage Spiritual—seeking comfort in spiritual beliefs during stressful times	Intraresident—declining health, possible cognitive impairment, socioeconomic factors, relocation trauma, death of a spouse Interresident—seeing decline of other residents, monitoring of neighbors with cognitive impairment Extraresident—physician consultation, diagnostic lab tests, transportation, shopping, anxiety regarding procedures, appointments	
Chiverton and Flannery, 1995	Flexible line of defense—cannot function optimally in individual cognitively impaired Normal line of defense—weakened by cognitive impairment, influenced by coping patterns, support systems Internal lines of resistance—may not rebound as quickly as cognitively intact individuals	Stress reduces cognitive ability. Psychological stress may disrupt ego structure and cognition. Indirect relationship between spiritual belief and sociocultural variables exists.		Internal environment—forces contained within the boundaries of the client system, including interpersonal factors Created environment—unconscious mobilization of all system variables—including basic structure, energy, factors toward system integration, stability, and integrity—may be unable to develop an unconsciously created environment

| Stuart and Wright, 1995 | Flexible line of defense—client's appraisal of the stressor and the range of available coping resources
Normal line of defense—usual wellness or state to which client has evolved over time | Created environment—psychological and sociocultural components of individuals
Lines of Resistance—coping mechanisms—cognitive, intrapsychic, and emotion-focused |
| Bueno and Sengin, 1995 | Physiological—e.g., breathing, gas exchange, exchange of food and nutrients, fluid and electrolyte balance, thermal regulation, cardiac function, and movement.
Psychological—mental and emotional process interrupted and potentially altered by illness or injury; management of fear, sadness, and psychosis, anxiety
Sociocultural variables—relationships, language, culture
Developmental—ability to conceptualize and respond to changes in health status, cognitive abilities, educational achievements, life experiences
Spiritual—religious beliefs and human values | |

Continued

TABLE 8-3

Definition of Terms—cont'd

Author	Lines of Defense and Resistance	Variables	Stressors	Environment
Rodriguez, 1995	Flexible line of defense—policies and procedures of department Normal line of defense—organizational structure of hierarchy of clinic staff Lines of resistance—senior management personnel	Physiological—individual or group physical structure Psychological—staff support esteem Sociocultural—interdepartmental relations, ethnicity Developmental—group beliefs that assist staff to cope with population morbidity and mortality	Intraclinical—staff selection, orientation training, employee health records, appropriate decision making, providing resident services, caring for clients Interclinical—activities involving coordinating services with other departments Extraclinical—areas such as long-term care protocols, ANA standards, establishing fees for service, working with nursing agencies, physical schedules	
Kelley and Sanders, 1995	Lines of resistance—resources comprised of characteristics that protect an organization by increasing its ability to prevent stressors from threatening ability of system or return it to a healthy state. Examples: organization's position in community; nursing system's position in organization; amount	Physiological variables—variables that imply or indicate overall health of nursing system, structure and processes that enable a nursing system or organization to accomplish mission or goals, size, number of employees and beds, types of service offered, urban or rural location, and composition of leadership team.		Internal—forces and stressors related to intrapersonal system, e.g., perceptions of one's role, length of time in that role, acceptability of role by others, and physical stamina required for the role Intranursing system—intraorganizational system: perception of nursing or organization regarding position in marketplace;

Psychological variables—characteristics of system that reveal personality of system, e.g., identity, channels and processes for communicating, leadership style, attitudes, cooperation, atmosphere

Sociocultural variables—social, cultural, economic, political, and technological viability of nursing system or organization and norms and values of nursing system or organization, e.g., loyalty, group affiliations, networks, economic and human resources, system or organization affiliations and values

Developmental variables—maturity level or degree to which organization has evolved, developed, or declined over time and as a result improved ability to accomplish mission; life patterns of nursing system; past experiences and history; previous demands

Spiritual variables—purpose, mission and philosophy of organizational system

or lack of trust, loyalty, cohesiveness, collaboration, and interaction among group members; economic position or financial viability of organization or nursing system; position in competitive marketplace, number, type, and mix of clients; available reputations of organization or nursing

Normal line of defenses—state of wellness considered "normal" for organization or nursing system; composite of how well goals and objectives are attained, financial outcomes achieved, quality service provided, productivity maintained; decision making; staff's morale; motivation levels; interactive processes; ethnicity; life-style; and quality of work

amount of change that has or has not occurred; social, cultural, and spiritual norms and values; structures and processes within systems, amount and type of resources available for accomplishing goals of systems

External—intersystem factors such as interpersonal conflicts resulting from competition for resources or markets

Extrapersonal factors—policies and procedures, job designs, standards, accreditation requirements, system design, social equity, interdepartmental stressors such as competition for market share and resources

Expected Outcomes of Nursing. Nursing outcomes as specified by Neuman (1995) are presented in Box 8-4.

Process Models

Neuman (1995) has proposed a nursing process format that includes diagnoses, goals, and outcomes. She does not state whether other disciplines following this model would use the same process that nursing uses. The nursing diagnosis is context-specific. That is, broad categories of variables are identified, but the specifics depend on the particular situation. The theories that guide the content of the process depend on the specifics of the particular client/client systems. Box 8-5 outlines the means for determining the appropriate database for establishing the nursing diagnoses.

BOX 8-4

Nursing Outcomes

1. Intervention using one or more of the three prevention modes—retaining system stability, attaining system stability, or maintaining system stability
2. Evaluation of outcome goals with reformulation of subsequent goals based on systemic feedback principles
3. Structuring of intermediate and long-range goals for nursing action in relation to short-term goal outcomes
4. Validation of the nursing process and feedback for further system input gathered from the client goal outcome

From Neuman, B.M. (1995). *The Neuman Systems Model* (3rd ed.). Norwalk, CT: Appleton & Lange.

BOX 8-5

The Database for Nursing Diagnosis

1. Identification and evaluation of potential or actual stressors threatening the stability of the client/client system (composite of physiological, psychological, socio-cultural, and spiritual variables)
2. Assessment of the condition and strength of basic structure factors and energy resources
3. Assessment of characteristics of the flexible and normal lines of defense, lines of resistance, degree of potential reaction, reaction, and/or potential for reconstitution following a reaction
4. Identification, classification, and evaluation of potential and/or actual intrapersonal, interpersonal, and extrapersonal interactions between the client and environment, considering all five variables (see Figure 8-1)
5. Evaluation of the influence of past, present, and possible future life process and coping patterns on client system stability
6. Identification and evaluation of actual and potential internal and external resources for an optimal state of wellness
7. Identification and resolution of perceptual differences between caregivers and client/client system

From Neuman, B.M. (1995). *The Neuman Systems Model.* (3rd ed.). Norwalk, CT: Appleton & Lange.

This database is used to determine variance from wellness through the following method (Neuman, 1995, p. 18):

- Synthesis of theory with client data to identify the condition from which a comprehensive diagnostic statement can be made. Goal prioritization is determined by client/client system wellness level, system stability needs, and total available resources to accomplish desired goal outcomes.
- Hypothetical goals and interventions postulated to reach the desired client stability or wellness level, that is, to maintain the normal line of defense and retain the flexible line of defense, thus protecting the basic structure.

Nursing goals are determined by negotiations with the client to prescribe change or goal outcomes in relation to the variance from wellness. Synthesizing theories with client data, nurses intervene through the strategies outlined in Box 8-5. These strategies are then negotiated with the client to promote retention, attainment, and maintenance of client system stability. The final phase of the nursing process labels nursing outcomes (see Box 8-4).

Using the NSM, Reed (1982, 1993) proposed a process for practice and research with families. Data about stressors that threaten the stability of family members or the family system were collected. The focus was on information about the flexible and normal lines of defense, the lines of resistance, and the basic family structure. The domains represented in this data collection are physiological, psychological, sociocultural, spiritual, and developmental. Reed proposes the type of data relevant to each domain and to the lines of defense and resistance. Additional research and development is required to clarify definitions of the concepts for practice purposes.

Practice Models

Although the NSM has been widely used in framing research related to practice issues, these studies for the most part represent individual efforts with limited generalizability to practice. Establishing research programs to develop and test middle-range theories will facilitate specifying practice models.

Implications for Administration

Several authors have reported ways in which the NSM applies to administration. Table 8-3 shows examples of how the concepts of the model have been operationalized in reference to administration. NSM-related literature has not discussed the validity of extending these person-centered concepts to organizations. Taylor (1989) has questioned the validity of such extensions in reference to Self-Care Deficit Nursing Theory. A similar discussion needs to occur for the NSM before the extension of the concepts from person to organization can be considered valid.

If the NSM is to structure practice within an organization, consideration must be given to the necessary antecedent knowledge. Nurses working from the NSM require an extensive understanding of system theory and stress theory. In addition, they require a foundational background in physiological, psychological, sociocultural, developmental, and spiritual concepts to enable them to determine the specific data to collect in relation to the elements of the NSM. These prerequisites are also required for making sense of that data within the context of the particular clinical situation. Instruments that suggest questions to be asked in data collection have been published in the literature. However, theories that hypothesize the relationships among the data items for nursing purposes have not been published. Nursing must develop theories and practice models within this broad conceptual framework.

Implications for Education

Additional development of the substantive structures of the concepts is required before developing continuing education programs for clinical practice can proceed.

STATUS OF THEORY DEVELOPMENT

The NSM can be approached from two perspectives: nursing and systems. The NSM is a model of the client or client system that links to the system context at the point of levels of prevention. The NSM appeals to many nurses interested in a model useful at the community level. From the perspective of developing nursing theory or science, the absence of a discipline-specific object limits the NSM.

Neuman described a partnership between nurse and client. Currently, however, her conceptualizations do not consider the nurse's role in the client system. The nurse elicits the client's view of stressors but remains separate from the client system. The systemic interactions between nurse and client are not yet described. The interaction of the two persons' systems should be a part of the model. Banathy noted that within system theory the relationship of the system and the environment is mutually interdependent. This requires viewing the system as a whole while also considering it an embedded part of its environment. This work has not been performed for the NSM. The incorporation of more classes of systems (client system, nurse-client system, healthcare economic system) would make the NSM more general and more applicable beyond nursing. However, the contribution of the NSM to the broader system needs to be clarified. Those scholars interested in working with the NSM should continue to develop stage 2 interpretation and application. Further work could include revisions of the original model and explicit linkages to the broader system within which the NSM exists, such as the healthcare delivery system.

NEXUS

The International Society for System Science (ISSS) has developed a model of the whole of systemic inquiry with two interrelated aspects: knowledge and action. They described knowledge as both philosophical (general) and theoretical (specific), whereas action is both methodology and praxis. Knowledge and action are constantly interrelated; inquiry proceeds from general principles to specific applications and then to applicable methodologies. Once the methodologies are realized, they then return to general principles, and the process repeats itself (ISSS). By its design, system theory is a model of the nexus proposed in this text.

REFERENCES

Ali, N.S. & Khalil, H.Z. (1989). Effect of psychoeducational intervention on anxiety among Egyptian bladder cancer clients. *Cancer Nursing, 12*(4), 236-242.

Ashby W. (1972). Systems and their informational measures. In G.J. Klir (Ed.), *Trends in General system theory.* New York: Wiley.

Banathy, B. (1999). A taste of systemics. The primer project. International society for systems studies. URL http://www.isss.org/tast.html.

Barker, E., Robinson, D., & Brautigan, R. (1999). The effect of psychiatric home nurse follow-up on readmission rates of clients with depression. *Journal of the American Psychiatric Nurses Association, 5*(4), 111-116.

Bass, L.S. (1991). What do parents need when their infant is a patient in the NICU? *Neonatal Network, 10*(4), 25-33.

Beynon, C. & Laschinger, K. (1993). Theory-based practice: Attitudes of nursing managers before and after educational sessions. *Public Health Nursing, 10*(3), 183-188.

Blank, J.J., Longman, A.J., & Atwood, J.R. (1989). Perceived home care needs of cancer patients and their caregivers. *Cancer Nursing, 12*(2), 78-84.

Bowdler, J.E. & Barrell, L.M. (1987). Health needs of homeless persons. *Public Health Nursing, 4*(3), 135-140.

Bowman, A.M. (1997). Sleep satisfaction, perceived pain and acute confusion in elderly clients undergoing orthopaedic procedures. *Journal of Advanced Nursing, 26*(3), 550-564.

Breckenridge, D.M. (1997a). Patient perceptions of why, how, and by whom dialysis treatment modality was chosen. *ANNA Journal, 24*(3), 313-319.

Breckenridge, D.M. (1997b). Decision regarding dialysis treatment modality: A holistic perspective. *Holistic Nursing Practice, 12*(1), 54-61.

Brown, K.C., Sirles, A.T., Hilyer, J.C., & Thomas, M.J. (1992). Cost-effectiveness of a back school intervention for municipal employees. *Spine, 17*(10), 1224-1228.

Bueno, M.M., Redeker, N., & Norman, E.M. (1992). Analysis of motor vehicle crash data in an urban trauma center: Implications for nursing practice and research. *Heart & Lung, 21*(6), 558-567.

Bueno, M.M. & Sengin, K.K. (1995). Neuman Systems Model for critical care nursing: A framework for practice. In B.M. Neuman (Ed.), *The Neuman Systems Model.* (3rd ed.). Norwalk, CT: Appleton & Lange.

Carrigg, K.C. & Weber, R. (1997). Development of the Spiritual Care Scale. *Image, 29*(3), 293.

Carroll, T. (1989). Role deprivation in baccalaureate nursing students pre and post curriculum revision. *Journal of Nursing Education, 28*(3), 134-139.

Chiverton, P. & Flannery, J.C. (1995). Cognitive impairment: Use of the Neuman Systems Model. In B.M. Neuman (Ed.), *The Neuman Systems Model.* (3rd ed.). Norwalk, CT: Appleton & Lange.

Clark, C.C., Cross, J.R., Deane, D.M., & Lowry, L.W. (1991). Spirituality: Integral to quality care. *Holistic Nursing Practice, 5*(3), 67-76.

Collins, M.A. (1996). The relation or work stress, hardiness, and burnout among full-time hospital staff nurses. *Journal of Nursing Staff Development, 12*(2), 81-85.

Courchene, V.S., Patalski, E., & Martin, J. (1991). A study of the health of pediatric nurses administering Cyclosporine A. *Pediatric Nursing, 17*(5), 497-500.

Decker, S.D. & Young, E. (1991). Self-perceived needs of primary caregivers of home-hospice clients. *Journal of Community Health Nursing, 8*(3), 147-154.

Emery, F. (1969). *Systems Thinking.* Baltimore: Penguin Books.

Fawcett, J. (1995). Constructing conceptual-theoretical-empirical structures for research: Future implications for use of the Neuman systems model. In B. Neuman (Ed.), *The Neuman Systems Model.* (3rd ed.). Norwalk, CT: Appleton & Lange.

Flannery, J. (1995). Cognitive assessment in the acute care setting: Reliability and validity of the Levels of Cognitive Functioning Assessment Scale (LOCFAS). *Journal of Nursing Measurement, 3*(1), 43-58.

Freese, B., Beckman, S. Boxley-Harges, S. Bruick, C., Harris, S., Hermiz, M., Meininger, M., & Steinkeler, S. (1998). Betty Neuman Systems Model. In A. Marriner-Tomey & M.R. Alligood (Eds.), *Nursing Theorists and Their Work.* St. Louis: Mosby.

Gavigan, M., Kline-O'Sullivan, C., & Klumpp-Lybrand, B. (1990). The effect of regular turning on CABG patients. *Critical care nursing quarterly, 12*(4), 69-76.

Gellner, P., Landers, S., O'Rourke, D., & Schlegel, M. (1994). Community health nursing in the 1990s—Risky business? *Holistic Nursing Practice, 8*(2), 15-21.

Gigliotti, E. (1999). Women's multiple role stress: Testing Neuman's flexible line of defense. *Nursing Science Quarterly, 12*(1), 36-44.

Grant, J.S. & Bean, C.A. (1992). Self-identified needs of informal caregivers of head-injured adults. *Family Community Health, 15*(2), 49-58.

Hainsworth, D. (1996). The effect of death education on attitudes of hospital nurses toward care of the dying. *Oncology Nursing Forum, 23*(6), 963-967.

Hanson, M.J. (1999). Cross-cultural study of beliefs about smoking among teenaged females. *Western Journal of Nursing Research, 21*(5), 635-651.

Hazzard, M.E. (1971). An overview of system theory. *Nursing Clinics of North America, 6*(3), 385-393.

Heffline, M.S. (1991). A comparative study of pharmacological versus nursing interventions in the treatment of postanesthesia shivering. *Journal of Post Anesthesia Nursing, 6*(5), 311-320.

Hinds, C. (1990). Personal and contextual factors predicting clients' reported quality of life: Exploring congruency with Betty Neuman's assumptions. *Journal of Advanced Nursing, 15*(4), 456-462.

ISSS Primer Project Group. The four domains. URL http://www.isss.org/primer/4domains.htm.

Kelley, J.A. & Sanders, N.F. (1995). A systems approach to the health of nursing and health care organizations. In B.M. Neuman (Ed.), *The Neuman Systems Model* (3rd ed.). Norwalk, CT: Appleton & Lange.

Klir, G.J. (1972). Preview: The polyphonic general system theory. In G.J. Klir (Ed.), *Trends in General system theory*. New York: Wiley.

Koku, R. (1992). Severity of low back pain: A comparison between participants who did and did not receive counseling. *AAOHN Journal, 40*(2), 84-89.

Lazarus, R. (1981). The stress and coping paradigm. In B.C. Eisendorf, D. Cohen, A. Kleinman, & P. Maxim (Eds.), *Models for Clinical Psychopathology*. New York: SP Medical and Scientific Books.

Lazlo, E. (1972). *The systems view of the world: The natural philosophy of the new development in the sciences*. New York: Braziller.

Leja, A.M. (1989). Using guided imagery to combat post-surgical depression. *Journal of Gerontological Nursing, 15*(4), 6-11.

Loescher, L.J, Clark, L., Atwood, J.R., Leigh, S., & Lamb, G. (1990). The impact of the cancer experience on long-term survivors. *Oncology Nursing Forum, 17*(2), 223-229.

Louis, M. (1995). The Neuman model in nursing research: An update. In B. Neuman (Ed.), *The Neuman Systems Model*, (3rd ed.). Norwalk, CT: Appleton & Lange.

Lowry, L.W. & Anderson, B. (1993). Neuman's framework and ventilator dependency: A pilot study. *Nursing Science Quarterly, 6*(4), 195-200.

Lowry, L.W., Walker, P.H., & Mirenda, R. (1995). Through the looking glass back to the future. In B. Neuman (Ed.), *The Neuman Systems Model* (3rd ed.). Norwalk, CT: Appleton & Lange.

Mackenzie, S.J. & Laschinger, H.K. (1995). Correlates of nursing diagnosis quality in public health nursing. *Journal of Advanced Nursing, 21*(4), 800-808.

Maligalig, R. (1994). Parents' perceptions of the stressors of pediatric ambulatory surgery. *Journal of Post Anesthesia Nursing, 9*(5), 278-282.

Mannina, J. (1997). Finding an effective hearing testing protocol to identify hearing loss and middle-ear disease in school-aged children. *Journal of School Nursing, 13*(5), 23-28.

Marsh, V., Beard, M., & Adams, B. (1999). Job stress and burnout: The mediational effect of spiritual well-being and hardiness among nurses. *Journal of Theory Construction and Testing, 3*(1), 13-19.

Montgomery, P. & Craig, D. (1990). Levels of stress and health practices of wives of alcoholics. *The Canadian Journal of Nursing Research, 22*(2), 60-70.

Neuman, B.M. (1974). The Betty Neuman Health-Care Systems Model: A total person approach to client problems. In J.P. Riehl & C. Roy (Eds.), *Conceptual Models for Nursing Practice*. New York: Appleton-Century-Crofts.

Neuman, B.M. (1982). *The Neuman Systems Model: Application to nursing education and practice*. Norwalk, CT: Appleton-Century-Crofts.

Neuman, B.M. (1989). *The Neuman Systems Model*. (2nd ed.). Norwalk, CT: Appleton & Lange.

Neuman, B.M. (1990). Health as a continuum based on the Neuman Systems Model. *Nursing Science Quarterly, 3*(3), 129-135.

Neuman, B.M. (1995). *The Neuman Systems Model*. (3rd ed.). Norwalk, CT: Appleton & Lange.

Neuman, B.M. (1996). The Neuman Systems Model in research and practice. *Nursing Science Quarterly 9*(2), 67-70.

Neuman, B. & Koertvelyessy, A. (1986, August). *The Neuman Systems Model and nursing research*. Paper presented at the Nursing Theory Congress, Toronto, Canada.

Neuman, B.M. & Young, R.J. (1972). A model for teaching total person approach to patient problems. *Nursing Research, 21*(3), 264-269.

Putt, A.M. (1978). *General system theory applied to nursing.* Boston: Little, Brown.

Radwanski, M. (1992). Self-medicating practices for managing chronic pain after spinal cord injury. *Rehabilitation Nursing, 17*(6), 312-317.

Reed, K.S. (1982). The Neuman systems model: A basis for family psychosocial assessment and intervention. In B. Neuman (Ed.), *The Neuman Systems Model: Application to nursing education and practice.* Norwalk, CT: Appleton-Century-Crofts.

Reed, K.S. (1993). *Betty Neuman: The Neuman Systems Model.* Newbury Park, CA: Sage.

Rodrigues-Fisher, L., Bourguignon, C., & Good, B.V. (1993). Dietary fiber nursing intervention: Preventing constipation in older adults. *Clinical Nursing Research, 2*(4), 464-477.

Rodriguez, M. (1995). The Neuman Systems Model adapted to a continuing care retirement community. In B.M. Neuman (Ed.), *The Neuman Systems Model.* (3rd ed.). Norwalk, CT: Appleton & Lange.

Sabo, C.E. & Michael, S.R. (1996). The influence of personal message with music on anxiety and side effects associated with chemotherapy. *Cancer Nursing, 19*(4), 283-289.

Selye, H. (1974). *Stress without distress.* New York: J.B. Lippincott.

Silva, M.C. (1986). Research testing nursing theory: State of the art. *Image, 18*(1), 1-11.

Sirles, A.T., Brown, K., & Hilyer, J.C. (1991). Effects of back school education and exercise in back injured municipal workers. *AAOHN Journal, 39*(1), 7-12.

Smith, M.C. & Edgil, A.E. (1995). Future directions for research with the Neuman Systems Model. In B. Neuman (Ed.), *The Neuman Systems Model.* (3rd. ed.). Norwalk, CT: Appleton & Lange.

Speck, B.J. (1990). The effect of guided imagery upon first semester nursing students performing their first injections. *Journal of Nursing Education, 29*(8), 346-350.

Stuart, G.W. & Wright, L.K. (1995). Applying the Neuman Systems Model to psychiatric nursing practice. In B.M. Neuman (Ed.), *The Neuman Systems Model.* (3rd ed.). Norwalk, CT: Appleton & Lange.

Taylor, S. (1989). An interpretation of family within Orem's general theory of nursing. *Nursing Science Quarterly, 2*(3), 131-137.

Vaughn, M. Cheatwood, S., Sirles, A.T., & Brown, K.C. (1989). The effect of progressive muscle relaxation on stress among clerical workers. *AAOHN Journal, 37*(8), 302-306.

von Bertalanffy, L. (1968). *General system theory.* New York: Braziller.

Waddell, K.L. & Demi, A.S. (1993). Effectiveness of an intensive partial hospitalization program for treatment of anxiety disorders. *Archives of psychiatric nursing, 7*(1), 2-10.

Ziemer, M. (1983). Effects of information on post-surgical coping. *Nursing Research, 32*(5), 282-287.

CHAPTER

9

Modeling Nursing From a Transaction Systems Perspective

KING'S CONCEPTUAL SYSTEM and THEORY of GOAL ATTAINMENT

Key Terms

human interaction, p. 237
interpersonal systems, p. 236
personal systems, p. 236
social systems, p. 236
transaction, p. 237

Imogene King recognized the need for a frame of reference for nursing (1964, 1968). Using a general system theory approach, she formulated the systems framework to provide a way to select, organize, and develop concepts for nursing. In 1971, King authored *Toward a Theory of Nursing*. In 1981 she theorized a conceptual framework of dynamic interacting systems. This was further developed to King's Conceptual System (King, 1981, 1992). The Theory of Goal Attainment and several other theories were derived from the conceptual system (King, 1997a). In 1997, King noted that the only changes to the conceptual system were the additions of the concept of coping to the personal system and the concept of human beings as spiritual.

King's theoretical system comprises three components: (1) a conceptual system constructed of interacting systems, (2) a transaction process model and (3) a middle-range Theory of Goal Attainment. The language of goal attainment and systems is familiar to

BOX 9-1

King's Central Questions

SET 1

- What are some of the social and educational changes in the United States that have influenced changes in nursing?
- What basic elements are continuous throughout these changes in nursing?
- What is the scope of the practice of nursing, and in what kind of settings do nurses perform their functions?
- Are the current goals of nursing similar to those of the past half century?
- What are the dimensions of practice that have given the field of nursing a unifying focus over time?

SET 2

- What kind of decisions are nurses required to make in the course of their roles and responsibilities?
- What kind of information is essential for them to make decisions?
- What are the alternatives in nursing situations?
- What alternative courses of action do nurses have in making critical decisions about another individual's care, recovery, and health?
- What skills do nurses now perform and what knowledge is essential for nurses to make decisions about alternatives?

From King, I.M. (1971). *Toward a theory for nursing: General concepts of human behavior*. New York: John Wiley and Sons, Inc.

many nurses. The concept of health is defined by growth, development, and functioning in social roles. King's theory has strong human action and interpersonal components.

THE STARTING POINT OF THE MODELING PROCESS

King anticipated that a conceptual framework would generate a general theory for nursing (1971). She began with the belief that essential characteristics or properties of nursing have persisted despite changes in the world. She explored questions about changes in nursing and factors that influenced them, the scope of practice and practice settings, goals of nursing, and the unifying dimensions of practice. This led King to select universal ideas—man, social systems, health, perception, and interpersonal relations—as the bases for her conceptual work.

The organization of the body of knowledge for nursing also stimulated her work. King considered nursing a process in which nurses assist individuals to meet their basic needs; perform activities of daily living; cope with health and illness; or attain, maintain, and restore health. The development of these concepts and universal ideas constitute King's Conceptual System.

King's early questions about nursing and its place in society illustrate her process for furthering her work. The initial questions led her to others directly related to the structure and content of nursing. These are presented in Box 9-1. Reflection on these questions led King to identify the key concepts of her conceptual system. Development of the framework of systems led to the Theory of Goal Attainment and the transaction process model to explain how the interrelated systems functioned. The outcome of King's models is goal attainment.

King has called information-processing systems with instant communication a hallmark of contemporary society. Humans communicate and interact in small groups within their nations' social systems. The personal, interpersonal, and social systems in King's Conceptual System represent "interconnected links for information processing in a high-tech world of healthcare and nursing and provides an approach to structure a world community of human beings" (King, 2001, p. 276). The Howland Systems Model (1976) and the Howland and McDowell conceptual framework (1964) influenced King's development of a schematic representation of nursing.

Phenomenon of Concern

King initially selected four universal ideas—social systems, health, perception, and interpersonal relations—as the conceptual bases of the nursing dimensions. The goal of nursing is to "help individuals and groups attain, maintain, and restore health. If this is not possible, nurses help individuals die with dignity" (1981, p. 13). Nurses' major functions are those of the nursing process. Health is "dynamic life experiences of a human being, which implies continuous adjustment to stressors in the internal and external environment through optimum use of one's resources to achieve maximum potential for daily living" (King, 1981, p. 5).

King's Theory of Goal Attainment describes nurse-patient interactions that lead to goal achievement (1981). The theory essentially models nurse-patient transactions wherein goals are set and met (King, 1995). King (1981) presented a schematic diagram of a Theory of Goal Attainment that she now calls "erroneous" (personal communication, January 5, 2001). Her changed perspective reflects her belief that nursing knowledge must constantly be modified by updating earlier concepts (King, 1975). The schematic had included process elements (agreeing to means, exploring means, and mutual goal setting) as well as perception and communication. The transaction process is described later in this chapter.

King was moved to "focus on knowledge development as an information-processing, goal-seeking, and decision-making system" (2001, p. 277). Her philosophical position is rooted in general system theory and centers on humans and their environments. Several middle-range theories have been developed from King's interacting systems framework, such as Brooks and Thomas' theory of perceptual awareness (1997), Frey's theory of families, children, and chronic illness (1995), and Sieloff's theory of departmental power (1995b).

King began by reflecting on defining the nursing act as a human act. She considered nursing as action rather than intervention and the nursing process as a "series of these actions" (King, 1997a, p. 15).

DESCRIPTION OF KING'S THEORETICAL SYSTEM
Philosophical Perspectives

The basic abstraction of nursing is the phenomenon of man and his world (King, 1971). The focus of nursing is "human beings interacting with their environment leading to a state of health for individuals, which is an ability to function in social roles" (1981, p. 143).

The dynamics of nursing are a "constant restructuring of relationships between the nurse and patient to cope with existential problems" (King, 1971, p. 103).

King's work is based in and developed from the perspective of general systems with an emphasis on open systems. King identified general system theory as the philosophy of science that allowed her to study nursing as a whole system within the universe (1999). General system theory is also the ontology of King's Conceptual System. It provides not only the way of viewing reality but also the structure for languaging the concepts. She described three types of systems that interact between themselves and that interact as a whole with the environment. These are **personal, interpersonal, and social systems** (Figure 9-1).

The philosophical assumptions of the conceptual system define human beings as open systems in interaction with the environment. Human beings and environment constitute a whole. King described human beings as "social, sentient, rational reacting, perceiving, controlling, purposeful, action-oriented, time-oriented and spiritual beings" (1999, p. 293). King considers personalism and realism to be foundational to her conceptual system (1981). However, the relationship of these philosophies to general system theory is not established.

Nursing is concerned with helping patients in the realm of existential problems—that is, problems arising from or associated with the conditions of living. The nature of human beings is not highly developed in King's writings. However, focusing on human nature as an essential part of King's system, Whelton (1999) presented a cogent analysis of the philosophical core. Concepts of human nature Whelton identifies as Aristotelian and Thomistic

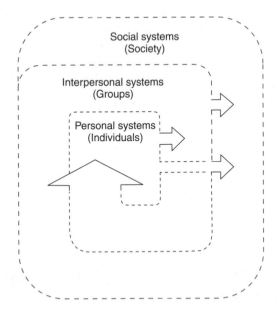

FIGURE 9-1 A conceptual system for nursing: dynamic interacting systems. (Copyright Imogene King.)

include the integration of material and principle and powers and capabilities for human acts. These concepts are described in Chapter 5. Within this philosophical tradition, human action involves knowledge and choices. When two people meet in any situation, some kind of action is involved (King, 1999). When the two persons are nurse and patient, the action is interaction. A transaction occurs when mutual understanding, goals, and agreement on methods are achieved.

King focused on individual perception as the means whereby a person experiences her or his environment. The transaction process begins with perceiving an event or object and then interacting with it. **Transactions** are interactions that have temporal and spatial dimensions in which "human beings communicate with environment to achieve goals that are values" within a shared frame of reference that consists of facts, beliefs, experiences and preferences (King, 1981, p. 82). These concepts are congruent with a realist worldview.

DESCRIPTION OF MODEL AND THEORY

King's "conceptual system" is modeled in two primary diagrams: dynamic interaction systems and a process of **human interaction,** shown in Figures 9-1 and 9-2, respectively (1971, 1981). A now retracted model that attempted to tie the concepts together was included in her early work. The conceptual system model depicts individual systems in interaction with the interpersonal and social systems, the interpersonal systems in interaction with the personal and social systems, and all three systems as a whole. The dotted line indicates the openness of the systems to one another and to the environment. Concepts for each system are identified in Box 9-2.

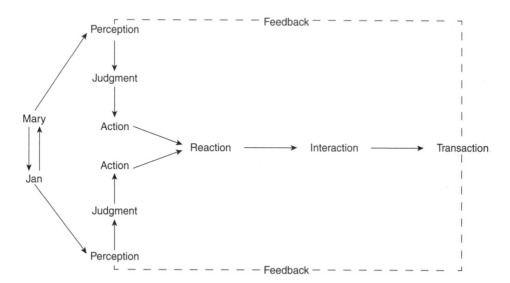

FIGURE 9-2 A model of transaction. (Copyright Imogene King.)

BOX 9-2

Concepts in the Systems Model

PERSONAL SYSTEMS (INDIVIDUALS)	INTERPERSONAL SYSTEMS
Perception	Role
Self	Interaction
Body Image	Communication
Growth and Development	Transaction
Time	Stress
Space	Coping

RESEARCH DERIVED FROM KING'S CONCEPTUAL SYSTEM AND THEORY OF GOAL ATTAINMENT

King approaches knowledge development through both inductive and deductive methods and views the world from a wholistic perspective. Refinement in the General Systems Framework and the Theory of Goal Attainment have continued as more has become known through research and practice.

Research Instruments

Two published instruments developed using King's Conceptual System and the Theory of Goal Attainment are the Family Needs Assessment Tool (FNAT), developed by Rawlins, Rawlins, and Horner (1990), and the Measure of Goal Attainment by King (1988). To measure the perceived needs of family members of chronically ill children, Rawlins, Rawlins, and Horner (1990) developed the FNAT so that parents' actual needs could be identified from the needs health professionals perceived that the parents had. The FNAT consists of four sections, representing service needs (14 items), information needs (28 items), obstacles to treatment (12 items), and a demographic survey. Modest instrument stability was indicated by test/retest scores. Factor analysis established a strong foundation for construct validity for the FNAT. This instrument is useful for identifying major needs of parents of chronically ill children (Table 9-1).

King (1988) developed the Measure of Goal Attainment to document nursing care and conduct research related to the Theory of Goal Attainment. The measure is a criterion-referenced instrument in that it ascertains an individual's status in relation to a defined performance area. Specifically, the scale assesses patients' functional abilities to perform activities of daily living. The instrument consists of three scales: physical abilities, behavioral response, and goals. Three subscales are embedded in each of the three scales: personal hygiene, containing eight items; movement, containing six items, and human interaction, containing 12 items. The instrument takes approximately 15 minutes to complete. Nurses can use the resulting data for setting goals with patients and for measuring goal attainment by assessing the differences between the scores on goals set and goals attained. The Measure of Goal Attainment has adequate levels of content validity. King (1988) claims that decision validity is also present but fails to offer specific evidence of how she determined this finding. Interrater reliability for this instrument is strong.

TABLE 9-1

Research Instruments Based on King's Conceptual System and Theory of Goal Attainment

Instrument/Description	Study/Year	Reliability and Validity
Family Needs Assessment Tool 54 items	Rawlins, Rawlins, and Horner, 1990	Content validity was established through a literature review, a parent panel, and two nurse experts. A sample of 1,494 families with chronically ill children completed the FNAT. Test/retest reliability with a two-week interval was 0.77. Factor analysis on service needs and information needs items yielded nine interpretable factors that explained 79.6% of variance. Factors included the following: healthcare information, growth and development information, day-respite care, special therapy services, information about child's psychosocial needs, information about meeting education needs, counseling or psychological support services, hygiene information, and material health support. Factor analysis for obstacles to treatment subscale yielded four factors that accounted for 52.1% of variance. They were the following: discourteous treatment, problems with appointments, questions about prescribed care, and overall hassles of office/clinic visits. A second order factor analysis to confirm hypothesized needs extracted three factors, information (60% of variance in parent need scores), obstacles to treatment (26.68% of variance), and special services (11.25% of variance).
Measure of Goal Attainment 4-point scale	King, 1988	An initial draft was reviewed by graduate students for clarity and consistency. Content validity was established by two specialists (CVI = 0.88). Interrater reliability was established with two nurses with master's degrees who evaluated 20 patients (total score agreement = 85%, physical ability subscale = 83%, behavior response = 84%, goal attainment = 87%). Item agreement ranged from 63% to 100%. A second sample of 20 patients was evaluated by BS nurses (r = 0.99 for total scale, with subscale correlations ranging from 0.92 to 0.99).

Nurses rate a patient's functional ability on a scale of 1 to 4, with a score of 1 indicating complete dependence in performing an activity of daily living and a score of 4 indicating independence. Scoring for the Measure of Goal Attainment is accomplished by taking the score of the baseline performance on the selected activity and the score selected for the goal to be attained by the patient and examining the difference. For example, if the patient were initially unable to bathe himself on baseline assessment, he would receive a score of 1. A feasible goal might be bathing alone after assistance with entering the bathtub or shower—a score of 3, according to the scale criteria. If the patient were actually able to achieve that goal, the item would be scored a +2. If the patient did not attain the goal and continued to be totally dependent, the difference between the goal of 3 and the score of 1 is −2. When a goal is achieved, the score is 0, which indicates congruence between the set goal and the attained goal. King (1988) suggests converting the raw scores to percentage scores.

Review of Related Research

King's Conceptual System and the Theory of Goal Attainment have been used as theoretical perspectives for a number of research studies. Several studies are based on middle-range theories derived from King's Conceptual System. King's Conceptual System has been used to guide research with families, women's health, health promotion, chronic illness, and clinical decision making. King's Theory of Goal Attainment has guided research on adolescents, on postoperative patients, and in multicultural settings. Examples of studies from each of these areas are provided in the following paragraphs. Table 9-2 summarizes the research studies.

Families. Although King's Conceptual System initially focused on individuals, family systems can be viewed as basic structural and functional units that are both social and interpersonal. As a result, King's framework has served in conjunction with other family theories as a guide for research focusing on families. Studies by Hobdell (1995) and Doornbos (1995) exemplify this concept. Work by Frey (1995) on chronic illness also deals with family dynamics.

In a study of the loss of an "ideal" child, Hobdell (1995) assessed the likelihood of parents of children with neural tube defects accurately perceiving their children's cognitive development. Using King's concept of perceptions as being subjective and personal representations of reality, Hobdell hypothesized that chronic sorrow would influence parental perceptions of cognitive development. Indeed, she found some parents inaccurately perceived their children's cognitive development. This supports the concept of subjectivity influencing perception within personal systems.

To test a middle-range theory of family health derived from King's Conceptual System, Doornbos (1995) examined the family health impact of living with a young, chronically mentally ill family member. Doornbos proposed that the family composed an interpersonal system influenced by stressors, coping, perceptions of the patient's health, and time since diagnosis of mental illness. Findings led Doornbos to propose that family health was an outcome of family coping, particularly in terms of access to services, age of respondent, and stressors. Stressors were mediated by the family's perception of the patient's health and the time since mental illness diagnosis. Poorer perception of patient health and recent diagnosis increased stress levels. Findings from this study support King's assertion that family members seek assistance from a healthcare system when they are no longer able to cope with a health problem. Additionally, King's Conceptual System suggests that unique perceptions of life events and the individual interpretations attributed to those events influence response. This concept is supported by the influence of perception of the patient's health and time since diagnosis on family members' stress levels.

Women's Health. Sharts-Hopko (1995; Sharts-Engel, 1987) explored factors related to perceived health status during menopause. Menopause was viewed as a developmental process occurring within an open systems framework in which individuals have unique

Text continued on p. 246

TABLE 9-2

Selected Research Studies Using King's Framework

Study/Year	Purpose	Methods	Findings
FAMILIES			
Doornbos, 1995	This predictive correlational study explored the influence of having a chronically mentally ill family member on family health.	A nonprobability sample of 84 family members having a chronically mentally ill relative completed measures for stressors [Family Inventory of Life Events and Changes Scale (FILE)], coping [Family Crisis Oriented Personal Scales (F-COPES)], patient function [Progress Evaluation Scale (PES)], and family adjustment [Family APGAR, FACES III, FACES III Adaptability Scale, and Family Environment Scale (FES)].	Stepwise multiple regression revealed that family health was related to the number of family stressors (as associated with perception of patient health and time since diagnosis), family coping strategies (particularly in terms of mobilizing the family to seek out and use community resources), and age of respondent.
Hobdell, 1995	The study explored the relationship between chronic sorrow and accuracy parental perception of cognitive development of children with neural tube defects.	Parents of 69 children with neural tube defects responded to measures of sorrow (Adapted Burke Questionnaire and direct question). Child cognitive development was measured with the Slosson Intelligence Test. Parental perception of child cognitive development was measured by Minnesota Child Development Inventory or Minnesota Infant Development Inventory.	Both mothers and fathers exhibited chronic sorrow and inaccurate perceptions of cognitive skills.
WOMEN'S HEALTH			
Sharts-Engel, 1987 Sharts-Hopko, 1995	The studies explored factors related to women's perceived health status through menopause.	Two hundred forty-nine women aged 40 to 55 years responded to Life Experiences Survey, Index of Sex Role Orientation, Menopause Symptom Checklist, and Perceived Health Status Instrument. Pearson correlations and hierarchical regression were used for analysis.	Menopausal stage, life change, sex role orientation, menopausal symptoms experienced, perception of mothers menopause, and timing of menopause explained 43% of perceived health status.

Continued

TABLE 9-2			
Selected Research Studies Using King's Framework—cont'd			
Study/Year	Purpose	Methods	Findings
HEALTH PROMOTION			
Martin, 1990	The study investigated knowledge and attitudes about prostate and testicular cancer following an educational program.	Four hundred forty-eight men completing a cancer awareness program responded before and after the program to investigator-developed questionnaires to measure previous experience with cancer, early detection practices, and knowledge about male-specific cancers.	Subjects' mean scores improved by 23% following attendance at the male cancer awareness sessions. Before the program, few men participated in early detection practices (7% self-examination and 27% yearly physical examination). Following the program, subjects perceived detection behaviors as important.
CHRONIC ILLNESS			
Frey, 1995	The study tested a theory of family, children, and chronic illness derived from King's Conceptual System.	Fifty children aged 10 to 16 years with diabetes mellitus and 39 children with asthma and their parents formed a convenience sample. Parents completed FACES III, Coping Health Inventory for Children, Family Inventory of Life Events and Changes, Family Inventory of Resources for Management, and Norbeck Social Support Questionnaire. Children completed FACES III, the Denyes Self-Care Practice Instrument (DSCPI), Diabetes or Asthma Self-Care Practice Instrument (DiSCPI or ASCPI), Denyes Health Status Instrument (DHSI), Self-Perception Profile for Children (SPPC), and Brief Symptom Inventory (BSI).	Asthmatic children tended to have fewer family resources and greater stressors. Diabetics had their illness for fewer years; experienced greater illness support; were more active in illness management; and experienced greater social acceptance, behavioral competence, self worth, and perception of health. Health predictors derived from multiple regression for the diabetic group included the following: general health and illness management behaviors, age at diagnosis, duration of illness, family cohesion and adaptability, mother's social support, and child's satisfaction with social support. Health predictors for asthmatics were family adaptability, cohesion, coping, resources, stressors, and social support.

| Frey, 1996 | The study examined the relationships of general health behavior, illness management behavior, and indicators of health and illness across five samples of youths with diabetes or asthma. | General health management was measured by DSCPI, DISCPI or ASCPI, responsibility of care, and satisfaction with responsibility. Health was measured with SPPC, BSI, and DHSI. Illness control was measured by glycosylated hemoglobin (Ghb) or Pulmonary Function Tests (PFTS) and duration and perception of disease severity. | General health behaviors were related to illness management behaviors. Diabetics with higher levels of general health behaviors reported greater functional status and positive perceptions of health. Youths exhibiting higher levels of general health behaviors had higher perceptions of health status and physical and mental status. In diabetic youth, illness management related to perception of health. Diabetic youths with better physical and mental status also had better functional status and higher perception of health. |

DECISION MAKING

| Brooks and Thomas, 1997 | The study explored characteristics of clinical decision making of senior baccalaureate students. | Eighteen senior nursing students from three programs participated in structured interviews that focused on a clinical situation vignette. Content analysis was used to identify theoretical categories. | An interrelationship existed between perception and judgment occurring within intrapersonal characteristics of self. All responses were derived from personal knowing or understanding of clinical situation from the unique perspective of the self. Intrapersonal factors included the following: experience, personal values and beliefs, beliefs regarding pain, sources of intrapersonal knowledge, culture and lifestyle, religion, and personal knowledge. |

GOAL ATTAINMENT

| Caris-Verhallen, Kerkstra, van der Heijden, and Bensing, 1998 | The study explored communication between nurses and older adults in two care settings. | One hundred eighty-one videotaped encounters involving 47 nurses and 109 patients were analyzed for characteristics of communication patterns. Communication patterns for home care patients versus nursing home patients were compared. | Socioemotional communication identified the following: social behavior (small talk and joking) and affective (verbal attentiveness of nurse). Task-related communication identified the following: technical care, hygienic care, and psychosocial care. Nurses of institutionalized older adults used more social behaviors. Home care nurses used more affective and counseling behaviors. No differences in communication about lifestyle and emotional topics were discovered. |

Continued

TABLE 9-2

Selected Research Studies Using King's Framework—cont'd

Study/Year	Purpose	Methods	Findings
GOAL ATTAINMENT—cont'd			
Froman, 1995	This exploratory study examined the perceptual congruency between patient and nurse perception of illness, nursing care, and patient-care satisfaction.	A convenience sample of 40 client-nurse pairs completed the Perceptual Congruency Questionnaire. Clients completed the Patient Satisfaction with Care Scale.	There were significant differences between client and nurse perceptions of the illness and the nursing care required. However, when congruency existed, patients were more satisfied with care.
Hanna, 1994	This exploratory descriptive study investigated adolescent perceptions about personal and interpersonal oral contraceptive benefits and barriers.	Twelve adolescent females seeking oral contraceptives for first time responded to a decisional balance sheet and participated in a structured interview on contraceptive benefits and barriers. Content analysis was used to discern common elements.	Twenty-five descriptions reflected perceived benefits, whereas 19 indicated perceived barriers to oral contraceptives. Thirty-one additional descriptions were obtained through structured interviews. Benefits most often mentioned were pregnancy prevention and personal responsibility. Most frequently mentioned barriers were side effects and disapproval by others.
Hanucharurn-kul and Vinya-nguag, 1991	This experimental study tested the use of a nurse-patient interaction intervention on outcomes of postsurgical patients.	Forty surgical patients were randomly assigned to an experimental or control group. The experimental group participated in self-care through nurse-patient interaction, whereas controls received usual care. Variables measured included postoperative pain, ambulation, complications, length of postoperative stay, and patient satisfaction.	Pain sensation, distress, and use of analgesics was lower for the experimental group. Ambulation on the first three postoperative days was higher for the experimental group. Complications, particularly abdominal distention, were substantially fewer. The experimental group stay was four and half days; the control group stay was six days. The experimental group's satisfaction scores were significantly higher.

Kameoka, 1995	This study explored specific factors interfering with nurse-patient interactions.	The study analyzed nurse-patient interactions with data derived from nonparticipant observations on two orthopedic wards in Japanese hospitals. Nineteen process recordings were examined.	Three factors interfered with nurse-patient interactions: (1) differences of perceptions and inadequate communication between nurse and patient, (2) one-sided nurse-patient relationship, and (3) lack of concern for patient and lack of special knowledge of nursing.
Long, Kee, Graham, Saethang, and Dames, 1998	The study attempted to identify the association of selected characteristics with medication compliance in older hemodialysis patients and to assess the effectiveness of teaching intervention on compliance.	The study was initiated with 26 subjects. Subjects initially responded to the Iowa Self-Assessment Inventory. Medications were checked initially, two weeks later, and two weeks after the teaching intervention. Teaching consisted of an individualized medication teaching session, in which each drug was discussed, and written information given to patient.	The study had an 80% attrition rate with only five subjects in the final sample. Medication compliance rates were very low both before and after teaching. Average compliance rates did not significantly associate with economic resources, education, number of medications, trusting others, mobility, gender, social support, or age.
Spees, 1991	This descriptive study investigated patient and family knowledge of medical terminology.	Twenty-five hospitalized patients and 25 family members responded to a 50-item questionnaire on common medical terminology.	Patient scores ranged from 30 to 50. Family scores ranged from 38 to 50. Only 9 terms were correctly identified by all participants. Nurses overestimated comprehension of terms.

perspectives. The initial study (Sharts-Engel, 1987) revealed slightly poorer perceptions of heath and lower life satisfaction associated with later menopausal stages. Women experiencing more life change had lower perceptions of health. In regression analysis (Sharts-Hopko, 1995), significant characteristics contributing to health status of menopausal women included current life change, perceptions of one's mother, perceptions of one's life partner, symptoms, perceived timing of menopause, and education level. Findings supported King's Conceptual System. King suggested that individual systems have unique perspectives within a context of personal systems that change with growth and development. Health is related to the way individuals deal with these developmental changes. Sharts-Hopko (1995) demonstrated that a changing internal environment and interaction with the external environment impacted the health of women undergoing menopause.

Health Promotion. Using the goal of health maintenance derived from King's Conceptual System, Martin (1990) investigated the impact of a male-specific cancer self-awareness program on knowledge and attitudes of participants. Subjects indicated limited participation in early detection of male-specific cancers prior to the program but after the program could express the importance of detection behaviors. Knowledge level regarding male-specific cancers significantly increased following the program. A limitation of the study was that no mechanism for long-term follow-up determined whether actual practices changed. King specified that the goal of nursing is to help maintain health of individuals. Martin also failed to address the study implications for King's theory. Although these factors are limiting, this study supported the concept of nursing providing education programs to maintain patient health.

Chronic Illness. Frey (1995) used the King's framework as a guide for development of a middle-range theory of families, children, and chronic illness. Using children diagnosed with asthma or diabetes, Frey found a different pattern of predictors for health outcomes for the two groups. Health outcomes for diabetic youths were related to general health, illness management behaviors, age at diagnosis, and duration of illness. Children with diabetes tended to better manage their disease than children with asthma, for whom family health variables influenced outcomes. Variables for children with asthma included adaptability, cohesion, coping, resources, stressors, and child support. This study supported King's concept of multidimensionality of health, particularly in terms of functional role. Findings led Frey to suggest that a theory of family, children, and chronic illness must consider how family factors influence illness management and general health behaviors and how illness management influences illness status.

Using a composite of five samples of children with chronic illness and their families, Frey (1996) investigated health behaviors, illness management, and outcomes. She found that youths with asthma and diabetes exhibited behaviors that promote general health (such as good nutrition, exercise, sleep, and stress management) also better managed their illness. General health indicators were most related to health rather than illness. However, illness management behaviors, such as treating hypoglycemia or avoiding triggers for asthma attacks, were associated with high perceptions of health. Evidence of general health maintenance affecting chronic illness management supported King's Conceptual System. Thus nurses should focus on general wellness as well as specific illness management; both are essential to health.

Clinical Decision Making. Brooks and Thomas (1997) sought to validate Brooks' Theory of Intrapersonal Perceptual Awareness, a middle-range theory derived from King's framework. Brooks' model proposed that the nurse is a whole person who engages in clinical situations as a whole. Brooks and Thomas describe the state of wholeness as "everything the nurse is intrapersonally, as a perceiving, judging, sensing, intuiting, thinking, feeling, believing, and valuing person" who makes decisions (p. 52). Brooks and Thomas' theory extends King's concept of perception to include intuition, perception, judgment, and decision making in the personal system. To validate this middle-range theory, Brooks and Thomas (1997) identified and classified factors integral to decision making by senior baccalaureate students. In a structured interview, student responses to a clinical vignette revealed diversity in the ways students viewed the situation. Student views of the vignette were highly individualized reflections of unique personal knowing or understanding. This supported the central premise of nurses as whole persons. Perception and judgment occurred intrapersonally as well as interpersonally. However, the interactivity of perception and judgment within the personal system made separating the two difficult. This study supported adding the concept of perception and judgment as an interactive process into King's system framework. However, the decision-making aspects of King's Conceptual System were not supported because King's decision-making focus is the observable aspects of clinical situations. Brooks and Thomas focus on the individualized perceptual awareness in intrapersonal decision making.

Goal Attainment. Use of the Theory of Goal Attainment derived from King's Conceptual System has been the topic of several recent studies of transaction. Transactions are interchanges between nurses, patients, and families and are used to attain goals (King, 1997b). The Theory of Goal Attainment reflects the interactive nature of nurse-patient relationships and suggests that more goals will be attained through transactions involving mutual goal setting and jointly establishing strategies to achieve goals. Studies using goal attainment as a theoretical basis include those dealing with health promotion, chronic illness, care satisfaction, postoperative recovery, and elder care. Interactions have been examined with other cultural groups as well. Examples of these studies are presented below.

Froman (1995) examined the congruency of patient and nurse perceptions of illness, care needed, and patient satisfaction with care. She hypothesized that nurses' and patients' shared perceptions would lead to patient satisfaction. Unfortunately, patients and nurses significantly differed in perceptions of illness and required care. However, congruency correlated with patient satisfaction, which supported the Theory of Goal Attainment.

In her study of adolescents requesting oral contraceptives, Hanna (1993) tested King's concept of nurse-patient transactions. The theoretical framework for the study was augmented by Rosenstock's Health Belief Model (Hanna, 1993, 1995). The transactional intervention involved action and reaction, disturbance, and mutual goal setting. Hanna discussed the benefits and barriers of oral contraceptives and agreed with adolescents on tactics to avoid pregnancy. Adolescents receiving the intervention were significantly more likely to be adherent 3 months later. This finding supported King's concept that transactions can shift perceptions and subsequently alter behaviors.

In a related study, Hanna (1994) explored adolescent perceptions of benefits and barriers to using oral contraceptives. Both personal and interpersonal factors were considered. Pregnancy prevention was the primary personal and interpersonal reason for requesting contraceptives. Other considerations included taking responsibility and seeking the approval of others. Personally, many adolescents feared side effects, whereas interpersonally they feared others' disapproval. This study supports King's concept of a dynamic interaction between personal, interpersonal, and social systems. A nursing implication is that nurses can potentially influence the transaction by exchanging perceptions and negotiating a particular outcome.

Long, Kee, Graham, Saethang, and Dames (1998) explored medication compliance of older hemodialysis patients, focusing on the need for mutual goal transactions. Investigators proposed that sharing medical information would contribute to effective health maintenance and mutual goal transaction. The purpose of the study was twofold: to examine characteristics associated with medication compliance and to assess a transactive teaching program on self-administering medication. Medication compliance behaviors both before and after teaching were substantially lower than expected. Unfortunately, the attrition rate in this study was 80%, which left only five subjects. The Iowa Self Assessment Inventory had not been previously validated for use with minority respondents, and this fact may also have limited the study. These factors limited support for the Theory of Goal Attainment.

Spees (1991) used King's Theory of Goal Attainment to frame assessment of patient and family understanding of medical terminology. Spees proposed that family members constituted an interpersonal system that would interact to meet its basic needs. This proposition reflects the Theory of Goal Attainment. Communication was viewed as the key for increased understanding of illness and as a mechanism for stress reduction. Findings indicated that nurses overestimated patient and family knowledge of medical terminology and that family members and patients were similarly familiar with the terminology. A shortcoming of this study was Spees' failure to tie findings back to the Theory of Goal Attainment. However, limited understanding of medical terminology could impede nurse-patient interactions and prevent successful transactions and goal attainment.

In an experimental study that tested a proposition from the combined frameworks of Orem and King, Hanucharurnkul and Vinya-nguag (1991) examined whether nurse-patient interactions led to goal attainment of self-care. Investigators proposed that nurse-patient interactions designed to promote patient participation in self-care would positively influence postoperative recovery and increase care satisfaction. Surgical patients undergoing pyelolithotomy or nephrolithotomy were assigned to either an experimental or control group. Self-care was promoted in the experimental group through the use of nurse-patient interactions in addition to routine care. Study findings supported the proposition—experimental group patients experienced less pain and distress, used fewer analgesics, ambulated more, had fewer complications, and reported higher satisfaction. Orem's claim that self-care was an important goal of nursing was supported, as was King's assertion that nurse-patient interactions facilitated goal achievement.

In the Netherlands, Caris-Verhallen, Kerkstra, van der Heijden, and Bensing (1998) studied nurse-patient communication in home care and in institutionalized settings. Drawing on the Theory of Goal Attainment, investigators conceived of the nurse-patient interaction as a dynamic reciprocal relationship that facilitates goal achievement. They found that conversations between nurses and patients were socioemotional in nature. Nurses employed social conversation and thus provided affective support. Nurses in institutional settings showed more social behaviors than nurses in home care, whereas home care nurses more often provided affective support such as concern and empathy. Home care providers also offered more counseling about medical conditions and nursing care. Findings support King's theory in that socioemotional communication is necessary to establish patient relationships. A methodological limitation of this study was the inability to clearly distinguish counseling behaviors of the nurse.

Kameoka (1995) used King's classification system of nurse-patient interactions to analyze interactions obtained through nonparticipant observation on two orthopedic wards in Japan. Differences in perceptions and inadequate communication between nurse and patient reflected mismatched between patient concerns and nurse perceptions. One-sided nurse-patient relationships reflected an inequality of power. One-sided relationships lead to nurse-directed rather than mutual decision making. Lack of concern for patients and lack of special nursing knowledge was exemplified by nurses neglecting patient problems and mutually sought alternatives. In this study, lack of essential elements suggested by King's Theory of Goal Attainment led to failed transactions, thus supporting the theory.

Research Summary. To summarize, King's Conceptual System and her Theory of Goal Attainment have theoretically framed a variety of studies in several cultural settings. Several studies (Brooks & Thomas, 1997; Doornbos, 1995; Frey, 1995; 1996; Sharts-Hopko, 1995) used the systems framework for middle-range theory development of a specific phenomenon. The development of middle-range theory from a broader conceptual model coheres with Fawcett's (1999) conceptual-theoretical-empirical structuring of research studies. Many of the recent studies specifically have used the aspect of goal attainment rather than the general systems framework. Although most of these studies have been descriptive, some notable exceptions exist. Using the systems framework, Martin (1990) demonstrated that a health promotion intervention could impact awareness, knowledge, and attitudes regarding male-specific cancers. Hanucharurnkul and Vinya-nguag (1991) established, consistent with the Theory of Goal Attainment, that nurse-patient interactions can positively influence postoperative recovery. Hanna (1993) verified achievement of correct oral contraceptive use in adolescents through transactions based on the Theory of Goal Attainment. These studies—the abstract Conceptual System and the middle-range Theory of Goal Attainment—demonstrate the usefulness of King's frameworks. However, additional empirical testing on the Theory of Goal Attainment as well as on other middle-range theories derived from King's Conceptual System. Future research could include the following:

- Further testing of developed middle-range theories
- Additional description of patient understanding of health, illness, and care interventions
- Description of specific elements of transaction that permit goal achievement for health promotion, disease prevention, and illness intervention
- Research based on systems theory

PRAXIS AND THEORY UTILIZATION: DESIGNING NURSING PRACTICE FROM THE PERSPECTIVE OF KING'S CONCEPTUAL SYSTEM AND THEORY OF GOAL ATTAINMENT

King's Conceptual System, Theory of Goal Attainment, and the associated research and development are significant contributions toward a providing a nursing-oriented theoretical perspective for nursing practice. In addition to exploring nursing situations, researchers have the opportunity to view from a nursing perspective the concepts and theories developed in other disciplines. Examples of this in the literature include empathy (Alligood, Evans, & Wilt, 1995) and space (Rooke, 1995).

An understanding of general system theory is foundational to practicing nursing from King's conceptual framework, in which nursing consists of three interlocking systems: personal, interpersonal, and social. Nurses also require an understanding of the concepts within each system. King (1997a) identified these concepts from a review of the nursing literature from 1923 to 1963 and deemed them essential knowledge for nursing as a discipline. Although King has initially defined some concepts, further explication of the substantive structure of each with accompanying theory development is essential for application to practice.

A major contribution of King's Conceptual System to nursing practice has been the Theory of Goal Attainment. The emphasis on mutual goal setting between patient and nurse makes nursing truly patient-centered. Other useful theories that have been derived from this include a theory of families, children, and chronic illness (Frey, 1995) and a theory of departmental power (Sieloff, 1995b).

The Variables of Concern for Practice

Practice with Individuals as Patient. The concepts in the systems model are identified in Box 9-2. Health's central place in King's conceptual framework demands a definition of health in order to guide practice. King (1981) defines health as "dynamic life experiences of a human being, which implies continuous adjustment to stressors in the internal and external environment through optimum use of one's resources to achieve maximum potential for daily living" (p. 5). Although she refers to group and community health, extending the definition of health to the individual is required. Winker (1995) calls for a new definition of health within King's conceptual framework. If nursing's goals are attaining, maintaining, and restoring health and if its concerns are with personal, interpersonal, and social systems, further explication of the construct and definition of health certainly is essential to practice.

Practice with Family as Patient. Several studies extend King's conceptual framework from the individual to the family. Gonot (1986) describes the family as an interpersonal system composed of a group of individuals interacting to meet their basic needs. The concepts applicable to the individual therefore also apply to the family. Family health is an additional concept. It is defined as "dynamic life experiences which imply continuous adjustment to stressors in the internal and external environment through optimum use of family resources to achieve maximum potential for daily living—health is the ability to function in social roles" (Gonot, 1986, p. 35). Thus the health of the family is a function of the family members' management of stressors. The environment is a suprasystem with which the family system interacts. Like Gonot, Wicks (1995) describes the goal of family nursing as family health again in terms of functioning. Frey (1995) describes family health in relation to structure and function—specifically adaptability, cohesion, coping, resources, and stressors. Building on Frey's work to study families of the young chronically mentally ill, Doornbos (1995) defined family health as "the ability of the family unit to adjust to stressors and to function in their social roles" (p. 198). She measured members' satisfaction with family functioning, cohesion, ability to adjust to stressors, and ability to manage conflict as indicators of family health.

Describing a Population for Nursing Purposes

No examples of describing a population for nursing purposes from the perspective of King's conceptual framework or the Theory of Goal Attainment were found in the literature reviewed.

Expected Outcomes of Nursing

The expected outcomes of nursing from the perspective of the Theory of Goal Attainment include mutual goal setting, transactions, and goal achievement. These are process outcomes. The content has not been specified, although elements of interest to nursing have been identified in the goal-oriented nursing record (King, 1984).

Process Models

Individuals. King asserts that the goal of nursing is helping "individuals and groups attain, maintain, and restore health" (1971, p. 84) The nursing process or method in practice is an interrelated system of actions consisting of assessing, diagnosing, planning, implementing, and evaluating. The content or theory associated with the process (King, 1996) includes perception, communication, and interaction of nurse and patient, decision making about goals and means to accomplish goals, transactions between nurse and patient, and evaluation of goal attainment. Effective nursing occurs as the nurse infers the needs and problems of patients from direct and indirect observation of patient behavior. Through a series of actions, interactions and reactions, analysis and interpretations, nurses infer patients' health statuses. Goals are mutually established, and a plan to achieve those goals is mutually agreed upon and implemented. Alligood's diagram (1995) of this process is depicted in Figure 9-3.

In support of nursing from this perspective, King (1981) developed a patient database. This database subsequently was used to develop categorizations of the North American Nursing Diagnosis Association (NANDA) nursing diagnoses according to the systems and concepts of King's conceptual framework (Coker, Fradley, Harris, Tomarchio, Chan, & Caron, 1995; Fawcett, Vaillancourt, & Watson, 1995). The database consists of data health information available to any healthcare professional. The work associated with this framework has not yet progressed to theoretical direction for specifying the nursing questions about the data collected. The parameters of what constitutes "a problem" have not been specified beyond a mutual decision between nurse and patient/patient that one or more health related problems exist. A problem is considered solved when the mutually determined goal has been achieved. Identifying the concepts associated with the process of mutual goal setting and their relationships have been identified in the Theory of Goal Attainment. The concepts associated with the content of this process for nursing purposes have not been specified. This is a prerequisite to developing a schema for nursing diagnoses. Research is required to validate the "fit" between King's conceptual framework and the NANDA categorization. Although King has suggested a patient database and has specified a theory base for the process, a theory base for the content of the nursing process has yet to be fully developed for nursing purposes and published.

King and her colleagues (1984) have developed a goal-oriented nursing record. The content for this record is derived from King's 1981 database. The record provides the means for recording goals, the patient and nurse actions necessary to attain the desired

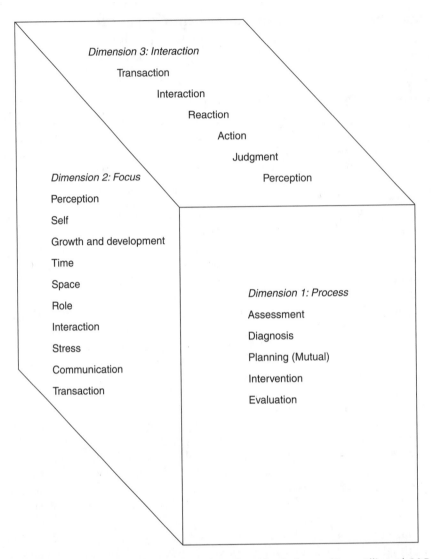

FIGURE 9-3 Three dimensional nursing process based on King's theory. (From Alligood, M.R. (1995). Theory of Goal Attainment: Application to adult orthopedic nursing. In M.A. Frey & C.L. Sieloff (Eds.), *Advancing King's systems framework and theory of nursing.* Thousand Oaks, CA: Sage.)

goals, and evaluation of the extent of goal achievement. The record has helped nurses practice from this perspective. Fawcett, Vaillancourt and Watson (1995) describe development of a record with the acronym SOGIE, which stands for *subjective, objective, goal, implementation of nursing actions, and evaluation.* This record also reflects the Theory of Goal Attainment.

Families. Gonot (1986) describes the direction the Theory of Goal Attainment provides for the processes of nursing with the family as patient. The focus is on the family as an interpersonal system, the individuals as subsystems, and the environment as the suprasystem. Data about interactions, perception, communication, transaction, role, stress, and growth and development are collected. The synthesis of assessment data and the discipline's knowledge base generates relevant diagnoses. Intervention begins when the nurse begins to interact with the family, forming an interpersonal system different from the interpersonal system of the family. Interaction clarifies the concerns and goals of the family, airs the nurses' perceptions, establishes shared goals, and identifies the means for achieving the goals. The nurse acts as an educator, mediator, facilitator, and resource person. Family health is achieved as family members engage in goal-directed behavior leading to transactions.

Practice Models

Continuing development of theories derived from King's conceptual framework and related research programs are necessary to the development of practice models. Existing theories include a theory of family health (Wicks, 1995), a theory of families, children, and chronic illness (Frey, 1995) and theory development in relation to the health of families with young chronically mentally ill children (Doornbos, 1995).

Implications for Administration

King's Conceptual System and, more specifically, the Theory of Goal Attainment have organized the development of systems of nursing service in a number of settings (Tritsch, 1998; Laben, Sneed, and Seidel, 1995; Messmer, 1995; Hampton, 1994). Fawcett, Vaillancourt, and Watson (1995) describe in detail the integrating of King's framework in nursing practice, first ensuring that the philosophies of the nursing departments reflected the framework, continuing through to developing an education program, a recording system, and patient-care standards. Mutual goal setting is reflected not only in patient care but also in nurse-to-nurse actions.

An organization wishing to structure nursing practice from the perspective of King's Conceptual System must first decide on a definition of health. Will it be as King has defined it, with health limited to role function? Will it be as Winker (1995) expanded it, "the ability of the individual to create meaningful symbols based on either biological or human values within his or her cultural and individual value systems" (p. 42)? The latter moves the practice of nursing from the goal of helping "individuals maintain their health so they can function in their roles" to "restoring or maximizing health through the mutual identification of symbols and the meaning attached to them, allowing maximum expression in life or death" (King, 1981, pp. 3-4). However, neither definition differentiates nursing from other professions, such as social work, that also may lay claim to the same goals as part of their domains. Additional theory development is required to differentiate the goal of nursing.

Sieloff (1995a), working from King's conceptual framework, extends the concept of health to social systems. She proposes health of a social system can be defined as "the dynamic experiences of a social system, which implies continuous adjustment to stressors in the internal and external environment through optimum use of the system's resources to achieve maximum potential" (p. 139). The attributes that indicate the health of the system include openness, self-regulation, negentropy, differentiation, integration, and goal directedness. Research is required to further define health of a social system, particularly nursing, and to determine the validity of the attributes suggested and which contribute the greatest variance to the health of the social system. Sieloff proposes that development of such theory would provide nurse administrators with a nursing rather than a business administration basis for decision making.

Sieloff (1995b) also has developed a theory of departmental power that may be useful to nurse administrators. This theory, derived from King's Conceptual System, attempts to increase a nursing department's power capacity and actualized power. In the theory it is "a nursing department's control of the effect of environmental forces, its position and role within a health care suprasystem, and its resources contribute to its power capacity" (p. 60). Actualizing power capacity depends on clearly defined department goals, the chief nurse executive's recognition of power as important, knowledge of power, and skill in using power.

Implications for Education

Practicing nursing from the perspective of King's Conceptual System and the Theory of Goal Attainment requires a background in general systems theory. In addition, theory related to the concepts identified in Box 9-1 needs to be developed from a nursing perspective and incorporated as such into nursing education programs.

STATUS OF THEORY DEVELOPMENT

Although the Theory of Goal Attainment is theoretically derived from the conceptual system, the linkages that would allow the discipline to develop from this model are not explicit. The Theory of Goal Attainment has been used and developed. Its appeal lies in the identification of concepts familiar to most nurses. The meaning of the many dimensions or characteristics of human beings as personal systems has yet to be developed.

Hanucharurnkul (1989) compared King's and Orem's work. She noted the similarities in views of the nature of nursing and suggested that they could be used together to "make nursing theory more complete" (p. 371). Both are developed within personalist and realist worldviews. Both view human action as requiring knowledge and choice. Many of the concepts are more highly developed by Orem. The transaction model is more developed within King's work, though the object of the transaction is not as clearly defined.

It is interesting to compare Neuman and King, since both based their work on the general system theory. Neuman's model is more detailed, places emphasis on the person-environment interaction, and the processes the individual uses to protect and defend against stressors. King put greater emphasis on the interaction of levels of systems and process for functioning within these through the establishing of goals. The ubiquity of systems theory can both strengthen and limit research.

Carter and Dufour (1994) responded to critiques of King's work. King had been criticized for using the terms *theory and paradigm*. Carter and Dufour determined a "need for consistent use of theoretical terminology in nursing in general and for use consistent with the theorist's intent" (p. 132). This is a valid caution; however, it is not always possible to know a theorist's intent. Rather, the theorist should present the definition of terms as she or he uses them. It is not reasonable to expect a consistent use of terms—not only within nursing but in other disciplines as well—with so many varying definitions.

Much still could be done to relate the theoretical system to others systems. Most of the theory and research development has been stage 2, interpretation and application (Banathy, 1996). As Chapter 8 noted, this is a reasonable expectation of systems theory work.

NEXUS

King's Conceptual System and the Theory of Goal Attainment that is derived from it have provided a mechanism for bringing the concept of nurse-patient interactions into practice. These concepts are useful in working with individuals, couples, and groups. King suggests that people who work toward goal achievement spend their time constructively (personal communication, October 29, 2000). Conceptual System and Theory of Goal Attainment have proven useful not only in practice and education but also in guiding research. Noting the variety of titles given to her work, King has stated that her theoretical system should be called King's Conceptual System, Theory of Goal Attainment, and Transaction Process Model (personal communication, October 29, 2000).

REFERENCES

Alligood, M.R. (1995). Theory of Goal Attainment: Application to adult orthopedic nursing. In M.A. Frey & C.L. Sieloff (Eds.), *Advancing King's systems theory framework and theory of nursing*. Thousand Oaks, CA: Sage.

Alligood, M.R., Evans, G.W., & Wilt, D.L. (1995). King's interacting systems and empathy. In M.A. Frey & C.L. Sieloff (Eds.), *Advancing King's systems theory framework and theory of nursing*. Thousand Oaks, CA: Sage.

Banathy, B. (1996). A taste of systemics: The primer project. International society for systems studies. URL http://www.isss.org/tast.html.

Brooks, E. & Thomas, S. (1997). The perception and judgment of senior baccalaureate student nurses in clinical decision making. *Advances in Nursing Science, 19*(3), 50-69.

Caris-Verhallen, W., Kerkstra, A., van der Heijden, P., & Bensing, J. (1998). Nurse-elderly patient communication in home care and institutional care: an explorative study. *International Journal of Nursing Studies, 35*(1/2), 95-108.

Carter, K.F. & Dufour, L.T. (1994). King's theory: Critique of the critiques. *Nursing Science Quarterly, 7*(3), 128-133.

Coker, E., Fradley, T., Harris, J., Tomarchio, D., Chan, V., & Caron, C. (1995). Implementing nursing diagnoses within the context of King's conceptual framework. In M.A. Frey & C.L. Sieloff (Eds.), *Advancing King's systems theory framework and theory of nursing*. Thousand Oaks, CA: Sage.

Doornbos, M. (1995). Using King's Conceptual System to explore family health in the families of the young chronically mentally ill. In M.A. Frey & C.L. Sieloff (Eds.), *Advancing King's systems theory framework and theory of nursing*. Thousand Oaks, CA: Sage.

Fawcett, J. (1999). *The relationship of theory and research* (3rd ed.). Philadelphia: F.A. Davis.

Fawcett, J.M., Vaillancourt, V.M., & Watson, C.A. (1995). Integration of King's Framework into nursing practice. In M.A. Frey & C.L. Sieloff (Eds.), *Advancing King's systems framework and theory of nursing*. Thousand Oaks, CA: Sage.

Frey, M. (1995). Toward a theory of families, children, and chronic illness. In M. Frey & C. Sieloff (Eds.), *Advancing King's systems framework and theory of nursing*. Thousand Oaks, CA: Sage.

Frey, M. (1996). Behavioral correlates of health and illness in youths with chronic illness. *Applied Nursing Research, 9*(4), 167-176.

Froman, D. (1995). Perceptual congruency between patients and nurses. In M.A. Frey & C.L. Sieloff (Eds.), *Advancing King's systems framework and theory of nursing*. Thousand Oaks, CA: Sage.

Gonot, P.W. (1986). Family therapy as derived from King's conceptual model. In A.L. Whall (Ed.), *Family therapy for nursing: Four approaches*. Norwalk, CT: Appleton-Century-Crofts.

Hampton, C.C. (1994). King's Theory of Goal Attainment as a framework for managed care implementation in a hospital setting. *Nursing Science Quarterly, 7*(4), 170-173.

Hanna, K. (1993). Effect of nurse-patient transaction on female adolescents' oral contraceptive adherence. *Image, 25*(4), 285-290.

Hanna, K. (1994). Female adolescents; perceptions of benefits of and barriers to using oral contraceptives. *Issues in Comprehensive Pediatric Nursing, 17*(1), 47-55.

Hanna, K. (1995). Use of King's Theory of Goal Attainment to promote adolescents' health behavior. In M.A. Frey & C.L. Sieloff (Eds.), *Advancing King's systems framework and theory of nursing*. Thousand Oaks, CA: Sage Publications, Inc.

Hanucharurnkul, S. (1989). Comparative analysis of Orem's and King's theories. *Journal of Advanced Nursing, 14*(5), 265-372.

Hanucharurnkul, S. & Vinya-nguag, P. (1991). Effects of promoting patients' participation in self-care on postoperative recovery and satisfaction with care. *Nursing Science Quarterly, 4*(1), 14-20.

Hobdell, E. (1995). Using King's interacting systems framework for research on parents of children with neural tube defects. In M.A. Frey & C. L. Sieloff (Eds.), *Advancing King's Systems Framework and Theory of Nursing*. Thousand Oaks, CA: Sage.

Howland, D. & McDowell, W. (1964). A measurement of patient care: A conceptual framework. *Nursing Research, 13*(4), 320-324.

Howland, D. (1976). An adaptive health systems model. In H.H. Werley et. al. (Eds.), *Health systems research: The systems approach*. New York: Springer.

Kameoka, T. (1995). Analyzing nurse-patient interactions in Japan. In M. Frey & C. Sieloff (Eds.), *Advancing King's Systems Framework and Theory of Nursing* (pp. 251-260). Thousand Oaks, CA: Sage.

King, I.M. (1964). Nursing theory: problems and prospects. *Nursing Science, 1*(3), 394-403.

King, I.M. (1968). A conceptual frame of reference for nursing. *Nursing Research, 17*(1), 27-31.

King, I.M. (1971). *Toward a theory for nursing: General concepts of human behavior*. New York: John Wiley and Sons, Inc.

King, I.M. (1975). A process for developing concepts for nursing through research. In P.J. Verhonick (Ed.), *Nursing research*. Boston: Little, Brown.

King, I.M. (1981). *A theory for nursing: Systems, concepts, process*. New York: John Wiley and Sons.

King I.M. (1984). Effectiveness of nursing care: Use of a goal-oriented nursing record in end-stage renal disease. *American Association of Nephrology Nurses and Technicians Journal, 2*(2), 11-17.

King, I.M. (1988). Measuring health goal attainment in patients. In C. Waltz & O. Strickland (Eds.), *Measurement of Nursing Outcomes: Measuring Patient Outcomes*. New York: Springer.

King, I.M. (1992). King's Theory of Goal Attainment. *Nursing Science Quarterly, 5*(1), 19-26.

King, I.M. (1995). The Theory of Goal Attainment. In M.A. Frey and C.L. Sieloff (Eds.), *Advancing King's Systems Framework and Theory of Nursing*. Thousand Oaks, CA: Sage.

King, I.M. (1996). The Theory of Goal Attainment in research and practice. *Nursing Science Quarterly, 9*(2), 61-66.

King, I.M. (1997a). Reflections on the past and a vision for the future. *Nursing Science Quarterly, 10*(1), 15-17.

King, I.M. (1997b). King's Theory of Goal Attainment in practice. *Nursing Science Quarterly, 10*(4), 180-185.

King, I.M. (1999). A Theory of Goal Attainment: philosophical and ethical implications. *Nursing Science Quarterly, 12*(4), 292-296.

King, I.M. Personal communication. October 29, 2000.

King, I.M. (2001). Worldview: Conceptual system and middle-range Theory of Goal Attainment. In M. Parker (Ed.), *Nursing theories and nursing practice*. Philadelphia: F.A. Davis.

Laben, J.K., Sneed, L.D., Seidel, S.L. (1995). Goal Attainment in short-term group psychotherapy settings. *Advancing King's systems framework and theory of nursing*. Thousand Oaks, CA: Sage.

Long, J., Kee, C., Graham, M., Saethang, T., & Dames, F. (1998). Medication compliance and the older hemodialysis patient. *ANNA Journal, 25*(1), 43-49.

Martin, J.P. (1990). Male cancer awareness: Impact of an employee education program. *Oncology Nursing Forum, 17*(1), 59-64.

Messmer, P.R. (1995). Implementation of theory-based nursing practice. *Advancing King's Systems Framework and Theory of Nursing.* Thousand Oaks, CA: Sage.

Rawlins, P., Rawlins, T., & Horner, M. (1990). Development of the family needs assessment tool. *Western Journal of Nursing Research, 12*(2), 201-214.

Rooke L. (1995). The concept of space in King's Conceptual System: Its implications for nursing. In M.A. Frey & C.L. Sieloff (Eds.), *Advancing King's systems framework and theory of nursing.* Thousand Oaks, CA: Sage.

Sharts-Engel, N. (1987). Menopausal stage, current life change, attitude toward women's roles and perceived health status among 40- to 50-year old women. *Nursing Research, 36*(6), 353-357.

Sharts-Hopko, N. (1995). Using health, personal, and interpersonal system concepts within King's Conceptual System to explore perceived health status during menopause transition. In M. Frey & C. Sieloff (Eds.), *Advancing King's systems framework and theory of nursing.* Thousand Oaks, CA: Sage.

Sieloff C.L. (1995a). Defining the health of a social system within Imogene King's framework. In M. Frey & C. Sieloff (Eds.), *Advancing King's systems framework and theory of nursing.* Thousand Oaks, CA: Sage.

Sieloff C.L. (1995b). Development of a theory of departmental power. In M. Frey & C. Sieloff (Eds.), *Advancing King's systems framework and theory of nursing.* Thousand Oaks, CA: Sage.

Spees, C. (1991). Knowledge of medical terminology among patients and families. *Image, 23*(4), 225-229.

Tritsch, J.M. (1998). Application of King's Theory of Goal Attainment and the Carondelet St. Mary's case management model. *Nursing Science Quarterly, 11*(2), 69-73.

Whelton, B.J. (1999). The philosophical core of King's Conceptual System. *Nursing Science Quarterly, 12*(2), 158-163.

Wicks, M.N. (1995). Family health as derived from King's framework. In M. Frey & C. Sieloff (Eds.), *Advancing King's systems framework and theory of nursing.* Thousand Oaks, CA: Sage.

Winker, C.K. (1995). A systems view of health. In M. Frey & C. Sieloff (Eds.), *Advancing King's systems framework and theory of nursing.* Thousand Oaks, CA: Sage.

Modeling Nursing From an Adaptation Perspective

ROY'S ADAPTATION MODEL

Key Terms

adaptation, p. 263
cognator, p. 261
contextual stimuli, p. 261
focal stimulus, p. 261
regulator, p. 261
residual stimuli, p. 261

First published in 1970, Roy's conceptual work focused on the person, the recipient of care, as an adaptive system. Roy believed that adaptation could consider the wholistic person (Roy & Roberts, 1981). Work done by Roy and by others has moved dynamically from the logical middle in recent years. The philosophical, research, and practice dimensions have been expanded and refined. In 1991, Roy and Andrews published a "definitive statement" that synthesized the work of key authors. Roy and Andrews intended this synthesis to become the only text needed; all others became outdated. In 1997, Roy proposed additional major changes to her work, including an expanded definition of adaptation, revised philosophical and scientific assumptions, and an explicit statement on cosmology.

THE STARTING POINT OF THE MODELING PROCESS

Roy began theory work as a graduate student at the University of California-Los Angeles. She later used that work as the conceptual framework for the curriculum at Mount Saint Mary's College (Phillips, Blue, Brubaker, Fine, Kirsch, Papazian, Riester, & Sobiech, 1998). Roy credits Dorothy Johnson, a nursing scholar and theorist at UCLA, with motivating her to develop her conceptualizations. Roy and Roberts believed that nursing needed to identify the nature of its service to develop a unique body of knowledge (1981).

Reason for Theory Development

Roy's goal was to develop theory that would demonstrate nursing's impact on the health status of the population (Roy & Roberts, 1981). Her recent work has been motivated by challenges she has faced in the past decade. She redefined the concept of adaptation as the object of nursing in a way that would position nurses as major social forces in the next century (1997). This reflects growing concern within nursing for models, theories, and knowledge specific to the field and valuable to society.

In her recent expression of the cosmology, Roy argued that the development of nursing science and practice depended on the inclusion of views of rationality and progress in science of the person and environment. Roy recognized the difficult but necessary challenge of consistently articulating a value-based wholism and a view of persons as purposive participants in their own and their environmental well-being. Nurses who act from such a viewpoint will be a major social force in the future.

Phenomenon of Concern

Roy and Roberts identified three major units that need to be addressed in any nursing model (1981, p. 23):

- A description of the person who receives nursing care
- A statement of the goal or purpose of nursing
- A delineation of nursing intervention of activities of the nurse

Roy's conceptualizations about these elements constitute the central focus of Roy's Adaptation Model (RAM), as shown in Figure 10-1. When Roy began her conceptualizing, adaptation as a response to stress was a new concept popular in the contemporary culture. It presented a way of viewing the person as more than biological. Roy used these foundational concepts from Helson (1964) in developing her conceptual framework for nursing.

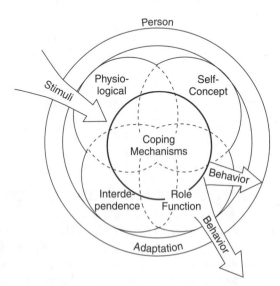

FIGURE 10-1 The Roy Adaptation Model. (From Roy, C. & Andrews, H. (1999). *The Roy Adaptation Model.* (2nd ed.). Stamford, CT: Appleton & Lange.)

The goal of nursing is to promote patient adaptation in regard to the modes of adaptation, thus promoting wellness. Nursing intervention occurs in the context of the nursing process, mobilizing regulator activity and cognator ability in order to assist the individual to integrate and adapt to his or her environment. As the term would suggest, **regulators** are those natural (physiological, biochemical) processes that serve to regulate human functioning. **Cognators** involve conscious awareness and choice, processes the individual uses to create the future. A **focal stimulus** is a person's most pressing internal or external stimulus. **Contextual stimuli** are all other stimuli present in a situation that contribute to the focal stimulus. **Residual stimuli** are internal or external environmental factors but are not the center of a person's attention or energy (Roy & Andrews, 1991).

DESCRIPTION OF ROY'S THEORETICAL SYSTEM
Philosophical Perspectives

The Focus of Nursing. The focus of nursing is the person as adaptive system. The patient is identified as a wholistic adaptive system, with coping mechanisms of cognator and regulator subsystems maintaining adaptation in regard to the four adaptive modes: the physiological (physical, for collectives), the self-concept (group identity for collectives), role function (for individuals and collectives) and interdependence (pertaining to both) (Roy & Andrews, 1999) (Figure 10-2). The identification of the modes of adaptation and

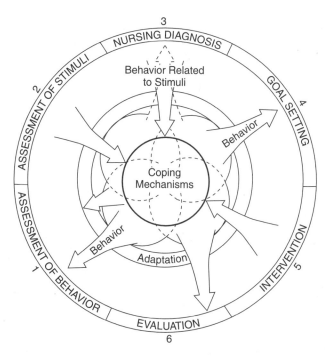

FIGURE 10-2   The nursing process as it relates to Roy's description of the person. (From Roy, C. & Andrews, H. (1999). *The Roy Adaptation Model.* (2nd ed.). Stamford, CT: Appleton & Lange.)

the mechanisms of regulators and cognators reflect the person's wholism and response to stressors. The person, as a biopsychosocial being, is characterized as a summation of parts into a whole. The current conceptualization of adaptation implies a view of the person as unitary and complex, in a mutual relationship with the world and a god-figure.

Cosmology and Ontology. Roy (1997) introduced the discussion of cosmology into her adaptation model, clarifying the place of the individual in relation to the universe and a god-figure. She holds to a cosmology that "sees God as intimately revealed in the diversity of creation, yet infinitely more than the whole creation." (p. 47). Roy's explanation of the "relationships between and among persons, universe, and God" are summarized in philosophical assumptions. Roy proclaims a "creation spirituality" wherein the person and the earth are at one with the earth and with the divine. These philosophical assumptions, presented in Box 10-1, are derived from this creation spirituality. Acceptance of this cosmology and ontology requires that the nurse base his or her care on human values. Rather than admonishing nurses to be value-neutral, they are now encouraged to acknowledge human values. The ontology of creation spirituality also forces one to act on behalf of the person and on the well-being of the earth and all creation.

The cosmology of the RAM necessitates reevaluation of previous work for congruence with the stated philosophy. This is a part of the backward and forward movement that occurs in a developing theoretical system (see Chapter 1). Roy's new material may lead to a reinterpretation of previous studies. If they are philosophically incongruent, the results of previous theoretical and empirical work might not fit this theoretical system.

Roy's ontology views nursing's concerns as the care and well-being of persons. Persons are coextensive with their physical and social environments. The value base of the discipline is rooted in beliefs about the human person, and nurses participate in actualizing the well-being of the human community (Roy, 1997). This stance views nursing within the context of adaptation and system theory.

Development of the RAM model adheres to Roy's belief that the person is the primary domain concept of nursing. Roy believes that a nursing ontology "rests upon the need for human meaning and articulation of values about the person" (1997, p. 45). She noted that "Helson's adaptation-level theory remains the parent theory for the origin of the Roy adaptation concept" (Roy & Andrews, 1999, p. 33). However, in the revised definition of adap-

---

BOX 10-1

Roy's Philosophical Assumptions for the 21st Century

- Persons have mutual relationships with the world and with a god-figure.
- Human meaning is rooted in an omega point convergence of the universe.
- God is intimately revealed in the diversity of creation and is the common destiny of creation.
- Persons use human creative abilities of awareness, enlightenment, and faith.
- Persons are accountable for the processes of deriving, sustaining, and transforming the universe.

From Roy, C. & Andrews, H. (1999). *The Roy Adaptation Model.* (2nd ed.). Stamford, CT: Appleton & Lange.

tation, Roy noted that "the notion from Helson that will remain useful in nursing assessment is that adaptation is a pooled effect of multiple influences . . . called focal, contextual, and residual stimuli" (1997, p. 45).

Description of Model and Theory

Adaptation Redefined. Roy (1997) redefined **adaptation** as "the process and outcome whereby the thinking and feeling person uses conscious awareness and choice to create human and environmental integration" (p. 44). Earlier, Roy had defined adaptation as a positive response to stimuli in persons coping with changing environments. This definition placed less emphasis on the cognator and regulator processes. For example, when Calvillo and Flaskerud (1993) examined the adequacy and scope of RAM, they did not mention either process.

The revised definition did not result from research but was a response to Roy's evolving worldview and perception of nursing's place within emerging social contexts. In redefining the object of her theory, Roy was aware of the impact on earlier studies. She believed that the redefined definition maintained continuity with the past while providing direction for the future. Again, only evaluation of previous studies can confirm this belief.

Scientific Assumptions. The revised "scientific assumptions for the 21st century" combine "expanded notions of systems and adaptation into one set of assumptions" (Roy, 1997, p. 45). These are presented in Box 10-2. These assumptions focus more on the human-environment relationship and meaning of relationships than they originally did. The models presented in Figures 10-1 and 10-2 are likely to be modified in the near future. Although Roy predicts the development of the cognator and regulator inner dynamics, the assumptions hint that cognators will be the dominant dynamic structure.

Model and Theory. The Roy Adaptation Model (Roy & Andrews, 1991), Theory of Person as an Adaptive System, (Roy & McLeod, 1981) and Theory of Adaptive Modes (Roy & Roberts, 1981) are the core of Roy's theoretical system. The RAM and associated

---

BOX 10-2

Roy's Scientific Assumptions for the 21st Century

- Systems of matter and energy progress to higher levels of complex self-organization.
- Consciousness and meaning constitute person and environment integration. Awareness of self and environment is rooted in thinking and feeling.
- Human decisions are accountable for the integration of creative processes.
- Thinking and feeling mediate human action.
- System relationships include acceptance, protection, and fostering of interdependence.
- Person and the earth have common patterns and integral relations.
- Person and environment transformations are created in human consciousness.
- Integration of human and environment meanings result in adaptation.

From Roy, C. & Andrews, H. (1999). *The Roy Adaptation Model*. (2nd ed.). Stamford, CT: Appleton & Lange.

theories are highly developed and complex. The models that represent the theories are presented in Figures 10-1 and 10-2. These models are congruent with Roy's redefinition of adaptation. The revised assumptions underlying the RAM encourage nurses to view the RAM more expansively, and with this value-based concept of adaptation, change their views of self as nurse. The need for more attention to the cognators and regulators (Roy, 1997) also means that the interpretations of research and practice model development need to consider the "cosmogenic" features of the redefined adaptation. That is, a full explanation of the meaning of research resulting from the RAM should include value-based wholism and purposive participation.

RESEARCH DERIVED FROM THE ROY ADAPTATION MODEL

The RAM focuses on wholism, in which the system is more than the sum of its parts. Humans are viewed as constantly changing. Phenomena investigated using the RAM have included studies about basic life processes, adaptation in normal and illness-related transitions, and nurse interventions to increase adaptation. Investigators have focused on objective observation in which they institute controls over data collection. Analysis methods have been primarily quantitative rather than qualitative, with some exceptions.

Research Instruments

The RAM has underpinned several research instruments related to adaptation. Five instruments were derived from the role function mode of the RAM: the Inventory of Functional Status After Childbirth (IFSAC), the Inventory of Functional Status-Antepartum (IFSAP), the Inventory of Inventory of Functional Status—Fathers (IFS-F), the Inventory of Functional Status—Cancer (IFS-CA), and the Inventory of Functional Status-Caregiver of a Child in a Body Cast (IFSCCBC). Four of the functional status inventories—the IFSAC, the ISFAP, the IFS-F, and the IFS-CA—measure functional status during normal life transitions or, in the case of the IFS-CA, during serious illness (Fawcett, 2000). Functional status was considered a multidimensional reflection of a person's actual performance in their usual role-related activities during a life transition or serious illness (Fawcett, 2000). Common to all the functional status scales is their focus on primary activities such as personal care, secondary activities such as household or occupational tasks, and tertiary activities such as social or community duties.

Using the RAM and other theories, Zhan and Shen (1994) developed the Self-Consistency Scale (SCS) to measure coping in the aging process. Table 10-1 provides an overview of these instruments. Although several measures of functional status have been developed, their use to date primarily is limited to research programs of their creators.

Inventory of Functional Status after Childbirth. Fawcett, Tulman, and Myers (1988) developed the IFSAC to describe five dimensions of functional status following childbirth—infant care responsibilities, household activities, social and community activities, self-care activities, and occupational activities. The four-point scale on self-care activities and occupational activities ranges from "never" to "all of the time." The remaining three subscales range from "not at all" to "fully." Because some of the specified activities do not apply to all women (for example, not all women cared for pets), means are calculated for each subscale and the total score for comparison. The higher the IFSAC score, the better the functional status.

TABLE 10-1

Research Instruments Using the Roy Adaptation Model

Instrument/Description	Study/Year	Reliability and Validity
Inventory of Functional Status After Childbirth (IFSAC) 36 items with 5 subscales 4-point Likert scale responses	Fawcett, Tulman, Myers, 1988	Content validity was established with a panel of seven professionally educated women who had given birth within the past year. Following instrument modification, average congruency was 96.7%. A sample of 76 women having either vaginal births or cesarean sections completed the IFSAC 6 to 10 weeks postpartum. Internal consistency for total scale = 0.76 with subscales ranging from 0.56 (self-care activities) to 0.98 (occupational activities). Test/retest reliability ($\underline{n}$ = 18) over 4 to 7 days ranged from 0.48 (household activities) to 0.93. No differences were demonstrated in scores of women with vaginal versus cesarean births. Construct validity correlating IFSAC subscales demonstrated low to moderate correlations ($\underline{r}$ = 0.02 to 0.53), which indicated some degree of scale uniqueness but with covariance of scales in some instances.
Inventory of Functional Status—Antepartum (IFSAP) 44 items with 6 subscales 4-point Likert scale responses	Tulman, Higgins, Fawcett, Nunno, Vansickel, Haas, and Speca, 1991	Content validity was established using 10 pregnant women and yielded an average congruency of 92.6%. Internal consistency for total scale was not reported but ranged from 0.57 (Personal Care Activities) to 0.87 (Educational Activities). Test/retest reliability using a 6- to 14-day time interval ranged from 0.27 (Personal Care Activities) to 0.93 (Childcare Activities) and was 0.90 for total scale. Construct validity demonstrated some interscale correlations, but the contrasted groups technique was able to differentiate functional status of pregnant and nonpregnant women as well as pregnant women with and without activity restrictions.
Inventory of Functional Status—Fathers (IFS-F) 51 items with 6 subscales	Tulman, Fawcett, and Weiss, 1993	Content validity was determined using eight expectant fathers and six new fathers. The resulting average congruency score was 86%. The sample of 125 expectant fathers and 57 new fathers was used for reliability and validity testing. Internal consistency ranged from 0.54 (Household Activities) to 0.75 (Social and Community Activities). Construct validity indicated very low correlations among subscales, with the exception of Household Activities and Childcare Activities ($\underline{r}$ = 0.69).
Inventory of Functional Status Cancer (IFS-CA) 39-item, 4-point Likert scale Pencil and Paper Questionnaire	Tulman, Fawcett, and McEvoy, 1991	A sample of 16 women receiving chemotherapy for breast cancer served as content experts. Content validity was established at 98.5% with an average congruency procedure. A convenience sample of 100 women completed IFS-CA. Internal consistency for the total IFS-CA = 0.59, Household and Family Activities = 0.74, Social and Community Activities = 0.82, Personal Care Activities = 0.56, and Occupational Activities = 0.59. Four- to 7-day test/retest reliability evaluated with 17 women ranged from 0.43 (Personal Care Activities) to 0.96 (Occupational Activities) and 0.91 for total IFS-CA. Construct validity was evaluated using subscale correlations that ranged from 0.33 to 0.62, which indicated some scale covariance, particularly between Household and Family Activities and Social and Community Activities. Two groups—one currently receiving therapy and one who had completed treatment—were contrasted. As predicted, functional status was higher for women who had completed treatment.

Continued

TABLE 10-1

Research Instruments Using the Roy Adaptation Model—cont'd

Instrument/Description	Study/Year	Reliability and Validity
Inventory of Functional Status—Caregiver of a Child in a Body Cast (IFSCCBC)	Newman, 1997	A three-round expert review using parents caring for children in body cast established content validity with average congruency score of 90%. A sample of 105 parents caring for children in body cast was use to establish internal consistency reliability and construct validity. Item to subscale correlations ranged from 0.63 to 0.88; subscale to total scale correlations ranged from 0.14 to .75. Construct validity was tested by calculating Pearson Correlations between subscales. Correlations ranged between −0.31 to 0.79. The greatest magnitude of overlap (0.79) was between Personal Care Activities and Occupational Activities. Otherwise most of correlations were relatively low, which indicated independence of subscales.
Self-Consistency Scale (SCS) 27 item, 4-point Likert scale	Zhan and Shen, 1994	Content validity was established via literature and expert panel review. Following pilot testing with small group, 130 hearing-impaired older adults responded to the SCS, the Visual Analog Scale-A Sense of Self (VAS), and the Geriatric Depression Scale (GDS). Internal consistency for total scale was 0.89. Convergent validity established correlating SCS scores to VAS, which resulted in $r = 0.60$ ($p < 0.01$). Divergent validity was established using SCS and GDS, which resulted in the anticipated negative correlation ($r = -0.57$; $p < 0.01$). Factor analysis revealed two factors—Self-Knowledge and Stability of Self-Concept, which accounted for 44% of variance.

Content validity for the scale was strong. Internal consistency ratings were strong for infant care and occupational activities but were below 0.70 for self-care activities, household activities, and social and community activities. However, Popham's average congruency procedure, which was used for calculation, yields lower reliability ratings than other procedures do. Internal consistency for the total scale sufficiently met standards for new scale development. Test/retest reliability was strong, despite lower stability scores for the household activity subscale. Construct validity testing failed to reveal predicted differences between the vaginal and cesarean birth groups, but subscale correlations indicated that the IFSAC was multidimensional, despite some shared variance in subscales.

Inventory of Functional Status—Antepartum Period. As a counterpart to the IFSAC, Tulman, Fawcett, and McEvoy (1991) developed the IFSAP, a 44-item questionnaire, to assess functional status during pregnancy. The six subscales measure the extent to which pregnant women maintain their usual household, social and community activities, childcare, personal care, occupation, and educational activities. The mean score for each subscale indicates functioning status. Higher scores indicate greater functional status.

Content validity using the average congruency scores was strong. Internal consistency was variable. Personal Care Activities rated lowest. A Fisher's z transformation, which was used to estimate internal consistency, yields lower reliability estimates. No internal consistency reliability was reported for the total IFSAP. Subscales such as the Childcare Activities Scale indicated great stability in test/retest assessments, whereas others such as the Personal Activities Subscale demonstrated low reliability. Construct validity demonstrated some dependence between subscales, but the IFSAP could differentiate between functional status of pregnant and nonpregnant women. The IFSAP also detected differences in functional status between women with no pregnancy restrictions and those with various restrictions. These findings indicate that the IFSAP is a potentially useful assessment.

Inventory of Functional Status—Fathers. Tulman, Fawcett, and Weiss (1993) developed the IFS-F as a counterpart to the IFSAC and to measure fathers' changes in household, social and community, childcare, personal care, occupation, and educational activities. The IFS-F also measures the degree to which fathers assume infant-care responsibilities during pregnancy and the postpartum period. This 51-item questionnaire is scored by calculating the mean score for each subscale. As with the other functional status scales, higher scores indicate better function. Strong content validity was established. Again, however, internal consistency reliabilities using Fisher's z transformations for the subscales are low, and the total scale reliability is not reported. Construct validity evaluated by correlation of the subscales indicated that most of the subscales are independent, except the Social and Community Activities Subscale and Childcare Activities.

Inventory of Functional Status—Cancer. Tulman, Fawcett, and McEvoy (1991) developed the IFS-CA as a measure of functional status in women with cancer. The IFS-CA is a 39-item, 4-point scale in which assessment of primary, secondary, and tertiary role behaviors are measured with four subscales. The first subscale, Household and Family Activities, consists of 15 items and reflects performance of secondary role activities. The second subscale, Social and Community Activities, has six items and measures tertiary role behaviors. The Personal Activities subscale consists of 10 items measuring primary role behaviors such as bathing, eating, and dressing. The Occupational Activities subscale, representing secondary role performance, has eight items measuring the amount of work accomplished at a job. Fawcett, Sidney, Riley-Lawless, and Hanson (1996) modified the IFS-CA for use with multiple sclerosis patients by substituting the words "multiple sclerosis" for "cancer." The acronym used for the modified instrument was IFS-MS.

Content validity for instrument items was strong. Subscale reliability was sufficient for three subscales, but the total scale internal consistency and the Personal Care Activities Subscale fell below acceptable reliability standards. Short-term test/retest reliability was adequate, particularly considering that functional status may change with time for women undergoing chemotherapy. Initial evaluation of construct validity findings indicated the IFS-CA could differentiate between groups in active chemotherapy and those who had completed chemotherapy.

Inventory of Functional Status—Caregiver of a Child in a Body Cast. Newman (1997) created the IFSCCBC by drawing items from the IFSAC and IFSAP. The 49-item instrument has six subscales related to household activities, social and community activities, care of child in body cast activities, care of other children, personal care activities, and occupational activities. Content validity established by a series of expert parent panels was adequate. Internal consistency was adequate for a new instrument. The scale has multidimensional elements with some overlap between personal care and occupational activities.

Self-Consistency Scale. To better measure self-consistency in older adults Zhan and Shen (1994) used the RAM and other theories as the basis for the Self-Consistency Scale (SCS). The SCS is a 27-item, 4-point Likert scale with a total score range from 27 to 108. Items reflect self-esteem, private consciousness, social anxiety, and stability of self-concept. Zhan and Shen indicate that the scale was tailored for use with older adults by including large print and simple items relating to older people with altered health. Internal consistency reliability levels were within acceptable ranges for a new instrument. Convergent, divergent, and construct validity using factor analysis were all well supported.

Review of Related Research

Well over 100 studies using the RAM have been published in the past ten years. This number is greater than the number of research studies that used other theoretical frameworks. The quantity of published studies indicates the ease with which nurses can conceptually use an adaptation model as a research guide. Many physiological, psychological, and functional modalities lend themselves to the concept of adaptation, and the RAM has proven to be a useful guide. Most of these studies reference the model as the theoretical framework for the study, but few specifically indicate theory testing as their function.

A strength of research efforts using RAM is the initiation of programs of research. In one of the most notable programs, Fawcett, Tulman, and others conducted a series of studies centered on aspects of childbirth. Subsequently, Samarel, Fawcett, and Tulman pursued a related program of research on facilitating adaptation in women with breast cancer. Another research program is Pollock's examination (1993) of adaptation to chronic illness. The following review explores studies from the established research programs and then provides overviews of selected adaptation studies from the broad range of completed research. Selection of these articles is not intended to negate other RAM research. There are simply too many articles to include them all. Table 10-2 presents a summary of the selected research studies.

Text continued on p. 286

TABLE 10-2

Selected Studies Using the Roy Adaptation Model

Study/Year	Purpose	Methods	Findings
CHILDBIRTH			
Tulman, Fawcett, Groblewski, and Silverman, 1990	This descriptive longitudinal study investigated functional status of women over 6-month period following delivery of healthy infants.	Ninety-seven subjects responded to the Inventory of Functional Status After Childbirth (IFSAC), the Postpartum Self-Evaluation Questionnaire (PSQ), and the Infant Characteristics Questionnaire (ICQ) at 3 weeks, 6 weeks, 3 months, and 6 months postpartum.	Significant improvements in functional status occurred between 3 and 6 weeks and between 3 and 6 months. Infant care responsibilities were assumed most rapidly, followed by household activities. Personal self-care activities had been fully resumed by only 20% of women at 6 months. At 3 weeks physical energy, vaginal delivery, and nature of occupation influenced functional status. Physical energy, parity, maternal confidence, a temperamentally predictable infant, education, and father participation later influenced functional status.
Tulman and Fawcett, 1990	The study focused on employment of women for 6 months postpartum.	Eighty-three women served as a subset for this aspect of the Tulman, Fawcett, Groblewski, and Silverman (1990) study.	Employment steadily increased post delivery, and 58% were working at the 6-month period. Employed mothers were more likely to report recovery of usual energy levels by 6 months, less fussy babies, greater husband involvement in childcare, and better relationships with husbands.
Tulman, Morin, and Fawcett, 1998	The study investigated the relationship of prepregnancy weight and weight gain during pregnancy to functional status, physical symptoms, and physical energy.	A secondary analysis of data from 222 pregnant women who completed IFSAP, Symptom Checklist, and question regarding physical energy during each trimester of pregnancy was completed.	Women gaining excessive weight during pregnancy had lower levels of functional status ($M = 2.30$) than those not gaining excess weight ($M = 2.430$) ($t = 2.47$, $p = 0.014$). No differences in energy or physical symptoms were found.

Continued

TABLE 10-2

Selected Studies Using the Roy Adaptation Model—cont'd

Study/Year	Purpose	Methods	Findings
CHILDBIRTH—cont'd			
Fawcett, Pollio, Tully, Baron, Henklein, and Jones, 1993	This intervention study investigated the effects of incorporating information about cesarean sections in standard childbirth preparation classes on maternal reactions to unplanned cesarean sections.	Seventy-four women in the experimental group received cesarean information, and 48 in the control group received standard childbirth preparation information. Following delivery, participants responded to Pain Intensity Scale, Distress Scale, Self-Esteem Scale, IFSAC, Feelings about Baby Scale, Relationship Change Scale, and Perception of Birth Scale 1 to 2 days postpartum and at 6 weeks.	Perception of the birth experience was not different between the two groups. No differences in pain intensity or physical distress were found. The experimental group experienced a change in pain intensity over time, whereas the control group had small decline. Groups did not significantly differ on self-esteem, functional status, feelings about the baby, and changes in quality of marital relationship.
Fawcett and Weiss, 1993	This exploratory study examined cultural influences on response to cesarean birth in Caucasian, Hispanic, and Asian women.	The sample consisted of 15 women from each culture (Caucasian, Hispanic, and Asian) who responded to Perception of Birth Scale and an open-ended questionnaire within 1 to 3 days of giving birth.	Caucasian and Hispanic women expressed more physiological needs than Asian women did. Hispanic women were the only group to express self-concept need due to surprise at having cesarean deliveries. All groups expressed a need to be with partners and infants, and all expressed role function needs. Although many women felt nothing more could have improved the experience, some women wanted more support and care from their health professionals.

Reichert, Baron, and Fawcett, 1993	The study compared findings of three qualitative studies about women's responses to planned and unplanned cesarean sections.	Data from three studies conducted between the years 1973 to 1990 using a similar questionnaire were subjected to content analysis to identify women's responses to open-ended questions. The adaptive modes (physiological, self-concept, role function, and interdependence) of the RAM were used to categorize responses.	In the first study there were more ineffective than effective adaptive responses. Mothers reported ineffective responses of extreme fatigue, disappointment about not having a vaginal delivery, delayed assumption of parenting responsibilities, and delayed contact with newborn. Mothers in the second study had more adaptive responses but continued to have ineffective responses similar to those of first study. In third study, the physiological and role function modes had more ineffective responses, but self-concept and interdependence mode had more adaptive responses. However, ineffective responses were again similar to those in first study.
Fawcett, Tulman, and Spedden, 1994	The study compared the reactions of women having vaginal births after previously delivering by cesarean sections.	Twelve to 24 hours post-delivery, 32 women having vaginal births after prior cesareans responded to Perception of Birth Scale and Birth Experience Questionnaire. A chi square determined delivery differences. Content analysis was used for open-ended responses.	Women reported moderately positive perceptions of experience of vaginal delivery and had more adaptive responses to vaginal delivery than to the previous cesarean delivery. Decision making for vaginal birth was based on recommendations from external sources beyond women's control.
BREAST CANCER			
Samarel, Fawcett and Tulman, 1993	This pilot study investigated influence of cancer support groups with coaching on adaptation of women with breast cancer.	Sixty-four women with breast cancer were randomly assigned to a cancer support group (CSG) with coaching, CSG with no coaching, or no CSG. Symptom distress was measured by Symptom Distress Scale (SDS), emotional distress measured with Profile of Mood States Linear Analog Self-Assessment (POMS-LASA), and functional status measured with IFS-CA.	There were no significant differences in baseline measures of the 3 groups. Although the MANOVA indicated significant differences in symptom distress, emotional distress, and functional status, univariate F's did not reveal significant differences among groups. Intervention, methods, and instrumentation were judged appropriate for a major study.

Continued

TABLE 10-2

Selected Studies Using the Roy Adaptation Model—cont'd

Study/Year	Purpose	Methods	Findings
BREAST CANCER—cont'd			
Samarel, Fawcett and Tulman, 1997	This major study investigated the effects of CSGs on adaptation and symptoms of women with breast cancer.	One hundred eighty-one women with newly diagnosed breast cancer were randomly assigned to CSG with coaching, CSG without coaching, or control group. Data were collected using SDS, POMS-LASA, IFS-CA, and Relationship Change Scale at baseline. These instruments were administered after treatment and 8 weeks later. Repeated measures MANOVA were used for analysis.	No differences were found in symptom distress, emotional distress, or functional status. In the CSG with coaching, significant improvement in relationship quality was present following treatment, but improvements were not sustained at the eight-week measure.
Samarel, Fawcett Krippendork, Piacentino, Eliasof, Hughes, Kowitski, and Ziegler, 1998	The study investigated the influence of support group intervention and education with coaching on adaptation of women with breast cancer.	Seventy women undergoing treatment for breast cancer were interviewed regarding adaptation level, view of illness, physical and emotional effects of illness, and effects of participating in research. Data were analyzed via content analysis.	Seventy-three percent of women indicated their attitude toward breast cancer improved, reflected a theme of cure, and emphasized positive feelings. Research participation was positive, with women indicating greater adaptation, appreciating opportunity to verbalize, and receiving educational information. Support groups facilitated physiological adaptation by handling symptoms and promoting greater understanding. Self-concept responses reflected a reduction of stress and fear. Downward comparison enhanced well-being, and group participation facilitated normalization. Role function mode responses reflected women either returning to routine duties or electing to participate in fewer usual activities. The interdependence mode revealed improved relationships with significant others.

Citation	Description	Methods	Findings
Tulman and Fawcett, 1996	This pilot study explored the relationship of depression, interpersonal relationships, and immune status to functional status of women with breast cancer.	Fourteen women responded to IFS-CA, Beck Depression Inventory, and Psychosocial Adjustment to Illness Scale (PAIS) at 1, 7, and 13 months following diagnosis. Immune status was measured each time with absolute counts of natural killer, CD4, and CD8 cells from venous blood samples.	Women undergoing chemotherapy had lower functional status than those not undergoing chemotherapy. Women with lower depression scores had higher functional status. Women with better interpersonal relationships had higher levels of functional status.
Mock, Burke, Sheehan, Creaton, Winningham, McKenney-Tedder, Schwager, and Liebman, 1994	This experimental study examined the effects of a nursing rehabilitation program on adaptation of women with breast cancer.	Fourteen women receiving chemotherapy randomly were assigned to experimental or usual care group. The experimental group participated in a structured exercise program and support group meetings. Subjects completed the Karnofsky Performance Status Scale, 12-minute Walking Test, PAIS, Brief Symptom Inventory, Tennessee Self-Concept Scale, Body Image Visual Analogue Scale, and Symptom Assessment Scale at baseline, midway, and at the completion of chemotherapy.	The experimental group increased level of walking, whereas the control group decreased. Both groups experienced lower levels of psychosocial adjustment over chemotherapy but had higher levels at its end. Emotional distress decreased for the experimental group and increased in the control group. Self-concept remained constant for both groups over the course of the study. Body satisfaction remained constant in the experimental group but decreased in the control group. Fatigue and difficulty sleeping were present in both groups but was greater in the control group. Participants reported that the rehabilitation program had positive effects.
Mock, Dow, Meares, Grimm, Dienemann, Haisfield-Wolfe, Quitasol, Mitchell, Chakravarthy, and Gage, 1997	This experimental study evaluated the effects of a walking program on women with breast cancer who were receiving radiation therapy.	A two group pretest, posttest design was used. Forty-six subjects were assigned to either an experimental or control group. Subjects completed 12-minute Walking Test, Symptom Assessment Scale, and Piper Fatigue Scale at the beginning and end of radiation therapy. At mid-therapy, subjects were assessed for fatigue and symptoms again. The experimental group was taught a walking exercise program following the initial evaluation.	MANCOVA using baseline data as covariates and subsequent post hoc testing revealed that the exercise group significantly increased their performance on 12-minute walking test. Walkers demonstrated decreases in the following: fatigue, sleep difficulties, anxiety, depression, and body dissatisfaction. Emotional distress decreased in the exercise group while increasing in the control group.

Continued

TABLE 10-2

Selected Studies Using the Roy Adaptation Model—cont'd

Study/Year	Purpose	Methods	Findings
BREAST CANCER—cont'd			
Young-McCaughan, 1996	The study described current sexual functioning in women with breast cancer, comparing women with and without pharmacological manipulation.	Sixty-seven women responded to mailed questionnaire regarding menopausal symptoms and the Derogatis Sexual Functioning Inventory. Thirty women received neither chemotherapy nor endocrine therapy; 8 women received both; 12 women received only endocrine therapy; and 17 received only chemotherapy.	Controlling for endocrine therapy, the 25 women receiving chemotherapy were more likely to report menopausal symptoms, sexual dysfunction, and negative body image. When chemotherapy was controlled, the twenty women undergoing endocrine therapy did not have menopausal symptoms nor sexual dysfunction more often than those not undergoing endocrine therapy. Sixteen percent of women did not use measures to decrease sexual dysfunction. More than half were never asked about sexual issues by their healthcare providers.
CHRONIC ILLNESS			
Courts and Boyette, 1998	This descriptive study compared anxiety, depression, and psychosocial adjustment of patients on home hemodialysis (HD), incenter hemodialysis, and peritoneal dialysis (PD).	Fifteen males receiving either home HD, in-center HD, or PD completed the Clinical Anxiety Scale, Generalized Contentment Scale, Hemodialysis Stressor Scale, PAIS-SR, and a psychosocial interview. Five males were in each group.	Home HD patients experienced the lowest levels of anxiety, and PD experienced greatest levels. Home HD patients had lowest depression levels while in-center HD patients had the highest level. Home HD patients experienced higher levels of psychosocial adjustment to illness and perceived the fewest stressors than the other groups.
Fawcett, Sidney, Riley-Lawless, and Hanson, 1996	This exploratory study examined the effects of alternative therapies on symptoms severity and functional status of respondents with multiple sclerosis.	Sixteen respondents completed telephone interviews and mailed questionnaire regarding functional status, Multiple Sclerosis Alternative Therapies Questionnaire, and severity of multiple sclerosis symptoms. The 13 alternative therapies used included homeopathy, massage, nutrition, and counseling.	Milder symptoms were associated with greater functional status ($r = -0.51$). Severity of symptoms improved with alternative therapies ($t(15) = 6.45, p = 0.0005$). Content analysis of open-ended responses focused on beneficial effects of therapy, need to pace oneself, change in self-perception, and spiritual aspects of self.

Jackson, Strauman, Frederickson, and Strauman, 1991	This descriptive study evaluated the biopsychosocial effects of interleukin-2 therapy.	Forty-five patients with cancer that was not treatable with conventional therapies were measured for physiological toxicities, severity of illness, emotional concerns, symptom distress, quality of life, and financial data. Measures recorded before treatment, during leukopheresis, during interleukin-2, and at 1 month and 6 months.	Only 28 patients were still in the study at the last data collection. Physiological toxicities were worst during treatment and diminished with protocol changes. Severity of illness and symptom distress were greatest during treatment, and diminished after treatment. Emotional concerns diminished following treatment. Nursing care was the most expensive component of treatment.
Frederickson, Strauman, and Strauman, 1991	The study tested the RAM by examining biopsychosocial adaptation of cancer patients.		Perception of symptoms positively correlated with psychosocial adaptation ($r = 0.60$; $p < 0.001$). Perception was a greater factor in determining adaptation than was actual physiological status.
McGill and Paul, 1993	The study examined the relationship of hope and functional status of older adults with and without cancer.	Sixty-eight older adults with cancer and 88 people living in the community completed instruments on functional status and hope.	Physical health, income, and education level were related to hope. Declining physical health and lower socioeconomic level were associated with decreased hope. Cancer diagnosis did not diminish hope levels.
Pollock, 1986	This descriptive correlational study identified factors associated with physiological and psychological adaptation.	Three groups ($n = 20$ each) of adults with diagnoses of diabetes, hypertension, or rheumatoid arthritis responded to adaptation instruments (diabetes, hypertension, or arthritis), Health-Related Hardiness Scale (HRHS), and Psychosocial Adjustment to Illness (PAIS).	Of the three groups, significant correlations between physiological and psychological adaptation and hardiness in the diabetic group were found ($r = 0.43$; $p < 0.5$; $r = 0.62$; $p < 0.5$). Hardiness was not a factor in the arthritis group. In the hypertension group, hardiness was related to physiological but not psychological adaptation ($r = 0.39$, $p < 0.5$).

Continued

TABLE 10-2

Selected Studies Using the Roy Adaptation Model—cont'd

Study/Year	Purpose	Methods	Findings
CHRONIC ILLNESS—cont'd			
Pollock, 1989	This descriptive study investigated variables related to physiological adaptation in diabetic patients.	Thirty adults with diabetes completed the Stress Questionnaire and Revised Ways of Coping Checklist, HRHS, and Physiological Adaptation to Diabetes Scale. Correlations and multiple regression were used to determine relationships.	Responses to the Stress Questionnaire were grouped into the anticipatory category, which incorporated the concepts of threat and challenge, and the outcome category, consisting of harm and benefit. Diabetic patients who perceived illness as a threat or challenge were more likely to use emotion-focused coping techniques. Hardy individuals perceived illness as a potential harmful or beneficial factor. Hardy individuals tend not use emotion-focused coping strategies. Variables explaining 56% of the variation in physiological adaptation included outcome appraisal, a mixed focus coping pattern, hardiness, patient education, and emotion-focused coping.
Pollock, Christian, and Sands, 1990	This comparative study examined physiological and psychological adaptation of adults with three different diagnoses of chronic illness.	Two hundred eleven adults with arthritis, multiple sclerosis (MS), or hypertension completed a diagnosis specific adaptation instrument, the Mental Health Index (MHI), HRHS, and Margin in Life Scale (MIL), which measures ability to tolerate change.	Although psychological adaptation was similar for the three diagnostic groups, physiological adaptation varied. Patients with arthritis were more dependent on their medications and were less likely to be involved in regular physical activities than adults with hypertension. Patients with arthritis experienced less psychological distress than those with MS, but they were less likely to be involved in health-promoting activities.
NEONATAL ADAPTATION			
Shogan and Schumann, 1993	The study examined the influence of changes in environmental lighting on oxygen saturation of very low birth weight neonates.	Twenty-seven sleeping infants were exposed to lighting levels beginning at 100-foot candles, decreasing to 5-foot candles and then returning to 100-foot candles. Oxygen saturation was recorded at 1 and 5 minutes after lighting level changes.	Lowering lighting did not influence oxygen saturation at 1 and 5 minutes. Increasing lighting generated a 4% to 7% decrease in oxygen saturation within one-minute after change.

Garcia and White-Traut, 1993	The study examined the effect of two interventions on preterm infants experiencing apneic episodes.	A convenience sample of 14 nonventilated preterm infants were compared to determine the effectiveness of taste/smell or tactile stimulation during apneic episodes. Tactile stimulation consisted of rubbing infants' legs during apnea. Taste/smell was administered by rubbing with lemon-glycerine swab. Infants received each intervention twice.	Fifty six observations (28 for each group) were recorded for 14 infants. Infants receiving taste/smell intervention required intervention for a shorter period before reinstitution of respirations. When taste/smell intervention was used, infants were able to retain baseline sleep state, whereas tactile intervention moved infants from sleep to alert state.
Kitchin and Hutchinson, 1996	The study described touching during preterm infant resuscitation.	Ten videos of preterm infant resuscitation were analyzed.	Human and mechanical touching occurred. Both human touch and mechanical touch were associated with tasks, protective functions, and accidental touching.
CHILDREN AND ADOLESCENTS			
Bournaki, 1997	The study described behavioral and heart rate response to venipuncture.	Ninety-four children between 8 and 12 years of age had heart rate and behavioral responses recorded during venipuncture. Parents completed survey on temperament and Modified Child Rearing Practices Report. Children completed Child Medical Fears Scale, Revised Fear Survey Schedule for Children, Adolescent Pediatric Pain Tool, a visual analog scale for pain, and a word list for pain quality. Child Distress Scale, pulse oximeter measure, behaviors, and heart rate during venipuncture were observed.	Low sensory thresholds were associated with greater pain intensity. As perception of pain intensity increased so did behavioral and heart rate responses. Age and threshold explained 12% of variance in heart rate. Age, medical fears, distractibility, and threshold explained 6% of variance in heart rate and pain quality.
Corser, 1996	The study described sleep patterns for 1- and 2-year-olds admitted to the PICU. It compared patterns to those before illness and determined the time required to return to normal sleep patterns.	Twelve children aged 1 or 2 were assessed for original sleep patterns, observed for sleep length and disturbances, and evaluated for return to original sleep patterns. Caregiver activities were rated while children were in PICV.	Average sleep time for children in PICU was 453 minutes with nine awakenings during a 12-hour night. Sleep periods averaged 52 minutes. Sleep time decreased with light, noise, caregiver activity, and pain. Children received significantly less sleep and had more awakenings when sleeping in the PICU. Sleep patterns returned to original levels by 3½ weeks after discharge.

Continued

TABLE 10-2

Selected Studies Using the Roy Adaptation Model—cont'd

Study/Year	Purpose	Methods	Findings
CHILDREN AND ADOLESCENTS—cont'd			
Russell, Reinbold, and Maltby, 1996	The study investigated the nature of transition for adolescents with cystic fibrosis moving to adult care programs.	Seven adolescents and eight parents were interviewed using semistructured and open-ended questions. The adaptive modes of the RAM were initially used to categorize data.	Adolescents increased self-identity and independence with disease management and other life events. Adaptive tasks for parents included giving up some control, although they were often hesitant to do so and felt excluded. Situational transition was found to be difficult due to lack of planning and coordination. Chronic illness served as more of an undercurrent with treatment routines arranged around other life activities.
FAMILY ADAPTATION			
Bokinskie, 1992	This quasiexperimental study tested the influence of family conferences on the anxiety levels of family members.	Twenty-two family members of the neuroscience intensive care unit (NICU) admissions completed state anxiety scale 24 hours before infant transfer from Neuro Intensive Care and 24 hours following transfer to a rehabilitation unit. Experimental group participants ($n = 15$) were a part of a family conference prior to transfer.	ANCOVA using pretest anxiety scores demonstrated significant differences in anxiety levels between the two groups ($F_{2,1} = 30.77$, $p = 0.001$). Family members participating in family conferences had lower levels of anxiety following the conference.
Fisher, 1994	This descriptive study identified the needs of parents with children in pediatric intensive care.	Fifteen mothers and fifteen fathers of 30 PICU patients responded to a modified version of the Critical Care Family Needs Inventory.	The top five needs were the following: knowing prognosis, knowing why things are done, feeling there is hope, knowing child is being treated for pain, and knowing child may be able to hear even if not awake.

Gagliardi, 1991	The study described experiences of having a child with Duchenne muscular dystrophy.	Three families with boys diagnosed with Duchenne muscular dystrophy were followed through 10 weekly family visits. Data were collected through participant observation and in-depth interviews.	Themes related to recognizing the disease were organized under three major headings—disillusionment, working through the disease, and achieving resolution—were identified. Disillusionment involved realizing the impossibility of living a normal life, physical deterioration, physical pain, self-awareness, and social confirmation of the impossibility of normalcy. Working through the disease was characterized by family adaptation to the disability and self-imposition of boundaries creating a smaller world. Achieving resolution involved letting go or hanging on and a hope that disabilities would be better socially tolerated in the future.
Komelasky, 1990	The study evaluated the effectiveness of structured home visitation on parental anxiety and CPR knowledge of parents with apnea-monitored children.	A treatment group ($n = 12$) receiving home visits was compared to a control group ($n = 11$) on state anxiety and CPR knowledge retention. Comparisons were made before and after treatment.	In general, both groups exhibited moderately low levels of state anxiety, and no significant differences between treatment and control groups following home visitation were found. No significant differences were found in CPR knowledge retention.
Niska, Lia-Hoagberg, and Snyder, 1997	This ethnographic study identified parental concerns of new Mexican-American parents.	Twenty-six families were followed longitudinally with eight home visits over first 6 months of the infants' lives. Interviews from each home visit were transcribed and subjected to content analysis.	Illness of infant was the major concern of most parents. Providing for material needs, threatened job loss, infant diet, concerns about rearing infant, future threats to infant, and lack of assistance in parenting were also important concerns.

Continued

TABLE 10-2

Selected Studies Using the Roy Adaptation Model—cont'd

Study/Year	Purpose	Methods	Findings
FAMILY ADAPTATION—cont'd			
Niska, 1999	The study evaluated the similarity in ways nurses and Mexican-American couples enhanced family processes of nurturing, support, and socialization. Evaluated the acceptability of nursing interventions to enhance family processes.	Twenty-three families participating in the original study were contacted and responded to 20 examples of family-enhancing interventions that were printed on index cards. Participants stacked cards according to whether the behavior was similar to Mexican-American parenting behaviors. This was followed by a similar process that assessed the acceptability of the intervention. One week later, participants commented on findings of the card sorting.	In family nurturing, 61% to 70% of the families indicated nursing techniques to enhance family nurturing were similar to those used by their own parents. Most accepted (87%) was the technique of the nurse assisting family members who wished to be caretakers. Three methods of facilitating family socialization were rated similar to current practices of Mexican-American families (ranging from 43% to 78%). Acceptability of these practices ranged from 78% to 96%. For family support, 83% to 100% of the 14 behaviors were rated similar, and 35% to 96% of the behaviors were considered acceptable.
PERIOPERATIVE			
Leuze and McKenzie, 1987	The study developed a perioperative assessment using the RAM and evaluated the circulating nurse's psychosocial knowledge when the assessment was used.	A random sample consisted of 20 patients (10 control and 10 experimental) scheduled for surgery. Investigators completed RAM perioperative assessments for the experimental group and attached them to the OR charts that would be reviewed by the circulating nurses. Thirty minutes following surgery, circulating nurses caring for study patients completed evaluation checklists assessing their patient knowledge.	Nurses caring for patients with completed RAM-based assessments demonstrated greater knowledge of psychosocial and physiological aspects of the patient.

Takahashi and Bever, 1989	This exploratory study identified characteristics of perioperative assessments performed on ambulatory surgery and day-of-surgery admission patients.	Data were collected using observation of perioperative nurses' preoperative assessments, chart audits, and self-reported questionnaires completed by nurses. Forty-eight assessments were observed.	The following assessment behaviors were observed 80% of the time: self-introduction; verification of operative procedure and site; documentation of allergic reactions; informing patients before activities; communicating information obtained from assessment to other care providers; and documenting patient consent, medication history, and indicators of mental-emotional state. The following assessments were observed less than 20% of the time: giving postoperative instruction, discussing physiological status with patient, determination of patient substance abuse, taking vital signs, soliciting information on cultural practices or religious beliefs, communicating psychosocial behaviors, ensuring waiting area quiet, receiving verbal report from preoperative area, and reporting deviations of diagnostic studies to other care providers.
Gaberson, 1991	This pilot study evaluated the effectiveness of humorous distraction on preoperative anxiety.	Fifteen preoperative same-day surgery patients were divided into three groups: control, music only group, and music plus humorous distraction. Treatment occurred during a 20-minute wait in the day surgery waiting area. Anxiety was measured using visual analog scale.	No significant differences found among the groups, but the control group evidenced the highest anxiety levels. A moderate treatment effect was found.
Gaberson, 1995	This major study evaluated effectiveness of humorous distraction on preoperative anxiety.	Forty-five preoperative same-day surgery patients were divided into three groups. Treatment protocol and measurement were the same as in the pilot study.	Although anxiety levels were highest for control group, no significant differences were found between the groups.

Continued

TABLE 10-2

Selected Studies Using the Roy Adaptation Model—cont'd

Study/Year	Purpose	Methods	Findings
PERIOPERATIVE—cont'd			
Meeker, 1994	The study determined the impact of structured preoperative treatment program on atelectasis and patient satisfaction.	Ninety-five patients received standard informal patient education, and 49 received structured teaching program. Atelectasis was measured by chest x-ray report or physician notation. Satisfaction was measured using Patient Satisfaction Inventory.	Although class evaluations indicated most felt well prepared for surgery and had decreased anxiety, there were no differences in episodes of atelectasis or in patient satisfaction with teaching.
THEORY TESTING			
Hammer, 1996	The study tested the RAM proposition related to the interdependence of nurse and patient. It was proposed that perceived control over visitation would influence adequacy of seeking and receiving affection.	Sixty medical surgical intensive care patients were assessed for severity of illness, perceived control over visitation, hardiness, state anxiety, and length of stay (LOS). Path analysis was used to test the proposed model.	Only 18% of the variance in the model predicting LOS was explained by the variables severity of illness, anxiety, hardiness, and patient control over visitation. Hardiness was associated with patient control over visitation but was significant only at the 0.1 level. Other paths between severity of illness and LOS, hardiness and LOS, severity of illness and anxiety, and anxiety and LOS were not supported.

Lévesque, Ricard, Ducharme, Duquette, and Bonin, 1998	This cross-sectional study developed a theoretical model derived from the RAM and assessed the findings of five studies for empirical verification of the model.	An aposteriori approach was used to analyze five studies within the perspective of the conceptual elements of the RAM. In the first study, 265 caregivers living with a demented relative completed the Revised Memory and Behavior Problems Checklist, Interpersonal Relationship Inventory (IPRI), Indices of Coping Responses, and Brief Symptom Inventory (BSI). In the second study, 200 informal caregivers for psychiatrically ill relatives completed the Social Behavior Assessment Scale, IPRI, Indices of Coping Responses, and Psychiatric Symptoms Index. In the third study, 163 caregivers of mentally ill persons at home completed the Social Behavior Assessment scale, IPRI, Indices of Coping Responses, and the Psychiatric Symptoms Index. In the fourth study, 1564 nurses working in geriatric long-term facilities completed the Nursing Stress Scale, Work Relationship Index, Indices of Coping Responses, and the Psychiatric Symptoms Index. In the fifth study, 135 community-dwelling older couples responded to the Geriatric Social Readjustment Rating Scale, IPRI, F-Copes, and Psychiatric Symptoms Index.	LISREL was used for path analysis. The initial fit was not acceptable, so an exploratory search for a model commenced. In the exploratory model, variance of the psychological distress was explained for 17% of professional caregivers and 56% of caregivers to psychiatrically ill relatives. In the modified model, the contextual stimulus of social support directly and positively affected the focal stimulus of perceived stress. Perceived stress triggered passive avoidance coping strategies, which were positively linked to psychological distress. No linkage between gender and available or enacted social support and perceived stress was found. No linkage between active coping strategies and psychological distress was found. New paths indicated that available or enacted social support and passive/avoidance coping strategies directly and positively affected active coping strategies. Conflicts were demonstrated to have a direct, positive effect on passive coping strategies. Conflicts and perceived stress had a direct, positive link to psychological distress.

Continued

TABLE 10-2

Selected Studies Using the Roy Adaptation Model—cont'd

Study/Year	Purpose	Methods	Findings
THEORY TESTING—cont'd			
Ducharme, Ricard, Duquette, Lévesque, Lachance, 1998	The follow-up study to Lévesque, Ricard, Ducharme, Duquette, and Bonin (1998) tested a longitudinal model derived from the RAM on the psychosocial determinant of adaptation in four target groups.	In the first study, 161 informal caregivers of psychiatrically ill patients, 111 informal caregivers of demented relatives, 498 professional caregivers of older adults, and 98 older spouses completed measures on perceived stress, conflicts, social support, coping strategies, psychological distress, and life satisfaction at two points in time. The second measure occurred between 6 and 48 months.	LISREL was used to analyze the model. The initial fit was not acceptable, so an exploratory search for modified model commenced. At initial measure, the model indicated many patterns of relationships of informal caregivers. Positive relationships between social support and stress were found. Stress triggered passive avoidance strategies, which were positively related to psychological distress. Unhypothesized links were found between available social support and passive avoidance strategies that influenced active coping and psychological distress. Models explained between 25% and 49% of psychological distress. The stability of model was assessed at second measure and accounted for 24% to 39% of variance in psychological distress. Older caregivers failed to provide an adequate fit. All links present at the initial measure were present at the second measure. Confirmatory longitudinal analysis was not achieved. Exploratory longitudinal analysis indicated that variance explained by models ranged from 32% to 47%. Increased conflict and passive avoidance coping increased psychological distress. Reciprocal effects between (1) psychological distress and conflict level, (2) psychological distress and passive avoidance coping strategies, and (3) active coping strategies and perceived stress were demonstrated.

Nuamah, Cooley, Fawcett, and McCorkle, 1999

The study tested a RAM-based theory of health-related quality of life in cancer patients.

Investigators conducted a secondary analysis of 375 cancer patients who completed the Symptom Distress Scale, the Center for Epidemiological Studies—Depression Scale, and the Enforced Dependency Scale. Baseline measures were made and then repeated three months later.

Structural equation modeling was used to test the model. Health-related quality of life was found to be defined by affective status, functional status, and physical symptoms but somewhat less by social support, which indicates that all four response models are not related.

At baseline a model fit regarding the influence of environmental factors on quality of life was achieved ($\chi^2 = 140.97$, $\underline{df} = 32$, $\underline{p} < 0.001$; goodness of fit = 0.945; adjusted goodness of fit = 0.866, comparative fit index = 0.809). Hospitalization, complications, and stage influenced illness severity. Environmental stimuli of adjuvant treatment, severity, marital status, race, age, income, and gender influenced health-related quality of life as measured by symptom distress levels, functional status, and depression levels. Environmental factors accounted for 59% of variance in quality of life at baseline. At three months, these factors and the baseline quality of life status influenced the second measure of quality of life ($\chi^2 = 262.92$, $\underline{df} = 64$, $\underline{p} < 0.001$; goodness of fit = 0.919; adjusted goodness of fit = 0.848; comparative fit index = 0.835).

Childbirth. Tulman, Fawcett, Groblewski, and Silverman (1990) investigated changes in functional status in 97 mothers of healthy babies for 6 months after delivery. Functional status represented the role function mode of the RAM. The physiological mode was measured by health variables; self-concept was measured by psychosocial variables; and interdependence mode was measured by family variables. Although functional status improved over the 6-month postpartum period, none of the mothers had fully assumed functional activities after 6 months, particularly in terms of self-care. Factors influencing resumption of activity included physical energy, type of delivery, prior occupation, maternal confidence, support from husband, education, infant temperament, and parity. The relationship found between functional status (role function mode) and variables in the physiological self-concept, and interdependence adaptive modes and contextual stimuli is congruent with Roy's conception of a complex system necessary for adaptation. However, these relationships were not consistent over time.

Using a subset of subjects from this longitudinal study, Tulman and Fawcett (1990) examined maternal employment patterns for 6 months following childbirth. Over half of mothers were employed within 6 months after delivery. Although employed mothers engaged in more roles, employed and unemployed mothers were similar in many respects. Multipara mothers appeared better able to manage work following delivery than primiparas. This led investigators to suggest that previous adaptation to multiple roles of homemaker, mother, and employee might influence adaptation.

Cesarean births served as the subject for a series of studies using the RAM. Fawcett, Pollio, Tully, Baron, Henklein, and Jones (1993) investigated the effects of cesarean birth information given in childbirth preparation classes on mothers' postpartum reactions to unplanned cesarean deliveries. The RAM model proposition that management of contextual stimuli promotes adaptation was not supported. The intervention failed to create any differences between women receiving cesarean birth information and those who did not. Investigators postulated that the experimental and control protocols were not sufficiently different and thus did not yield significant differences.

A subsequent study by Fawcett and Weiss (1993) examined crosscultural adaptation to cesarean birth. No substantial differences between the cultural groups were found. Women from all three groups exhibited a moderate level of global adaptation. This suggests that the adaptive modes of the RAM are useful in different cultural groups.

Reichert, Baron, and Fawcett (1993) compared the findings of three studies regarding women's responses to planned and unplanned cesarean sections. Content analysis was directly tied to the adaptation modes of the RAM. Although women had both adaptive and ineffective responses, findings suggested that women who delivered by cesarean sections required sensitive care that considered special needs for information, the presence of partners, and early and sustained contact with their newborns. The self-concept and interdependence modes as proposed by the RAM facilitated adaptive responses.

Fawcett, Tulman, and Spedden (1994) explored vaginal delivery by women who previously had cesarean sections. Although experiences were moderately positive, ineffective adaptive responses included pain, fatigue, fear of failure, wanting to give up, and worry about the newborn. However, more adaptive responses, including excitement, relief, confidence, control, and interdependence, were also noted. Women valued the active participation, shorter recovery time, and the presence of the partner for entire experience. Findings of this study contrasted those of the Reichert, Baron, and Fawcett (1993) in that it did not find adaptive responses in the physiological, interdependence, and self-concept modes. This study demonstrated the influence of type of delivery on adaptation and provided a basis for directing interventions toward the physiological, and interdependence modes of adaptation.

Finally, Tulman, Morin, and Fawcett (1998) tested the RAM proposition that focal and contextual stimuli influence responses. In this instance investigators proposed that the focal stimuli of weight before and during pregnancy and the contextual stimuli of parity and pregnancy trimester would influence pregnant women's physical energy and functional response to physical symptoms. Excessive weight gain was found to affect third trimester functional status. This outcome partially supports the RAM proposition that focal and contextual stimuli influence role function responses. The focal stimuli of weight before pregnancy failed to influence physical symptoms and physical energy during pregnancy. However, the focal stimuli of excessive weight gain during pregnancy influenced role function, lending some support to the RAM. Further research needs to be completed to clarify the role of focal stimuli in generating role outcomes.

The composite of these childbirth studies reveals that adaptation occurs to varying degrees. Return to a normal functional status, even 6 months after childbirth, was not always achieved (Tulman, Fawcett, Groblewski, & Silverman, 1990). Mixed findings for the role contextual variables played in adaptation were exhibited. Fawcett, Pollio, Tully, Baron, Henklein, and Jones (1993) found that a contextual variable of information giving failed to influence adaptation, whereas Tulman, Fawcett, Groblewski, and Silverman (1990) found that contextual variables interrelated with other adaptive modes and influenced functional status. Tulman, Morin, and Fawcett (1998) did not find that focal stimuli uniformly influenced functional role status, nor did they find consistent relationships between the coping systems over time. This may suggest a need for a longitudinal approach in future investigations. The RAM's adaptive modes were reflected in crosscultural groups (Fawcett & Weiss, 1993). However, different responses were found in the Reichert, Baron, and Fawcett comparison (1993) of planned and unplanned cesarean births and in the Fawcett, Tulman, and Spedden study (1994) of women undergoing vaginal births after previously giving birth by cesarean section. Although the interdependence and self-concept modes significantly influenced adaptation in women having planned or unplanned cesarean births, the physiological, self-concept, and interdependence modes did not promote adaptation in women undergoing vaginal births following cesarean sections.

Breast Cancer. As part of a continuing program of research, Samarel and Fawcett (1992) and Samarel, Fawcett, and Tulman (1993, 1997) completed a series of studies on strategies to enhance adaptation for women with breast cancer. In the first study, Samarel and Fawcett (1992) initially proposed a framework for research that involved modifying traditional support groups for women with breast cancer. Drawing on successful models from childbirth and diabetes education, Samarel and Fawcett (1992) added coaching by a significant other to breast cancer support groups. Considering the RAM, investigators proposed that level of distress from diagnosis and treatment of breast cancer (physiological mode), the level of emotional distress (self-concept mode), functional status (role function), and relationships with others (interdependence mode) work together to influence adaptation. Investigators targeted the intervention of breast cancer support groups (a focal stimulus) as a mechanism for managing stimuli to facilitate adaptation. A preliminary pilot study of six subjects indicated that participants were able to learn the skills and techniques for adaptation to chronic illness. This evaluation permitted modification of strategies for some support sessions.

Samarel, Fawcett, and Tulman (1993) subsequently conducted a pilot study to determine the feasibility of a major study about the influence of coaching groups on adaptation. This study compared three treatments: participation in a cancer support group with coaching intervention, participation in a support group without coaching, and no participation in a support group. Although significant differences between the groups were not found, the study methods, instrumentation, and intervention were found to be appropriate for a major study.

In their major study regarding adaptation of women with breast cancer, Samarel, Fawcett, & Tulman (1997) found that cancer support groups (CSGs) with coaching resulted in better relationships with significant others but did not decrease symptoms or emotional distress or improve functional status. Changes in relationship were not sustained 8 weeks after intervention. Findings led investigators to question the credibility of Roy's model in explaining the effects of social support for women with breast cancer.

Samarel, Fawcett, Krippendorf, Piacentino, Eliasof, Hughes, Kowitski, and Ziegler (1998) tested the influence of a support group on adaptation in breast cancer patients. Investigators hypothesized that the focal stimulus of a support group and education for women with breast cancer along with contextual stimuli of demographics and cancer treatment variables would influence adaptation. This study provided a different picture of the influence of the support group intervention and education provision for breast cancer patients. Most women perceived the support group and educational interventions as effective. Most indicated positive attitudinal changes and reported adaptive changes in physical functioning, self-concept, role functioning, and support systems. The Samarel, Fawcett, and Tulman (1997) study focused on quantitative findings from the investigator's perception of what was important. However, the interviews in this study reflected the women's perspectives, thus broadening perspective on this topic. The study reaffirmed the idea that focal stimuli influence adaptation.

Tulman and Fawcett (1996) examined biobehavioral correlates of functional status following a diagnosis of breast cancer. A pilot study of 14 women found that chemotherapy patients tended to have lower functional statuses than patients who did not receive chemotherapy. Women with better interpersonal relationships had higher levels of functional status at 1 and 7 months after diagnosis. The pilot study indicated that design changes were needed to investigate linkages between behavioral and immunological variables. Subject recruitment for the pilot study was difficult because some feared having a venous blood sample drawn. Additionally, the Beck Depression Inventory did not measure situational depression associated with breast cancer diagnosis. Lymphocyte function rather than lymphocyte count needed to be measured to accurately assess the variables of study.

Three other studies of women with breast cancer used the RAM as the conceptual framework for the research. Mock, Burke, Sheehan, Creaton, Winningham, McKenney-Tedder, Schwager, and Liebman (1994) examined the effects of a nursing rehabilitation program on the physical and psychosocial adaptation of women receiving chemotherapy for breast cancer. The RAM led investigators to accurately surmise that a rehabilitation program that includes a walking exercise program and a support group would facilitate physiological and psychosocial adaptation. In a subsequent study, Mock, Dow, Meares, Grimm, Dienemann, Haisfield-Wolfe, Quitasol, Mitchell, Chakravarthy, and Gage (1997) found similar positive effects of exercise on physical functioning and symptom intensity for breast cancer patients receiving radiation therapy. Both studies clearly linked their variables to the RAM and directly linked study variables and empirical indicators. Additionally, both studies supported intervention that positively influenced physiological and psychosocial adaptation. The interaction of the physiological and psychological modes supports the RAM's concept of an integrated biopsychosocial person.

Young-McCaughan (1996) explored sexual functioning in breast cancer patients receiving adjuvant therapy. The RAM was used to examine long-term effects of cancer treatment and subsequent attempts for adaptation. Chemotherapy was found to generate menopausal symptoms and sexual dysfunction, but endocrine therapy was not found to produce greater symptoms. Their healthcare providers asked fewer than 20% of women about sexual issues. This study provided a description of adaptation for women undergoing treatment for breast cancer. Although this study was framed using the RAM, research findings were not discussed in light of the model.

Finding of studies using the RAM in promoting adaptation for women with breast cancer provide mixed support. In the studies by Fawcett, Tulman, and others, social support was not found to significantly influence adaptation in breast cancer patients. However, in studies by Mock, Burke, Sheehan, Creaton, Winningham, McKenney-Tedder, Schwager, and Liebman (1994) and Mock, Dow, Meares, Grimm, Dienemann, Haisfield-Wolfe, Quitasol, Mitchell, Chakravarthy, and Gage (1997), a physiological (walking) and psychosocial support program (support group) significantly impacted adaptation. Successful interventions promoting adaptation, such as those found by Mock and colleagues (1994, 1997), raise further research questions, including the optimum timing and intensity for walking, what factors facilitate adherence to walking programs, and whether similar programs would work for patients with other types of cancer.

Chronic Illness. Pollock (1993) developed a program of research examining adaptation to chronic illness. In a series of five studies, three focused on adaptation to specific chronic illnesses, and two were comparative studies of patients with chronic health problems. The adaptation to chronic illness model, which used the concept of focal, contextual, and residual stimuli derived from the RAM, theoretically framed the studies. This model clarified concepts and specified relationships for chronic illness (Pollock, 1993).

Initially, Pollock (1986) studied physiological and psychological responses to chronic illness in adults who had been diagnosed with diabetes mellitus, hypertension, or rheumatoid arthritis in the previous year. She found that the greatest relationship in physiological and psychological adaptation was associated with the characteristic of hardiness in adults with diabetes. In her 1989 study, Pollock subsequently found that adult diabetics who believed they could influence events, who were committed to health-related knowledge, who viewed health changes as challenges, and who appraised their illnesses as potentially beneficial or harmful adapted better. Perception of illness and coping strategies were important. This second study provided evidence for a framework of adaptation for patients with diabetes.

In the third of the study series, Pollock, Christian, and Sands (1990) compared the psychological and physiological adaptation of adults with three types of chronic illnesses:

rheumatoid arthritis, hypertension, and multiple sclerosis. Psychological adaptation was independent of the type of chronic illness. However, differences in physiological adaptation were exhibited. Hardiness promoted both physiological and psychological adaptation.

The two remaining studies were unpublished but were considered in Pollock's research program (1993). Pollock's studies occurred over a 7-year period and included 597 adults with chronic illnesses. From this composite perspective Pollock concluded that hardiness, the ability to tolerate stress, and participation in health promotion activities contributed positively to physiological and psychological adaptation. Although specific diagnoses such as multiple sclerosis and rheumatoid arthritis might limit physiological adaptation, persons with various diagnoses of chronic illness experienced most psychosocial adaptation when they were able to tolerate stress. Perception of disability was an important mediating factor in psychosocial adaptation. Based on the findings from these collective studies, Pollock concluded that the middle-range model for adaptation to chronic illness, which was partially derived from the RAM, was supported. Interventions for chronic illness should focus on contextual stimuli, which can mediate changes.

The RAM has been used as a framework for studying adaptation to other chronic illnesses. An exploratory study by Fawcett, Sidney, Riley-Lawless, and Hanson (1996) examined the impact of alternative therapies on the adaptation of 16 patients with multiple sclerosis. Respondents reported significant improvement in symptom severity following alternative therapies. This preliminary study supported the RAM proposition that focal stimuli (alternative therapies) influence adaptation responses. Additionally, the strong relationship between symptom severity (physiological mode response) and functional status (role function response mode) reflects the RAM notion of the interrelatedness of the response modes.

Several studies using the RAM as a theoretical guide specifically considered cancer and cancer therapies. McGill and Paul (1993) found that failing physical health decreased a sense of hope in patients with or without cancer. In a pair of related studies, Jackson, Strauman, Frederickson, and Strauman (1991) and Frederickson, Jackson, Strauman, and Strauman (1991) studied the adaptation of patients receiving aggressive cancer treatment programs for cancers beyond cure with conventional therapies. Their goal was to focus on wholistic needs and aspects of care. In a study focusing on factors important in treatment with interleukin-2, Jackson, Strauman, Frederickson, and Strauman (1991) found that physiological toxicities increased over treatment but that alterations in therapy could mediate malaise and hypotension. As therapy continued, illness severity increased. It then decreased after therapy. Patients experienced diminished quality of life during treatment phases. Greater quantities of nursing care were required for patients in their third treatment.

Frederickson, Jackson, Strauman, and Strauman (1991) focused specifically on testing the RAM by examining the relationship between psychosocial adaptation and physiological symptoms and related distress. Investigators found that perceived physiological adaptation rather than actual physiological state related to psychosocial adaptation. These findings supported the RAM. Perception affected the interpretation, translation, and alteration of physiological stimuli. Physiological stimuli mediated and translated the cognator (coping system) depending on patient self-perceptions. The tenet that individuals form an integrated biopsychosocial whole was also confirmed.

In a small study of three types of dialysis patients, Courts and Boyette (1998) found the greatest level of psychosocial adjustment in patients receiving home hemodialysis. These patients experienced less anxiety and depression and perceived fewer stressors than their counterparts. Flexibility was perceived to be a key in adaptation and is consistent with the wholistic approach proposed by the RAM.

A summary of finding on adaptation to chronic illness affirms the RAM concept of the person as a biopsychosocial integrated whole (Jackson, Strauman, Frederickson, & Strauman, 1991; Frederickson, Jackson, Strauman, & Strauman, 1991; Courts & Boyette, 1998). The series of studies by Pollock and others (1986, 1990, 1993) provided a basis for the development of a middle-range model specifically explaining adaptation to chronic illness and suggested potential interventions to facilitate adaptation. Focal stimuli were found to influence adaptation responses (Fawcett, Sidney, Riley-Lawless, & Hanson, 1996). In general, these studies support the use of the RAM to explain adaptation to chronic illness and to facilitate adaptive interventions. Research opportunities exist for studying adaptation in other chronic conditions and the possible influence of comorbid conditions. Numerous studies could be directed toward nursing interventions that facilitate adaptation from a wholistic, biopsychosocial persective.

Preterm Infant Adaptation. Several researchers have investigated the influence of focal and contextual stimuli on physiological adaptation of preterm infants. In the following examples, the RAM guided the conceptualization of research variables. The findings from these studies supported RAM concepts of physiological adaptation.

Shogan and Schumann (1993) examined the effects of environmental lighting on the oxygen saturation of preterm infants in neonatal intensive care (NICU). Focal stimuli were related to the NICU environment, whereas contextual stimuli were related to infant prematurity. Physiological adaptation as evidenced by oxygen saturation was the variable of concern. Although lowering lights did not improve infants' oxygen saturation, increased lights significantly decreased oxygen saturation by 4% to 7% at 1 and 5 minutes. Rapidly increasing lighting serves as an environmental stressor that healthcare providers can potentially eliminate. This study supports the RAM conception of focal stressors and their impact on physiological adaptation.

Another focal stimulus that is a stressor for preterm infants is apnea. When monitor alarms indicate apnea, the traditional intervention is to provide tactile leg stimulation until the episode ends. Unfortunately, this intervention wakes the infants into alertness. Garcia and White-Traut (1993) compared use of a taste/smell intervention to traditional tactile methods and found that the apnea episode ended sooner and did not change sleeping state. This study supported the facilitation of physiological adaptation through focal stimuli changes.

Kitchin and Hutchinson (1996) explored the focal stimulus of touch during resuscitation of preterm infants. Investigators sought to assess behaviors and stimuli that might influence adaptation. Two types of touch—human touch and mechanical touch—were discovered in the 10 videos of preterm infant resuscitation. Human task touch occurred to ensure the infant's survival and was performed alone or in combination with equipment. Examples of this type of touch included restraining or repositioning during a procedure or during cardiopulmonary resuscitation. Protective human touch shielded the infant from injury and was smooth, gentle, and caring. Accidental, inadvertent touching, such as brushing or poking the infant, had poor results. Mechanical touch was related to tasks such as endotracheal intubation or oxygen administration. Accidental mechanical touch comprised equipment poking or dragging along the infant. Investigators were able to descriptively delineate touching behaviors that can influence adaptive responses of infants during resuscitation. The failure to tie the description back to the RAM weakened the study, but investigators were able to recommend that touching behaviors during infant resuscitation be reviewed to maximize outcomes.

Findings of neonatal studies indicated that physiological adaptation is influenced by focal stimuli. The stimuli included environmental lighting (Shogan & Schumann, 1993); taste, smell, and tactile stimulation during apneic episodes (Garcia & White-Traut, 1993); and touching during resuscitation (Kitchin & Hutchinson, 1996). A concern of these studies was the adverse physiological adaptation that occurred in light of harsh focal stimuli. Research directed toward the impact of neonatal focal stimuli and at interventions that promote adaptation and decrease the effects of unwanted focal stimuli could reduce these concerns.

Adaptation of Children and Adolescents. The RAM has been used in evaluation of needs and adaptation of children aged from 1 to 17 years of age. It has proven useful in the following studies.

Corser (1996) examined sleep-wake patterns of 1- to 2-year-old children admitted to the pediatric intensive care unit (PICU). Corser identified environmental stimuli associated with sleeping and waking and compared the current patterns with those before the illness. The balance of rest and activity was perceived as necessary to physiological integrity. Sleep patterns before illness were found to be similar to those for other healthy children. Children admitted to the PICU experienced significant sleep loss and frequent awakenings that disrupted rapid eye movement sleep. Increased light, noise, caregiver activities, and pain decreased the amount of sleep time. Following discharge, it took more than 3 weeks for children to return to sleep patterns consistent with previous habits. This study supported Roy's proposed linkage between environmental stimuli and adaptive behaviors.

Bournaki (1997) used the RAM to study school-aged children's responses venipuncture. In addition to behavioral measurements of temperament and fear, adaption to pain was measured by changes in heart rate and responses about the location, intensity, and quality of pain. Children with lower pain tolerance experienced increased pain and had higher heart rates and more behavioral response. Only a small percentage of variation of behavioral and heart rate responses was explained by the variables of age, temperament, threshold, distractibility, and medical fears. Therefore the study only offered limited support for the RAM, but it supported the need for aggressive assessment and management of pediatric pain.

Russell, Reinbold, and Maltby (1996) investigated the experience of adolescents with cystic fibrosis transferring to an adult healthcare. The RAM was selected to guide the study because of its focus on the continuing adjustment of individuals, families, groups, and communities. Semi-structured and open-ended questions on the interview guide were based on the RAM's four modes of adaptation. Investigators found that both adolescents and parents underwent role transitions. Adolescents completed developmental tasks of becoming more independent from parents and planning for the future. Managing their cystic fibrosis facilitated greater independence. Parents sometimes felt excluded when physicians consulted with the adolescents alone. They were hesitant to relinquish control.

Adaptation to chronic illness was a less predominant theme unless the patient experienced a high number of acute episodes with the cystic fibrosis. Transfer to adult programs for treatment was congruent with developmental transitions and could be facilitated through planning by healthcare providers. Although the RAM guided this study, investigators did not discuss their findings in light of the model. However, their findings indicated that adaptation to a new care system occurred in both the patient and the parents.

These studies on adaptation of children and adolescents all supported the RAM. Corser's study (1996) linked environmental stimuli to adaptive behaviors of changing sleep patterns. Bournaki's findings (1997) on pain reaction provided limited support for the RAM and suggested that other factors could also affect adaptation to painful stimuli. Russell, Reinbold, and Maltby's descriptive study (1996) discovered that both parents and adolescent adapted to the cystic fibrosis patients' transfer to adult care. Each of these studies is descriptive, and none specifically intended to test theory. Future research can expand to other areas, such as adolescent adaptation, intervention studies, and theory testing.

Family Adaptation. Adaptation of families has been a concern of several studies using the RAM as a theoretical guide. Studies focus on needs or stimuli to promote adaptation. Fisher (1994) identified needs of parents in a pediatric intensive care unit. Knowledge needs were particularly important for parents. These included knowing the prognosis, knowing why things were done, knowing that child was being treated for pain, and knowing that child might still be able to hear even if not awake. Feeling that there was hope was a critically important need.

Komelasky's intervention study (1990) of parental adaptation evaluated the impact of home visits on retention of cardiopulmonary resuscitation (CPR) knowledge in parents who monitored their infants' apnea. Home visits manipulated the focal stimulus of parental need to learn CPR and monitor use. The visits were also considered contextual and residual because they assisted parents in coping with the monitoring process. Home visits were not found to significantly reduce anxiety or to promote retention of CPR knowledge. One potentially problematic area of this study is that differences in the gain scores between the first and second testing were assessed. Use of gain scores to assess differences is less reliable because of the potential correlation between measurement error at each testing (Crocker & Algina, 1986). Therefore it is less likely that differences between groups would be discovered even if they existed.

In another family intervention study, Bokinskie (1992) examined the effects of a family conference on anxiety levels of family members of patients in neurointensive care units. Family conferences reduced fragmentation of information and significantly reduced the anxiety level of family members. This intervention facilitated an adaptive response to stressors, thus supporting the RAM.

Gagliardi (1991) described the experiences of family members having a child with Duchenne muscular dystrophy. As a part of analysis, Gagliardi matched the major stages and related themes to Roy's model. Recognition of themes of disillusionment and societal confirmation of the impossibility of normalcy were related to the physiological and self-concept modes. Themes of family dynamics and a smaller world, exemplified by the family's withdrawal into themselves as the muscular dystrophy progressed, were related to Roy's role modes. The final stage with themes of letting go, hanging on, or believing in change exemplified interdependence in Roy's model. In this instance, the adaptive responses of the RAM and the observed findings were closely related.

Niska, Lia-Hoagberg, and Snyder (1997) conducted a qualitative study describing parental concerns of first-time Mexican-American parents. The concept of individual and family adaptive systems was derived from the RAM. Salient concerns included potential infant illness, providing for infant material needs, future threats to the infant, access to knowledge about child rearing, lack of parenting assistance, and threatened job loss. Nurses can facilitate Mexican-American parental adaptation by addressing parental concerns. This study helped to support the RAM applicability to multicultural groups.

Niska (1999) followed this study with another that assessed the similarity of nursing interventions to existing ways Mexican-American couples enhanced family processes such as nurturing, support, and socialization. An acceptable way of promoting nurturing was to allow willing family members to care for one another. Unacceptable behaviors included perceiving the nurse as an outsider, maintaining tight family boundaries, or preferring old habits. Three acceptable ways of enhancing socialization were inviting the family to attend a neighborhood meeting, helping the family register for community programs, and inviting the family to make use of the healthmobile. All participants agreed that family support through conversation and emotional support was a function common to both the nurse and the family. Offering additional resources and helping families to understand emotions could acceptably enhance family support. Once again, these findings suggest that nurses must attend to changes within and among family members and the environment. This is congruent with Roy's contention that nurses must assess family patterns and that they must enhance processes of nurturing, support, and socialization.

Gagliardi's description (1991) of family adaptation supported the interconnectedness of stimuli and modes of adaptation. Niska, Lia-Hoagberg, and Snyder (1997) and Niska (1999) suggested multicultural applications of the RAM. Bokinskie (1992) demonstrated that family conferences facilitated adaptation as exhibited by reduced parental anxiety. The finding contrasted with the findings of Komelasky's study (1990), in which home visits failed to influence anxiety levels or parents' CPR knowledge. There is evidence that adaptation occurs within a family system; however, interventions need to be planned appropriately and measures evaluated carefully to facilitate and accurately assess adaptation.

Adaptation of Surgical Patients. The RAM has guided assessment and interventions with surgical patients and their families. Leuze and McKenzie (1987) developed a surgical assessment tool based on Roy's four adaptive modes. They compared knowledge of surgical patients in nurses using the assessment tool to those using standard assessment techniques. Nurses who completed assessments based on the RAM demonstrated greater knowledge of patients' psychosocial needs than those who used the routine assessment. This was one of the first perioperative uses of the RAM.

In a similar manner, Takahashi and Bever (1989) used the adaptive modes of the RAM to develop a Perioperative Observation/Chart Audit Tool and a Perioperative Nursing Care Questionnaire to identify perioperative nursing assessment characteristics. Five of the nine most commonly observed areas fell into the documentation category. This indicated the importance of legal ramifications associated with perioperative practice. Eight of the 14 assessment activities observed less than 20% of the time related to the biological/physical category, which indicates a dependence on physical assessments performed in the preoperative holding area and inadequate time for nursing assessments.

Gaberson (1991, 1995) conducted a pilot study and a major study assessing the influence of humorous distraction on preoperative anxiety. The RAM suggested that anxiety was common before surgery. Although the pilot did not demonstrate significant differences in anxiety for subjects receiving humorous distraction, a moderate effect was calculated. Unfortunately, humor and music tapes were not found to significantly reduce anxiety, although the control group did exhibit a higher level of anxiety.

Meeker (1994) proposed that a structured preoperative educational intervention would influence postoperative patient outcomes of atelectasis and patient satisfaction. Meeker proposed that preoperative education identified and controlled stimuli that affect individual adaptation in the four adaptive modes suggested by the RAM. Education was conceived as helping individuals cope and manage individual adjustment. Although participants reported that the classes decreased anxiety and that they felt well prepared for surgery, no differences in incidence of atelectasis or in satisfaction with education were reported. However, instruments used to measure satisfaction may not have been sufficiently sensitive to differentiate degrees of satisfaction. Moreover, the group that received patient education classes already exhibited a higher risk for developing postoperative respiratory complications. Thus the lack of significant findings may be attributable to these factors rather than to a weakness in the RAM.

In summary, the adaptive modes of the RAM usefully guided systematic assessments of perioperative patients (Leuze & McKenzie, 1987; Takahashi & Bever, 1989). These studies support the wholism suggested by the RAM. Other nursing practice areas certainly could benefit by systematic application of the RAM to patient assessment. The intervention studies by Gaberson (1991, 1995) and Meeker (1994) did not fare as well in supporting the RAM. These studies failed to demonstrate that the RAM guided interventions influenced patient outcomes. However, both studies had identifiable difficulties with instrumentation.

Theory Testing. Two studies specifically conducted to test the RAM are those of Hamner (1996) and Lévesque, Ricard, Ducharme, Duquette, and Bonin (1998). Using a proposition from the RAM, Hamner (1996) proposed a model of a patient's length of stay (LOS) in intensive care. Hamner proposed that freedom of communication patterns would positively influence the adequacy of seeking and receiving affection. The model suggested that as severity of illness increased, patient control over visitation would decrease and anxiety would increase. This increased LOS. Higher levels of hardiness increased perceived control over visitation, generating a decreased length of stay. Although severity of illness, anxiety, hardiness, and patient-controlled visitation were shown to influence LOS, the remaining elements of the model did not exhibit the proposed effects.

Lévesque, Ricard, Ducharme, Duquette, and Bonin (1998) proposed a model derived from the RAM and then tested it with an aposteriori analysis of five completed studies. The model proposed that three contextual stimuli (gender, conflicts, and available social support) would influence the focal stimulus of perceived stress. This focal stimulus would then trigger active or passive coping mechanisms and ultimately would facilitate adaptation or nonadaptation in the self-concept mode. Findings indicated support for only one proposition of the RAM—that contextual stimuli influence focal stimuli and result in the promotion or hindrance of adaptation. The remaining two propositions were not found to be true. Passive coping strategies directly triggered active strategies.

Ducharme, Ricard, Duquette, Lévesque, and Lachance (1998) examined this derived model in a follow-up longitudinal study. Investigators initially proposed that the contextual stimuli of conflicts would increase the focal stimulus of perceived stress, whereas social support would reduce stress. The focal stimulus of stress would stimulate coping strategies, which could promote positive or negative adaptations. The exploratory longitudinal analysis found that people using active coping strategies during the second time measure may have initially used passive or avoidance strategies. If people experienced high levels of distress at the initial measure, they tended to perceive conflict in their support relationships and were more likely to use passive and avoidance coping strategies at the second measure. The reverse was true for caregivers experiencing less distress on the initial measure.

This study's findings indicated that the derived model was stable over time but lacked consistency in patterns of relationships between the studies. Few significant proposed relationships were found. Investigators attribute the lack of significant linkages and differences between studies to the nature of stress and the difference in stress exposure for participants in each of the four studies. In other words, stressors faced by older adult spouses are different from those of family caregivers of patients with dementia or from those of professional caregivers. Differences for the timing of the second measure also existed. The time ranged from 6 to 48 months. The RAM was supported in that the focal stimulus of perceived stress triggered coping strategies. Additionally, the study's longitudinal approach enabled exploration of the circular nature of the RAM, in which variables mutually affect one another over time. Positive links between passive avoidance strategies, conflicts, and psychological distress were established. This supports the RAM concept that cognator mechanisms and contextual stimuli can influence adaptation.

Nuamah, Cooley, Fawcett, and McCorkle (1999) proposed a theory derived from the RAM on health-related quality of life in cancer patients. In this model, health-related quality of life was represented by the four response modes Roy identified: physiological, self-concept, interdependence, and role function. A strength of this study is the clarity with which the middle-range concepts were derived from the RAM and the identification of the empirical indicators to measure middle-range concepts. Three propositions were tested: (1) "the four response modes are interrelated" (p. 231), (2) environmental stimuli influence the biopsychosocial response modes, and (3) biopsychosocial responses following diagnosis predict biopsychosocial responses 3 months later. Findings failed to indicate the interrelatedness of the four response modes, but the nature of measurement for these modes may have limited adequate exploration. However, environmental stimuli of receiving adjuvant cancer treatment and severity of disease did influence biopsychosocial responses. Investigators suggested that nurses assess the needs and demands of cancer patients receiving adjuvant therapies and intervene to manage symptoms. They further suggest that research using the RAM should assess environmental stimuli that could be amenable to nursing intervention, such as nutrition and smoking cessation.

Findings from these studies (Hamner, 1996; Lévesque, Ricard, Ducharme, Duquette, & Bonin, 1998; Ducharme, Ricard, Duquette, Lévesque, & Lachance, 1998; Nuamah, Cooley, Fawcett, & McCorkle, 1999) not only provide some support for the RAM but also introduce some intriguing possibilities about the direct and indirect connections between focal and contextual stimuli and adaptive responses. A strength of the studies by Lévesque, Ricard, Ducharme, Duquette, and Bonin (1998) and Ducharme, Ricard, Duquette, Lévesque, and Lachance (1998) is the pooling of data from several studies to provide more cohesive findings. These studies pave the way for further theory-testing studies that could validate theories or offer new insight into model reconceptualization. Further research is needed to examine indicators of adaptation as well as the influence of various stimuli on adaptation.

Research Summary. Research using the RAM has primarily used the framework to guide variable selection and methods of study, but studies specifically testing the model— such as those described in the preceding section—have been completed. Investigators find the model easily applicable to their research, as is demonstrated by the large number of published studies that use the RAM. The RAM often is used in conjunction with other models—usually nonnursing models—as a basis for proposed research. Although several instruments have been developed to measure adaptation, they are only infrequently used by investigators other than their creators. Despite some programs of established research, only a few studies specifically identify model testing as a research aim. Findings from these studies have offered mixed support for the RAM. To continue model development, additional middle-range theory development must be derived from the theoretical system of the RAM, and further studies must specifically test model propositions. Support for model propositions has been mixed; focal and contextual stimuli have not consistently influenced functional roles. These findings indicate a need for further research and probably for further model refinement.

PRAXIS AND APPLICATION: DESIGNING NURSING PRACTICE PROGRAMS WITHIN THE THEORETICAL SYSTEM OF THE ROY ADAPTATION MODEL

Practicing nursing from the perspective of the RAM requires that nurses' goals are promoting and facilitating adaptation and that nurses agree with Roy's definition of adaptation. This definition addresses the relationship between the person and his or her environment. Underlying this revised definition of adaptation is the change in systems theory, including the ability of all matter and energy to self-organize and to progress to higher levels of complex organization. This thinking replaces the previously held notion that the system maintains itself. Roy and Andrews (1991) propose that nursing knowledge development occurs in one of three ways: nursing conceptual model development, theory construction, and research to test and develop new theories. The conceptual model identifies the variables with which nursing is concerned and suggests the ways in which these variables are linked together and influence each other. The processes of theory construction, testing through research, and development of new theories enriches the knowledge base about the substantive structure of the concepts of the model and, in turn, enriches the content associated with the processes of nursing. Collaboration between researchers and practitioners facilitates these processes.

The Variables of Concern for Practice

Individuals. The variables of concern for practice include the person with innate and acquired coping mechanisms, response behaviors that show coping mechanism activity, and an adaptation level at which a person responds positively. In addition, the environmental variables of focal, contextual, and residual stimuli remain important. Two categories of coping mechanisms, the cognator subsystem and the regulator subsystem, control the human system. The regulator subsystem responds automatically through neural, chemical, and endocrine function. The cognator subsystem responds through perceptual/ information processing, learning, judgment, and emotion. The adaptative modes are physiological, self-concept, role function, and interdependence (Roy & Andrews, 1991).

Families. It has been suggested that the family, as an adaptive system, may be the recipient of nursing care (Roy & Roberts, 1981; Roy, 1983). Roy and Roberts (1981) suggest that the family maintains itself in regard to the physiological, self-concept, role function, and interdependence modes. If it is viewed as an adaptive system, it is viewed as a unit. However, in cases in which the RAM has been used in relation to families, the focus tends to be on the individual persons making up the unit rather than on the unit as a whole. Schultz (1987) states that "if families, groups, organizations and communities as interactional units with a plurality of persons as components are conceptually appropriate extensions of the concepts of patient and person in nursing, then all other domain concepts including all steps in the nursing process need to be specified to reflect these extended definitions" (p. 79). Additional concept formalization and development of the constructs' substructure remains crucial to extending the concepts beyond the single person to the family, both in theory and in practice. The need for additional development also applies to using the RAM in communities and other groups.

Describing a Population for Nursing Purposes

It should be possible to use concepts associated with the RAM to describe a population for nursing purposes. For example, the adaptive modes could be used to describe subsets of a population of interest to nursing. This has yet to be done.

Expected Outcomes of Nursing

The expected outcomes of nursing center on promotion of adaptation, and they include increasing a person's adaptive responses and decreasing the ineffective responses (Roy, 1984). In recent writings Roy (1997) describes nursing as "acceptance, protection, and fostering of person and environment integral relationships" (p. 47). From this description, one could infer that an expected outcome of nursing would be an integrated person-environment relationship. This relationship needs to be defined further to be useful to practitioners.

Process Models

The processes of nursing within the RAM reflect problem solving—gathering data, identifying capacities and needs, establishing goals, implementing approaches for care, and evaluating outcomes of the care (Andrews & Roy, 1986; Roy & Andrews, 1991). The specific focus is on assessing behavior, collecting data, and interpreting it in relation to factors that affect adaptation, goal setting, and intervention to promote adaptive abilities. Roy has recently added that the nurse is also concerned with person-environment integration (Roy, 1997). Behavior is all the responses of the human adaptive system, including capacities, assets, knowledge, skills, abilities, and commitments. The nurse evaluates the effectiveness of behavior in terms of adaptation or nonadaptation. The patient's perception is important in deciding whether a behavior is adaptive, nonadaptive, or ineffective. A typology of indicators of positive adaptation for some of the behaviors has been developed along with a typology of commonly recurring adaptation problems (Roy & Andrews, 1991). Continuing development of the model should address criteria for differentiating adaptive and nonadaptive behavior and for developing a categorization or taxonomy of such behavior.

The nurse first collects data in relation to the four adaptive modes: physiological-physical, self-concept–group identity, role function, and interdependence. Roy and her colleagues have identified specific data to be gathered for each mode (Roy & Andrews, 1991, Cho, 1998).

The second step in the nursing process involves identifying internal and external stimuli that influence behaviors. In consultation with persons involved in the situation and through perceptive observation, measurement, and interviewing, the nurse classifies stimuli as internal or external. Stimuli are classified as one of the following:

- Focal: Most immediate; for example, a pathological condition
- Contextual: All stimuli that are evident in a situation but that are not focal stimuli
- Residual: Stimuli that indeterminately affect behavior.

When a residual stimulus demonstrably influences behavior, it is reclassified as focal or contextual. Common stimuli affecting adaptation have been identified through research framed from the perspective of the RAM and through articulation of the RAM with other theoretical formulations (Sato, 1984). These include such influences as culture, family, and developmental stage.

The third step in the nursing process is interpreting the data and formulating descriptive or diagnostic statements. These statements include identified behaviors and significant stimuli and thus specifically direct nursing intervention. Roy and Andrews (1999) have proposed a classification system that allows for linking of commonly recurring adaptation problems with the diagnostic classification system of the North American Nursing Diagnosis Association.

The fourth step of the nursing process involves establishing goals or behavioral outcomes of nursing care. In general, nursing intervention seeks to maintain and enhance adaptive behavior and/or to change ineffective behavior. Goals refer to specific objectives to be achieved and have three parts: the behavior to be observed, the means for detecting the behavior change, and the time frame. Patients should be involved in establishing the goals. It is important to note that the RAM defines behavior very broadly as "actions and reactions under specified circumstances" (Andrews & Roy, 1986, p. 32). Behavior may be external, as when a person laughs or cries, or it may be internal, such as a physiological response (e.g. elevated blood pressure). Therefore a goal could be that within 1 week a person will have mastered injecting insulin and will return to a blood pressure of 120/80 mm Hg within 15 minutes of the injection.

The fifth step is intervention to promote adaptation by changing the stimuli or strengthening the adaptive processes. Stimuli may be managed by altering, increasing, decreasing, removing, or maintaining them. Nurses must first select the stimuli to be changed. In consultation with the persons involved, nurses list stimuli affecting behavior, identify the relevant coping processes, and consider whether the consequences of changing each stimulus would be desirable. The most appropriate intervention is selected, and the means of achieving it are determined and implemented.

The final step in the nursing process is evaluating the effectiveness of the intervention and determining whether the desired goal(s), have been achieved. This is accomplished through observation, measurement, and interview. If goals have not been met, nurses assess reasons for the failure.

Although the nursing process has been specified as a problem-solving process and although the end result of such a process is usually visualized as a definition of the problem with proposed solutions, the picture becomes very different when the pieces of the puzzle are put together in different ways. The process definitely is not linear, and more than one course of action might be appropriate. Roy (1997) has suggested that nurses look at human experience from a variety of perspectives as the experience changes with variations in stimuli and responses, much like the changing patterns of a kaleidoscope (p. 41).

Practice Models

Pollock, Frederickson, Carson, Massey, and Roy (1994) analyzed research they conducted as individual authors using the RAM. From a synthesis of their findings they developed several middle-range theories that could become practice models after further testing and development. Their analysis has identified support for moving beyond disease-specific nursing interventions to considering psychosocial factors in promoting adaptation.

A second group of researchers, who did not use the RAM to guide their original investigations, subsequently analyzed five longitudinal studies within the perspective of the conceptual elements of the RAM (Lévesque, Ricard, Ducharme, Duquette, & Bonin, 1998). From this analysis they constructed a theoretical model and tested it through structural equation analyses. Their findings indicate the importance of exploring patients' perception of environmental stimuli, because factors such as social support may hinder rather than facilitate adaptation. In addition, passive/avoidance coping strategies should be examined and assessed regularly. The work of this group also precedes describing practice models as they pursue the development and evaluation of nursing interventions that focus on conflicts, perceived stress, and coping strategies in a variety of clinical populations.

Implications for Administration

Nursing agencies interested in implementing theory-based practice have found the RAM useful. Mastel, Hammond, and Roberts (1982) describe the use of the RAM as a framework for practice in an orthopedic setting. This is one of the earliest published reports of the process of implementing a nursing conceptual model in an organization. It describes the process of model implementation, and demonstrates the recording system to support such practice.

Rogers, Jones, Clarke, Mackay, Potter, and Ward (1991) describe the integration of the RAM into the structuring of nursing practice in a 125-bed specialty hospital. Concepts derived from the model were incorporated into the philosophy of nursing and the components of the mission statement relative to nursing practice. The model was used for developing standards related to nursing assessment, care planning, implementation of nursing care, evaluation of nursing care and professional development, and accountability. Job descriptions were revised to reflect the nature of nursing practice from the perspective of the model. This included an expectation that the values and beliefs espoused by the registered nurse as guiding practice were consistent with the RAM. This involved a major reconceptualization of the nurse's responsibilities from performing a variety of tasks to practicing nursing within a particular theoretical framework. The criteria for performance as measured by the performance appraisal system were revised to make explicit expectations about use of the RAM in nursing practice. The quality-monitoring program was analyzed to determine consistency with and reflection of the RAM. Unsurprisingly, the major emphasis in the quality-monitoring program was on the physiological mode, and further development of monitoring specifications for the self-concept, role-function, and interdependence modes were needed.

Weiss, Hastings, Holly, and Craig (1994) reported on a study designed to examine the utility of the RAM as a framework for nursing practice within a hospital setting. They found varying levels of knowledge about the model and integration of the model into practice among the participating nurses. This depended in part on the place of the practitioner in relation to the clinical ladder system, level of involvement with nursing models, shared beliefs with other model supporters, and the environment in which the model implementation occurs. The perceived value of the model varied. Those who found the model useful supported its utility for organizing thoughts about patient care and directing the nursing process. They commented on its comprehensiveness and wholistic nature. As in other writings about model implementation (see Chapters 5 and 7), nurses recognized a unique body of nursing knowledge and role in patient care.

Roy and Andrews (1999) describe the process of implementing the RAM in a regional medical center. Using the RAM to frame the implementation process, this group followed an interesting path, which consisted of the following:

- Assessing behavior and stimuli within the environment in relation to the staff and the implementation process.
- Identifying internal system forces and external events that facilitated model implementation and that reinforced the need for model based practice.
- Developing outcome statements or goals arising from the descriptions of the ineffective behaviors and their influencing factors to predict the outcomes of implementation and identified intervention strategies to achieve the goals.
- Conducting education programs for managers to facilitate model implementation.
- Incorporating accountability for successful implementation into performance expectations for managers.
- Developing model-based nursing process tools, including an assessment tool and documentation system using strategies similar to those described by Rogers, Jones, Clarke, Mackay, Potter, and Ward (1991).
- Revising job descriptions and performance appraisal tools to reflect the model. In keeping with using the model as the overall framework for the implementation process, the job descriptions reflected the physiological, self-concept, role function, and interdependent modes of the RAM.
- Implementing a four-step staff development (clinical ladder) program based on increasing expertise in application of the model.
- Instituting ongoing evaluation of the implementation process and using the results to modify and further develop the ongoing process.

The literature, which includes many examples of RAM applications, evidences the model's usefulness to practitioners (Phillips, Blue, Brubaker, Fine, Kirsch, Papzian, Riester,

& Sobiech, 1998). However, additional development in relation to the model is required to further explicate the meaning of creating human and environmental integration. The model requires further development if nurses are to define their primary practice roles as acceptance, protection, and fostering of person and environment.

Implications for Education

Nurses practicing from the perspective of the RAM require in-depth knowledge of the sciences and theories underlying the four modes of adaptation—physiological, interdependence, role functioning, and self-concept. Additionally, they require prior knowledge of adaptation. They must be able to synthesize data from a variety of sources to understand it in relation to adaptation. Fully functioning from this perspective would probably require at least baccalaureate-level preparation or intense continuing education in a practice setting.

STATUS OF THEORY DEVELOPMENT

The development of the RAM is a good illustration of the dynamic movement along the continuum from philosophy to models. The RAM and theories of person as adaptive system and of adaptive modes have been developed into a complex theoretical system. The work completed since 1970 was synthesized in 1991 into what was called the "definitive statement" of the RAM. The physiological mode of adaptation, with its emphasis on regulator and cognator processes, is highly developed. It needs to be integrated into this new value-based wholism and purposive participation.

Roy has not yet developed the concept of nurse as adaptive system in conjunction with the patient as adaptive system. This would add an important dimension to Roy's conceptualizations. Given the concept of patient as adaptive system and participant in adaptive processes, one might ask how the nurse interacts, what actions are appropriate for nurses, and what nursing looks like.

 NEXUS

The RAM significantly contributed to the theory of nursing, to the guidance of nursing research, and to nursing practice. The concept of adaptation is broadly based and easily applicable within multiple clinical settings. The extent of the research conducted using the RAM speaks to its ability to facilitate conceptualization of variables within nursing practice. The RAM has also generated middle-range theories. Initial theory development studies have generated provocative discussions of adaptation and the mechanisms that influence it.

REFERENCES

Andrews, H.A. and Roy, C. (1986). Essentials of the Roy Adaptation Model. East Norwalk, CT: Appleton-Century-Crofts.

Bokinskie, J. (1992). Family conferences: A method to diminish transfer anxiety. *Journal of Neuroscience Nursing,* 24(3), 129-133.

Bournaki, M. (1997). Correlates of pain-related responses to venipuncture in school-age children. *Nursing Research,* 46(3), 147-154.

Calvillo, E.R. & Flaskerud, J.H. (1993). The adequacy and scope of Roy's Adaptation Model to guide crosscultural pain research. *Nursing Science Quarterly* 6(3), 118-129.

Cho, J. (1998). *Nursing manual assessment tool according to the Roy Adaptation Model.* Glendale, CA: Polaris.

Corser, N. (1996). Sleep on 1- and 2-year old children in intensive care. *Issues in Comprehensive Pediatric Nursing, 19*(1), 17-31.

Courts, N. & Boyette, B. (1998). Psychosocial adjustment of males on three types of dialysis. *Clinical Nursing Research, 7*(1), 47-63.

Crocker, L. & Algina, J. (1986). *Introduction to classical and modern test theory.* Orlando: Harcourt Brace Jovanovich.

Ducharme, F., Ricard, N., Duquette, A., Lévesque, L., & Lachance, L. (1998). Empirical testing of a longitudinal model derived from the Roy adaptation model. *Nursing Science Quarterly, 11*(4), 149-159.

Fawcett, J. Tulman, L., & Myers, S.T. (1988). Development of the inventory of functional status after childbirth. *Journal of Nursing-Midwifery, 33*(6), 242-260.

Fawcett, J., Pollio, N., Tully, A., Baron, M., Henklein, J., & Jones, R. (1993). Effects of information on adaptation to Cesarean birth. *Nursing Research, 42*(1), 49-53.

Fawcett, J. & Weiss, M.E. (1993). Crosscultural adaptation to Cesarean birth. *Western Journal of Nursing Research, 15*(3), 282-297.

Fawcett, J., Tulman, L., & Spedden, J.P. (1994). Responses to vaginal birth after Cesarean section. *Journal of Obstetric, Gynecologic, and Neonatal Nursing, 23*(3), 253-259.

Fawcett, J., Sidney, J., Riley-Lawless, K., & Hanson, M.J. (1996). An exploratory study of the relationship between alternative therapies, functional status, and symptom severity among people with multiple sclerosis. *Journal of Holistic Nursing, 14*(2), 115-129.

Fawcett, J. (2000). *Measuring functional status.* Unpublished manuscript, University of Massachusetts-Boston.

Fisher, M.D. (1994). Identified needs of parents in a pediatric intensive care unit. *Critical Care Nurse, 14*(3), 82-90.

Frederickson, K., Jackson, B., Strauman, T., & Strauman, J. (1991). Testing hypotheses derived from the Roy Adaptation Model. *Nursing Science Quarterly, 4*(4), 168-174.

Gaberson, K. (1991). The effect of humorous distraction on preoperative anxiety: A pilot study. *AORN Journal, 54*(6), 1258-1264.

Gaberson, K. (1995). The effect of humorous and musical distraction on preoperative anxiety. *AORN Journal, 62*(5), 784-791.

Gagliardi, B. (1991). The impact of Duchenne muscular dystrophy on families. *Orthopaedic Nursing, 10*(5), 41-49.

Garcia, A. & White-Traut, R. (1993). Preterm infants' responses to taste/smell and tactile stimulation during an apneic episode. *Journal of Pediatric Nursing, 8*(4), 245-252.

Hamner, J. (1996). Preliminary testing of a proposition from the Roy Adaptation Model. *Image, 28*(3), 215-220.

Helson, H. (1964). *Adaptation level theory.* New York: Harper and Row.

Jackson, B., Strauman, J., Frederickson, K., & Strauman, T. (1991). Long-term biopsychosocial effects of interleukin-2 therapy. *Oncology Nursing Forum, 18*(4), 683-690.

Kitchin, L. & Hutchinson, S. (1996). Touch during preterm infant resuscitation. *Neonatal Network, 15*(7), 45-51.

Komelasky, A. (1990). The effect of home nursing visits on parental anxiety and CPR knowledge retention of parents of apnea-monitored infants. *Journal of Pediatric Nursing, 5*(6), 397-392.

Leuze, M. & McKenzie, J. (1987). Preoperative assessment: Using the Roy Adaptation Model. *AORN Journal, 46*(6), 1122-1134.

Lévesque, L., Ricard, N., Ducharme, F. Duquette, A., & Bonin, J. (1998). Empirical verification of a theoretical model derived from the Roy Adaptation Model: Findings from five studies. *Nursing Science Quarterly, 11*(1), 31-39.

Mastel M.P., Hammond H, & Roberts, M.P. (1982). Theory into hospital practice: A pilot implementation. *The Journal of Nursing Administration, 12*(6), 9-13.

McGill, J. & Paul, P. (1993). Functional status and hope in elderly people with and without cancer. *Oncology Nursing Forum, 20*(8), 1207-1213.

Meeker, B. (1994). Preoperative patient education: Evaluating postoperative patient outcomes. *Patient Education and Counseling, 23*(1), 41-47.

Mock, V., Burke, M., Sheehan, P., Creaton, E., Winningham, M., McKenney-Tedder, S., Schwager, L., & Liebman, M. (1994). A nursing rehabilitation program for women with breast cancer receiving adjuvant chemotherapy. *Oncology Nursing Forum, 21*(5), 899-908.

Mock, V., Dow, K., Meares, C., Grimm, P., Dienemann, J., Haisfield-Wolfe, M., Quitasol, W., Mitchell, S., Chakravarthy, A., & Gage, I. (1997). Effects of exercise on fatigue, physical functioning, and emotional distress during radiation therapy for breast cancer. *Oncology Nursing Forum, 24*(5), 991-1000.

Newman, D. (1997). The inventory of functional status-caregiver of a child in a body cast. *Journal of Pediatric Nursing, 12*(3), 142-147.

Niska, K., Lia-Hoagberg, B., & Snyder, M. (1997). Parental concerns of Mexican-American first-time mothers and fathers. *Public Health Nursing, 14*(2), 111-117.

Niska, K. (1999). Family nursing interventions: Mexican-American early family formation. *Nursing Science Quarterly, 12*(4), 335-340.

Nuamah, I., Cooley, M., Fawcett, J., & McCorkle, R. (1999). Testing a theory for health-related quality of life in cancer patients: A structural equation approach. *Research in Nursing and Health, 22*(3), 231-242.

Phillips, K., Blue, C., Brubaker, K., Fine, J., Kirsch, M., Papazian, K., Riester, C., & Sobiech. (1998). Sister Callista Roy: Adaptation Model. In A. Marriner-Tomey & M. Aligood (Eds.), *Nursing theorists and their works.* (4th ed.). St. Louis: Mosby.

Pollock, S. (1986). Human responses to chronic illness: Physiologic & psychosocial adaptation. *Nursing Research, 35*(2), 90-95.

Pollock, S. (1989). Adaptive responses to diabetes mellitus. *Western Journal of Nursing Research, 11*(3), 265-280.

Pollock, S., Christian, B., & Sands, D. (1990). Responses to chronic illness: Analysis of psychological & physiologic adaptation. *Nursing Research, 39*(5), 300-304.

Pollock, S. (1993). Adaptation to chronic illness: A program of research for testing nursing theory. *Nursing Science Quarterly, 6*(2), 86-92.

Pollock, S.E., Frederickson, K., Carson, M.A., Massey, V.H. & Roy, C. (1994). Contributions to nursing science: Synthesis of findings from adaptation model research. *Scholarly Inquiry for Nursing Practice, 8*(4), 361-372.

Reichert, J.A., Baron, M., & Fawcett, J. (1993). Changes in attitudes toward Cesarean birth. *Journal of Obstetric, Gynecologic, and Neonatal Nursing, 22*(2), 159-167.

Rogers, M., Jones, L., Clarke, J., Mackay, C., Potter, M. & Ward, W. (1991). The use of the Roy Adaptation Model in nursing administration. *Canadian Journal of Nursing Administration, 4*(6), 21-26.

Roy, C. (1970). Adaptation: A conceptual framework for nursing. *Nursing Outlook, 18*(3), 43-45.

Roy, C. (1983). The Roy adaptation model. In I. Clements & F. Roberts, (Eds.), *Family health: A theoretical approach to nursing care.* New York: Wiley.

Roy, C. (1984). *Introduction to nursing: An adaptation model.* (2nd ed.). Englewood Cliffs, NJ: Prentice-Hall, Inc.

Roy, C. (1997). Future of the Roy model: Challenge to redefine adaptation. *Nursing Science Quarterly, 10*(1), 42-48.

Roy, C. & Andrews, H. (1991). *The Roy Adaptation Model: The definitive statement.* Norwalk, CT: Appleton-Lange.

Roy, C. & Andrews, H. (1999). *The Roy Adaptation Model.* (2nd ed.). Stamford, CT: Appleton & Lange.

Roy, C. & McLeod, D. (1981). Theory of the person as an adaptive system. In C. Roy & S. Roberts (Eds.), *Theory construction in nursing: An adaptation model.* Englewood Cliffs, NJ: Prentice-Hall.

Roy, C. & Roberts, S. (1981). *Theory construction in nursing: An adaptation model.* Englewood Cliffs, NJ: Prentice-Hall.

Russell, M., Reinbold, J., & Maltby, H. (1996). Transferring to adult health care: Experiences of adolescents with cystic fibrosis. *Journal of Pediatric Nursing, 11*(4), 262-268.

Samarel, N. & Fawcett, J. (1992). Enhancing adaptation to breast cancer: The addition of coaching to support groups. *Oncology Nursing Forum, 19*(4), 591-596.

Samarel, N., Fawcett, J., & Tulman, L. (1993). The effects of coaching in breast cancer support groups: A pilot study. *Oncology Nursing Forum, 20*(5), 795-798.

Samarel, N., Fawcett, J., & Tulman, L. (1997). Effect of support groups with coaching on adaptation to early stage breast cancer. *Research in Nursing and Health, 20*(1), 15-26.

Samarel, N., Fawcett, J., Krippendorf, K., Piacentino, J., Eliasof, B., Hughes, P., Kowitski, C., & Ziegler, E. (1998). Women's perception of group support and adaptation to breast cancer. *Journal of Advanced Nursing, 28*(6), 1259-1268.

Sato, M.K. (1984). Major factors influencing adaptation. In C. Roy (Ed.), *Introduction to nursing: An adaptation model.* (2nd ed.). Englewood Cliffs, NJ: Prentice Hall.

Schultz, P.R. (1987). When client means more than one: Extending the foundational concept of person. *Advances in Nursing Science, 10(1),*71-86.

Shogan, M. & Schumann, L. (1993). The effect of environmental lighting on the oxygen saturation of preterm infants in the NICU. *Neonatal Network, 12*(5), 7-13.

Takahashi, J. & Bever, S. (1989). Preoperative nursing assessment. *AORN Journal, 50*(5), 1022-1035.

Tulman, L. & Fawcett, J. (1990). Maternal employment following childbirth. *Research in Nursing & Health, 13*(3), 181-188.

Tulman, L., Fawcett, J., Groblewski, L. & Silverman, L. (1990). Changes in functional status after childbirth. *Nursing Research, 39*(2), 70-75.

Tulman, L., Higgins, K., Fawcett, J., Nunno, C., Vansickel, C., Haas, M.B., & Speca, M.M. (1991). The inventory of functional status—antepartum period: Development and testing. *Journal of Nursing-Midwifery, 36*(2), 117-123.

Tulman, L., Fawcett, J., & McEvoy, M.D. (1991). Development of the inventory of functional status—cancer. *Cancer Nursing, 14*(5), 254-260.

Tulman, L., Fawcett, J., & Weiss, M. (1993). The inventory of functional status—fathers: Development and psychometric testing. *Journal of Nursing-Midwifery, 38*(5), 276-282.

Tulman, L. & Fawcett, J. (1996). Biobehavioral correlates of functional status following diagnosis of breast cancer: Report of a pilot study. *Image, 28*(2), 181.

Tulman, L., Morin, K., & Fawcett, J. (1998). Prepregnant weight and weight gain during pregnancy: Relationship to functional status, symptoms, and energy. *Journal of Obstetric, Gynecologic, and Neonatal Nursing, 27*(6), 629-634.

Weiss, M.E., Hastings, W.J., Holly, D.C., & Craig, D.I. (1994). Using Roy's adaptation model in practice: Nurses' perspectives. *Nursing Science Quarterly, 7*(2), 80-86.

Young-McCaughan, S. (1996). Sexual functioning in women with breast cancer after treatment with adjuvant therapy. *Cancer Nursing, 19*(4), 308-319.

Zhan, L. & Shen, C. (1994). The development of an instrument to measure self-consistency. *Journal of Advanced Nursing, 20,* 509-516.

Modeling Nursing From the Perspective of Health

PENDER'S HEALTH PROMOTION MODEL

Key Terms

cognitive-perceptual factors, p. 315
modifying factors, p. 315

Pender's Health Promotion Model (HPM) deals with a phenomenon of concern to many nurses, but it is not itself a model of nursing. It is one of the more popular models in use by nurses. Its midlevel of abstraction and narrower concept make it easier to use and understand than the more complex nursing theoretical systems.

Pender began her work, first published in 1982, with the belief that nurses are responsible for "care that results in better health and more productive living for individuals and families" (p. 182). From this belief, the HPM, a wholistic predictive model of health-promoting behavior, was developed. The model was revised in 1987 and again in 1996. Pender's scholarly work encouraged a focus on health rather than disease.

THE STARTING POINT OF THE MODELING PROCESS

The starting point for Pender's HPM was existing psychological theory. Pender identified a number of theories and models as foundational to understanding motivation for health behavior (Box 11-1). The HPM creatively synthesizes social cognitive theory and expectancy-value theory and focuses on health promotion by maintaining conditions of healthy interactions between the self and the environment. All the models and theories identified as foundational to or necessary for understanding the HPM relate to personal behavior or change within a social environment.

Reason for Model Development

The purpose of Pender's book, and by inference, the reason for developing the model was "(1) to provide nurses with a conceptual framework for understanding the many factors

BOX 11-1

Theories and Models Foundational for Understanding Motivation for Health Behavior

- The Health Promotion Model
- Protection Motivation Theory
- Theory of Reasoned Actions
- Theory of Planned Behavior
- Social Cognitive Theory (Self-efficacy)
- The Theory of Interpersonal Behavior
- Cognitive Evaluation Theory
- The Interaction Model of Patient Health Behavior
- Relapse Prevention

From Pender, N.J. (1996). *Health promotion in nursing practice*. (3rd ed.). Stamford, CT: Appleton & Lange.

that affect the health behaviors of individuals and families, and (2) to present specific nursing strategies for providing preventive and health-promotion services to patients" (Pender, 1982, p. viii). The 1996 revisions intended to increase utility of the model for prediction and intervention in health behaviors. Pender's continued development of and work with the HPM is motivated by the belief that health promotion and disease prevention should be the primary focus in healthcare and that health promotion and disease prevention should be central to any transformations of the healthcare system.

Phenomenon of Concern

The HPM is concerned specifically with health promotion as a behavior of the nurse or other provider. It is based on concepts of *health, health protection*, and *motivation for health behavior* of the person being served. Health is an evolving concept, a wholistic experience, and a multidimensional approach for human beings as competent personal care and meaningful relationships facilitates the actualization of both inherent and acquired potential. The HPM's desired outcome is a view of health as a dynamic process inherent in the lives of individuals, families, and communities. Conceptualization of health and wellness as primary and positive concepts could lead competence models rather than illness models in healthcare. Although the HPM is not uniquely designed for nursing, it describes one aspect of the object of nursing. From its original conceptualization, development has embellished the model and its practical application.

DESCRIPTION OF PENDER'S THEORETICAL SYSTEM
Philosophical Perspectives

The HPM, presented at a mid-level of abstraction, is not linked to any specific philosophy of science, nature, or person or to any more general theory of nursing. However, the philosophical foundations of the HPM can be inferred. The HPM integrates concepts from expectancy-value theory and social cognitive theory, which consider personal behavior ra-

---

BOX 11-2

Assumptions of the Health Promotion Model

1. Persons seek to create living conditions through which they can express their unique human potential.
2. Persons have the capacity for reflective self-awareness, including assessment of their own competencies.
3. Persons value growth in positive directions and attempt to achieve personally acceptable balances between change and stability.
4. Individuals seek to actively regulate their own behavior.
5. Individuals, in all their biopsychosocial complexity, interact with the environment, progressively transforming the environment and being transformed over time.
6. Health professionals constitute a part of the interpersonal environment, which exerts influence on persons throughout their life spans.
7. Self-initiated reconfiguration of person-environment interactive patterns is essential to changing behaviors.

From Pender, N.J. (1996). *Health promotion in nursing practice.* (3rd ed.). Stamford, CT: Appleton & Lange.

---

tional and economical. Pender views environmental events, personal factors, and behavior as reciprocal determinants of health. Human beings have the basic capabilities of symbolization, forethought, vicarious learning, self-regulation, and self-reflection. The HPM is based on assumptions, listed in Box 11-2, that reflect nursing and behavioral science perspectives and the patient's active role. The patient shapes and maintains health behaviors and modifies the environmental context for health behaviors (1996). The HPM's ontology reflects these assumptions in terms of the person's views and relationships to the environment.

Description of Model and Theories

The HPM, shown in Figure 11-1, is "a competence- or approach-oriented model" (Pender, 1996, p. 53). It depicts the multidimensional nature of persons interacting with their environments as they pursue health. The model contains three major categories: individual characteristics and experiences, behavior-specific cognitions and affect, and behavioral outcome. The model depicts the variables and interrelationships and identifies the theoretical underpinnings. Although the model has been used to frame research, no named theories have been advanced. Pender (1996) has not specifically identified any constructs or propositions, despite the many inferred relationships between elements of the model.

Figure 11-1 identifies the major concepts of the model. Individual characteristics and experiences are unique and personal and impact subsequent action. This includes prior related behavior and personal factors. Behavior-specific cognitions and affect are important for motivation and provide focal points for intervention. These include perceived benefits of action, perceived barriers to action, perceived self-efficacy, activity-related affect, interpersonal influences, and situational influences. The third category, behavioral outcome, is the health-promoting behavior directed toward attaining positive health outcomes. Commitment to a plan of action and immediate competing demands and preferences are two variables that influence this outcome.

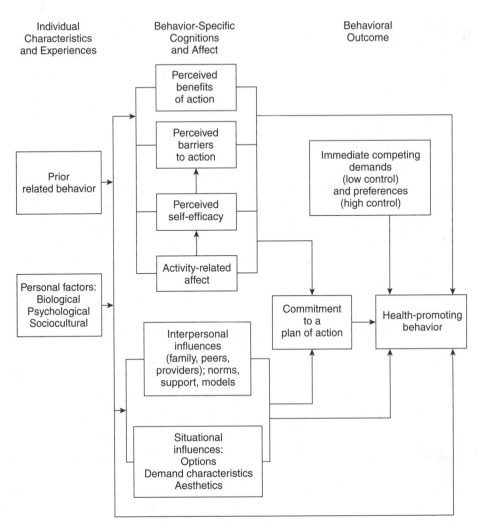

FIGURE 11-1   Pender's Health Promotion Model (From Pender, N.J. (1996). *Health promotion in nursing practice.* (3rd ed.). Stamford, CT: Appleton & Lange.)

Pender (1990) proposed a five-dimension classification system for the way people express health (Box 11-3). This framework for studying health complements the HPM in that it gives content to one of its major elements.

RESEARCH DERIVED FROM PENDER'S HEALTH PROMOTION MODEL

The concept of health promotion has important associations in healthcare and has figured prominently in many nursing studies. Pender's HPM often has theoretically framed these investigations. Modes of scientific inquiry have incorporated both quantitative and qualitative studies, but most research is quantitatively oriented.

BOX 11-3

Classification System for Expressions of Health

Affect

Serenity	Harmony	Vitality	Sensitivity
Calm	Close to god-figure	Energetic	Aware
Relaxed	Contemplative	Vigorous	Connected
Peaceful	At one with the universe	Zestful	Intimate
Content		Alert	Loving
Comfortable		Fit	
Glowing		Buoyant	
Happy		Exhilarated	
Joyous		Powerful	
Pleasant		Courageous	
Satisfied			

Attitudes

Optimism	Relevancy	Competency
Hopeful	Useful	Purposive
Enthusiastic	Contributing	Initiating
Open	Valued	Self-motivating
Reverent	Caring	Innovative
Trustful	Committed	Masterful
	Involved	Challenged

Activity

Positive Life Patterns	Meaningful Work	Invigorating Play
Eating a healthy diet	Setting realistic goals	Having meaningful
Exercising regularly	Varying activities	hobbies
Managing stress	Undertaking challeng-	Engaging in satisfying
Resting adequately	ing tasks	leisure activities
Avoiding harmful substances	Assuming responsibility	Planning energizing
Building positive relationships	for self	diversions
Seeking and using health	Collaborating with	
information	coworkers	
Monitoring health	Receiving intrinsic or	
Coping constructively	extrinsic rewards	
Maintaining a health-		
strengthening		

Aspirations

Self-Actualization	Social Contribution
Growth or emergence	Enhancement of global harmony and interdependence
Personal effectiveness	Preservation of the environment
Organismic efficiency	

Accomplishments

Enjoyment	Creativity	Transcendence
Pleasure from daily	Maximum use	Freedom
living	of capacities	Expansion of consciousness
Sense of achievement	Innovative contribution	Optimized harmony between
		man and environment

From Pender, N.J. (1996). *Health promotion in nursing practice*. (3rd ed.). Stamford, CT: Appleton & Lange.

Research Instruments

Two instruments have been developed specifically to address health promotion. The Health-Promoting Lifestyle Profile (HPLP), (Walker, Sechrist, & Pender, 1987) was revised and subsequently named the Health-Promoting Lifestyle Profile II (HPLP II) (Walker & Hill-Polerecky, 1999). The Exercise Benefits/Barriers Scale (EBBS) (Sechrist, Walker, & Pender, 1987) also measures health promotion. Many health promotion studies have used the HPLP as a measure of health-promoting behaviors, but more recent studies use the HPLP II. A summary of the psychometric characteristics of these instruments can be found in Table 11-1.

Health Promotion Lifestyle Profile. To measure health-protecting and health-promoting behaviors that constitute a health-promoting lifestyle, Walker, Sechrist, and Pender (1987) developed the HPLP, which derived items from the Lifestyle and Health Habits Assessment. The 48 reported health behaviors are rated on a 4-point Likert scale with options ranging from *never, sometimes, often,* and *routinely.* The six subscales represent specific health-protecting and health-promoting behaviors suggested by the HPM and include self-actualization, health responsibility, exercise, nutrition, interpersonal support, and stress management. Investigators reverse score negatively stated items and then calculate the mean responses for each subscale and total scale. Subscale and total scale scores can range from 1 to 4. Although calculating mean scores for each subscale and the total scale is the recommended method of scoring, some investigators have used summed scores for their statistical analysis. Reliability and validity for the HPLP was strong for the total scale, despite more modest subscale ratings. The subscale ratings, however, were within acceptable parameters. In their study of African-American women, Ahijevych and Bernhard (1994) noted that readability and applicability of the HPLP instrument might have affected its reliability and validity in use with a diverse sample. Although they did not assess validity, Ahijevych and Bernhard found high internal consistency for the total HPLP at 0.95. Subscale reliabilities were lower, ranging from 0.72 for the nutrition subscale to 0.89 for the self-actualization subscale.

Translations of the HPLP have been made to Spanish and Arabic. Walker, Kerr, Pender, and Sechrist (1990) completed the initial psychometric evaluation for the Spanish language version and found the instrument culturally relevant. Although factor analysis demonstrated that factors were similar to that of the English language version, items failed to load onto the factors as clearly on the Spanish language version. Reliability was strong for the total scale but more modest for the subscales.

Kuster and Fong (1993) conducted additional psychometric evaluation of the Spanish language version using a predominantly Central-American sample. Although the total scale reliability was strong, subscale scores—with the exceptions of self-actualization and health responsibility—were lower than 0.80. Stability (test/retest) was lower than the sampled tested by Walker, Sechrist, and Pender (1987). However, the retested sample for this study was small. Kuster and Fong's findings resembled the reliability findings of Kerr and Ritchey (1990) in their study of migrant farm workers. Reliability for the Spanish language version of the HPLP in the Kerr and Ritchey study was 0.90 for the total scale, with subscales ranging from 0.53 to 0.84. Thus although overall scale reliability is strong, subscale scores indicate that further work on the Spanish language HPLP is needed. However, it should be noted that few Spanish language instruments to measure health behaviors are available.

TABLE 11-1

Research Instruments Based on Pender's Health Promotion Model

Instrument/Description	Study/Year	Reliability and Validity
Health-Promoting Lifestyle Profile (HPLP) 48-item, 4-point Likert scale	Walker, Sechrist, and Pender, 1987	Modifications were made in a pilot study of nursing students, and four experts completed content validation. Using a scale with 107 items and 10 perceived subscales, item analysis, factor analysis, and reliability analysis were completed with 952 adults. Items depressing internal consistency or found to be highly intercorrelated were deleted. Principal axis factoring with oblique rotation resulted in a six-factor, 48-item scale that explained 38.9% of the variance. Internal consistency of the 48 item scale was 0.922 and ranged from 0.70 to 0.90 for the six subscales. Test/retest reliability for 63 adults with a two-week intervening time interval was $r = 0.926$ for that total scale and ranged from 0.808 to 0.905 for subscales.
HPLP—Spanish Language Version	Walker, Kerr, Pender, and Sechrist, 1990	The Spanish version of the HPLP was administered to 485 Mexican-Americans from both rural and metropolitan areas. Principal components factor analysis with oblique rotation extracted six components that explained 45.9% of variance. Items from the stress management subscale failed to clearly load onto that factor. Internal consistency for total scale was 0.94, with subscales ranging from 0.70 to 0.87. Test/retest reliability for 53 adults with a two-week intervening time interval was $r = 0.87$ for total scale and ranged from 0.73 to 0.85 for subscales.
	Kuster and Fong, 1993	Researchers tested the HPLP–Spanish version with a Central-American sample of 106 adults. Internal consistency reliability for total scale was 0.94 and ranged from 0.64 to 0.89 for subscales. Stability with two week interval tested with 17 subjects was $r = 0.71$ for total scale and ranged from 0.59 to 0.78 for subscales. Means and standard deviations were similar for this sample and for other Spanish-speaking samples.
HPLP II 52-item Likert scale	Walker and Hill-Polerecky, 1999	A sample of 712 adults responded to HPLP II. Factor analysis confirmed six established dimensions of HPLP II. Convergent validity was demonstrated by correlation with Personal Lifestyle Questionnaire ($r = 0.678$) and divergent validity with nonsignificant correlation to social desirability. Concurrent validity was confirmed by correlation with perceived health and quality of life, with correlations ranging from 0.269 to 0.491. Internal consistency validity was 0.943 for total scale, with subscales ranging from 0.793 to 0.872. Stability was assessed with 3-week test/retest, resulting in a correlation of 0.892 for total scale.

Continued

TABLE 11-1

Research Instruments Based on Pender's Health Promotion Model—cont'd

Instrument/Description	Study/Year	Reliability and Validity
Exercise Benefits/Barriers Scale (EBBS) 43-item, 4-point Likert scale	Sechrist, Walker, and Pender, 1987	The original 65-item instrument was analyzed for content validity by four nurse researchers, and all items were retained. A sample ($N = 650$) completed the EBBS, and four items were subsequently deleted because the corrected item total correlations indicated no contribution to internal consistency. Fifteen items were deleted due to redundancy as determined by high item-intercorrelations of greater than 0.60. Principal components factor analysis with varimax rotation yielded a 9-factor solution explaining 64.9% of variance. Factors included the following: life enhancement, physical performance, psychological outlook, exercise milieu, social interaction, time expenditure, preventive health, physical exertion, and family encouragement. A second order principal components factor analysis with oblique rotation extracted two factors (benefits and barriers), which accounted for 47.4% of the variance. Internal consistency for the 43-item instrument was 0.952; for the 29-item benefits scale = 0.953; for the 14 item barriers scale = 0.866. Two-week test/retest reliability from sample of 63: Total instrument = 0.889; benefits scale = 0.893; and barriers scale = 0.772.

Haddad, Al-Ma'aitah, Cameron, and Armstrong-Stassen (1998) tested an Arabic language version of the HPLP using 950 Jordanian adults. Principal components factor analysis with oblique rotation revealed six factors accounting for 39.3% of variance. Although similarities to findings using the English language version existed, the findings were not identical. Although self-actualization, health responsibility, and exercise extracted in the factor analysis were similar to the English version, nutrition, interpersonal support, and stress management subscales were less defined. Initial levels of internal consistency reliability and construct validity were demonstrated, but further testing was recommended. Some adaptation based on cultural considerations might be necessary.

Walker and Hill-Polerecky (1999) revised the HPLP to include 52 items on the total scale. The Health-Promoting Lifestyle Profile II (HPLP II)'s six subscales measure dimensions of spiritual growth, interpersonal relations, nutrition, physical activity, health responsibility, and stress management. The instrument is considered more adequate than its predecessor in measuring health-promoting behavior.

Exercise Benefits/Barriers Scale. Sechrist, Walker, and Pender (1987) developed the Exercise Benefits/Barriers Scale (EBBS) to measure perceived benefits and perceived barriers of exercise, a behavior consistent with a health-promoting lifestyle. The EBBS is a 43 item, 4-point Likert scale that consists of two subscales—a 29-item benefits scale and a 14-item barriers scale. The total instrument's potential scores range from 43 to 172. The benefits scale scores range from 29 to 116 and the barriers scale from 22 to 56. To score the instrument, items on the barrier scale are reverse-coded. The initial psychometric evaluation study had adequate sample size for instrument length and was conducted methodically. Findings for reliability and validity indicate the instrument is internally consistent, remains reasonably stable over short time spans, and possesses adequate construct validity. The EBBS is a useful measure of patient perceptions of benefits and barriers to exercise, and nurses can use it to assess patient perceptions of exercise and willingness to exercise regularly. As model testing continues, the EBBS also may assist in research.

Review of Related Research

A large number of research studies have been conducted using the HPM as a basis to guide discovery. Many of these research studies speculate about the effects of modifying factors and cognitive-perceptual factors in determining participation in health promotion activities. **Modifying factors** are demographic characteristics—such as age, income, gender, education, and ethnicity—that impact health promotion participation. **Cognitive-perceptual factors** are motivational mechanisms such as patients' perceptions of the importance of health and self-efficacy. Perceived control of health, health definition, health status, benefits of health-promoting behaviors, and barriers to health-promoting behaviors also fall in this category. Pender's original conceptualization (1987) of the HPM proposed that cognitive-perceptual factors directly influenced participation in health-promoting behaviors. Pender posited that demographical, biological, interpersonal, situational, and behavioral modifying factors would not only directly influence cognitive perception but also would indirectly influence health promotion. In the revised HPM, both cognitive-perceptual factors and modifying factors influence health-promoting behaviors (Pender, 1996). Table 11-2 summarizes the studies discussed in the following paragraphs.

Text continued on p. 329

TABLE 11-2

Selected Research Studies Using Pender's Health Promotion Model

Study/Year	Purpose	Methods	Findings
DETERMINANTS OF HEALTH PROMOTION BEHAVIORS AND HEALTH STATUS			
Duffy, 1988	The study analyzed impact of health locus of control, self-esteem, and health status for impact on health-promoting lifestyle activities of midlife women.	Two hundred sixty-two women between ages 35 to 65 years responded to Multidimensional Health Locus of Control Scale (MHLC), Rosenberg Self-Esteem Scale, Health Perceptions Questionnaire (HPQ), and HPLP. Stepwise multiple regression was completed, using the total health promotion score, modifying demographic variables, MHLC, Health Perception Questionnaire subscale scores, and total Rosenberg Self-Esteem Score. Canonical correlation was used to examine the relationship between predictor variables and health promotion subscale scores.	Twenty-five percent of the variance in health promotion scores was explained by chance health locus of control, self-esteem, current health, health worry/concern, post-high school education, and internal health locus of control. Two canonical covariates explained 72.8% of variance in subscale scores of HPLP. Internal health locus of control, self-esteem, current health status, and future health status accounted for 36.3% of variance in self-actualization, interpersonal support, and exercise subscales of HPLP. Age, negative chance of health locus of control, health worry/concern, and negative prior health status explained 36.5% of health responsibility, nutrition, and stress management subscales.
Duffy, 1989	The study investigated the influence of health locus of control, self-esteem, and health promotion activities on health status of employed women aged 21 to 65 years.	The sample consisted of 420 employed women who completed MHLC, Rosenberg Self-Esteem Scale, Ware's Health Perception Questionnaire, and the HPLP. Hierarchical multiple regression analysis was used to identify health determinants.	A diagnosed problem and level of household income initially accounted for 17.3% of variance in health status. Major variables of study were then added to regression equation in stepwise fashion. Internal health locus of control, self-actualization, negative chance health locus of control, negative health responsibility, and exercise explained an additional 15.4% (total 32.7%) of variance in health status.

| Duffy, 1993 | The study determined the degree to which selected health components from Pender's HPM explained health promotion behaviors of older adults. | The sample consisted of 477 persons aged 65 and older. Variables measured included the following: age, gender, race, educational level, marital status; individual perceptions of health locus of control, self-esteem, and health status. Health promotion practices measured included the following: nutrition, exercise, stress management, interpersonal support, self-actualization, and health responsibility. Canonical correlation analysis was used to test the hypothesis. | The first canonical correlation was 0.57 and explained 61% of variance. Subjects who indicated good health status had high self-esteem and believed health was under their control. The second correlation was 0.51 and explained 19.6% of variance. Males with higher incomes and self-esteem but poor health were less likely to engage in frequent exercise and good nutrition. The third correlation was 0.24 and explained 7.8% of variance. Older subjects with higher incomes and who were married and less likely to leave control of health to chance tended to engage in health promotion practices of exercise, health responsibility, and stress management. |
| Duffy, 1997 | The study was based on the revised HPM. It determined the degree to which selected modifying factors, locus of control, self-efficacy, and health status explained participation in health promotion practices. | The sample was composed of 397 Mexican-American women who completed mailed packets containing Multidimensional Health Locus of Control (MHLC), Health Perceptions Questionnaire (HPQ), the Self-Efficacy scale, and the Health-Promoting Lifestyle Profile (HPLP). Analysis was conducted using canonical correlation. | Three canonical correlations were significant (0.68, 0.39, and 0.26) but the third covariate accounted for a small portion of variance. The first covariate, accounting for 73% of variance, indicated women's beliefs that they were personally competent and in control of their health, had a good health outlook both currently and for the future, and were more likely to engage in six health-promoting activities. The second covariate, accounting for 15% of variance, demonstrated that younger, more educated women who believed they controlled health and felt past, current, and future health was good were more likely to engage in exercise. |

Continued

TABLE 11-2

Selected Research Studies Using Pender's Health Promotion Model—cont'd

Study/Year	Purpose	Methods	Findings
DETERMINANTS OF HEALTH PROMOTION BEHAVIORS AND HEALTH STATUS—cont'd			
Fleetwood and Packa, 1991	The study determined knowledge of coronary artery disease (CAD) risk factors, health-promoting behaviors, and relationships of health-promoting behaviors to health locus of control, value of health, and risk factor knowledge.	A convenience sample of 520 military officers completed a knowledge questionnaire for CAD, a CAD risk appraisal, the HPLP, the MHLC, and an adaptation of the health value survey. Pearson correlations and one-way ANOVA followed by Bartlett Box F test and Scheffe procedure were used for analysis.	Significant relationships ($p < 0.05$) existed between health-promoting lifestyle and internal locus of control ($r = 0.22$), chance locus of control ($r = -0.17$), health value ($r = 0.20$), and knowledge of CAD ($r = 0.20$). Knowledge of CAD was significantly related to internal locus of control ($r = 0.14$) and chance locus of control ($r = -0.09$). Internal locus of control was related to health value ($r = 0.13$) and chance locus of control ($r = -0.41$). Chance locus of control was related to control by powerful others ($r = 0.22$). Individuals with the best health-promoting lifestyle profiles believed that health was controllable, either by self or others ($F(7,512) = 3.898, p < 0.5$).
Gillis, 1994	The study determined relationships between health-promoting lifestyles of adolescent females and cognitive-perceptual variables.	The sample consisted of 184 adolescent females in grades 7 through 12 and their parents. Variables included HPLP, Health Conception Scale, Health Subscale, and General Self-Efficacy subscale. Stepwise multiple regression with backward elimination was used for analysis.	There was a weak association between health-promoting lifestyles of adolescents and mothers ($r = 0.28, p < 0.01$) and fathers ($r = 0.16, p < 0.05$). Variables of health conception, functional health, clinical health, self-efficacy, health status, and ethnicity explained 41% of variance in adolescent participation in health-promoting lifestyles.
Stuifbergen and Becker, 1994	The study examined predictors of participation in health-promoting lifestyles in persons with disabilities.	A sample of 117 adults with disabilities completed instruments measuring definition of health, self-efficacy, perceived health status, demographical and disability-related measures, and the HPLP.	Most felt that their health was good or excellent (75%). Cognitive-perceptual variables (self-rated abilities, self-efficacy, and definition of wellness) and modifying factors (dependence on mechanical assistance and gender) accounted for 50% of variance in health-promoting activities.

MODEL TESTING

| Frank-Stromborg, Pender, Walker, and Sechrist, 1990 | This descriptive, correlational, ex post facto study tested the usefulness of the HPM in explaining the occurrence of health-promoting behaviors of ambulatory cancer patients. It determined the extent to which cognitive-perceptual factors and modifying factors explained the occurrence of health-promoting behaviors. | A sample of 385 ambulatory cancer patients receiving outpatient chemotherapy or radio-therapy responded to scales measuring four of seven cognitive-perceptual factors, including importance of health, perceived health control, definition of health, perceived health status, reaction to diagnosis of cancer questionnaire, and the HPLP. | Regression analysis revealed 23.5% of variance in health-promoting lifestyle was explained by three cognitive/perceptual and four modifying factors. Cognitive-perceptual factors of positive health conception, health rating, and feelings of control over health accounted for 15.8% of variance, and modifying factors of educational level, age, family income, and employment status added an additional 7.7%. A second regression incorporated illness-specific variables and accounted for 24.7% of variance in health promotion participation. Four cognitive-perceptual variables and two modifying factors influenced health-promoting lifestyles. Confrontation of cancer diagnosis accounted for 3.9% of variance. Canonical correlation produced two sets of canonical variates that accounted for 44.4% of shared variance. |
| Johnson, Ratner, Bottorff, and Hayduk, 1993 | The study tested the HPM and determined whether LISREL was capable of suggesting modifications to the HPM. | The National Survey of Health Practices and Consequences database was used for analysis. The database consisted of 3025 adults aged 20 to 64 years. Demographical data, indicators for the three cognitive-perceptual factors, and indicators for health-promoting behaviors were extracted from the database. | Initial tests indicated that the model failed to fit the data. Modifying factors for health promotion influenced behaviors through other mechanisms than those specified in model. The model was modified to reflect the direct effect of the factors of sex, age, income, marital status, and body mass on selected health promotion behaviors, A marginal fit was achieved; however, the modified model failed to explain variation in participation in health-promoting activities. |

Continued

TABLE 11-2

Selected Research Studies Using Pender's Health Promotion Model—cont'd

Study/Year	Purpose	Methods	Findings
MODEL TESTING—cont'd			
Lusk and Kelemen, 1993	The study measured the components of the HPM in preparation for testing the larger model.	Ninety-eight metal shop workers completed scales measuring benefits and barriers to hearing protection use, value of outcomes of using hearing protection, health conception, self-rated subindex of health, and the HPLP.	Benefits of hearing protection were related to use of protection ($r = 0.29$, $p < 0.01$) and were deterred by barriers ($r = -0.23$, $p < 0.05$). Hearing protection was used to keep noise out and increase sense of well-being ($r = 0.23$, $p < 0.05$; $r = 0.24$, $p < 0.05$). Health-promoting factors of self-actualization and stress management influenced workers' use of hearing protection ($r = 0.33$, $p < 0.01$; $r = 0.31$, $p < 0.01$). Regression revealed that 24% of variance of hearing protection use was predicted by benefits, self-actualization, and interpersonal support. Interpersonal support diminished protection use.
Lusk, Ronis, Kerr, and Atwood, 1994	The study tested the HPM, using it as a causal model to predict use of hearing protection by workers.	A sample of 561 workers responded to the MHLC, Perceived Self-Efficacy, Clinical Health Subscale, Nonclinical Health subscale, Self-Rated Health Subindex of Philadelphia Geriatric Center Multilevel Assessment Instrument, Benefit and Barrier Subscale, Value of Outcome Scale, and measures of situational factors and use of hearing protection. Structural equation modeling was completed for both the theoretical path model and two exploratory path models.	Theoretical model fit well and explained 49% of workers' hearing protection use. Direct effects included value of use, few barriers, high self-efficacy, and low health competency. In the first exploratory model, explaining 52.7% of variance, additional direct paths to protection use included blue-collar job category and situational factors. In the second exploratory model, explaining 50.7% of protection, all original predictors as well as job category and situational factors directly related to protection use.

Lusk, Ronis, and Baer, 1997	The study tested the HPM as a causal model to predict hearing protection use by male and female blue-collar workers.	A sample of 253 women and 251 men were measured for situational factors, cognitive-perceptual factors, definition of health, health status, self-efficacy, benefits, barriers, and hearing protection use. Analysis was conducted using structural equation modeling with EQS, followed by factor analysis.	Predictors accounted for 64.1% for variance in use of hearing protection for men, 47% for women, and 52.3% for the combined group. Men's causal path of hearing protection use was indirectly affected by situational factors and age and was directly affected by barriers, self-efficacy, and value of use. For women, protection use was indirectly associated with situational factors and minority status and was directly associated with barriers, self-efficacy, and place of employment.
Lusk, Ronis, and Hogan, 1997	The study tested the HPM as a causal model to understand hearing protection use by construction workers.	A sample of 359 construction workers were assessed for noise exposure, interpersonal influence (social support, interpersonal norms, interpersonal support), situational factors, control, health definition, health status, self-efficacy, benefits and barriers to use, and hearing protection use. Structural equation modeling using EQS was followed by confirmatory factor analysis to test theoretical and exploratory model.	The theoretical model, which proposed direct paths from cognitive-perceptual factors to health-promoting behaviors and direct paths from modifying factors to cognitive-perceptual factors, accounted for 36.3% of hearing protection use. The exploratory model, accounting for 50.6% of variance for hearing protection use, indicated that three cognitive-perceptual factors and two modifying factors (interpersonal influence and noise) influenced hearing.
Pender, Walker, Sechrist, Frank-Stromborg, 1990	The study tested the ability of the HPM to explain health-promoting lifestyles of employees and investigated the usefulness of the HPM in predicting future health-promoting behaviors.	The sample consisted of 589 health promotion program enrollees who responded to cognitive-perceptual measures of importance of health, perceived control of health, perceived self-efficacy, perceived personal competence, definition of health, and perceived health status. Participants also completed measures for behavioral factors and the HPLP. Measures were taken at one and three months. Hierarchical multiple regression was used to predict the influence of cognitive/perceptual variables and modifying factors on health-promoting lifestyles.	Regression revealed that cognitive-perceptual variables of definition of health (wellness), health status, and control of health (by powerful others and chance) and modifying factors of gender, age, and phase of exercise accounted for 31% of health promotion participation. Three months later, 25% of the variance was accounted for by wellness, health status, internal control, control by others, personal competence, gender, age, and phase of exercise. Canonical correlation assessed the extent to which the six health-promoting dimensions contributed to lifestyle. Sixty-two percent of the variance was explained.

Continued

TABLE 11-2

Selected Research Studies Using Pender's Health Promotion Model—cont'd

Study/Year	Purpose	Methods	Findings
MODEL TESTING—cont'd Ratner, Bottorff, Johnson, and Hayduk, 1994	The study tested a causal model of cognitive-perceptual and modifying factors on health-promoting lifestyles. It also examined the influence of gender.	Data from the National Survey of Personal Health Practices and Consequences (1979 to 1980) were used. A sample of 3025 adults aged 20 to 64 years was examined. Indicators for cognitive-perceptual variables of health control, self-efficacy, and health status were identified. Factors congruent with health-promoting lifestyle were identified. Modifying demographics were identified. Stacked analysis using LISREL was completed to discern gender differences on the causal model.	The initial model was found to be poor fit for both men and women. The model was modified to allow for additional interactions. Only limited variance was explained by these models. In addition to the influence of sex and marital status, education was found to be an important indicator for women's nutrition. Body mass index explained men's nutritional behavior; health control was related to exercise engagement for women; greater self-efficacy was related to taking responsibility for health in men; health responsibility was related to exercise for men. As men age, they perceive less control over health.
Ratner, Bottorff, Johnson, and Hayduk, 1996	The study used multiple indicators to test the multidimensionality of two concepts of the HPM.	A subsample of 197 males was analyzed. Measures included the following: Health Locus of Control, Health Conception Scale, reported age, health status, and exercise. Three models were constructed and tested. LISREL was used to test three causal models.	The first model, using single indicators for health promotion, fit the data. Successive models that used two indicators for each concept and one that used three indicators per concept demonstrated poorer fits with the model. The model that used three indicators failed.
Weitzel, 1989	The study tested the HPM by examining the health behaviors of blue-collar workers.	A sample of 179 blue-collar workers completed the MHLC, value survey, Multilevel Assessment Instrument, General Self-Efficacy Scale, and HPLP.	Participation in health-promoting behaviors was determined by health status, self-efficacy, health value, and education, which accounted for 20% of variance. Health status was a significant predictor of self-actualization, health responsibility, exercise, nutrition, interpersonal support, and stress management. Psychological factors consistently had more predictive power than demographical modifying factors for total HPLP and individual subscales did.

HEALTH-PROMOTING PRACTICES

Ahijevych and Bernhard, 1994	The study examined health-promoting behaviors of African-American women ages 18 to 65.	One hundred eighty-seven African-American women completed the HPLP and furnished saliva samples for cotinine analysis to confirm smoking status.	Moderate participation in health-promoting activities was reported (HPLP mean = 2.55). The highest subscale means were for self-actualization (2.89) and interpersonal support (2.90), whereas the lowest subscale mean was for exercise (1.95). Significant correlations were found between health promotion and the following: years of education ($r = 0.19$, $p = 0.009$), number children in home ($r = -0.16$, $p = 0.05$), income level ($r = 0.25$, $p = 0.001$), employment status ($r = 0.22$, $p = 0.006$), and medical diagnosis ($r = 0.21$, $p = 0.004$). Income explained 12% of variance in health promotion. Presence of a medical diagnosis (4.3%), and employment status (2.3%) also explained some variation.
Ali, 1996	The study identified predictors of osteoporosis prevention behaviors.	Two hundred thirty-three college students completed questionnaires on lifestyle habits and osteoporosis prevention behaviors, exercise participation, calcium intake, Exercise Benefits and Barriers, General Self-Efficacy, Health Locus of Control, a health value survey, knowledge of healthy behaviors, and perceptions of current body weight.	Although 88% exercised, only 3% did so regularly. Sixty-two percent exercised irregularly, and 35% exercised only when they consumed a large number of calories. Thirty-six percent of variance in calcium intake was attributed to perception of barriers to calcium intake, skipping meals, and knowledge of healthy behaviors. Internal health locus of control and perceptions of barriers to exercise participation explained only 8% variance in exercise.
Foster, 1992	This descriptive correlational study investigated the relationship of health-promoting behaviors to life satisfaction and current health status.	One hundred African-American adults aged 60 to 89 years responded to the HPLP, Current Health Scale, a modified version of Life Satisfaction Index, and Two-Factor Social Position Index Scale.	Life satisfaction was positively correlated with current health status ($r = 0.58$, $p = 0.001$), health-promoting activities ($r = 0.32$, $p = 0.001$), age ($r = 0.23$, $p = 0.05$), and socioeconomic status ($r = 0.27$, $p = 0.0l$). An inverse relationship between health activities and smoking ($r = 0.22$, $p = 0.01$) was found. No association between current health and health-promoting activities was found.

Continued

TABLE 11-2

Selected Research Studies Using Pender's Health Promotion Model—cont'd

Study/Year	Purpose	Methods	Findings
HEALTH-PROMOTING PRACTICES—cont'd			
Riccio-Howe, 1991	This descriptive correlational study investigated factors associated with adolescent safety belt use.	Three hundred twenty 11th and 12th grade adolescents completed questionnaires that assessed seat belt use and benefits and barriers to use, accident locus of control (ALOC), and a revised health value scale.	Students who learned to drive before implementation of mandatory seat belt laws had a lower rate of use. Higher seat belt use occurred if adolescents sat in the front seat or if parents or friends used belts. Females perceived more benefits of use, whereas males perceived more barriers. Benefits promoted use, and barriers deterred use.
Riffle, Yoho, and Sams, 1989	This descriptive correlational study examined relationships among health-promoting behaviors, social support, and self-reported health.	One hundred thirteen Appalachian adults aged 55 years or older responded to the HPLP, the Older American Resources and Services (OARS) questionnaire, and the Personal Resource Questionnaire (PRQ2)	Health-promoting activities were positively associated with social support ($r = 0.2968$, $p < 0.0008$). Health-promoting activities were positively associated with self-reported health ($r = 0.2205$, $p < 0.0103$). Self-reported health was not related to social support. Thirteen percent of variance in health-promoting behaviors was attributable to social support and perceived health status.
Serafine and Broom, 1998	The study determined factors that predicted attendance at preterm birth prevention classes.	One hundred three pregnant women at low-risk for preterm birth participated. Thirty-seven women attended preterm birth class. All participants answered the Fetal Health Locus of Control Scale, Health Value Scale, a perceived barrier scale, and opened-ended questions regarding class participation.	Two predictor variables accounted for 30% of variance between women who attended or did not attend class. Attendees were more likely to have planned to attend and perceived fewer barriers to class attendance. Predicted group membership using those variables improved from 36% to 68% for women attending and from 64% to 85% for those not attending.

Speake, Cowart, and Stephens, 1991	The study compared health beliefs and lifestyle practices of rural and urban older adults.	Three hundred forty-three volunteers aged 55 to 93 from rural and urban locations completed the MHLC, three questions on perceived health status, and the HPLP.	Small percentages of variance in HPLP subscales were predicted by the variables of education, income, residence, health status, internal health locus of control, chance health locus of control, and powerful others health locus of control. Variances for predictions of health promotion subscales included the following: stress management (8%), exercise (9%), nutritional lifestyle practices (13%), health responsibility (13%), self-actualization (21%), and interpersonal support (13%).
Telleen, 1993	The study compared health-promoting practices of pregnant and nonpregnant women.	One hundred pregnant and 93 nonpregnant women of childbearing age responded to the HPLP.	The HPLP total score and subscale score means ranged from 2.46 to 3.31 on a 4-point scale. Health-promoting behaviors for pregnant and nonpregnant women were different only with regard to nutrition ($t = 3.06$, $p = 0.003$).
EXERCISE			
Desmond, Conrad, Montgomery, and Simon, 1993	The study identified factors associated with physical activity of male white- and blue-collar workers.	A convenience sample of 325 male workers were evaluated for physical activity (work, sports, and leisure), health status, self-efficacy, and perceived barriers. Correlation and regression were used to evaluate factors influencing activity.	Job category and self-efficacy accounted for 30% of variance for all physical activity. Fifty-six percent of variance in occupational activity was explained by income and job activity. Six percent of variance in sports activity was attributable to perceived health status. Perceived self-efficacy and job category accounted for 13.5% of variance in leisure activity.
Bonheur and Young, 1991	The study examined differences in self-esteem and perceived benefits and barriers between exercisers and nonexercisers.	Exerciser ($\underline{n} = 57$) and nonexerciser ($\underline{n} = 48$) college student groups completed instruments measuring exercise intensity, the Exercise Benefits and Barriers Scale (EBBS), and a self-esteem inventory.	Exercisers exhibited a greater degree of self-esteem ($t = -3.38$, $\underline{df} = 100.3$, $p < 0.001$), perceived greater benefits of exercise ($t = -6.11$, $\underline{df} = 101.6$, $p < 0.000$), and fewer perceived barriers to exercise ($t = 3.56$, $\underline{df} = 87.6$, $p < 0.000$). Stepwise regression revealed that self-esteem, perceived benefits, and perceived barriers accounted for 32% of difference in exercise participation.

Continued

TABLE 11-2

Selected Research Studies Using Pender's Health Promotion Model—cont'd

Study/Year	Purpose	Methods	Findings
HEALTH-PROMOTING PRACTICES—cont'd			
Garcia, Broda, Frenn, Coviak, Pender, and Ronis, 1995	The study investigated the influence of gender and developmental differences in exercise belief and exercise behaviors of youths.	The sample consisted of 286 racially diverse youth in grades 5, 6, and 8. Youths were measured for exercise (Child/Adolescent Exercise Log), Rosenberg Self-Esteem Scale, Children's Self-Efficacy Survey, self-schema (Me Now and Future Scale), and the Children's Perceived Benefits/Barriers to Exercise Scale. Path analysis was used to test causal model.	In the causal model, gender and access to facilities explained 19.3% of variance in exercise participation. In exploratory path analysis, 32% of variance in exercise benefits/barriers was explained by developmental stage, perceived health status, exercise self-efficacy, social support for exercise, and exercise norms.
Gillis and Perry, 1991	The study examined differences in physical activity and health-promoting behaviors of midlife women participating or not participating in a structured exercise program.	An experimental group of 52 women who completed a 12-week program of physical activity were compared to 40 control group women for well-being, self-esteem, health locus of control, HPLP, and health perceptions. Measures were completed before the program, following program completion, and 6 months later. Repeated measures ANOVA (2×3) and stepwise regression were used for analysis.	The exercise group demonstrated greater increases over time in health-promoting areas of exercise (Time 2: $F_{(1,90)} = 15.87$; $p < 0.000$; Time 3: $F_{(1,90)} = 15.55$; $p < 0.000$) and stress management (Time 2: $F_{(1,90)} = 2.29$; $p < 0.04$). In the exercise group, regression indicated that wellbeing, exercise, and stress management accounted for 52% of variance in program adherence.

Neuberger, Kasal, Smith, Hassanein, and DeViney, 1994

The study determined factors that predicted exercise behavior and aerobic fitness in patients with arthritis.

One hundred outpatients with arthritis completed the EBBS, Arthritis Impact Measurement Scale, Stanford 7-day Recall of Physical Activity interview, a bicycle ergometer test, and a body mass index calculation. Path analysis was used to test the causal model.

Poor perceived health status was associated with greater severity of arthritis, longer time since diagnosis, less education, and higher pain scores. Better perceived health status was associated with older age and higher income levels. Modifying factors accounted for 26% of variance in health status score and 18.4% of perceived benefits of exercise score. Lower perceived benefits of exercise were associated with higher arthritis scores, longer arthritis duration, and less education, whereas higher perceived benefits were associated with previous exercise. Modifying factors contributed to 15.6% of variance in perceived benefits to exercise. Longer duration of arthritis, higher arthritis scores, higher body mass index scores, and fewer years of education were associated with more perceived barriers. The model accounted for 20% of variance in composite exercise scores. Perceived benefits of exercise were associated with exercise participation. Poorer health status and higher perceived barriers were associated with lower exercise participation.

HEALTH-PROMOTING INTERVENTIONS

Campbell and Kreidler, 1994

This phenomenological study evaluated personal responsibility for health-promoting behaviors and perceptions of wellness of older adults participating in a community-based health promotion program.

Thirty-three patients were interviewed during their participation in a community-based health promotion program that aimed to maintain patients' independence by improving lifestyle practices. Interventions consisted of structured educational programs, health assessments, and home visits aimed at healthy lifestyle choices.

Patients viewed themselves as not well and felt that their physicians were key to indicating their level of health status. Mobility was of key importance to a sense of wellness. Themes of depression and hopelessness emerged for less mobile individuals.

Continued

TABLE 11-2

Selected Research Studies Using Pender's Health Promotion Model—cont'd

Study/Year	Purpose	Methods	Findings
HEALTH-PROMOTING INTERVENTIONS—cont'd			
Frenn, Borgeson, Lee, and Simandl, 1989	This qualitative study examined factors that cardiac rehabilitation patients viewed as enabling or disabling health-promoting lifestyle changes.	Six men and four women who were part of an outpatient cardiac rehabilitation program were interviewed about program and lifestyle changes. Audiotapes were transcribed and were analyzed with the grounded theory method.	The cardiac events precipitated patients' needs to change. In health protection patients felt change was necessary or were afraid not to change. In health promotion, changes made were to enjoy life. Individualized factors of program, family/friends, self-perceptions, presence or absence of barriers, and lifestyle experience either enabled or disabled change forces. Lifestyles were repatterned by changing beliefs, attitudes, and anticipations.
Richter, Malkiewicz, and Shaw, 1987	The study examined differences in health promotion behaviors in nursing students in three different health education programs.	Group 1 ($n = 21$) enrolled in a 10-week Health-Promoting Behaviors course; Group 2 ($n = 20$) enrolled in a personalized health assessment experience; and Group 3 ($n = 27$), a control group, enrolled in an adult health nursing course. Before intervention and 6 months after intervention, participants completed the Lifestyle Assessment Questionnaire (LAQ) and physiological measures of pulse, blood pressure, height, and weight.	The only significant differences between groups were found on the exercise subscale of the LAQ ($F = 5.24$, $p < 0.01$) and heart rate LAQ ($F = 7.35$, $p < 0.01$). The mean exercise score increased slightly for the group enrolled in the health promotion course. The mean heart rate increased more for the control group than for the other groups.

Many of the systematic studies measure the cognitive-perceptual factors that Pender identified. The Rokeach Values Survey or a modification of the Health Value Scale is frequently used as a measure of importance of health. Control of health is often measured by the Multidimensional Health Locus of Control Scales (MHLC). Other instrument choices have included the Accident Locus of Control Scale (ALOC) and the Children's Health Locus of Control Scale. Perceived self-Efficacy has been measured with the General Self-Efficacy subscale of the Self-Efficacy scale. The Laffrey Health Conception Scale has measured health definition. Perceived health status often is measured with the Current Health Status Scale or the Health Scale, which is a subscale of the Multilevel Assessment Instrument. Although they have been inconsistently studied, a variety of instruments have measured perceived benefits and perceived barriers. The EBBS has been used for exercise benefits and barriers. Others have used investigator-developed scales specific to hearing protection, safety belt use, or health promotion for individuals with disabilities.

Several research programs centered on health promotion have determined health promotion and status indicators and have tested the HPM's ability to predict health-promoting behaviors. Additional studies have focused on crosscultural groups or on groups of persons ranging in age from adolescents to older adults. Although many studies have used the HPLP, they were not necessarily based on the HPM. In the following discussion, priority was given to studies that composed a program of research. The following studies successfully incorporated the HPM into variable selection, measurement, and evaluation. Table 11-2 summarizes the research studies included in the following discussion.

Determinants of Health Promotion Behaviors and Health Status. Several investigators (Duffy, 1988, 1989, 1993, 1997; Fleetwood & Packa, 1991; Gillis, 1994; Stuifbergen & Becker, 1994) have assessed determinants of health-promoting behaviors for different groups of various ages and affiliations. Sample age groups ranged from adolescents to older adults, and group affiliations included women, nursing students, and white- and blue-collar workers.

To examine determinants of health-promoting behaviors and health status, Duffy (1988) conducted a major research program in which she analyzed the impact of health locus of control, self-esteem, and health status on health-promoting lifestyle activities of 262 midlife women. Subjects who reported high self-esteem, current good health, high internal locus of control, and low chance health locus of control had high scores on the HPLP subscales of self-actualization, nutrition, exercise, and interpersonal support. Participants who were older, had high health worry/concern scores, reported lower past health status, and had low chance health locus of control scores demonstrated high HPLP subscale scores for health responsibility, nutrition, and stress management elements of health promotion. Findings supported Pender's HPM, which suggests that individual perceptions of health locus of control, self-esteem, and health status influence health promotion behaviors.

In a subsequent analysis, Duffy (1989) examined health status determinants of employed women aged 21 to 65. She found that employed women who rated their overall health status as good typically had good household incomes and no diagnosed health problems. Their health promotion scores indicated high internal locus of control, high self-actualization, high levels of exercise, and low health responsibility. Once again, these findings tentatively supported Pender's suggestion that health locus of control, health promotion activities, and health status are related. The women's self-actualization was congruent with

Pender's conceptualization that health promotion is a method of sustaining or increasing well-being.

Duffy (1993) investigated the degree to which selected components of Pender's model explained health promotion practices of persons aged 65 and over. Older healthy persons had high esteem and internal locus of control with regard to health issues and reported using five of six health promotion strategies. These typically included nutrition, exercise, stress management, health responsibility, and self-actualization. They less often relied on interpersonal support. Men with higher incomes and high self-esteem did not tend to use health promotion practices as often as women did. Pender's HPM was partially supported by this study in that internal locus of control, high self-esteem, and positive health status related to health promotion practices. However, with the exception of a relationship of income to exercise and stress management to health responsibility activities, the predicted relationships of demographic characteristics and health promotion practices were not found. In other words, this study failed to demonstrate that many of the modifying factors indirectly influenced health-promoting activities, as Pender's HPM had suggested.

In a final study, Duffy (1997) examined the degree to which modifying demographic factors, cognitive-perceptual factors, and health status influenced Mexican-American women in the six health promotion activities proposed by the revised HPM. Factors of age; education; internal sense of control; personal competence; and perception of past, present, and future health status were important in determining the level of participation in health promotion activities. In this study, marital status and household income did not impact health promotion practices. However, the modifying factors of age and education were only small factors in determining health promotion activities, which led Duffy to conclude that the HPM should be modified to reflect the minor role of demographic variables.

Fleetwood and Packa (1991) investigated determinants of health-promoting behaviors in military personnel. They were specifically interested in subjects' knowledge about coronary artery disease (CAD) and related risk reduction behaviors. Subjects with greater knowledge about cardiac risk factors participated in more health-promoting behaviors. Those with the highest participation in health-promoting behaviors believed that health was controllable, either by self or by others.

Gillis (1994) examined determinants of health-promoting lifestyles in adolescent females. Only a weak relationship between the health-promoting practices of either parent and those of the adolescent existed. Definition of health, self-efficacy, perceived health status, and ethnicity predicted adolescent participation in health-promoting lifestyles.

Using a population that has been traditionally overlooked in health promotion, Stuifbergen and Becker (1994) examined predictors of health-promoting lifestyles in persons with disabilities. Adults with disabilities were more likely to engage in health-promoting activities if they were female, possessed a high sense of self-efficacy, had a wellness-oriented definition of health, and required less mechanical assistance with daily activities. This study confirmed the value of using the HPM to explain health behaviors of disabled individuals. Cognitive-perceptual factors accounted for at least half of the variance associated with health promotion behaviors. This finding is particularly significant for patients with disabilities because attitudinal factors can be changed.

In summary, study findings revealed that cognitive-perceptual variables often influenced health-promoting behaviors (Duffy, 1988, 1993; Gillis, 1994; Stuifbergen & Becker, 1994).

However, the role of modifying factors was less clear. Duffy (1993, 1997) found that modifying factors played only a minor role in determining health-promoting behaviors. Pender (1996) subsequently revised the role of modifying factors in her model. The variety of people included in the samples—including women (midlife, and employed versus unemployed), older adults, Mexican-Americans, adolescents, and persons with disabilities—is a clear strength of all these studies of health promotion determinants.

Model Testing. Several investigators have aimed health promotion studies at specifically testing the HPM. Cognitive-perceptual or modifying factors' direct or indirect influence on health-promoting behaviors is a central issue. Findings from some of these studies contributed toward further refinement and revision of the HPM.

Pender, Walker, Sechrist, and Frank-Stromborg (1990) investigated the HPM's success in explaining health-promoting lifestyles among employees. Investigators also wanted to determine whether the HPM would predict future health-promoting lifestyles. Those who tended to engage in health-promoting lifestyles tended to be older, female, and self-confident in managing life situations. They tended to define health as possessing high level wellness and believed that their personal health was good and was affected by significant others but not by chance. This study supported the HPM in that cognitive-perceptual factors, health definition, perceived control, and perceived health status influenced health promotion activities. However, not all cognitive-perceptual factors impacted behaviors. Moreover, some modifying factors—gender, age, and phase of exercise program—influenced behaviors more directly than Pender had anticipated.

Frank-Stromborg, Pender, Walker, and Sechrist (1990) also studied application of the HPM to ambulatory cancer patients. Investigators found that better educated, older, wealthier patients who held a wellness orientation, rated their personal health status as high, expressed a belief that health was self-controlled, and worked outside the home were more likely to participate in health-promoting activities. When illness factors were included in the regression, reaction to cancer diagnosis accounted for additional variance in health-promoting lifestyles. Once again, modifying factors—particularly education and age—modestly but directly contributed to participation in health-promoting behaviors.

Weitzel (1989) tested the HPM with a group of blue-collar workers. Both cognitive-perceptual factors (which Weitzel termed psychological variables) and modifying factors of education and income contributed modestly to health-promoting behaviors. The strongest indicators of blue-collar male participation in health-promoting behaviors were feelings of good health status and strong senses of self-efficacy. For the most part, this group of blue-collars workers exhibited a high internal locus of control with regard to their health. However, because the study accounted for little variance, Weitzel concluded that other factors must be considered in explaining health promotion participation.

Using the HPM, Lusk and Kelemen (1993); Lusk, Ronis, Kerr, and Atwood (1994); Lusk, Ronis, and Baer (1997); and Lusk, Ronis, and Hogan (1997) conducted a series of studies predicting workers' use of hearing protection. Hearing protection was considered a good measure of participation in a health-promoting activity because subjects worked in noisy areas and because hearing protection use requires personal responsibility. In a preliminary study used to prepare for causal model testing of the HPM, Lusk and Kelemen (1993) found that only half the workers used hearing protection. Lusk and Kelemen concluded that workers who used hearing protection did so because of perceived benefits, the self-efficacy of use, the perceived value of eliminating noise, increased senses of wellbeing, and use of health-promoting behaviors of self-actualization and stress management.

In a subsequent study by Lusk, Ronis, Kerr, and Atwood (1994), the HPM guided development of a causal model predicting workers' use of hearing protection. The model hypothesized that use of hearing protection was influenced directly by cognitive-perceptual factors (perceived control of health, health definition, and perceived benefits) that in turn were influenced directly by modifying factors (situation, gender, age, education, and job category). The investigators hypothesized that modifying factors indirectly influence hearing protection use. This model was a good fit for the data, but the exploratory models demonstrated a slightly better fit. Low perceived health competence, high self-efficacy, high value of use, and low perceived barriers increased workers' likelihood of hearing protection use. Education level was associated with higher health competence but lower use of hearing protection. Exploratory analyses established additional direct paths, including modifying factors of situation and job category, to hearing protection use. Thus the HPM can predict use of protective behaviors, despite the unexpected direct linkages of modifying factors.

Using the HPM, Lusk, Ronis, and Baer (1997) specifically addressed the use of hearing protection in a group of male and female blue-collar workers. Proposing that cognitive-perceptual factors would directly influence hearing protection use and that modifying factors would directly influence cognitive-perceptual factors and indirectly influence hearing protection use, investigators tested the proposal through structural equation modeling. Although two cognitive-perceptual factors of barriers and self-efficacy directly explained use of hearing protection for both males and females, other gender-associated differences surfaced. Situational factors indirectly explained hearing protection use for both genders. However, male workers' perceived value of use directly influenced their choice to use protection, whereas increasing age indirectly influenced use. For females, plant site was directly associated with protection use, whereas minority status decreased use. As with the prior studies, the HPM provided a predictive theoretical model. However, some modifying factors directly influenced hearing protection use.

In a follow-up study, Lusk, Ronis, and Hogan (1997) used the HPM as a causal model to predict construction workers' use of hearing protection. The initial confirmatory test supported the proposed theoretical model of hearing protection use was supported. The cognitive-perceptual factors of benefits, barriers, self-efficacy, and perceived health influenced construction workers' use of hearing protection. Exploratory analysis of the model followed the confirmatory analysis and indicated that protection use was tied directly to the cognitive-perceptual factors of value of use, barriers, and self-efficacy and the modifying factors of interpersonal modeling and noise exposure. Both the theoretical model and the exploratory models supported the HPM. Significantly, the exploratory model's indication of the direct influence of modifying factors on health promotion was congruent with Pender's revised HPM, which theorizes a direct relationship between modifying factors and participation in health promotion behaviors.

Not all studies have found the HPM an adequate explanation of participation in health promotion activities. Johnson, Ratner, Bottorff, and Hayduk (1993) tested the HPM using a causal model containing three of the cognitive-perceptual factors—perceived health control, perceived self-efficacy, and perceived health status—that Pender proposed as influences on participation in health-promoting behaviors. Investigators used structural behavioral modeling to simultaneously test multiple variables that potentially accounted for participation in health-promoting behaviors. Findings of the initial causal model indicated that the HPM did not fit the data. Modifying factors for health promotion influenced behaviors through other mechanisms than those specified in the model. Although a marginal fit was discovered following causal model modification, the modified model did not explain differences in health-promoting behaviors. Authors suggested that the HPM must be reevaluated. However, a criticism of this study is that only three of the seven cognitive-perceptual factors associated with the HPM were included.

Ratner, Bottorff, Johnson, and Hayduk (1994) investigated the interaction effects of gender within the HPM. Investigators hypothesized that cognitive-perceptual variables of control of health, self-efficacy, and health status would directly influence self-actualization, health responsibility, exercise, nutrition, and interpersonal support. Additionally, they hypothesized that gender would influence the effects of marital status on perceived control of health, self-efficacy, perceived health status, self-actualization, nutrition, and interpersonal support. Although gender significantly mediated health-promoting behaviors, researchers found the HPM a poor fit. Participation in a health-promoting lifestyle was deemed a complex group of numerous interactions that needed to be delineated.

In a follow-up study to test the dimensionality of two concepts—perceived health control and definition of health—Ratner, Bottorff, Johnson, and Hayduk (1996) examined multiple indicators. Investigators proposed that if health promotion is a multidimensional concept, then using summed, unidimensional indicators will lead to association with other model concepts. Therefore researchers tested three models: one using single indicators for concept measurement, one double indicators, and the final one triple indicators. The key concepts for which indicators were derived included age, perceived control of health, perceived health status, definition of health, and exercise. The single indicator model, testing the influence of age on exercise with health control, health status, and health definition as intervening variables achieved a good fit with the data. However, addition of other indicators diminished the fit, with the second model achieving a poor fit and the triple indicator model failing to fit.

In summary, the model testing studies also found that modifying factors such as age, gender (Pender, Walker, Sechrist, & Frank-Stromborg, 1990), and education (Frank-Stromberg, Pender, Walker, & Sechrist, 1990; Lusk, Ronis, Kerr, & Atwood, 1994) directly influenced participation in health-promoting activities. Weitzel (1989) suggested that additional factors also accounted for health promotion participation. A strength of the HPM is that cognitive-perceptual factors consistently influenced participation in health-promoting activities (Frank-Stromborg, Pender, Walker, & Sechrist, 1990; Lusk, Ronis, & Baer, 1997; Lusk, Ronis, & Hogan, 1997; Pender, Walker, Sechrist, & Frank-Stromborg, 1990). Perhaps the greatest exceptions to this finding are the studies by Johnson, Ratner, Bottorff, and Hayduk (1993) and Ratner, Bottorff, Johnson, and Hayduk (1994), which suggested that health promotion participation is complex and is not fully explained by variables in the HPM. Ongoing further refinement is necessary to bolster initial support for the HPM.

Health-Promoting Practices. A number of descriptive studies have described the health-promoting practices of various groups. Groups include the elderly, adults, pregnant women, and selected ethnic groups. Speake, Cowart, and Pellet (1989) examined the relationship between healthy lifestyle and perceived health status and locus of control in a healthy group of older adults. Participants, particularly Caucasians and those with more education, possessed high degrees of internal locus of control over health issues. Most participants rated their heath as good or excellent and generally felt their health had been stable over the past 6 months. This finding was particularly true for younger, married, educated, female Caucasians. Perceived health status and internal locus of control were associated with older adults who engaged in more health-promoting activities. This study supports the HPM's theoretical proposition that modifying factors of gender, race, level of education, and age are associated with differences in the cognitive-perceptual factors of locus of control and perceived health status. Subsequently, cognitive-perceptual factors of locus of control and health status were associated with health-promoting lifestyle practices.

In a subsequent study Speake, Cowart, and Stephens (1991) studied the influence of urban or rural residence on older adults' health promotion lifestyle practices. When income and level of education were controlled, investigators discovered that place of residence did not generate differences in health-promoting behaviors. Low income negatively influenced health practices, whereas higher levels of education had a positive influence. Other factors influencing health-promoting behaviors included internal locus of control and perceived health status. It should be noted that in both studies (Speake, Cowart, & Pellet, 1989; Speake, Cowart, & Stephens, 1991), factors of education, income, and locus of control influenced health-promoting behaviors but explained only a small percentage of the variation. These findings indicate that other predictors need to be investigated for their contribution to explaining health promotion practices. Pender's HPM indicates that other cognitive-perceptual factors are also associated with health promotion. It is important to consider these factors as well.

Riffle, Yoho, and Sams (1989) also investigated health-promoting behaviors—specifically, Appalachian older adults' relationship between health behaviors, perceived social support, and self-reported health. Older adults engaging more health-promoting behaviors also reported a higher perceived health status, and those with higher levels of social support engaged in more health-promoting behaviors. Once again, higher levels of education and income positively influenced participation in health-promoting activities. Participants tended to participate less often in self-care activities such as screening and health education. The HPM was supported in that cognitive-perceptual factors of perceived health and social support influenced participation in health-promoting activities. However, these factors only explained a small portion of variance in participation in a health-promoting lifestyle.

Two studies specifically addressed health-promoting practices of African-Americans. Both are important because relatively few investigations have been conducted on non-Caucasian ethnic groups and health promotion. Ahijevych and Bernhard (1994) examined health-promoting practices of African-American women between the ages of 18 and 65 years. Self-actualization and interpersonal support were the strongest areas of health-promoting activity, and exercise was the lowest. Higher levels of income, the presence of a medical diagnosis, and employment positively influenced participation in health-promoting behaviors. Findings from this study differed from others in that exercise participation figured less significantly, but women in this study assumed more health responsibility and sought professional assistance when needed. Participants in other studies tended to be white, more educated, and wealthier. Findings indicated that women responded differently to diagnosed illness than the HPM would indicate. According to the HPM, illness does not have motivational significance for health-promoting behaviors. In this study women with a diagnosed illness tended to participate in more health-promoting behaviors.

Foster (1992) analyzed the relationships between health-promoting behaviors, perceived current health status, and life satisfaction of older African-American adults. Participants reporting greater life satisfaction also indicated greater participation in health-promoting activities and higher socioeconomic status. Those engaging in a higher number of health-promoting activities were less likely to smoke. One finding inconsistent with the HPM was that current health status was not associated with health promotion participation.

Telleen (1993) compared health promotion practices of pregnant and nonpregnant women. The researcher hypothesized that pregnancy would be a modifying factor that would influence health-promoting activities. Both groups of women had moderate participation in health promotion activities. However, pregnant women demonstrated significantly better nutritional practices than nonpregnant women did. Pregnancy as a modifying factor for health participation affected only nutritional practices.

Four studies used the HPM to predict participation in specific health-promoting activities: seat belt use (Riccio-Howe, 1991), osteoporosis prevention (Ali, 1996), contraceptive use (Felton, 1996) and attendance at preterm birth prevention classes (Serafine & Broom, 1998). Using the HPM, Riccio-Howe proposed that adolescent perception of importance of health, locus of control for accidents, and an understanding of the benefits and barriers of seat belt use would cue safety belt use. Findings partially supported the proposed model in that the proposed cues to action modified behavior. Friend or parents use of safety belts and perception of benefits of safety belts positively influenced safety belt use. Adolescents who perceived many barriers to use tended not to use safety belts. Locus of control and health value did not influence safety belt behaviors. Support for the HPM was offered by the finding that cues to action, benefits, barriers, situation, and interpersonal factors influence choices about seat belt use. The finding that a high value on health and high locus of control failed to influence participation in seat belt use did not support the HPM.

Ali (1996) examined the usefulness of the HPM in determining predictors of osteoporosis prevention behaviors of young women. Using the HPM, she hypothesized that cognitive-perceptual variables of perception of benefits and barriers to calcium intake, exercise participation, self-efficacy, control of health, and importance of health would positively influence preventive activities. Women reporting the lowest calcium consumption commonly skipped meals, consumed a large number of caffeinated drinks, were overweight, felt health was controlled by others, and perceived barriers to calcium intake and regular exercise. Conversely, women with higher calcium intakes tended to be more pleased with their body weights, believed that they controlled their health, valued health, knew about health behaviors, and perceived that benefits for calcium intake and exercise existed. Health promotion variables contributed to the prediction participation in behaviors that prevent osteoporosis and explained more than a third of the variance in calcium intake but only a limited amount of variance in exercise behaviors. Perceptions of benefits and barriers to calcium intake influenced behavior in a manner congruent with the HPM.

Felton (1996) differentiated characteristics of three groups of sexually active adolescents who used contraceptives consistently, used them intermittently, or did not use contraceptives. Guided by the HPM, Felton proposed that cognitive-perceptual variables of problem solving and self-image together with modifying factors of demographical characteristics, sexual history, and health promotion participation would explain contraceptive behaviors. Characteristics exhibiting the greatest discriminatory power were age at first coitus, prior pregnancy, and participation in health-promoting behaviors. Those who did not use contraceptives were different from consistent users in that nonusers had a higher pregnancy rate, were younger at first coitus, participated in fewer health-promoting activities, had fewer problem-solving skills, and were younger at the time of the study. Nonusers differed from intermittent users in that they were younger at first coitus, had lower self-images, and were more likely to be African-American. In this study, both modifying factors and cognitive-perceptual factors directly influenced contraceptive behavior. Health-promoting behaviors as suggested by the HPM discriminated between women using contraceptives and those who did not. Once again, modifying factors such as race and age played a direct role in predicting behaviors. Future research can be directed toward testing the theoretical linkages between variables of interest and concepts of the HPM.

Using the HPM, Serafine and Broom (1998) hypothesized that low-risk pregnant women who valued health, perceived the benefits of health-promoting activities, and perceived few barriers to health-promoting activities would be more likely to attend pregnancy-related education programs. Both the group that attended and the group that did not attend a class about premature birth prevention valued health. However, attendees perceived fewer barriers. Health locus of control did not predict attendance. Accordingly, Pender (1996) has indicated that locus of control does not always explain specific health behaviors.

To summarize, participation in health-promoting practices was determined by both modifying factors and cognitive-perceptual factors (Ali, 1996; Riffle, Yoho, & Sams, 1989; Speake, Cowart, & Pellet, 1989; Speake, Cowart, & Stephens, 1991; Riccio-Howe, 1991). However, almost every study found some notable exceptions to HPM concepts. The failure of cognitive and modifying factors to account significantly for differences commonly led researchers to conclude that unexpected, non-HPM predictors influence health promotion participation (Riffle, Yoho, & Sams, 1989; Speake, Cowart, & Pellet, 1989; Speake, Cowart, & Stephens, 1991). The relationship of illness to health promotion participation contradicted HPM concepts (Ahijevych & Bernhard, 1994). These studies collectively question the relationship of modifying factors to cognitive-perceptual factors and their direct or indirect relationship to the model.

Exercise. Five studies have specifically considered exercise as a health promotion activity. Bonheur and Young (1991) examined differences in self-esteem, perceived benefits of exercise, and exercise barriers for university students. Exercisers demonstrated higher self-esteem and perceived greater benefits and fewer barriers to exercise. These findings are congruent with the HPM. In a longitudinal study, Gillis and Perry (1991) compared differences in health-promoting behaviors and physical activity of middle-aged women by participation or nonparticipation in a structured exercise program. Unlike those of Bonheur and Young, the Gillis and Perry findings suggested that self-esteem did not significantly influence exercise participation over time. However, participating in a structured exercise program promoted greater participation in exercise and better stress management over time. Likewise, Pender's HPM predicts that self-efficacy, as a cognitive-perceptual variable, would promote exercise participation. The conflicting findings of these studies may suggest that multiple factors that influence health-promoting behavior and must be investigated further.

Comparing factors associated with exercise participation between white- and blue-collar workers, Desmond, Conrad, Montgomery, and Simon (1993) found the composite sum of all physical activity—comprised of work-related, sporting, and leisure activities—was associated with higher income and higher levels of self-efficacy. Higher levels of occupational activity were associated with higher income level. It should be noted that many blue-collar workers increased their base pay through overtime, which generated higher income. Workers with a higher perceived health status tended more often to participate in sports. Blue-collar workers participated in more leisure activities. Leisure activity participation was also associated with higher levels of self-efficacy. This study supports the HPM in that self-efficacy was associated with exercise. However, modifying factors such as income also demonstrated an influence.

Neuberger, Kasal, Smith, Hassanein, and DeViney (1994) investigated factors influencing exercise participation and aerobic fitness in outpatients with arthritis. The causal model predicted exercise participation but not aerobic fitness. Modifying factors such as age, education level, severity and duration of arthritis, and previous exercise influenced cognitive-perceptual factors of perceived health status, perceived benefits of exercise, and perceived barriers to exercise. In turn, these cognitive-perceptual factors explained 20% of exercise participation. This study demonstrated some support for the HPM; however, investigators indicated that the direct rather than indirect influence of modifying factors on health-promoting behaviors might account for a greater proportion of exercise variance.

Garcia, Broda, Frenn, Coviak, Pender, and Ronis (1995) investigated the influence of gender and developmental differences in exercise beliefs and prediction of exercise behaviors in youths enrolled in grades 5, 6, and 8. Researchers found that girls engaged in fewer leisure time activities than boys, reported poorer health status, and had poorer self-esteem. Male gender, fewer perceptions of barriers, and greater access by African-American youth to exercise facilities positively impacted exercise habits. Older youths were less likely than younger youths to report having support for exercise or exercise role models. This study indicates a need for and examination of direct and indirect variable influence on exercise in youths.

Studies of physical activity and health promotion result in a mixed picture of how modifying and cognitive factors influence participation. The studies by Bonheur and Young (1991) and Gillis and Perry (1991) exhibit conflicting findings. Modifying factors such as income (Desmond, Conrad, Montgomery, & Simon, 1993), age, education level, severity of illness (Garcia, Broda, Frenn, Coviak, Pender, & Ronis, 1995), and previous exercise demonstrated influence on physical activity levels.

Health-Promoting Interventions. A small number of studies focused on the influence of interventions aimed toward health-promoting practices. Richter, Malkiewicz, and Shaw (1987) compared nursing students engaged in three different educational programs on their participation in health-promoting activities six months after intervention. One group completed a health promotion course, one a clinical assessment with individualized consultation on health promotion activities, and the control group an adult health nursing course. An overall decrease in health-promoting behaviors occurred in all groups. The exercise score decreased most for the control and assessment groups. Heart rates also increased most in the control group. In this instance, the self-awareness Pender proposed as a health-promoting factor did not change behaviors when heavy course loads interfered with healthy activities.

Frenn, Borgeson, Lee, and Simandl (1989) qualitatively examined generation of lifestyle changes by patients participating in cardiac rehabilitation following an acute coronary event. Investigators discovered that enabling and disabling factors that promoted or prevented change were individualized. Repatterning was facilitated by changes in beliefs, attitudes, and plans. Two of the cognitive-perceptual factors that Pender theorized—health protection and health promotion—influenced both enabling and disabling lifestyle change. Pender's behavioral and situational variables, such as family, friends, and program influence, also were important in either generating or preventing lifestyle change.

Campbell and Kreidler (1994) also used a qualitative research approach to discover whether older persons who participated in structured health-promoting activities and follow-up home visits perceived themselves as more responsible for their health behaviors. They also examined whether older adults perceived themselves as well when they were able to function independently. The health-promoting interventions assumed that "wellness for older adults implied maintaining or improving the ability to function independently, despite disability or chronic illness, thus maintaining or improving quality of life" (p. 440). However, for older adults, mobility and freedom from pain were more associated with their perceptions of wellness than being able to function independently was. Older adults considered themselves healthy only if they were able to perform activities they perceived as worthwhile and were reasonably free of pain. In this sample most of the participants experienced at least one chronic illness and perceived themselves as unhealthy even when health providers perceived their wellness.

Campbell and Kreidler (1994) pointed out differences between their findings in a community outreach program and the HPM. Nurses who used the HPM considered patients to be well if they functioned independently, whereas patients considered themselves health if they were mobile and free from pain. Patients tended to leave responsibility for care to healthcare professionals rather than assume active roles. Chronic illnesses made patients feel unwell.

Intervention studies also produced mixed findings. Cognitive-perceptual variables such as health protection and health promotion influence exercise participation (Campbell & Kreidler, 1994; Frenn, Borgeson, Lee, & Simandl, 1989), but other factors, such as heavy work load, also play a role (Richter, Malkiewicz, & Shaw, 1987). Modifying factors such as chronic illness and mobility influenced participation in exercise as well (Campbell & Kreidler, 1994). The good news is that these interventions increased exercise participation; however, many other factors facilitated or diminished exercise participation.

Research Summary. In summary, tests of the HPM have yielded mixed support. In studies investigating the relationship of individual variables related to participation in health-promoting activities, only a portion of the variance has been explained (Duffy, 1988, 1989, 1993, 1997; Pender, Walker, Sechrist, & Frank-Stromborg, 1990). Multidimensional examinations of HPM concepts (Johnson, Ratner, Bottorff, & Hayduk, 1993; Ratner, Bottorff, Johnson, & Hayduk, 1994, 1996) generated little support for the HPM. These studies are criticized for incorporating only a limited number rather than all the cognitive-perceptual factor into the causal models. Moreover, measures selected to discern the cognitive-perceptual variables and health-promoting variables were somewhat constrained in the study by Johnson, Ratner, Bottorff, & Hayduk (1993) because the database did not permit specific instrument selection. Causal modeling studies by Lusk and others (1993, 1994, 1997, 1997) that used larger numbers of cognitive-perceptual factors proposed by the HPM yielded greater support for selected health promotion behavior participation, particularly when considered in light of Pender's modifications (1996) to the HPM. Revision of the HPM included identification of additional factors that directly influence engagement in health-promoting activities. These factors include activity-related affect, commitment to a plan of action, preferences, and immediate competing demand. The HPM has provided a useful way of thinking about motivation for participating in health promotion. Additional research should determine whether the model revisions adequately identify the predictors of individual health-promoting behaviors. Additional intervention research using the HPM as a basis is also needed.

PRAXIS AND THEORY UTILIZATION: DESIGNING NURSING PRACTICE PROGRAMS FROM THE PERSPECTIVE OF PENDER'S HEALTH PROMOTION MODEL

Pender's model has been used widely by researchers seeking to better understand health promotion and nursing's role in relation to the construct. This work has added significantly to the health promotion knowledge base and can help direct related nursing practice. Embedding this work in a major theoretical nursing perspective with explicit linkages would aid practitioners in incorporating health promotion into their total nursing practice. Pender's work is considered a middle-range theory, but practitioners might question exactly to what this middle refers.

The Variables of Concern for Practice

The variables of concern for practice are named in Figure 11-1. Much work remains to develop the substantive structure of these named concerns.

Describing a Population for Nursing Purposes

No references that describe populations using the HPM were found in the literature. The classification system for expressions of health (see Box 11-2) could form the basis for a population description.

Expected Outcomes of Nursing

The desired outcomes of nursing from the perspective of the HPM are commitment to a plan of action and health-promoting behavior.

Process Models

Pender proposes that the processes of nursing include assessment of health, health beliefs, and health behaviors; development of a health-protection-promotion plan; and modification of health-related lifestyle. These processes relate to individuals, families, and communities.

Assessment. Pender (1996) defines nursing assessment as "systematic collection of data about patient health status, beliefs, and behaviors relevant to developing a health-protection-promotion plan" (p. 116). These data form the basis for making decisions about strengths, problems, nursing diagnoses, desired outcomes, and interventions. A number of assessment tools are used and depend on a variety of patient characteristics, including cultural orientation and developmental stages. The goal of the assessment process is to identify health assets, lifestyle strengths, health-related beliefs, patients' at-risk beliefs and behaviors, and desired changes. The assessment tools selected are those deemed appropriate to the situation. A nurse using Pender's HPM presumably would make available to patients a collection of tools developed both by nurses and by other health-related professionals.

Since Pender views the family as the social structure in which health-related behaviors are learned, the family is also a unit of assessment. Pender suggests that individual and family assessments are interrelated. Family assessment includes both structural and functional components using a variety of tools that have been developed and reported in the literature of family-related disciplines. The nurse then chooses the most suitable tool to provide data for further decision making.

Community assessment is also an essential component of health assessment. This process includes collecting data to determine needs, opportunities, and resources for initiating community health action plans. Again, Pender suggests a number of instruments that can facilitate this data gathering. The time available and the purpose of the data determines the nature of the assessment.

Developing a Plan. Nurse and patients together identify the goals to be achieved and plans to accomplish these goals. Presumably, during the assessment process the nurse and the patient will develop a broadly based understanding of health stage and health behavior patterns, risk status, belief systems, and available options. Pender outlines nine steps that make up the health-planning process. These are summarized as follows (1996, p. 147):

1. Summarize data from the assessment
2. Reinforce the patient's strengths
3. Identify health goals and behavioral change options
4. Identify outcomes that will indicate goal achievement from the patient's perspective
5. Develop a behavior-change plan
6. Identify incentives for change
7. Consider environmental and interpersonal facilitators and barriers to change
8. Determine a time frame for implementing the plan
9. Commit to behavior change goals, including developing support needed to accomplish goals

Pender does not propose a comprehensive theoretical basis for these nine steps. Rather, these steps are derived from a variety of theoretical perspectives and use forms and procedures selected from a number of sources.

The Action Phase. In elaborating on the action phase, Pender again draws on a number of theoretical models and positions related to planned change. Behavioral change is patient-controlled and patient-directed. Nurses facilitate the change by providing a supportive climate, acting as a catalyst, assisting with various steps of the change process, and developing the patient's capacity for change. Specific strategies include consciousness raising, self-reevaluation, cognitive restructuring, reinforcement management, modeling, counterconditioning, and stimulus control.

Practice Models

Additional development is required before practice models can be described.

Implications for Administration

Health promotion is complex, and the literature associated with various aspects of health promotion is vast. Agencies that wish to adopt Pender's HPM must define for themselves health, health promotion, and motivation for health behavior so that they can select perspectives, data gathering tools, and strategies for change consistent with their conceptualizations.

Implications for Education

The HPM has been primarily a tool of research and, to a limited extent, practice. Bringing the HPM into a broader theoretical system would facilitate practical education and use.

STATUS OF THEORY DEVELOPMENT

The model will gain strength with the development of or linkage to philosophy, especially a philosophy of person. Pender focused her work on the definition of health and did not link it to any particular nursing theoretical system. She has recognized Orem's self-care conceptualizations, noting that "the nurse focusing on health promotion is primarily concerned with universal and developmental requisites, although health-deviation requisites . . . must be promptly attended to if they arise" (Pender, 1982, p. 99). She also articulates health promotion with Orem's "educative-developmental nursing system" (p. 100). In describing directions for research on self-care, Pender noted that Orem's theoretical work has been the driving force for empirical studies of the various dimensions of self-care and related nursing care systems. However, Pender does not attempt to integrate the two bodies of work. Pender does not cite the work of Orem and her colleagues in her conceptualizations (1990) about health and other dimensions of her work.

The HPM has great appeal to researchers and clinicians. The variables within the model are being tested empirically, and the outcomes of these studies have been used to modify the HPM. It would be helpful if the work on health promotion were developed in context of a general theory of nursing.

NEXUS

Health promotion has become an integral component of nursing practice. Much of the current thinking about health promotion has been influenced by Pender's model, which began emerging in the 1970s. To Pender's credit, the model has evolved through modifications based on research finding explicated in her most recent book (1996). Many descriptive studies exist, whereas few intervention studies have demonstrated the effectiveness of nursing interventions in promoting health activities. More theory-testing studies have been conducted for the HPM than for other theories. These studies have partially supported the HPM while also indicating the presence of other, still undiscovered factors that impact participation in health-promoting activities. Continued research needs to discern these factors. Further research also is needed to assess the efficacy of nursing interventions for health promotion.

REFERENCES

Ahijevych, K. & Bernhard, L. (1994). Health-promoting behaviors of African-American women. *Nursing Research, 43*(2), 86-89.

Ali, N. (1996). Predictors of osteoporosis prevention among college women. *American Journal of Health Behavior, 20*(6), 379-388.

Bonheur, B. & Young, S. (1991). Exercise as a health-promoting lifestyle choice. *Applied Nursing Research, 4*(1), 2-6.

Campbell, J. & Kreidler, M. (1994). Older adults' perceptions about wellness. *Journal of Holistic Nursing, 14*(4), 437-447.

Desmond, A., Conrad, K. Montgomery, A. & Simon, K. (1993). Factors associated with male workers' engagement in physical activity: White collar vs. blue-collar workers. *AAOHN Journal, 41*(2), 73-83.

Duffy, M. (1988). Determinants of health promotion in midlife women. *Nursing Research, 37*(6), 358-362.

Duffy, M. (1989). Determinants of health status in employed women. *Health Values, 13*(2), 50-57.

Duffy, M. (1993). Determinants of health-promoting lifestyles in older persons. *Image, 25*(1), 23-28.

Duffy, M. (1997). Determinants of reported health promotion behaviors in employed Mexican-American women. *Healthcare for Women International, 18*(2), 149-163.

Felton, G. (1996). Female adolescent contraceptive use or nonuse at first and most recent coitus. *Public Health Nursing, 13*(3), 223-230.

Fleetwood, J. & Packa, D. (1991). Determinants of health-promoting behaviors in adults. *Journal of Cardiovascular Nursing, 5*(2), 67-79.

Foster, M. (1992). Health promotion and life satisfaction in elderly Black adults. *Western Journal of Nursing Research, 14*(4), 444-463.

Frank-Stromborg, M., Pender, N., Walker, S., & Sechrist, K. (1990). Determinants of health-promoting lifestyle in ambulatory cancer patients. *Social Science Medicine, 31*(10), 1159-1168.

Frenn, M., Borgeson, D., Lee, H., & Simandl, G. (1989). Lifestyle changes in a cardiac rehabilitation program: The client perspective. *Journal of Cardiovascular Nursing, 3*(2), 43-55.

Garcia, A., Broda, M., Frenn, M., Coviak, C., Pender, N. & Ronis, D. (1995). Gender and developmental differences in exercise beliefs among youth and prediction of their exercise behavior. *Journal of School Health, 65*(6), 213-219.

Gillis, A. & Perry, A. (1991). The relationships between physical activity and health-promoting behaviors in midlife women. *Journal of Advanced Nursing, 16,* 299-310.

Gillis, A. (1994). Determinants of health-promoting lifestyles in adolescent females. *Canadian Journal of Nursing Research, 26*(2), 13-27.

Haddad, L., Al-Ma'aitah, R., Cameron, S., & Armstrong-Stassen, M. (1998). An Arabic language version of the health promotion lifestyle profile. *Public Health Nursing, 15*(2), 74-81.

Johnson, J., Ratner, P., Bottorff, J., & Hayduk, L. (1993). An exploration of Pender's health promotion model using LISREL. *Nursing Research, 43*(3), 132-138.

Kerr, M. & Ritchey, D. (1990). Health-promoting lifestyles of English-speaking and Spanish-speaking Mexican-American migrant farm workers. *Public Health Nursing, 7*(2), 80-87.

Kuster, A. & Fong, C. (1993). Further psychometric evaluation of the Spanish language health-promoting lifestyle profile. *Nursing Research, 42*(5), 266-269.

Lusk, S. & Kelemen, M. (1993). Predicting the use of hearing protection: A preliminary study. *Public Health Nursing, 10*(3), 189-196.

Lusk, S., Ronis, D., Kerr, M., & Atwood, J. (1994). Test of the health promotion model as a causal model of workers' use of hearing protection. *Nursing Research, 43*(3), 151-157.

Lusk, S., Ronis, D., & Baer, L. (1997). Gender differences in blue-collar workers' use of hearing protection. *Women & Health, 25*(4), 69-89.

Lusk, S., Ronis, D., & Hogan, M. (1997). Test of the health promotion model as a causal model of construction workers' use of hearing protection. *Research in Nursing and Health, 20*(3), 183-194.

Neuberger, G., Kasal, S., Smith, K., Hassanein, R, & DeViney, S. (1994). Determinants of exercise and aerobic fitness in outpatients with arthritis. *Nursing Research, 43*(1), 11-17.

Pender, N.J. (1982). *Health promotion in nursing practice.* Norwalk, CT: Appleton-Century-Crofts.

Pender, N.J. (1987). *Health promotion in nursing practice.* (2nd ed.). Norwalk, CT: Appleton-Century-Crofts.

Pender, N.J. (1990). Expressing health through lifestyle patterns. *Nursing Science Quarterly, 3*(3), 115-122.

Pender, N.J. (1996). *Health promotion in nursing practice*. (3rd ed.). Stamford, CT: Appleton & Lange.

Pender, N.J., Walker, S.N., Sechrist, K.R., & Frank-Stromborg, M. (1990). Predicting health-promoting lifestyles in the workplace. *Nursing Research, 39*(6), 326-332.

Ratner, P., Bottorff, J., Johnson, J. & Hayduk, L. (1994). The interaction effects of gender within the health promotion model. *Research in Nursing and Health, 17*(5), 341-350.

Ratner, P., Borrorff, J., Johnson, J., & Hayduk, L. (1996). Using multiple indicators to test the dimensionality of concepts in the health promotion model. *Research in Nursing and Health, 19*(3), 237-247.

Riccio-Howe, L. (1991). Health values, locus of control, and cues to action as predictors of adolescent safety belt use. *Journal of Adolescent Health, 12*(3), 256-262.

Richter, J., Malkiewicz, J., & Shaw, D. (1987). Health promotion behaviors in nursing students. *Journal of Nursing Education, 26*(9), 367-371.

Riffle, K., Yoho, J., & Sams, J. (1989). Health-promoting behaviors, perceived social support, and self-reported health of Appalachian elderly. *Public Health Nursing, 6*(4), 204-211.

Sechrist, K., Walker, S., & Pender, N. (1987). Development and psychometric evaluation of the exercise benefits/barriers scale. *Research in Nursing and Health, 10*(6), 357-365.

Serafine, M. & Broom, B. (1998). Predicting low-risk pregnant women's attendance at a preterm birth prevention class. *Journal of Obstetric, Gynecologic, and Neonatal Nursing, 27*(3), 279-287.

Speake, D., Cowart, M., & Pellet, K. (1989). Health perceptions and lifestyles of the elderly. *Research in Nursing and Health, 12*(2), 93-100.

Speake, D., Cowart, M., & Stephens, R. (1991). Healthy lifestyle practices of rural and urban elderly. *Health Values, 15*(1), 45-51.

Stuifbergen, A. & Becker, H. (1994). Predictors of health-promoting lifestyles in persons with disabilities. *Research in Nursing and Health, 17*(1), 3-13.

Telleen, T. (1993). Health promotion practices of pregnant and nonpregnant women. *Journal of Holistic Nursing, 11*(3), 237-245.

Walker, S., Sechrist, K., & Pender, N. (1987). The health-promoting lifestyle profile: Development and psychometric characteristics. *Nursing Research, 36*(2), 76-81.

Walker, S., Kerr, M., Pender, N., & Sechrist, K. (1990). A Spanish language version of the health-promoting lifestyle profile. *Nursing Research, 39*(5), 268-273.

Walker, S. & Hill-Polerecky, D. (1999). Psychometric evaluation of the health-promoting lifestyle profile II. Unpublished abstract.

Weitzel, M. (1989). A test of the health promotion model with blue-collar workers. *Nursing Research, 38*(2), 99-104.

CHAPTER 12

Modeling Nursing From the Perspective of Human Relations

PEPLAU'S THEORY of INTERPERSONAL RELATIONS

Key Terms

dimensions of relations, p. 348
nurse-patient relationship, p. 346
psychodynamic nursing, p. 346

Asked what motivated her to develop the Theory of Interpersonal Relations, Peplau responded:

> After my service in the Army Nurse Corps during World War II, it occurred to me that I knew things that would be worth knowing by other nurses. So I wrote the book [*Interpersonal Relations in Nursing,* 1952]. The book was very controversial at the time—publishers said no nurse should write such a book. Finally, Putnam published it, but they were very apprehensive. It was well received. It has never been revised. I think it was way ahead of its time. I have never really promoted my work. I never thought of myself nor spoke of myself as a theorist. My background in psychology included theory. I just wrote what I knew (personal communication, October 7, 1997).

The Theory of Interpersonal Relations (TIPR) is used primarily in psychoanalysis and psychotherapy. Some forms of nurse therapy, particularly in the practices of clinical specialists in psychiatric mental health nursing also have used the TIPR (Peplau, 1997).

THE STARTING POINT OF MODELING NURSING

Peplau (1992) identified the work of psychiatrist and psychoanalyst Harry Stack Sullivan as her starting point. Sullivan (1953) was noted for his Theory of Interpersonal Relations, which includes the impact of cultural forces on personality development. For example, Peplau uses Sullivan's modes of experiencing as one of her interpersonal constructs. Peplau advocated using knowledge from other disciplines and viewing nursing as applied science (1969). Her main interest was to derive constructs from clinical data and from other sciences to identify their congruence with nursing practice.

Peplau's work assumes the following (Peplau, 1952, p. xii):

1. The kind of person the nurse becomes make a substantial difference in what each patient will learn as he receives nursing care.
2. Fostering personality development toward maturity is a function of nursing and nursing education. Nursing uses principles and methods to guide the process toward resolution of interpersonal problems.

A third assumption, identified as "implicit," is "the nursing profession has legal responsibility for the effective use of nursing and for its consequences to patients" (Howk, Brophy, Carey, Noll, Rasmussen, Searcy, & Stark, 1998, p. 339).

Reason for Theory Development

The initial and continuing motivation for Peplau's work is improving nursing care, especially at the level of the nurse-patient interaction. She believed that interpersonal relationships belong at the center of the basic nursing curriculum (1952). Her work was meant to provide a conceptual framework basic to psychodynamic nursing. As noted earlier, Peplau wrote her 1952 book because she believed that she had something to share with nurses. She later clarified and applied the concepts but never revised the basic models or theory.

Phenomenon of Concern

Peplau was concerned with one aspect of nursing—how persons relate to one another. In Peplau's view, the center of nursing is the **nurse-patient relationship.** Therefore the concepts contained within her TIPR primarily explain the personal behavior of the nurse and patient in nursing situations and the psychosocial phenomena surrounding that behavior. Peplau believed that human behavior is characterized by purpose and goal seeking. Human needs are instinctual or acquired in the process of socialization. These needs drive human behavior toward purposeful goals.

DESCRIPTION OF PEPLAU'S THEORETICAL SYSTEM
Philosophical Perspectives

Peplau believed that nursing is both an art and a science. The art is in the use of self to enable, empower, and transform—that is, to produce favorable changes within patients. The self of the nurse is the primary instrument in psychodynamic nursing. The science explains and addresses the universals, the commonalities in patterns, and problems of humans as a group. She referred to this active, creative use of self for the good of the patient as **psychodynamic nursing.**

The TIPR concepts frame understanding of many of the dilemmas that patients experience within the domain of professional nursing practice. Peplau considered the domain of nursing practice congruent with the ANA definition, which identifies it as "the diagnosis and treatment of human responses to actual and potential health problems" (1994, pp. 6-8). The primarily subjective art of nursing seeks knowledge of the unique and highly personal variations of patterns of difficulty and behavior of individuals in their responses to actual and potential health problems. Nursing art illuminates the scientific understanding of the problem. Nursing science attempts to empirically explain and address the patterns of difficulty and problems in human behavior. Peplau often commented that nurses need to increase their understanding of a broad range of human problems and use both the art and science of nursing to understand the options available for practice. Peplau and others identified many concepts and constructs within the scope of the theory. Examples of this are seen in Figure 12-1 and Figure 12-2. Peplau referred to the TIPR as a body of knowledge and a source of theory (1997); however, she offered no general model or statement of the theory.

Description of Model and Theory

The main elements in a nurse-patient relationship are two persons, professional expertise, and patient need. The relationship is time-limited and therefore has starting and ending points that necessitate three phases: orientation, working, and resolution. The concepts of interpersonal relations explain psychosocial phenomena and the personal behavior of the nurse and patient in nursing situations. Three diagrams illustrate the framework of concepts. Figure 12-3 shows the changing aspects of nurse-patient relations. The overlapping phases in nurse-patient relationships are shown in Figure 12-4, and the phases and changing roles in nurse-patient relationships are presented in Figure 12-5. Peplau's most recent work did not include models *per se*, but she called the TIPR a useful theoretical framework (1992, 1997).

The use of self by the nurse in conjunction with the patient efforts produces the desired effects of developing personality and meeting human needs. Peplau was firm in her belief that, overall, much of nurses' work occurs during interaction with patients (1997). The nurse's roles were multiple and included that of stranger, resource person, teacher, leader, surrogate, counselor, consultant, tutor, safety agent, mediator, administrator, recorder, observer, and researcher. Peplau (1992) noted that the scope of theoretical constructs required for the practice of nursing is more comprehensive than she has presented. Peplau (1952) originally described four phases of the nurse-patient relationship—orientation, identification, exploitation, and resolution. Forchuk (1991) redefined these phases as orientation, working, and resolution. Peplau (1952) described the following concepts in her initial work:

- Instinctual and acquired human needs
- Energy and energy transformation
- Psychological experiences, such as frustration, conflict, anxiety, goals, and opposing goals
- Psychological tasks, such as learning to count on others, learning to delay satisfaction, identifying oneself, and developing skills in participation
- The interlocking operations of the nursing process: observation, communication, and recording

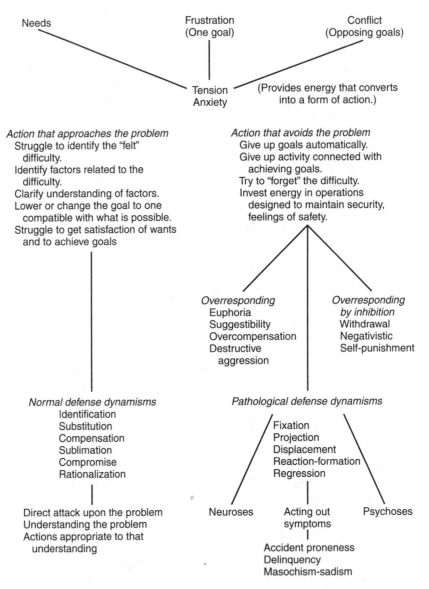

FIGURE 12-1 Transformation of energy into behavior. (From Peplau, H.E. (1991). *Interpersonal relations in nursing.* New York: Springer Publishing Company.)

Five **dimensions of relations** were added to Peplau's conceptualizations in 1992. These give a broader perspective to interpersonal relations and recognize many types of relations for many different purposes. These dimensions are the following (Peplau, 1992, p. 15):

- Their nature (named patterns or themes and variations)
- Their origin (history)

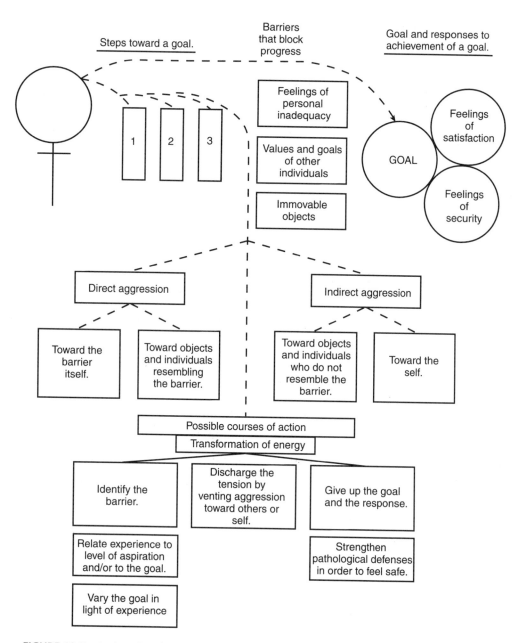

FIGURE 12-2 Actions involved in frustration. (From Peplau, H.E. (1991). *Interpersonal relations in nursing.* New York: Springer Publishing Company.)

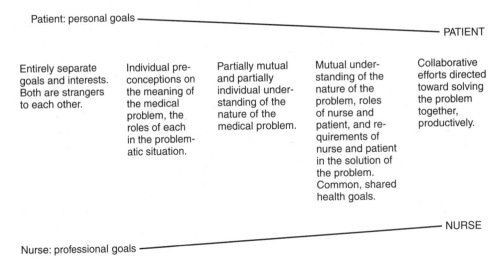

FIGURE 12-3   A continuum showing changing aspects of nurse-patient relations. (From Peplau, H.E. (1991). *Interpersonal relations in nursing.* New York: Springer Publishing Company.)

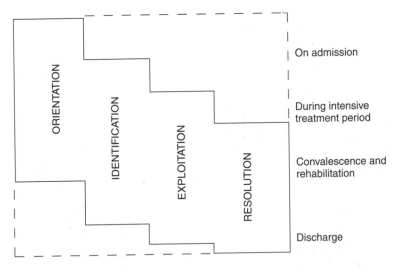

FIGURE 12-4   Overlapping phases in nurse-patient relationships. (From Peplau, H.E. (1991). *Interpersonal relations in nursing.* New York: Springer Publishing Company.)

- Their function (intent, motive, aim, goal, or purpose)
- Their mode (form, style)
- Their integrations (linkages with other persons' behavior).

In one way or another, interpersonal relations are a part of all nursing theoretical systems. Peplau's work was seminal and remains an important component of conceptualizations about nursing practice.

Nurse:	Stranger	Unconditional Mother Surrogate		Counselor Resource person Leadership Surrogate: Mother Sibling	Adult person
Patient:	Stranger	Infant	Child	Adolescent	Adult person
Phases in Nursing Relationship:	Orientation – – – – – – – – – – – Identification – – – – – – – – – – –				
	Exploitation – – – – – – – – – – –				
	– Resolution				

FIGURE 12-5　Phases and changing roles in nurse-patient relationships. (From Peplau, H.E. (1991). *Interpersonal relations in nursing.* New York: Springer Publishing Company.)

RESEARCH DERIVED FROM PEPLAU'S THEORY OF INTERPERSONAL RELATIONS

Discovery using the TIPR is a dynamic process in which both the nurse and the patient must be understood. Reality consists of individual conceptions that are contextual in nature and potentially conflict. The TIPR has guided qualitative research methods, such as observation and interviews. Quantitative research that uses selected measuring instruments such as those described in the following discussion also has been completed.

Research Instruments

Four research instruments have been developed to measure aspects of interpersonal relationships suggested by Peplau's theory, including the Social Interaction Inventory, a therapeutic behavior scale, the Empathy Construct Rating Scale, and the Relationship Form (Table 12-1). The earliest instrument development began in 1962, and the final instrument was developed in 1989, when Peplau's theory resurged in popularity. These instruments are explained in the following sections.

Social Interaction Inventory. Methven and Schlotfeldt (1962) designed the Social Interaction Inventory to determine the nature of the verbal responses that nurses use in emotionally laden situations. Investigators developed the inventory by observing and describing stressful occurrences in hospital situations. Nursing students and registered nurses generated potential responses to the described situations. The Social Interaction Inventory was derived from these situations and responses. The final format contained 30 situations that represented problems nurses encountered. Five types of replies are presented for each situation and are as follows:

- If the patient experiences an unmet need, the nurse conveys concern.
- If the patient experiences a problem, the nurse conveys sympathy and reassurance.
- If the patient experiences a problem, the nurse conveys an intent to investigate the problem.
- A patient expresses a need, but the nurse does not encourage him or her to verbalize it.
- A patient expresses a need, but the nurse rejects or denounces it.

TABLE 12-1

Research Instruments Using Peplau's Theory of Interpersonal Relations

Instrument/Description	Study/Year	Reliability and Validity
Social Interaction Inventory 30 items with five communication responses for each item	Methven and Scholtfeldt, 1962	Following development, the instrument was tested with 236 nurses: senior students ($n = 70$), graduate BS nurses ($n = 30$), graduate nurses with 2 years of college ($n = 15$), graduate nurses with 1 year of college ($n = 60$), and graduate diploma nurses ($n = 61$). The Social Interaction Inventory differentiated between the five groups in the hypothesized direction. Nurses with the most psychiatric training integrated throughout the curriculum selected the greatest number of therapeutic responses.
Therapeutic Behavior Scale 5-category rating scale	Spring and Turk, 1962	Instrument testing was completed with 24 nursing students and four staff nurses. Intrarater reliability had 95% agreement, and interrater reliability scores ranged form 89% to 100%. Internal consistency, as measured by Spearman Brown split-half coefficient, was 0.91. Construct validity was assessed by a known groups technique, in which practicing nurses received significantly higher therapeutic behavior scores than students ($t = 1.874$, $p < 0.05$). Correlation of therapeutic behavior scores with outside judges' ratings yielded correlations ranging from 0.42 to 0.59 ($p < 0.01$). Product-moment correlation between behavior scores and instructor rating was 0.58 ($p < 0.01$).

Empathy Construct Rating Scale (ECRS) 100-item, 6-point Likert scale	LaMonica, 1981	Students generated initial items, which an expert panel then evaluated for content validity. Additional items were added to the pool based on expert judgment. The final instrument had five subscales that consisted of 100 items: 46 representing lack of empathy and 54 representing well-developed empathy. Reliability was established for most (Form A) and least empathetic persons (Form B). Students ($\underline{N} = 103$) completed the ECRS. Coefficient alpha for Form A = 0.97 and for B = 0.98. Split-half reliability using Spearman Brown correction for Form A was $\underline{r} = 0.89$ and for Form B = 0.96. Multitrait-multimethod validity was established with Carkhuff's Index of Communication, California Psychological Inventory, Human-Heartedness Questionnaire, Chapin Social Insight Test, Philosophy of Human Nature, Vocabulary Test-GT, and Tennessee Self-Concept Scale. Instrument packets were completed by 300 registered nurses and nursing students, each of whom identified a peer and a patient who subsequently completed questionnaire packets (Total $\underline{N} = 900$). Principal components factor analysis with varimax rotation was used to analyze responses to all instruments. A 6-factor solution in which empathy subscales composed the initial factor emerged. Empathy, accounting for 48% of variance, did not share variance with any of the other derived factors. Subsequent principal component analysis of ECRS using subject, peer, and patient responses revealed two factors—Well-Developed Empathy and Lack of Empathy. The multitrait-multimethod matrix demonstrated discriminant validity between Empathy-self and Empathy-client.
Relationship Form One-page form delineating phases of nurse-patient relationship	Forchuk and Brown, 1989	Content validity was established through review by three mental health clinical nurse specialists and was reviewed by Peplau. Interrater reliability was established through clinician and CNS review of 32 randomly selected records and through rating the relationship phase of each record. With a 7-point rating scale, there was a 91% agreement within 1 point of each rating. Perfect agreement occurred 41% of the time and had a Kappa of 0.41.

Developers perceived that the first response of awareness and conveying concern is the most effective. The subsequent responses limit interaction. Scoring is accomplished by coding the type of response selected from the five options. Individual scores are then calculated to indicate the number of times each type of response was selected. Scores can range from 0 to 30 for each response type. Each participant has five scores.

Validity was established by using known groups technique in which investigators tested their predictions about how the groups would respond to the Social Interaction Inventory. Students, who were more informed about psychiatric nursing techniques than graduate nurses were, selected the greatest number of therapeutic responses. Methven and Schlotfeldt concluded that the Social Interaction Inventory could usefully evaluate verbal communication skills of students and practitioners. Despite the relatively early development of this inventory, only limited research measuring social interactions followed it.

Therapeutic Behavior Scale. The therapeutic behavior scale created by Spring and Turk (1962) was originally a 6-category scale designed to score observations of verbal interactions between psychiatric nurses and patients. The six categories included approach to patient, level at which interaction is responded to, topic, focus on patient versus therapist, consistency, and sentence structure. Testing found that five of the six of the categories—all but the sentence structure category—fit into a unidimensional scale. Scoring was accomplished by breaking the interaction into individual verbal units and rating each verbal unit as therapeutic (scored as a 1) or nontherapeutic (scored as 0) in each of the five categories. Each verbal unit could receive a score of 0 to 5. The ratings of individual verbal units were totaled and a mean score (the therapeutic behavior score) was derived. Intrarater, interrater, and internal consistency reliability were strong. Validity testing demonstrated that the five categories of the behavior scale were unidimensional and could yield a single therapeutic behavior score. Comparisons with outside judges and with instructor evaluations were within acceptable limits to establish validity. Again, this scale was developed at a time when nursing research was in its early stages. This instrument has subsequently experienced relatively little use.

Empathy Construct Rating Scale. LaMonica (1981) created the Empathy Construct Rating Scale (ECRS) to measure empathy through the use of positive and negative statements on the topic. The ECRS is a 100-item, 6-point Likert scale with item scores ranging from -3 to $+3$. To score it, investigators reverse the scores on negative scales and then add all items. Total scale scores range from -300 (lack of empathy) to $+300$ (well-developed empathy). Reliability and validity were well-established (see Table 12-1). Findings suggested that empathy existed as a whole entity that could not be further divided into subscales.

Relationship Form. Forchuk and Brown (1989) developed the Relationship Form to measure phases of the nurse-patient relationship as described by Peplau's theory. The 1-page format includes a brief summary of each phase and presents a pictorial guide to assist in monitoring the relationship. Initial content validity was established. Perfect-agreement interrater reliability was only 41% but rose to 91% when scores within one point of one another were included. The instrument was clinically useful in assessing nurse-patient relationships. Although initial measures of reliability and validity are adequate, further refinement is needed.

Review of Related Research

Research using Peplau's model began during the early 1960s, a time when using research to establish nursing practice was a relatively innovative idea. Early studies provided mixed findings of support for tenets of the TIPR. It is interesting to note that research efforts about interpersonal relationships in both psychiatric and nonpsychiatric patients and work roles are still guided by Peplau's conceptualizations. However, many of these conceptualizations have not been systematically investigated. This review will focus on recent, published research, beginning with the most cohesive program—Forchuk's examinations (1992, 1994, 1995a, 1995b, 1998) of nurse-patient relationships. Following nurse-patient relationships, the chapter will describe studies of depression, work roles, and medication compliance. Table 12-2 summarizes these studies.

Nurse-Patient Relationships. Studies on nurse-patient relationships encompass the work of Forchuk and that of others studying therapeutic relationships. Nurse-patient relationships have also been studied in nonpsychiatric patients (Vogelsang, 1990) and in patients with dementia (Middleton, Steward, & Richardson, 1999) or Alzheimer's disease (Williams & Tappen, 1999). Following development of the Relationship Form, Forchuk's initial work (1992) began by examining the length of the orientation phase of the nurse-patient relationship. Because Peplau established that the orientation phase represented the first stage of therapeutic work, Forchuk examined the factors influencing the time it took to establish trust, identify the roles of nurse and patient, and pinpoint relationship problems to improve. Number and length of hospitalizations factored in the length of the orientation process. Patients with the longest orientation phase had more and longer periods of hospitalization. Some patients who had moved to a working phase reverted to an orientation phase when a change of staff or worsening of psychiatric illnesses occurred.

In the next phase of research, Forchuk (1994) tested an aspect of the TIPR concerned with the orientation phase of nurse-patient relationships. Peplau proposed that characteristics of both the patient and the nurse influenced evolving therapeutic relationships. The nurse's positive preconceptions of the patient and the patient's positive preconceptions of the nurse facilitated development of therapeutic relationships and tended to shorten the orientation phase. Preconceptions developed early in the relationship and did not change substantially over the 6-month study. Other interpersonal relationships for patients influenced progress of therapeutic relationships. Anxiety on the part of the nurse or the patient did not significantly influence the therapeutic relationship. Combined nurse and patient variables influenced perceptions of evolving nurse-patient relationships. This study partially supported Peplau's proposal that certain factors influence development of therapeutic relationships. However, anxiety and the presence of other relationships may not influence formation of therapeutic relationships to the degree Peplau suggested.

In subsequent secondary analyses of the original prospective study, Forchuk (1995a, 1995b) examined factors influencing the progress of therapeutic relationships and uniqueness within nurse-patient relationships. Patients with previous lengthier hospital stays tended to spend more time in the orientation phase. Shorter orientation periods were associated with longer meetings and a greater total time per month spent in meetings. Progress in therapeutic relationships occurred more quickly when nurses were older and had more nursing experience, particularly in psychiatric nursing. More meeting time per

Text continued on p. 363

TABLE 12-2

Selected Research Studies Using Peplau's Framework

Study/Year	Purpose	Methods	Findings
NURSE-PATIENT RELATIONSHIPS			
Forchuk, 1992	This retrospective record review examined the length of orientation phase of patients and nurses in a community mental health program.	Seventy-three patient charts were reviewed and rated by an investigator using the Relationship Form. Most common diagnoses included schizophrenia and depression.	Fifteen patients were still in the orientation phase after 1 year. The length of orientation ranged from 1 to 23 months, with an average of 5.9 months. The number and length of psychiatric hospitalizations was significant in determining the length of the orientation phase. Thirty patients reverted from the working phase to the orientation phase with a change of staff or worsening psychiatric illness.
Forchuk, 1994	The study tested Peplau's theory of influences during the orientation phase of the nurse-patient relationship.	A prospective, longitudinal design was used to identify factors related to the development of therapeutic nurse-patient relationships. Independent variables of preconceptions, interpersonal relationships, and anxiety, and dependent variables of development of therapeutic relationship were measured at initiation, at 3 months, and at 6 months. One hundred twenty-four nurse-patient dyads began the study. Fifty-seven remained at 3 months, and 38 remained at 6 months.	Fifty-one of 94 nurse-patient dyads completed orientation. Thirty others discontinued the relationship while still in orientation, and 13 remained in orientation after 6 months. Preconceptions of both the nurse and the patient most were significantly related to the development of therapeutic relationship ($r = 0.37$ patient and 0.31 nurse, $p < 0.05$). Combined nurse and patient variables explained over 60% of the variance in perceptions of the evolving therapeutic relationship.

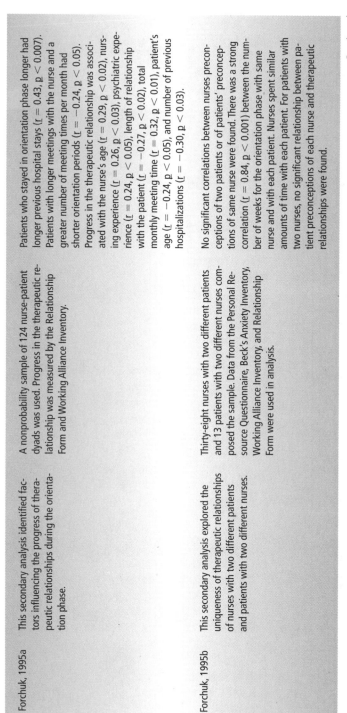

| Forchuk, 1995a | This secondary analysis identified factors influencing the progress of therapeutic relationships during the orientation phase. | A nonprobability sample of 124 nurse-patient dyads was used. Progress in the therapeutic relationship was measured by the Relationship Form and Working Alliance Inventory. | Patients who stayed in orientation phase longer had longer previous hospital stays ($r = 0.43$, $p < 0.007$). Patients with longer meetings with the nurse and a greater number of meeting times per month had shorter orientation periods ($r = -0.24$, $p < 0.05$). Progress in the therapeutic relationship was associated with the nurse's age ($r = 0.29$, $p < 0.02$), nursing experience ($r = 0.26$, $p < 0.03$), psychiatric experience ($r = 0.24$, $p < 0.05$), length of relationship with the patient ($r = -0.27$, $p < 0.02$), total monthly meeting time ($r = 0.32$, $p < 0.01$), patient's age ($r = -0.24$, $p < 0.05$), and number of previous hospitalizations ($r = -0.30$, $p < 0.03$). |
| Forchuk, 1995b | This secondary analysis explored the uniqueness of therapeutic relationships of nurses with two different patients and patients with two different nurses. | Thirty-eight nurses with two different patients and 13 patients with two different nurses composed the sample. Data from the Personal Resource Questionnaire, Beck's Anxiety Inventory, Working Alliance Inventory, and Relationship Form were used in analysis. | No significant correlations between nurses preconceptions of two patients or of patients' preconceptions of same nurse were found. There was a strong correlation ($r = 0.84$, $p < 0.001$) between the number of weeks for the orientation phase with same nurse and with each patient. Nurses spent similar amounts of time with each patient. For patients with two nurses, no significant relationship between patient preconceptions of each nurse and therapeutic relationships were found. |

Continued

TABLE 12-2

Selected Research Studies Using Peplau's Framework—cont'd

Study/Year	Purpose	Methods	Findings
NURSE-PATIENT RELATIONSHIPS—cont'd			
Forchuk, Westwell, Martin, Azzapardi, Kosterewa-Tolman, and Hux, 1998	This qualitative study identified factors that influence movement from the orientation phase to the working phase of therapeutic relationships in tertiary psychiatric settings.	Unstructured interviews were conducted with 10 newly formed nurse-patient dyads. Patients were interviewed two to nine times. The dyad was considered to have moved out of orientation to working phase based on agreement of patient, nurse, and clinical specialist. Audio-taped interviews were transcribed and analyzed.	Factors that facilitated movement from the orientation to working phase included planned therapeutic interaction meetings (able to talk and be listened to, able to be with same nurse), events outside of formal meetings (nurse follow-through with planned actions), and attitudes of the nurses (friendly, trusting, interested, genuine). Hampering factors included lack of availability of nurse, sense of distance and/or inequity, differences in realities and values of nurses and patients, and mutual withdrawal in relationships that were not progressing. In progressing relationships, the nurse was viewed as close, genuine, trusting, friendly, and sociable. The nurse was not viewed as a friend. In extended orientation relationships, there was mutual avoidance, not talking, and not listening. Nurses were not perceived as real persons.
Middleton, Steward, and Richardson, 1999	The study investigated the perceptions of formal caregivers on special care dementia units compared to traditional long-term care units.	Thirty-nine special care staff (SC) and 38 traditional (T) unit staff responded to a questionnaire regarding caregiving relationships, disruptive behavior, job characteristics, and job satisfaction.	SC staff experienced more disruptive behavior exposure ($M = 79.87$, $SD = 23.57$) than T staff ($M = 62.89$, $SD = 28.07$; $p < 0.05$) but exhibited less distress over the disruptive events (SC = $M = 46.30$, $SD = 15.96$) ($M = 54.03$, $SD = 14.48$; $p < 0.005$).

Vogelsang, 1990	This intervention study examined the impact of ambulatory surgery patients' continued contact with a familiar nurse form before admission to discharge.	A convenience sample of 40 women—20 in experimental and 20 in control groups—participated. The experimental group received contact from same nurse before admission, at postoperative awakening, and at discharge from the postanesthesia care unit. Interviews were conducted 3 to 5 days after discharge.	Contact group members reported greater readiness to return home (t = 3.75, p < 0.005). Seventy-five percent were ready to be discharged, compared to 45% of the control group. The contact group also reported greater satisfaction with nursing care (t = 3.1, p < 0.01); 80% believed that care was excellent, compared to 40% of the control group.
Williams and Tappen, 1999	The study examined the feasibility of developing a therapeutic relationship with patient with moderate- to late-stage Alzheimer's Disease (AD).	Researchers analyzed the transcripts of 42 residents' sessions conducted by 4 advanced practice nurses (APNs). APNs met with participants 3 times per week for 16 weeks. Recording occurred during the first, eighth, and sixteenth weeks.	During the orientation phase, patients verbalized trust and distrust. During the working-identification phase, patients verbalized emotion, feeling, satisfaction and enjoyment of interaction, and affection for the nurse. During the working-exploitation phase, patients described specific emotional events and desired continued relationships with nurses. During the resolution-titling phase, patients expressed sadness at ending the relationship.

Continued

TABLE 12-2

Selected Research Studies Using Peplau's Framework—cont'd

Study/Year	Purpose	Methods	Findings
DEPRESSION Beeber and Caldwell, 1996	The study examined clinical data from a pilot intervention program to identify pattern integrations in reciprocal interactions between nurse and patients experiencing depression.	Data were gathered from the clinical interactions of the investigators with six women over four months. Each woman participated in four to 15 intervention sessions. Through collaborative relationships with two primary care providers, patients were referred to two psychiatric mental health clinical specialists for assessment and intervention. Intervention consisted of interpersonal relationships in which other strategies such as health practices, cognitive interventions, and social network changes—were used. Analysis was derived from 42 hours of taped intervention sessions.	Clusters of behaviors constituting patterns for patients were identified and paired with nurse responses. Consistent core elements were reviewed to discover the nature of reciprocity between the nurse and patient. The most commonly observed pattern integration was "helpless persons and helper nurse," a complementary form of interaction. Patients perceived that they were unable to solve own problems and therefore relied on the nurse. Mutual patterns were demonstrated by helper-helper roles, in which the nurse directed the patient to do certain things and the patient was helpful in return. The alternating form of pursuer-distancer was embodied by either the patient or nurse alternating pursuit or maintaining distance in relationships or therapeutic issues. Antagonistic patterns occurred in poor fits between patient and nurse. The patient portrayed herself as cold, rejecting, and critical, while the nurse remained engaged in the relationship, even when the patient denied the value of therapeutic work.

Beeber and Charlie, 1998	This study evaluated a primary care intervention measure for its ability to decrease depressive symptoms.	Thirty-three women with depression participated in eight therapeutic sessions based on the TIPR. Before and after intervention, they responded to the Beck Depression Inventory, Describe Yourself Inventory (self-esteem), and Tilden's Interpersonal Relationship Inventory. Intervention consisted of assessment (thoughts, feelings, actions, and body), development of a problem statement and targeted outcomes, contract agreement, and sessions with a psychiatric mental health advanced practice nurse.	Depression was significantly reduced (BDI $M = 23.3$; $SD = 9.32$; Post $M = 7.03$; $SD = 6.23$; $t = 8.76$, $df = 29$, $p = 0.000$). Increases in efficacy and self-esteem were not significant. No difference in social self-esteem was found. Satisfaction with interpersonal relations also increased, but it did not increase significantly.
WORK ROLE			
Morrison, Shealy, Kowalski, LaMont, and Range, 1996	The study operationalized Peplau's work roles of psychiatric staff nurses.	One-to-one interactions of 30 psychiatric staff nurses with 62 patients were taped. Tapes were transcribed, and content was analyzed to identify role behaviors, describe work roles, and compare work roles with Peplau's conceptualized roles.	Primary work roles on the adult unit most often included counselor, resource person, and surrogate. On the adolescent unit primary roles included counselor, surrogate, resource person, and friend.
MEDICATION COMPLIANCE			
Lund and Frank, 1991	This descriptive study compared nurses' and patients' perceptions about medication compliance and reasons for noncompliance.	The sample consisted of 25 adult psychiatric patients and 25 registered nurses who completed an investigator-developed medication compliance questionnaire.	Compliance ratings by nurses and patients were similar, which indicated similar perceptions. Veteran nurses believed noncompliance to be greater than nurses in practice for less than 5 years. Patients and nurses offered different reasons for noncompliance. Almost half of the nurses believed that patients did not perceive a need for medications. Although some responses were congruent, patients offered reasons for noncompliance—ranging from lack of medication effectiveness to lack of transportation to pharmacy— that were not identified by nurses.

Continued

TABLE 12-2

Selected Research Studies Using Peplau's Framework—cont'd

Study/Year	Purpose	Methods	Findings
PARENTING ROLES Jacobson, 1999	This descriptive study investigated the experiences of parenting with a group of parents identified as having positive parenting process.	Sixteen parents of children who had graduated from high school were interviewed regarding perceptions of positive parenting. Audiotapes were analyzed using the Parse method.	Parents expressed that "[c]larity and continuity in positive outcomes of parenting arise as contentment with life, and efforts to achieve independence are balanced with maintaining connectedness with others" (p. 242). Parents' self-expectations are described by the phrase "parental guidance leads to integrity and communication of values through actions and interactions with others" (p. 242). Interpersonal strategies were expressed in the sentiment that "maintaining family integrity based on values takes priority in achieving positive parenting" (p. 242).

month also facilitated progress. Hindrances to progress in the relationship included shorter time knowing the patient and greater number and duration of previous hospitalizations.

Examining uniqueness within relationships, Forchuk (1995b) found that the same nurse working with two different patients had different preconceptions regarding each and thus had different patient relationships in terms of bond, task, and goals. Patients treated by two nurses had different preconceptions and different therapeutic relationships with each nurse. Patients who formed new relationships with a second nurse tended to develop working relationships in less than 3 months. A combination of nurse and patient factors influenced the quality of therapeutic relationships, and relationships tended to be unique.

In the most recent step, Forchuk, Westwell, Martin, Azzapardi, Kosterewa-Tolman, and Hux (1998) identified influences on movements of nurse-patient dyads from the orientation phase to the working phase. Progress in therapeutic relationships was facilitated by the positive nature of planned therapeutic sessions, nurse activities between sessions on behalf of the patient, and the nurse's attitude. Hindrances included perceived unavailability of the nurse, lack of communication, sense of inequity of relationships, mutual withdrawal, and differences in values and realities between patient and nurse. Validation of Peplau's TIPR was established in that patients valued therapeutic relationships and could identify new phases of the relationship.

Forchuk's findings confirmed the complexity of developing therapeutic nurse-patient relationships. She and others have attempted to systematically test Peplau's formulations about therapeutic relationships. Her findings support Peplau's contention that characteristics of both the nurse and the patient influence the relationship. However, Forchuk's studies did not support Peplau's suggestion that factors such as anxiety would influence therapeutic relationships. Some factors that facilitated therapeutic relationships, such as length of meetings, amount of meeting time per month, and lack of progress with a particular therapy dyad are modifiable and have implications for practice.

In a study of nonpsychiatric patients, Vogelsang (1990) also focused on interpersonal relationships between nurses and women undergoing ambulatory surgery. Vogelsang proposed that continued contact in the interpersonal process would result in appropriate nursing care, in which health goals could be outlined and achieved through the patient's interaction with a consistent nurse. Patients with continued contact expressed greater readiness for discharge and greater satisfaction with care, thus supporting Peplau's contentions about the importance of interpersonal relationships.

Noting the lack of knowledge in long-term care regarding the development of therapeutic relationships, Middleton, Steward, and Richardson (1999) studied perceptions of staff members on special care units caring specifically for dementia patients and of staff on regular long-term care units. Although the TIPR suggests that therapeutic relationships can improve interactions with others, staff caring for older adults on a long-term basis had little if any preparation for developing therapeutic relationships. Therefore the TIPR contextualized this study rather than guided specific study variables. Findings indicated that although special care units experienced significantly more disruptive behavior, special care staff experienced less distress in handling the behavior than other long-term care workers. The fact that almost half the special care staff considered being hit part of their jobs may account for their lower distress. Investigators suggested that the TIPR be used for further staff development in the area of interpersonal relationships with dementia patients.

In order to investigate the possibility of developing therapeutic relationships with dementia patients, Williams and Tappen (1999) applied the TIPR to interactions with Alzheimer's patients. A review of the session transcripts indicated that patients with even moderate or late Alzheimer's disease exhibited behaviors that demonstrated the phases of a therapeutic relationship suggested by the TIPR. Based on these findings, investigators challenged nurses to rethink assumptions that therapeutic relationships cannot be achieved with severely mentally impaired patients. Significantly, this study uses the TIPR on a different population and suggests a need for continued research on its use in interventions for patients with severe mental impairments.

Depression. Beeber (1996, 1998) and others began a series of pilot studies of depressed women. The first of these studies considered pattern integration, and the second symptom reversal. Pattern integrations are clusters of behaviors found in reciprocal interactions of nurses and patients. Pattern integrations may be associated with problems in the patients' lives and can lead to dysfunctional relationships for both the patient and the care provider. Analyzing audiotaped interpersonal intervention sessions, Beeber and Caldwell (1996) investigated the nature of pattern integrations of depressed young women who were referred from a primary care clinic to two psychiatric mental health clinical nurse specialists. The researchers developed a clinical intervention based on the TIPR.

Four patterns emerged and were identified according to their fit with categories identified by Peplau—complementary, mutual, alternating, and antagonistic. A complementary form of pattern integration was the helpless patient's reliance on the helper nurse to resolve difficulties. Nurses were viewed as the provider of answers, which matched the hypothesized need of nurses to be in control and the patient's need to accommodate others. Mutual pattern interactions consisted of the nurse helping the patient and the patient helping the nurse, which allowed the patient to avoid the anxiety of needing help. An alternate form of pattern integration is the pursuer-distancer relationship, in which the patient periodically distanced himself or herself from the nurse or from others in order to encourage that person to pursue him or her out of empathy. The antagonistic form occurred when a relationship was maintained in spite of a poor fit between patient and a nurse. The patient would continue the relationship while at the same time maintaining that it was not effective. Maintenance of the relationship would allow nurses to relieve personal anxiety over ineffectiveness. Beeber and Caldwell (1996) maintained that insight into pattern integrations could assist nurses to create more productive therapeutic relationships. The TIPR was demonstrated to be theoretically useful as a guide, as evidenced by the consistency of the identified patterns with those proposed in the TIPR.

In a study on reversing depressive symptoms of women in a primary care setting, Beeber and Charlie (1998) used an intervention based on the TIPR. They predicted that the intervention would reduce symptoms, increase performance self-esteem, increase social self-esteem, and increase satisfaction with interpersonal relations. The purpose of the pilot study was to test the feasibility of screening for depression and initiating intervention in a primary care setting. Using the TIPR as a guide, researchers established a therapeutic relationship to assess life transitions, investigate the role of depressive symptoms in anxiety management, and understand depressive symptoms in the context of self and relationships. One goal of the therapeutic relationship was to help women manage anxiety differently. Following therapeutic intervention, depression decreased significantly, but no significant differences for self-esteem and satisfaction with interpersonal relationships were found. Use of a therapeutic relationship in a primary care setting was demonstrated to be effective for reducing depression. However, the areas of self-esteem and satisfaction with interpersonal relationships were not as amenable to change in this study. Further investigation needs to be completed on the best use of therapeutic relationships in primary care settings.

Work Roles. Morrison, Shealy, Kowalski, LaMont, and Range (1996) conducted a qualitative study to operationalize Peplau's work roles of staff nurses in psychiatric settings. The observed roles of psychiatric nurses were compared to Peplau's conceptualizations of the roles. On adult units, the roles most often observed were those of counselor, resource person, surrogate, and stranger. Roles of teacher and friend occurred infrequently, and the leader role never emerged. On child and adolescent units, counselor remained the primary role; the roles of surrogate, resource person, and friend followed. Leader and stranger roles were not observed. One difficulty of the study was the inability to differentiate role behaviors. For example, it was hard to distinguish between the autocratic leader role, in which patients were told what to do, versus the surrogate role, in which advice was given. Congruent with Peplau's role conceptualizations, counselor was the central role found in psychiatric nursing practice. However, the surrogate role conceptualization was not upheld. Peplau contended that the surrogate role in nurses' relationships with patients was inappropriate except in cases in which patients were unable to perform activities of daily living or needed to develop social skills. In this study, the surrogate role figured prominently in nurses' activities.

Medication Compliance. Using Peplau's suggestion that the interpersonal process focuses on patients' self-repair and renewal in meeting physiological and interpersonal needs, Lund and Frank (1991) investigated nurse and patient perceptions about medication compliance and hypothesized that therapeutic relationships could establish common goals and better medication compliance. Nurses and patients similarly perceived the degree of medication compliance. However, nurses and patients attributed different reasons to noncompliance. Nurses' most common explanation was that patients did not see the need for medications. However, patients indicated reasons that included not believing the medication to be effective, growing tired of taking medication, liking the high feeling when they were not medicated, opposing medication for religious reasons, fearing poisoning their bodies, not having transportation to a pharmacy, and spouses opposing the medication. Medication compliance was found to be multidimensional and involving both patient and nurse interactions. Different perceptions about why medication was not taken may have generated a higher level of noncompliance.

Parenting. Jacobson (1999) proposed that parenting education and intervention fits within the TIPR in that the therapeutic roles Peplau attributes to nurses could guide nursing interactions with parents. Her qualitative description of positive parenting practices sought to facilitate communication between nurses and parents and suggested that this information would provide the clarity and continuity that Peplau considered essential to communication. Positive parenting was achieved by clarifying communication and showing mutual respect. Parents demonstrated a need for unconditional commitment while meeting new challenges. Interpersonal relationships and communication were viewed as central to families, and parallels between nurse-patient relationships and parent child relationships were drawn. This study makes a significant move by shifting Peplau's theory out of nursing and into family relationships. This research could be extended by exploring single parents' positive parenting practices.

Research Summary. Although Peplau's model for therapeutic relationships was initially developed during the 1950s, research has been slow to follow. It should be noted that some of the earlier measuring instruments in nursing were based on the TIPR and were developed in the 1960s, when few nurses undertook research efforts. Although a recent shift in research has focused more attention on a greater primary care orientation, earlier research centers around hospitalized populations. Forchuk developed the most continuous program of research that supports portions of Peplau's model—particularly in terms of the orientation and working phases. Additional work is clearly needed as concepts related to therapeutic relationships continue to influence nursing practice in both institutional and community settings.

PRAXIS AND THEORY UTILIZATION: DESIGNING NURSING PRACTICE FROM THE PERSPECTIVE OF PEPLAU'S THEORY OF INTERPERSONAL RELATIONS

Peplau has drawn attention to the rich resource of the practice arena for developing nursing knowledge, theory, and research. She considers nursing to be a maturing and educational instrument that fosters interactive processes associated with interpersonal relations and self-understanding of both the patient and the nurse. Interpersonal relationships and interpersonal processes are the central focus of nursing. Practice observations are the roots nursing knowledge development. These observations are "peeled out" (Reed, 1996, p. 31). That is, existing scientific theories, conceptual frameworks, and clinical knowledge are used to identify concepts that represent phenomena observed in practice. Tentative hypotheses can be formulated, validated with the patient, and tested in practice and in research programs (Reed, 1996).

Peplau's theory addresses the interpersonal relations component of nursing practice. The theory does not address physiological components of interest to nursing. These must be explored through other theories (Peplau, 1992). Peplau also contributes to uncovering the phenomena of concern to nursing by exploring the foundational constructs for practice that are associated with the TIPR. The characteristics, knowledge, and skills of both the nurse and the patient are components of concern to nursing. Information about these components is also required. They influence outcomes of nurse-patient actions and interactions. Thus the nurse is encouraged to know himself or herself and to be aware of the consequences of the nurse-patient interdependence in ongoing interpersonal transactions. Although it is particularly useful to nurses in psychiatric settings, this theory is useful to nurses in all settings, because the interpersonal process is a significant component of all nursing practice. Nurses using other nursing theories can also use the TIPR if their goals are congruent with Peplau's goal.

The Variables of Concern for Practice

The variables of concern for practice have been identified in the description of the model and theory. They include the phases of the relationship, roles of nurse and patient, needs, energy and energy transformation, psychological experiences, psychological tasks, nursing process operations, and the five dimensions of relations.

Describing a Population for Nursing Purposes

Without further development, the TIPR is limited in its usefulness to describe a population for nursing purposes, because it addresses only a portion of the concerns of nursing.

Expected Outcomes of Nursing

Forchuk and Voorberg (1991) identified the following expected outcomes of nursing when the TIPR was used to structure nursing practice in a community mental health program:
- Establishing a therapeutic nurse-patient relationship
- Enhancing current stages of patient learning
- Maintaining or improving coping effectiveness in activities of daily living
- Hospitalizing appropriately
- Reducing social isolation, thereby improving quality of life

Process Models

Individuals. Peplau's initial description (1992) of nursing processes include orientation, identification, exploitation, and resolution. Forchuk (1991) modified these stages to orientation, working, and resolution. Contending that certain transitions—such as changes in health, development, and personal and social events—cause anxiety central to the interpersonal process, Beeber (1998) added transition to the description. Anxiety can be mobilized to meet moderate challenges but inhibits more intense challenges. Peplau (1971) described four levels of anxiety: mild, moderate, severe, and panic. Certain transitions are predictable and can be "markers" useful to nursing in planning preventative intervention.

From Peplau's perspective, nursing is concerned with processes, patterns, and the problems that emerge from these processes and patterns (Peplau 1952, 1992). The processes include personality development, perceiving, language-thought processes, learning processes, and nursing therapeutic processes. Although they consist of separate acts, patterns share similar features and represent repeated behavior, such as withdrawal from an anxiety-laden situation. Pattern integration occurs in interpersonal situations. Categories of pattern integration include mutual patterns, in which both parties use the same pattern; complementary patterns, in which one person dominates; and antagonistic patterns, such as love-hate relationships (Peplau, 1992).

The problem-solving activity of nursing centers around the following three steps:
1. Exploring answers related to essential questions about the areas of concern (orientation)
2. Observing, analyzing, and interpreting patient behavior (working)
3. Working with the patient to develop personalities and skills appropriate to the situation, and/or to accomplish psychological tasks associated with forming and developing personality (resolution)

Each of these phases can be described in terms of purpose, dimensions, parameters, and cues (Peplau, 1992). In clinical practice, nurses contribute to nursing knowledge and advancement of this theory by being aware of the understandings perceived within each cell of Figure 12-6 and sharing this information with colleagues.

The areas of concern in the nursing process include the following: (1) human needs, (2) goal achievement and factors interfering with goal achievement, (3) the associated emotions and feelings, (4) behavior arising from goal achievement or lack of it, and (5) pa-

	Orientation	Working	Resolution
Purpose			
Dimensions			
Parameters			
Cues			

FIGURE 12-6   Phases of the nurse-patient relationship related to problem solving.

tients' defense mechanisms for handling those emotions and feelings. Understanding the *who, where, when,* and *what* of patient experience is essential to helping the patient to modify behavior. Assessing the patient's intellectual ability to know options available for change and how to bring about change is also important (Peplau, 1964).

Through the stimuli, messages, inputs, and cues that nurses send to patients in the interpersonal process, they influence and facilitate changes in patient behavior. The nurse not only observes behavior but also actively participates in the observation process. The behavior of both the observer and the observed becomes a part of the data on which decisions are made and courses of action are determined.

Drawing on Sullivan's work, Peplau (1992) suggests that nurses consider the phase of the "mode of experiencing" of the patient (p. 15). In the protaxic mode, patients may be so focused on the current moment that they cannot consider past or future events. The parataxic mode relates past and present events. In this mode, similarities between past events and/or persons influence the interpretation of current events and distort interpretation of the present. Peplau suggests that this can be resolved by helping the patient describe the similarity of and specify differences between the past and the present. In the syntactic mode, past, present, and future are linked.

Patterns are helpful to nurses in understanding and using the interpersonal process to change patient behavior. Patterns may be intrapersonal—that is, an attribute of one person. They may also be interpersonal, in which the interaction of each person's patterns and the relationship of these patterns are of interest.

Energy and energy transformation from the perspective of this theory are familiar concepts to many nurses. This energy is derived from anxiety and from biological needs (Peplau, 1992). Persons may engage in dysfunctional behaviors to reduce, relieve, or prevent more anxiety. These are termed "relief behaviors" (p. 17). Empathic processes transmit anxiety from one person to another; thus nurses must be aware of and able to control their own anxiety when working with patients. Beeber (1998) suggests that anxiety is a central concept within this theory.

Martin, Forchuk, Santopinto, and Butcher (1992) outline eight stages of learning that Peplau considers useful to nursing: observe, describe, analyze, formulate, validate, test, integrate, and utilize. Knowing the patient's stage of learning provides the nurse with a benchmark for designing strategies to teach new behaviors. According to the TIPR, the roles of the nurse include resource person, counselor, surrogate for another (such as a mother), and technical expert.

Extension to the Family. Forchuk and Dorsay (1995) suggest that the TIPR can be linked with family systems nursing theory (Wright & Leahey, 1994) because both theories are parts of interpersonal paradigms in which the interpersonal process is recognized as the essence of nursing. Within family systems nursing theory, both the family as a unit and the individuals who make up the unit are the concerns of nursing. The focus is on interactions and reciprocity (Wright & Leahey, 1994). Additional exploration of this link is important.

Practice Models

Beeber (1998) has begun a practice model for working with depressed patients. Beeber conceptualized depression as a health problem. This model directs the orientation, working, and resolution phases of nurse-patient contact for the advanced practice nurse. Beeber has added the dimension of transition to Peplau's work. A transition is a particular situation experienced when there is a need for changes in self and relations. These can be health-related, age-related, or based upon personal and social events. The need for change causes anxiety managed through security operations, which are "the thoughts, feelings, and actions developed to manage anxiety" (Beeber, 1998, p. 154).

Implications for Administration

Peplau's theory has been used extensively in nursing practice by individuals and by organizations interested in theory-based nursing, particularly in relation to psychiatric nursing. In 1991 Forchuk and Voorberg reported on the use of the theory in evaluating a community mental health program. The TIPR was used to structure practice, direct development of patient objectives, and develop instruments to measure outcomes of care.

Agencies that wish to practice from the TIPR should organize policies and procedures that foreground the interpersonal relation between nurse and patient or nurse and family system. As the nurse and patient interrelate, both change; development proceeds; and behavior is modified. Time becomes an element of consideration. Nurses establish specific interaction times with patients, and both nurse and patient know the times and purposes. Forchuk, Westwell, Martin, Azzapardi, Kosterewa-Tolman, and Hux (1998) found fewer satisfactory outcomes in relationships that took longer than 6 months to move from the orientation phase to the working phase. Factors that interfered with movement from one phase to another included unavailability of the nurse, patient, or both; superficial contact; and personal problems. Nurses who perceived themselves as superior to the patients or who did not view the patients as persons interfered with the movement between the stages. When the relationship did not progress, both the nurse and patient withdrew emotionally. The attention to nurse factors and to patient factors in the clinical setting impacts the attitude, focus, and behavior of the nurse.

Implications for Education

Education to practice from the perspective of TIPR should include studies in systems, communication, cybernetics, and roles. All of these are foundational to understanding interpersonal relations.

NEXUS

When asked about the future, Peplau replied:

The shift in emphasis will be from what nurses do to what nurses know. That's a paradigm shift of major proportions. Most of the emphasis in 1950s was on what nurses do . . . and it's only recently—starting with my book and others who put theory in the literature—now it's a question of what nurses know (1997).

The creation of Peplau's TIPR was groundbreaking, and the theory continues to influence research and practice. Much research remains to be completed in both psychiatric and healthy patient populations. Although the TIPR has been controversial, the practical nature of the theoretical propositions sometimes leads nurses to assume that they are true. Continued testing of constructs and of practice applications needs to be completed in the future to verify these assumptions.

REFERENCES

ANA (1994). *Nursing's social policy statement*. Kansas City, MO. Author.

Beeber, L.S. (1998). Treating depression through the therapeutic nurse-client relationship. *Nursing Clinics of North America, 33*(1), 153-157.

Beeber, L. & Caldwell, C. (1996). Pattern integrations in young depressed women: Part II. *Archives of Psychiatric Nursing, 10*(3), 157-164.

Beeber, L. & Charlie, M. (1998). Depressive symptom reversal for women in a primary care setting: A pilot study. *Archives of Psychiatric Nursing, 12*(5), 247-254.

Forchuk, C. (1991). Peplau's theory: Concepts and their relations. *Nursing Science Quarterly, 4*(2), 54-60.

Forchuk, C. (1992). The orientation phase of the nurse-client relationship: How long does it take? *Perspectives in Psychiatric Care, 28*(4), 7-10.

Forchuk, C. (1994). The orientation phase of the nurse-client relationship: Testing Peplau's theory. *Journal of Advanced Nursing, 20*(3), 532-537.

Forchuk, C. (1995a). Development of nurse-client relationships: What helps. *Journal of the American Psychiatric Nurses Association, 1*(5), 146-151.

Forchuk, C. (1995b). Uniqueness within the nurse-client relationship. *Archives of Psychiatric Nursing, 9*(1), 34-39.

Forchuk, C. & Brown, B. (1989). Establishing a nurse-client relationship. *Journal of Psychosocial Nursing, 27*(2), 30-34.

Forchuk, C. & Dorsay, J.P. (1995). Hildegard Peplau meets family systems nursing: Innovation in theory-based practice. *Journal of Advanced Nursing, 21*(1), 110-115.

Forchuk, C., Westwell, J., Martin, M., Azzapardi, W., Kosterewa-Tolman, D., & Hux, M. (1998). Factors influencing movement of chronic psychiatric patients from the orientation to the working phase of the nurse-client relationship of an inpatient unit. *Perspectives in Psychiatric Care, 34*(1), 36-44.

Forchuk, C. & Voorberg, N. (1991). Evaluation of a community mental health program. *Canadian Journal of Nursing Administration, 4*(2), 16-20.

Howk, C., Brophy, G.H., Carey, E.T., Noll, J., Rasmussen, L. Searcy, B., & Stark, N.L. (1998). Hildegard E. Peplau: Psychodynamic Nursing. In A. Marriner-Tomey & M.R. Alligood (Eds.), *Nursing theorists and their works*. St. Louis: Mosby.

Jacobson, G. (1999). Parenting processes: A descriptive explanatory study using Peplau's theory. *Nursing Science Quarterly, 12*(3), 240-244.

LaMonica, E. (1981). Construct validity of an empathy instrument. *Research in Nursing and Health, 4*(4), 389-400.

Lund, V. & Frank, D. (1991). Helping the medicine go down: Nurses and patients perceptions about medication compliance. *Journal of Psychosocial Nursing, 29*(7), 6-9.

Martin, M.L., Forchuk, C., Santopinto, M., & Butcher, H.K. (1992). Alternative approaches to nursing practice: Application of Peplau, Rogers, and Parse. *Nursing Science Quarterly* 5(2), 80-85.

Methven, D. & Scholtfeldt, R. (1962). A therapeutic behavior scale. *Nursing Research, 11*(2), 83-88.

Middleton, J., Steward, N., & Richardson, J. (1999). Caregiver distress related to disruptive behaviors on special care units versus traditional long-term care units. *Journal of Gerontological Nursing, 23*(3), 11-19.

Morrison, E., Shealy, A., Kowalski, C., LaMont, J., & Range, B. (1996). Work roles of staff nurses in psychiatric settings. *Nursing Science Quarterly, 9*(1), 17-21.

Peplau, H.E. (1952). *Interpersonal relations in nursing.* New York: G.P. Putnam's Sons.

Peplau, H.E. (1964). *Basic principles of patient counseling.* (2nd ed.). Philadelphia: Smith Kline & French Laboratories.

Peplau, H.E. (1971). Interpersonal relations in nursing: A conceptual framework of reference for psychodynamic nursing. New York: Springer Publishing Company.

Peplau, H.E. (1992). Interpersonal relations: Theoretical framework for application in nursing practice. *Nursing Science Quarterly, 5*(1), 13-16.

Peplau, H.E. Personal Communication. October 7, 1997.

Peplau, H.E. (1997). Peplau's Theory of Interpersonal Relations. *Nursing Science Quarterly, 10*(4), 162-167.

Reed, P.G. (1996). Transforming practice knowledge into nursing knowledge: A revisionist analysis of Peplau. *Image, 28*(1), 29-33.

Spring, R. & Turk, H. (1962). A therapeutic behavior scale. *Nursing Research, 11*(4), 214-218.

Sullivan, H.S. (1953). *Conceptions of modern psychiatry.* New York: Norton.

Vogelsang, J. (1990). Continued contact with a familiar nurse affects women's perceptions of the ambulatory surgical experience: A qualitative-quantitative design. *Journal of Post Anesthesia Nursing, 5*(5), 315-320.

Williams, C. & Tappen, R. (1999). Can we create a therapeutic relationship with nursing home residents in the later stages of Alzheimer's disease? *Journal of Psychosocial Nursing, 37*(3), 28-35.

Wright, L. & Leahey, M. (1994). *Nurses and families: A guide to family assessment and intervention.* (2nd ed.). Philadelphia: F.A. Davis.

Modeling Nursing from a Caring Perspective

WATSON'S TRANSPERSONAL NURSING and the THEORY of HUMAN CARING

Key Terms

Watson's early work (1979) presented nursing as an art and as a science of caring from a human science tradition. In 1985, she integrated science, art, ethics, and esthetics into the Theory of Human Caring. In a retrospective and prospective commentary about the Theory of Human Caring, Watson observed that her work is "both theory and beyond theory . . . it can be read as a philosophy, ethic, or even paradigm or worldview. It make(s) explicit that humans cannot be treated as objects, that humans cannot be separated from self, other, nature, and the larger universe" (1997, p. 50). Watson (1999) presented a transpersonal caring-healing model that she described as a transformative paradigm. She believes that this model is both nursing and beyond nursing—that is, as a way of living or being, it can transform the whole of healthcare. The caring-healing model she describes "requires a radical transformation of our consciousness, our cosmology, and our being in the universe" (1999, p. xxvi).

THE STARTING POINT OF THE MODELING PROCESS

In her 1997 retrospective, Watson noted that her work emerged from her "quest to bring new meaning and dignity to the world of nursing and patient care" (p. 49). She combined concepts from clinical nursing and empirical studies with her knowledge of the humanities. Strongly influenced by phenomenological psychology and existential philosophy, Watson's early work shifted toward a wholistic/humanitarian approach to developing theory (Conway, 1985). Watson began from a traditional science perspective, claiming that "[t]he scientific problem-solving method is necessary for the science of caring to study, guide, direct, and research knowledge and practice" (1979, p. 56). She identified basic assumptions and carative factors for the science of caring. In 1999, Watson reconceptualized nursing as transpersonal caring-healing manifested in a caring consciousness with an intent to care and heal. This moved her thinking to another dimension, leaving nursing scholars to ponder the effect of this reconceptualization on her earlier works and interpretations.

Reason for Theory Development

Committed to nursing's caring-healing role and mission, Watson proposed a "humanitarian, aesthetic, and spiritual" philosophy and science of caring (1997). Nursing science was to be developed within a human science context rather than the traditional natural or physical science view. From her initial focus to her recent work, Watson has been unwavering in her belief that caring remains the foundation for nursing and other health professions.

Phenomenon of Concern

According to Watson, the caring dimension is the primary phenomenon of concern for nursing. Watson's Theory of Human Caring described the caring phenomenon under the umbrellas of human science and art, which are intersubjective contexts that include the mutuality of the person/self of both the nurse and the patient and concepts such as phenomenal field, actual caring occasion, and transpersonal caring (1985). The Theory of Human Caring and the "caring-healing" model (1999) are the basis for a postmodern, transformative perspective of transpersonal nursing. By 1985, Watson was moving away from traditional science to view science, scientific development, and theory development as counterparts to art, the humanities, and philosophy. She wrote:

> I reject methods that ascribe an increasing degree of reality to numbers and factual information . . . I reject definitions and interpretations of science and scientific inquiry that bury the quest for discovery, beauty, creativity, and a higher sense of being-in-the-world. I want nursing to move beyond objectivism, verification, rigid operations, and definitions and concern itself more with meaning, relationships, context, and patterns (1985, p. 2).

This shift from science led Watson to view nursing as a metaphor and symbol manifested as the **sacred feminine archetype** (Watson, 1999). The sacred feminine archetype is considered "the very basis of reality" (Watson, 1999, p. 286). An archetype is "an enduring unconscious idea, image, original form or pattern in the human consciousness that is present and persists across time and across humanity" (p. 285). An archetype is more than a metaphor. In describing the sacred feminine archetype, Watson does not specifically define *sacred*. She describes the sacred in terms of spirit/spirituality, life's force and energy, soul, universal experience, the heavenly, the divine, the unitary, and the transcendent. *Feminine* is described as including feelings, receptivity, subjectivity/intersubjectivity, multiplicity, nurturing, cooperating, intuiting, relatedness, loving, caring, and peace. The feminine is not gender-specific. Men, too, can possess a feminine ontology; nonetheless, Watson identifies nursing issues with women's issues. This sacred feminine archetype provides the metaphors for understanding and shaping thought about nursing as transpersonal caring-healing. *Transpersonal* conveys a human-to-human connection in which both persons are influenced by the relationship. The persons engaged in transpersonal nursing are transformed, and nursing itself will be transformed as nurses take on these reconstructed ideas.

DESCRIPTION OF WATSON'S THEORETICAL SYSTEM
Philosophical Perspectives

Watson's description and discussion of postmodern nursing exemplifies movement from the starting point of traditional philosophy and science to a reconstructed philosophical and metaphorical description of nursing. Watson emphasized her changed worldview through her conceptualizations about nursing. In 1985, she defined nursing as a human science of persons and focused on human health-illness experiences that are mediated by professional, personal, scientific, esthetic, and ethical transactions with the nurse as an active coparticipant. Now Watson (1999) describes transpersonal caring-healing with a postmodern/transpersonal view of body and person. Nursing becomes the practice of transpersonal caring-healing; nursing arts of caring and healing "tap into feelings, emotions, inner processes, imagery, intuition and . . . consciousness" (p. 231). This reconstruction is viewed as a model for nursing, for all of healthcare, and, moreover, for humanity (Watson, 1999).

Cosmology and Ontology. Watson's thinking moved to acceptance of the idea of an evolving human consciousness integral to the universe and in harmony with the whole cosmos. Caring-healing is seen as a new cosmology that views the person-nature-universe as a connected whole, as a unitary consciousness—that is, a "consciousness of unity of **mindbodyspirit** and nature" (Watson, 1999, pp. 97-98). Watson believes that this cosmology of unity facilitates creative participation, which is characterized by ambiguity, paradox, connectedness, and freedom with the universe. It supports an epistemology open to multiple ways of being, knowing, and doing. The basic premises for the transpersonal-caring healing model are presented in Box 13-1. Watson asserted that this new cosmology is contained within the "sacred feminine archetype" (1999, p. 13).

Watson (1999) identified the ontology as a *relational ontology* grounded in the transpersonal. In the sacred feminine archetype ontology, two focal areas are considered important to nursing: the nature of being and the meaning of caring.

Nature of Being. Watson asserted in 1999 that the "postmodern/transpersonal view of body and person is still evolving" (p. 149). Within this ontology, the body is the lived body—the lived self, not "object but subject—embodied subjective world—a living, breathing subject" (1999, p. 131). She described the body as:

fully manifest as physical, present in the material, objective world. At the same time, it also manifests itself as fluid-like, as elemental vibrations of light and

---

BOX 13-1

Basic Premises for the Transpersonal-Caring Healing Model

- There is an expanded view of the person and what it means to be human—fully embodied, but more than body physical: and embodied spirit; a transpersonal, transcendent, evolving consciousness, unity of mindbodyspirit; person-nature-universe as oneness, connected.
- Acknowledgement of the human-environment energy field-life energy field and universal field of consciousness; universal mind (in Teilhard de Chardin and Bohm's sense of *mind*).
- Positing of consciousness as energy; caring-healing consciousness becomes primary for the caring-healing practitioner.
- Caring potentiates healing, wholeness.
- Caring-healing modalities (sacred feminine archetype of nursing) have been excluded from nursing and health systems; their development and reintroduction are essential for postmodern, transpersonal, caring-healing models and transformation.
- Caring-healing processes and relationships are considered sacred.
- Unitary consciousness as the worldview and cosmology, i.e., viewing the connectedness of all.
- Caring as a converging global agenda for nursing and society alike.

From Watson, J. (1999). *Postmodern nursing and beyond.* Edinburgh: Churchill Livingstone.

---

energy, as electrical currents. Each individual's energy field is in continuous interaction and exchange with the whole inner and external environment, one's non-physical energy field of existence. The mind, self, soul, spiritual and material are one (1999, p. 136).

Watson described humans as multisensory or extrasensory beings. "There is both an embodied consciousness and spirit and also a nonlocal, transcendent consciousness, which is capable of being connected with the universal sea of consciousness, across time and space" (p. 151).

Quantum thinking guides Watson's ontology. She states that "[q]uantum theory deals with *both particles and matter* that are *localized* in time and space, and also with *energy matter* that is *wave-like*, spread out and *nonlocalized*" (Watson, 1999, p. 107). Particle and wave phenomena are simultaneously present. Watson uses quantum theory in a metaphorical sense, not as in physics or mechanics. Watson (1988a) identified some basic principles that help with understanding the ontology through the metaphor of a holographic model. These are presented in Box 13-2.

The Meaning of Caring. A relational ontology requires caring. **Caring** is an essential part of life. It can be practiced intrapersonally, as within oneself, but, as Watson noted, "caring can be most effectively demonstrated and practiced interpersonally and transpersonally" (1999, p. 102). Interpersonal caring is a more traditional view in nursing and considers the nurse an active coparticipant. Transpersonal caring is more than interpersonal—both persons are influenced and changed by the relationship. Jensen, Bäck-Pettersson, and Segesten formulated the following definition of caring using Watson's conceptualizations: "caring

BOX **13-2**

Basic Principles within Holographic Thinking

- The whole is in the part.
- Humans are inseparably interconnected with one another and with the universe.
- Mind and consciousness are joined, and consciousness is communicated.
- Human consciousness is spatially extended, and consciousness exists through space.
- Human consciousness is temporally extended, and consciousness exists through time.
- Nonphysical consciousness dominates over physical matter.

From Watson, J. (1988a). New dimensions of human caring theory. *Nursing Science Quarterly, 1*(4), 178.

BOX **13-3**

Carative Components or Factors

- Formation of a humanistic-altruistic system of values
- Instillation of faith-hope
- Cultivation of sensitivity to oneself and to others
- Development of a helping-trust relationship
- Promotion and acceptance of expressing positive and negative feelings
- Systematic use of the scientific problem-solving method for decision making
- Promotion of interpersonal teaching-learning
- Provision for supportive, protective, and/or corrective mental, physical, sociocultural, and spiritual environments
- Assistance with gratification of human needs
- Allowance for existential-phenomenological forces

From Watson, J. (1979). *Nursing: The philosophy and science of caring.* Boston: Little, Brown.

consists of transpersonal intersubjective attempts to protect, enhance, and preserve humanity and human dignity by helping people to find meaning in their illness, suffering, pain, and existence" (1993, p. 98). The one-caring "helps another human being [the one-cared for] to gain self-knowledge, self-control, and self-healing" (Jensen, Bäck-Pettersson, & Segesten, 1993, pp. 98-99). Caring is guided by **carative components,** which were referred to as carative factors in earlier works. These are presented in Box 13-3 and are a part of the ontology of caring.

Description of Transpersonal Caring-Healing Model and Theory of Human Caring

Watson's 1999 treatise coalesced many of the concepts of caring into a Transpersonal Caring-Healing model (TCH). Watson suggests that the TCH model is the emerging nursing model because it is a "fuller completion of the model in which nursing has operated all

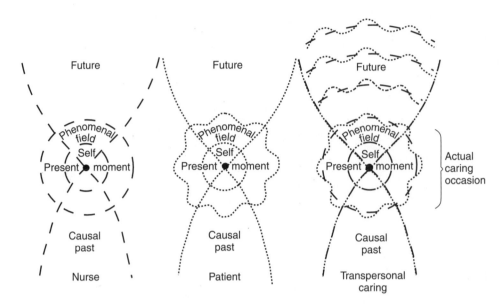

FIGURE 13-1 The caring field and caring moment. (From Watson, J. (1988). *Nursing: Human science and human care.* Sudbury, MA: National League for Nursing, Jones and Bartlett.)

along" (1999, p. xxi). Along with this model, Watson developed a theory of nursing as human science. To accommodate her views, Watson (1985) defined theory as "an imaginative grouping of knowledge, ideas, and experience that are represented symbolically and seek to illuminate a given phenomenon" (p. 1). This is now the Theory of Human Caring.

Transpersonal Caring-Healing Model. Caring requires two persons—one caring and one receiving care. They come together in a moment, simultaneously transcending the two and connecting to the human spirit realm. A basic premise of Watson's TCH is that the coming together of the nurse and patient in a caring connection has healing potential. This transpersonal caring generates and potentiates the self-healing processes. Nursing is described as a way of being that directs knowing and doing. Transcendence involves action and choice. The nurse moves to come together with the other, communicates caring, and assists in making choices about further action or doing. Nursing/caring/healing is lived. First and foremost, nursing is *being*—not *doing*. The caring field and caring moment are modeled in Figure 13-1. The TCH model is seen as a concrescence—that is, the growing together or coalescing of parts into a new whole. The transpersonal caring-healing field is the concrescence of the fields of the one caring and the one receiving care. A transpersonal caring relationship depends on a moral commitment to protect and enhance human dignity and on communication of the caring by maintaining the person as subject rather than an object. The relationship also depends on a newly created energy field—a caring field—at a focal point in time and space (Watson, 1988a). This moment is called the *caring moment*. This caring relationship has healing potential for both persons. Watson explains that "[t]ranspersonal recognizes that the power of love, faith, compassion, caring, community and intention, consciousness

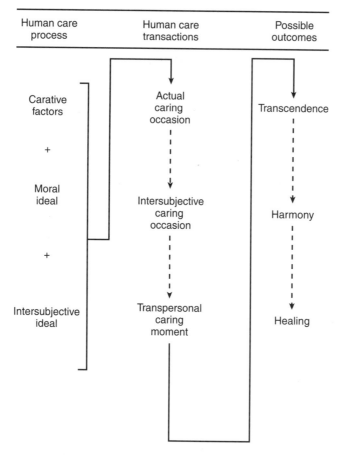

| Human care process | Human care transactions | Possible outcomes |

Carative factors

+

Moral ideal

+

Intersubjective ideal

Actual caring occasion

Intersubjective caring occasion

Transpersonal caring moment

Transcendence

Harmony

Healing

FIGURE 13-2 Watson's Theory of Human Care. (From Sourial, S. (1996). An analysis and evaluation of Watson's theory of human care. *Journal of Advanced Nursing, 24*(2), p. 401.)

and access to a deeper/higher energy source is as important to healing as are our conventional treatment approaches" (1999, p. 115).

Theory of Human Caring. Watson defines nursing as "a human science of persons and human health-illness experiences" (1985, p. 54). As she refined her conceptualizations, nursing became "a metaphor for the sacred feminine archetypal energy" (1999, p. 11) as "archetype and metaphor for woman and healer" (p. 14). She praised the ANA's 1995 revised definition of nursing—which includes attention to the full range of human experiences and responses, understanding of the subjective experience, and provision of a caring relationship that facilitates health and healing—as a more comprehensive definition than it had offered previously. Nursing becomes the practical art of transpersonal caring-healing. Watson refers to nursing in this light as *ontological artistry.* Sourial (1996) developed a model to illustrate the relationship of concepts within Watson's theory. This is shown in Figure 13-2. The human care processes are comprised of carative factors or components and moral and intersubjective ideals. This process is the basis for the transactions that begin in the actual caring occasion and move to transpersonal caring moment with healing as the desired outcome.

RESEARCH DERIVED FROM WATSON'S THEORY OF HUMAN CARING

Watson's method of knowing is most congruent with a critical theorist or constructivist orientation. According to Watson (1985), research methods need to fit the phenomena of study. The phenomenon of caring has challenged researchers who attempt to approach it quantifiably. Although some quantitative instruments that measure carative behaviors exist, many studies exploring the phenomenon of caring have used qualitative methods—particularly the phenomenological method. Watson indicated that phenomenological analysis describes human meanings of experiences unapproachable through the simplistic reduction found in traditional quantitative methods. One phenomenological method that Watson (1985) advocates is transcendental phenomenology, in which a poetic formulation interprets experiential evidence. In this method, the investigator writes poetry as a mechanism to penetrate the surface of the phenomenon and convey in a new language the experience being described. Poetry simply provides another mechanism for conveying the basic nature of the findings. Although it is expressively useful, it is not mandatory for use of Watson's theory.

Instruments

Although much of the caring research is phenomenological, some quantitative instruments the describe caring activities exist. Table 13-1 summarizes the research instruments.

Caring Behavior Inventory. In a multistep process, Wolf (1986) and Wolf, Giardino, Osborne, and Ambrose (1994) created the Caring Behavior Inventory (CBI). Originally a 75-item instrument of caring behaviors based on extensive literature review and nurse rankings, this instrument was reduced to 43 items rated on a 4-point Likert scale. Following content validation, reliability and validity were assessed with a group of nurses and patients (see Table 13-1). Wolf, Giardino, Osborne, and Ambrose (1994) present a strong case for both test-retest and internal consistency reliability. Additionally, the study provides evidence for construct validity established using the contrasted groups technique and a factor analysis. Contrasted groups of nurses were significantly different, and factor analysis indicated that the identified dimensions explained a substantial portion of the variance. The identified dimensions fit characteristics of caring as identified in Watson's theory.

Caring Behavior Assessment. Another instrument for measuring caring behaviors is the Caring Behavior Assessment (CBA) developed by Cronin and Harrison (1988). The CBA consists of a list of 61 items related to nurse caring behaviors that patients can rate on a 5-point Likert scale. The caring behaviors are congruent with Watson's carative factors. The 61 behaviors are divided into seven subscales, consisting of the following: (1) humanism/faith-hope/sensitivity, (2) helping/trust, (3) expression of positive/negative feelings, (4) teaching/learning, (5) supportive/protective/corrective environment, (6) human needs assistance, and (7) existential/phenomenological/spiritual forces. Although it is not specified in Cronin and Harrison's article, scoring is accomplished by adding the Likert ratings for items in each subscale and then dividing by the number of items in the scale. The lowest subscale score is 1, and the highest is 5. There is no score for the total

TABLE 13-1

Research Instruments Based on Watson's Transpersonal Nursing and Theory of Human Caring

Instrument/Description	Study/Year	Reliability and Validity
Caring Behavior Assessment (CBA) 61-item, 5-point Likert scale	Cronin and Harrison, 1988	Sixty-one nurse caring behaviors were grouped into seven subscales. Content validity was established by four content experts. Interrater reliability was assessed by a panel that rated the congruency of each behavior with the given subscale. Items with interrater reliability of less than 0.75 were recategorized. Internal consistency of subscales ranged from 0.66 to 0.90. Teaching-learning was strongest at 0.90, and expression of positive/negative feelings (alpha = 0.67) and existential phenomenological/spiritual forces (alpha = 0.66) were the lowest subscales.
Caring Behavior Inventory (CBI) 43-item, 4-point Likert scale	Wolf, 1986, 1994	A convenience sample of 97 registered nurses ranked 75 caring words on a 4-point Likert scale. Words with median ranks of 3.75 or lower were eliminated. The instrument was subsequently revised to include 43 items. Test-retest reliability was $\underline{r} = 0.96$, $\underline{p} = 0.000$, $\underline{rho} = 0.88$, $\underline{p} = 0.000$. Internal consistency reliability with nurses was 0.83, and with a combined sample of nurses and patients, internal consistency reliability was 0.96. Construct validity was established using a contrasted groups technique that compared 278 nurses to 263 patients and indicated that the groups were different ($\underline{t} = 3.01$, $\underline{df} = 539$, $\underline{p} = 0.003$). Factor analysis identified five dimensions that accounted for 56.8% of the variance. The five dimensions included the following: respectful deference to the other, assurance of human presence, positive connectedness, professional knowledge and skill, and attentiveness to the other's experience.

instrument. Evidence is offered only for content validity established by a panel of experts. Adequate interrater reliability is established; however, internal consistency reliability falls below acceptable levels on the two subscales of expression of positive/negative feelings and existential/phenomenological/spiritual forces. Although this instrument has been used in several caring studies (Cronin & Harrison, 1988; Parsons, Kee, & Gray, 1993; Marini, 1999), further work on instrumentation needs to be completed.

Review of Related Research

To gather research studies associated with Watson's transpersonal nursing and the Theory of Human Caring, a literature review was conducted using the Cumulative Index of Nursing and Allied Health Literature (CINAHL). The following three major types of articles were found: (1) those describing caring behaviors exhibited in nursing; (2) those describing human experiences associated with living in nursing homes, dealing with chronic illness, and living in a homeless shelter, and (3) a limited number of discussions dealing with caring outcomes. Table 13-2 summarizes caring studies that were guided by or that tested Watson's theory.

Text continued on p. 390

TABLE 13-2

Selected Research Studies Using Watson's Theory of Transpersonal Care

Study/Year	Purpose	Methods	Findings
NURSE CARING CHARACTERISTICS			
Brown, 1986	This qualitative study identified themes of patients feeling cared for by nurses.	Fifty patients aged 22 to 65 were asked to describe experiences in which a nurse cared for them. Critical incident reports were taped, transcribed, and analyzed.	Eight themes were identified. "Recognition of individual qualities and needs" involved nurses modifying care to meet unique needs. A "reassuring presence" was characterized by the nurse offering comfort and support. "Provision of information" reflected the nurse's actions to inform the patient. "Demonstration of professional knowledge and skill" resulted from the nurse taking immediate action in urgent situations. "Assistance with pain" was characterized by administering medications and modifying procedures to decrease pain. "Amount of time spent" related to the nurse spending extra time with the patient. "Promotion of autonomy" was characterized by making the patient feel in charge of decision making. "Surveillance" resulted from patient feeling under the nurse's watch.
Cronin and Harrison, 1988	This descriptive study of myocardial infarction patients identified nursing behaviors perceived as caring.	Twenty-two hospitalized patients were interviewed and completed the Caring Behaviors Assessment (CBA). Most important and least important caring behaviors were ranked based on mean scores. Subscales were ranked according to their mean scores.	Most important caring behaviors included the following: "know what they are doing" and "make me feel someone is there if I need them" ($M = 4.86$ for both items). The least important behavior was "visit me when I move to another hospital unit" ($M = 2.36$). Human needs assistance was the area in which patients felt the most need ($M = 4.6$). The least important area of need was expression of positive and negative feelings ($M = 3.80$).

Dennis, 1991	This qualified study examined the components of spiritual nursing care.	Ten nurses were interviewed about spiritual nursing care. The eight concepts from Watson's model were used to categorize the nurses' responses.	Spiritual nursing care has interdependent components that create nurse-person interactions. Self is the essence of who we are and resides in everyone. Persons are unique and create their own life experiences. Nurses must be committed and ready to be fully present to others. Everyone needs spiritual care, which is represented by a diverse spectrum. The process of spiritual nursing care reflects nurses' technical and intuitive skills and relies on experience. Varied goals range from healing to empowerment to finding meaning. Supportive environments influenced the amount of spiritual care given. The nature of the exchange between nurse and person was perceived as an intersubjective flow.
Dietrich, 1992	This phenomenological study examined caring practices, experience, and meanings of nurse-to-nurse caring, noncaring, and the environmental context.	Five registered nurses participated in in-depth, open-ended interviews. The investigator completed coding and content analysis of interview transcripts.	Nurse-to-nurse caring involved being sensitive, offering help, being open, being understanding, acknowledging coworkers' knowledge and skill, being supportive, and having camaraderie. Nurse-to-nurse noncaring consisted of lack of respect, lack of acknowledgement, and lack of camaraderie. Environmental contexts that facilitated caring included support from management. Caring was inhibited by limited time for interaction and perceptions of overwhelming workloads.
Jensen, Bäck-Pettersson, and Segesten; 1996	This qualitative study described the essential characteristics of excellent nurses as perceived by women undergoing treatment for breast cancer.	Ten women who underwent breast cancer surgery and remained in secondary treatment participated in semi-structured interviews regarding experiences with excellent nurses and caring situations.	Four concepts—competence, compassion, courage, and concordance—emerged. "Competence" referred to knowledge and practice skills about nursing, human interaction, and nursing care. "Compassion" related to the unconditional approach used by nurses and the interest nurses exhibited in managing patients' life situations. "Courage" referred to infusing hope and meaning with the nurse facing crises with patients. "Concordance" occurred when nurses inspired confidence, acted according to patient preferences, and maintained a sense of connectedness.

Continued

TABLE 13-2

Selected Research Studies Using Watson's Theory of Transpersonal Care—cont'd

Study/Year	Purpose	Methods	Findings
NURSE CARING CHARACTERISTICS—cont'd			
Kerouac and Rouillier, 1992	The study explored aspects of clinical and administrative caring in nursing.	Eight 2-hour group encounters with five head nurses were used for data collection. Activities of the group encounters included group discussion and exploration of the components of caring found in clinical and administrative nursing.	For head nurses, incorporating caring practices into nursing involved getting to know staff, appreciating staff strengths, and making assignments accordingly. Sharing difficult situations, role modeling caring behaviors, and responding to staff needs also were aspects of caring.
Lemmer, 1991	This qualitative study explored caring that was experienced by parents following a perinatal loss.	The sample consisted of 15 women and 13 men who had experienced perinatal loss either through stillbirth or neonatal death. Interviews were audiotaped and transcribed.	Parent descriptions included two major categories: "taking care of and caring for or about." Providing expert care and information were components of being taken care of. Providing emotional support; providing individualized, family-centered care; acting as a surrogate parent; facilitating the creation of memories; and respecting rights of the parents composed subcategories of "caring for or about."
Marini, 1999	This descriptive study identified nursing staff behaviors that indicated caring.	A convenience sample of 21 institutionalized older adults responded to 63-item Caring Behavior Assessment (CBA) Instrument.	The highest ranked subscale was human needs assistance ($M = 4.31$), followed by humanism/faith-hope/sensitivity ($M = 4.07$). Helping/trust ($M = 3.57$) ranked lowest.
McNamara, 1995	This qualitative study determined perceptions of perioperative caring behaviors by nurses.	Five perioperative nurses participated in semi-structured interviews that were transcribed and analyzed.	Themes of caring centered around humanistic caring by showing concern, communication, touch, and awareness of concerns. Caring behaviors changed from building a trusting relationship in the preoperative period to promoting safety and attending to physical needs during the intraoperative and postoperative periods.

Miller, Haber, and Byrne, 1992	This phenomenological study examined the experience of caring from the perspectives of patients and nurses.	Thirteen acute-care patients and 14 nurses participated in semistructured interviews about experience of caring.	Five parallel themes between patients and nurses emerged: "holistic understanding," "connectedness/shared humanness," "presence," "anticipating" and "monitoring needs," and "beyond the mechanical." Patient descriptions of caring involved a professional and personal sense of caring and connection. Nurses were courteous and always there to help but were also human. Nurses described caring as a way of being and established professional relationships that were also personal. They met patients' physical expectations, monitored patient conditions, and planned care so as to promote positive human outcomes.
Montgomery, 1992	This grounded theory study determined the spiritual connection in nurses' perceptions of caring.	Thirty-five nurses participated in semistructured interviews. Data were analyzed using interview transcripts, theoretical and methodological notes, and a constant comparative method.	The major emerging theme was spiritual transcendence, in which nurses described relationships with others as a force greater than oneself. Spiritual transcendence consisted of a caring connection within professional nursing relationships, as a source of energy and resource for the caregiver, and as an aesthetic of caring that guided the orchestration of caring experiences.
Parsons, Kee, and Gray, 1993	This study investigated perioperative patients' perceptions of caring behaviors and compared them to perceptions of patients experiencing myocardial infarction.	Nineteen perioperative patients responded to interview questions and completed a modified version of the CBA.	Patient perceptions of the most important caring behaviors of nurses were ranked. They included the following: knowing what they are doing, being kind and considerate, treating patients as individuals, reassuring, checking conditions closely, making patients feel that someone was there, doing what they said they would do, answering questions clearly, giving full attention; treating gently, being cheerful, and knowing how to handle equipment. The three subscales that were ranked as most important by both the myocardial infarction group and the perioperative group included the following: human needs assistance, teaching/learning; and humanism/faith-hope/sensitivity.

Continued

TABLE 13-2

Selected Research Studies Using Watson's Theory of Transpersonal Care—cont'd

Study/Year	Purpose	Methods	Findings
NURSE CARING CHARACTERISTICS—cont'd			
Ryan, 1992	The study determined most and least helpful nursing behaviors, as perceived by primary caregivers and hospice nurses.	Twenty primary caregivers and five hospice nurses completed a Q-sort that listed 60 caritive behaviors. They arranged the 60 cards into seven groups that ranged from most helpful to least helpful. Behaviors were then scored from 1 (least helpful) to 7 (most helpful).	The 10 most helpful behaviors identified by primary caregivers related to the following: patient psychosocial needs, patient physical needs, and caregiver psychosocial needs. Listening to the patient was ranked as most helpful behavior by primary caregivers. Hospice nurses ranked assuring the caregiver of the constant availability as the most helpful behavior.
Swanson-Kauffman, 1986	This qualitative study described the experiences and caring needs of women experiencing unexpected pregnancy loss.	Twenty women who had experienced spontaneous abortions before 16 weeks of pregnancy participated in two interviews regarding the pregnancy loss.	During the "knowing" phase, women wanted to be treated as persons experiencing loss within unique, personal contexts. "Being with" entailed feeling with the woman. "Doing for" was characterized by the woman's need to have others do for her during time of duress. "Enabling" was demonstrated by caring that facilitated woman's capacity to grieve and get through loss. "Maintaining belief" was represented by women's need to have others believe in their capacity to get through loss and to give birth in the future.
POPULATIONS NEEDING CARE			
Andershed and Ternestedt, 1999	This grounded theory study identified family member involvement in caring for dying relatives, developed theoretical understanding of family member involvement, and examined findings in light of two caring theories.	Six persons with dying spouses participated in interviews during the patient's final period of life and then 1 and 3 months after the patient's death. Patients died either in a surgical ward, an inpatient hospice ward, or a nursing home. The Glaser and Strauss constant comparative method was used for data analysis.	Three categories emerged. "To know" reflected caregivers' need to know more about the patient and was essential to further involvement in care. Knowing occurred through the patient, the staff, and through others. "To be" was a way of being present with the patient and being in the patient's world by knowing his or her needs and wishes. "To do" was a task-centered category that consisted of care actions or actions as spokespersons for the patient.

Martin, 1991	This qualitative study explored the experiences of adults with polycystic kidney disease.	Ninety-two participants were interviewed using a semistructured format.	Patients used multiple informal routes of seeking information—often not those of expert care providers. The diagnosis of polycystic kidney disease was not viewed as a "terrible" diagnosis. Divided views existed on the use of genetic screening. Knowledge of a polycystic kidney disease diagnosis would not influence family-planning decisions.
Nyman and Lützen, 1999	The study identified caring needs of rheumatoid arthritis patients.	Six women participated in a conversation guided by questions based on Watson's 10 carative factors. The sample was selected from women being treated with acupuncture for rheumatoid arthritis.	Discovered themes included the following: seeking help, searching for meaning (often between grief events and illness), uncertainty about day-to-day life, and fear of being disappointed in treatment.
Percy, 1995	This qualitative study described what homeless children living in shelter found meaningful.	Twelve children aged 6 to 12 used a camera to take pictures of what was special to them. During the initial interview, the word "special" was discussed, and children were given cameras. Follow-up interviews with each participant gave children an opportunity to view and describe their photographs. During the third interview, children ranked their five most special pictures.	Themes emerging from children aged 6 and 7 differed from those of children aged 9 to 12 years. Two themes of school-age children were having fun and special people. Preadolescent themes included feeling cared for and subthemes of belonging, trusting, relieving stress, and a special person's always being there.
Running, 1997	This qualitative study explored the experiences of adults aged 80 years and older who lived in a nursing home.	Six elders living in a nursing home took part in a "visit" process, in which weekly, unstructured interviews occurred over a 7-month period. Each resident was visited at least five times.	Individual vignettes of how persons came to be in a nursing home were shared. Findings focused on preserving individual stories rather than on categorizing composite commonalities.
Tracy, 1997	This hermeneutical, phenomenological study examined the experience of growing up with cystic fibrosis.	Ten adults participated in semistructured interviews about their experiences of growing up with cystic fibrosis.	Thematic findings included "being different," "don't call me terminal," "willpower," and "faith."
Weeks, 1995	The study examined the educational wants of prospective family caregivers of newly disabled adults.	Eighty-three prospective family caregivers responded to the Matthis Educational Wants of Family Caregivers of Disabled Adults Questionnaire.	The greatest interest in learning needs was about assisting the disabled adult and learning about health and human resources. Maintaining personal well-being was moderately important.

Continued

TABLE 13-2

Selected Research Studies Using Watson Theory of Transpersonal Care—cont'd

Study/Year	Purpose	Methods	Findings
OUTCOME STUDIES			
Duffy, 1992	This correlational study assessed the relationship of caring behaviors to hospitalized medical and surgical patient outcomes.	Eighty-six randomly selected patients responded to the Caring Assessment Tool, the Patient Satisfaction Visual Analog Scale, and the Sickness Impact Profile. The Medicus Patient Classification Tool measured required nursing hours per day. Nursing hours were multiplied by nursing hourly salary to calculate care cost.	As caring behaviors increased, patient satisfaction ($r = 0.46$, $p < 0.001$) also increased. No relationships between nurse caring behaviors and health status, length of stay, and cost of nursing care were found.
Leenerts, Koehler, and Neil, 1996	This descriptive survey obtained patient satisfaction and cost-effectiveness information related to use of the nursing caring partnership.	Seventy-five HIV positive patients who used the services of Caring Center responded to a 26-item questionnaire about satisfaction, hospitalizations, opinions about nursing care, cost effectiveness of care, and qualitative comments.	Patients indicated that nurses had increased their understanding of HIV/AIDS disease process, taught self-care skills to prevent hospitalization, and helped them follow their medical treatment plans, patients consulted nurses before primary care providers and received referrals to social service agencies. Cost savings for the third year were $1,590,384.

Neil and Schroeder, 1992	The study used focus groups to evaluate the Denver Nursing Project for Human Caring (DNPHC).	Fifty-one participants—including those with HIV, significant others, and clinic staff—responded to semistructured questions about services at the DNPHC. A total of eight focus groups were conducted.	Positive center aspects included caring behaviors, support groups, treatments, a nonclinical environment, and educational information. Areas for improvement included need for the following: longer clinic hours, emergency support, specialized support groups, varied support group meeting times, additional educational offerings, orientation and follow-up for new patients, improved social services, continuity of staff, publicity, and parking.
Schroeder and Maeve, 1992	The study evaluated nurse caring partnerships developed at the DNPHC.	A focus group was formed with nursing staff to elicit strengths and weaknesses of the program. Twenty nursing care records were randomly selected and reviewed for notation of carative factors (CF). Twenty-nine patients responded to a mailed survey. Three nurses and three patients gave narrative accounts of being in a Nursing Care Partnership (NCP).	Nurses highly valued partnerships as method to best interact with patients and to plan and coordinate care. Difficulties were having undisturbed time to plan care and role confusion. Limited documentation of carative factors was present. The most commonly documented CFs were the following: helping-trusting human care relationship; creative problem-solving caring process; supportive, protective and/or corrective mental, physical, societal, and spiritual environment; and medically supportive care. All respondents viewed the NCP program as supportive. Narrative accounts added further support for the value of NCPs.
Schroeder, 1993	The study examined the cost-effectiveness of the DNPHC caring program.	Using costs of HIV/AIDS care for Colorado and the US, the investigator computed costs for 240 patients in 1991 and 330 patients in 1992 who accessed the Caring Center.	Prevented hospital stays, shorter stays, complex medical treatments, and supported home deaths provided estimated savings of $785,744.00 for 1991 and $1,163,912.00 for 1992.

Nurses' Caring Behaviors. Caring behaviors of nurses have been the topic of a number of studies using Watson's Theory of Transpersonal Care. Some of these studies rely exclusively on Watson's theory as a guide; other studies, such as the one by Brown (1986), use several theorists' perspectives on caring to form a composite conceptualization.

Believing care to be the central focus of nursing, Brown (1986) gathered critical incidents from 55 hospitalized patients receiving care for medical and surgical problems. Brown used Watson's ten carative activities and caring concepts identified by other theorists to determine that caring was the central focus of nursing. Caring involved a process between nurse and patient, focusing on health attainment and maintenance or movement toward a peaceful death. Her qualitative analysis revealed eight major themes of care (see Table 13-2) and two patterns of care that were derived from the combined themes. These patterns included nurses' demonstration of professional knowledge and skill, surveillance, and reassuring presence. The second pattern related to nurses recognizing individual qualities and need, promoting autonomy, and spending time. This indicated that interactions were patient-focused rather than treatment-focused. Brown concluded that patients must first feel confident in the nurse's ability to provide physical care before more expressive caring concerns, such as listening and spending time, could be addressed. Although Brown's work was descriptive in terms of caring, relating the findings back to Watson's theory would have strengthened her study. Findings are congruent with Watson's carative factors of developing a helping trust relationship and providing a supportive, protective, and/or corrective mental, physical, sociocultural, and spiritual environment.

Ryan (1992) identified the most and least helpful caring behaviors exhibited by primary caregivers and hospice nurses in a hospice home care setting. Two of the helpful behaviors related to the physical needs of emergency management and comfort. Five behaviors were associated with patient psychosocial needs—listening to the patient, answering questions honestly, talking with patient to reduce fears, staying with the patient during difficult times, and assuring the patient that nursing services were always available. Three helpful behaviors related to the psychosocial needs of the caregiver. These included assuring nursing service availability, providing information needed for a death that occurs at home, and answering questions honestly. The highest ranked helpful behavior was listening to the patient, and the lowest ranked behavior was talking to the patient about guilt. This study supported Watson's contention that caring is central to nursing and, in this instance, to hospice nursing, in which both patients and primary caregivers receive care. Aspects of psychosocial care, including provision of information, active involvement of family in decision making, supportive environments, and trusting helpful relationships are related to Watson's carative factors. Increased awareness from both the patient's and the caregiver's perspectives of what is helpful in hospice care can assist in planning appropriate care.

Jensen, Bäck-Pettersson, and Segesten (1996) described essential characteristics of excellent nurses from the perception of 10 Danish women undergoing surgery and treatment for breast cancer. Critical caring factors were related to nurse competence in rendering care and their knowledge of human interactions. Nurses who acted from a humanistic and altruistic value system were called compassionate. Excellent nurses were perceived as genuine and respectful. Excellent nurses' ability to be near and act in an adequate manner during chaos indicated courage. Concordance was a crucial factor in establishing relationships with patients and in acting according to patient preferences to maintain harmonious relationships. Findings are congruent with Watson's identification that a humanistic and altruistic value system, courage, and the nature of the nurse patient relationship, in which nurses aid patients in integrating subjective, personal experiences with their objective views of the situation, are essential to caring.

Using a quantitative approach, Marini (1999) examined older adult perceptions of nurse caring behaviors. A small convenience sample of institutionalized older adults responded to a CBA that contained seven subscales related to carative behaviors. Behaviors perceived as most indicative of caring were assistance with human needs, such as nurses knowing what they were doing and calling the physician when necessary. The second most important subscale was related to humanism/faith-hope/sensitivity, which indicated the importance of being treated with respect and dignity. The study's value was limited by its small sample size and its failure to relate the findings back to Watson's Theory of Transpersonal Care.

Two studies specifically examined caring practices of perioperative nurses. One by Parsons, Kee, and Gray (1993) considered perceptions of surgical patients, whereas McNamara (1995) investigated nurses' perceptions. The study by Parsons, Kee, and Gray identified caring behaviors, weighted the importance of the behaviors, and compared behaviors identified by perioperative patients to those identified by patients experiencing a myocardial infarction. Based on the findings, investigators proposed that Watson's ten carative factors could be incorporated into nursing practice and were applicable regardless of the setting. Characteristics of caring were found to be important to perioperative patients—particularly in terms of attention to physical and emotional needs. Although rankings of the first three subscales of the CBA were similar for both perioperative and critical care patients, rankings differed in evaluating the importance of existential, phenomenological, and spiritual forces. This difference led investigators to conclude that these factors might be more important to critical care patients who faced more life-threatening problems. Caring factors were found in perioperative practice and were perceived as important to perioperative patients. This supported Watson's supposition.

McNamara's (1995) qualitative study of perioperative nurses examined perceptions of caring behaviors exhibited with conscious and unconscious patients in the perioperative period. Key elements of caring included showing concern for patients as unique humans, communicating, touching, and being sensitive to patients' experiences. Nurses demonstrated concern by providing spiritual and psychological supportive environments. During the preoperative period, caring behaviors focused on establishing trust. Caring behaviors shifted to providing safety and protection, which continued through the postoperative phase. Caring characteristics exhibited by nurses validated the dimensions of Watson's 10 carative factors. A limiting factor of this study was the very small sample size; only five nurses participated.

Using a caring framework that combined Watson's model with Leininger's model (1981), Swanson-Kauffman (1986) described perceptions of nurse caring by women who had unexpectedly lost a pregnancy. A central guiding thesis was Watson's contention that the personal dignity and worth of individuals must be recognized in the process of caring. Care for persons experiencing an unexpected pregnancy loss required supporting patients, attending to ongoing fears, and reassuring patients of their ability to get through the grieving process and to bear children in the future. Congruent with Watson's theory, Swanson-

Kauffman's findings indicated that nurse and patient interactions must focus on two persons striving to relate rather than maintaining separate roles.

Lemmer (1991) described carative behaviors of nurses as perceived by parents experiencing perinatal bereavement. Parents indicated that they were "taken care of" by nurses, which reflected the parents' ability to turn to nurses for knowledge and expertise to help regain control of the situation. Nurses were perceived as hands-on caregivers who attended to the woman's or the infant's condition and met comfort needs. Providing information was perceived as enormously important. Caring for or about the patients involved addressing emotional and affectional needs of the mothers, interpersonally interacting, and empathizing. Emotional support and family-centered care were hallmarks of this caring. Parents were concerned that their nurses lovingly care for their infants. Key behaviors by nurses included furnishing tangible evidence of the infants' lives through pictures and handprints. Respecting parents' rights, such as accommodating religious rites and providing privacy, were crucial. Noncaring behaviors were rooted in communication failures and time constraints. Patients' descriptions of the nursing behaviors reflected transactional caring as Watson suggested, and noncaring behaviors tended to occur more often in nurses not practicing from a transactional approach. A weakness of this study is its failure to discuss the findings in light of Watson's study.

Using Watson's theory as a basis, Cronin and Harrison (1988) examined indicators of caring as perceived by coronary care patients following myocardial infarctions. These patients found monitoring of their condition and demonstration of professional competence the most important indicators of caring. In general, attentiveness to human needs was found to be quite important. Although it was not identified as an important carative behavior during the early portion of the intensive care stay, expressions of positive and negative feelings became more important the longer the duration of the stay. This study supported Watson's contention that physiological needs must be met before more qualitative aspects of care become important.

Miller, Haber, and Byrne (1992) conducted a phenomenological study of acute-care patients and nurses about their perceptions of caring. Parallel descriptions of nurse caring were derived and indicated that caring nurses were individuals who connected with patients in professional and personal relationships that permitted monitoring and intervention. These findings were congruent with Watson's theory that patients value human care.

Most studies of nurse caring behaviors have focused on the actions of staff nurses. To gain a different perspective, Kerouac and Rouillier (1992) examined how head nurses can promote caring in their practices. This study was the outcome of a project designed to facilitate caring actions. A significant component discovered was that those nurses doing the caring also needed to receive care. The theoretical statement arising from the project study was "as caring is advocated by a facilitative nursing leader within a small group experience, nurses who benefit from the experience will exhibit caring behaviors toward their patients and peers and will interact in a healthy way within the organizational context" (p. 98). This study supports Watson's assumptions that caring is interpersonal, that it promotes growth, and that a caring environment can foster development. This study demonstrates the applicability of these ideas to the administrative level.

Dietrich (1992) also examined the environment of caring by exploring issues related to caring among nurses, identifying nurse-to-nurse caring and noncaring, and uncovering contextual factors that facilitated or inhibited caring among nurses. This study supported Watson's assumption that caring is interpersonal and demands connectedness, understanding, and support. Findings from this study are also congruent with those of Kerouac and Rouillier (1992) because both studies uncovered nurses' need to receive care in order to care for others.

Two studies (Dennis, 1991; Montgomery, 1992) examined the spiritual aspects of caring. Dennis undertook an exploratory study to discover nurses' descriptions of the components of spiritual care. She specifically used Watson's concepts of the spiritual aspects of human beings to frame and guide the study. Based on her findings, Dennis suggested that nursing is an art and a science that requires a wholistic view of care inseparable from other parts of nursing. Many of the components of transpersonal caring relationships that Watson describes were expressed in descriptions of spiritual care. Dennis (1991) asserts that two of Watson's tenets supported in this study of spiritual care are that the human soul can be undernourished and can need care and that transpersonal care is the core of nursing.

Montgomery (1992) examined a slightly different spiritual connection that focused on spirituality as a part of caring and derived a major theme of spiritual transcendence. In this spiritual transcendence, nurses connected with others at the level of the spirit, which permitted them to maintain involved professional relationships without succumbing to over-involvement. Spiritual transcendence in caring provided meaning for caregivers and helped to combat stressors. Finally, it better unified caring relationships. By focusing on the spiritual dimensions, Montgomery's study extends descriptions of nurse caring. In doing so, the study considers the concept of caring more wholistically.

To summarize, several studies discussed support aspects of Watson's Theory of Transpersonal Caring. Human care was found to be central and valued by patients (Miller, Haber, & Byrne, 1992). Studies upheld Watson's carative components of trust (Brown, 1986; McNamara, 1995), teaching/learning (Lemmer, 1991; Ryan 1992), provision of a supportive or protective environment (Cronin & Harrison, 1988; Lemmer, 1991; Ryan, 1992), humanistic value system (Jensen, Bäck-Pettersson, & Segesten, 1996; Marini, 1999), sensitivity to self and others (McNamara, 1995). These descriptive studies can provide insight about potential patient needs and concerns. Knowledge about these needs can be instrumental in assessing and planning care.

Studies about Caring Needs and Experiences of Specific Populations. Another way in which Watson's Theory of Transpersonal Care has influenced research is by philosophically supporting studies that investigate human experiences of residents in nursing homes, individuals coping with chronic diseases, and homeless children. These studies focus on caring needs experienced by different groups and suggest ways that caring might facilitate participants' well-being. These perceptions of caring are most commonly derived from the patients. One study, however, derived perceptions of caring from nurses. Two studies (Andershed & Ternestedt, 1999; Weeks, 1995) in this category focus on caring but examine family members who care for a relative who is disabled or is dying. These studies raise the issue of whether caring is unique to nursing.

Running (1997) described the experience of living in a nursing home for individuals 80 years of age or older. Running's "visit" method involves multiple weekly visits to residents for interviews. Rather than integrating and categorizing the stories to form a composite of the residents, researchers allow the stories to be presented as individual vignettes.

Through stories about why participants were in the nursing home and about how they coped with being there, investigators gained insights into the patients' experiences. Drawing conclusions and applying them elsewhere, however, was more difficult. Running ignores these aspects. Support for Watson's Theory of Transpersonal Caring might be derived from the fact that the individuality of the interactions is preserved in this technique. However, Watson's theory in this context is more related to the nature of the relationship between the resident and the investigator in the research process than in potential findings. Consequently, it is difficult to assess the support these insights collectively bring to Watson's theory or to provide comprehensive recommendations for future research.

Martin (1991) used Watson's theory to qualitatively explore the experiences of adults with polycystic kidney disease. Half of the sample was receiving dialysis, and the other half was not yet dialysis-dependent. Based on the findings, Martin recommended sensitivity to patients' needs for information. In congruence with Watson's theory, Martin suggested that nurses assist in searching for patients' personal meanings of polycystic kidney disease. Nurses need to work within the context of relationships and understand that genetic testing may frighten patients. Finally, sensitivity must be exercised in family planning decisions with patients.

Tracy (1997) conducted a phenomenological study of growing up with cystic fibrosis. The theme "being different" was exemplified by feelings of knowing that there was a difference from those without chronic illness but not feeling different than others with a chronic problem. Most thought of themselves as healthy. Tracy's phrase "Don't call me terminal" was characterized by participants' anticipated length of life and desire to not be treated as a statistic. "Willpower and faith" were focused on participants' willingness to focus on their goals and attempts not to become discouraged. Tracy derived several nursing implications based on findings and reflection on Watson's theory. Carative factors indicate that nurses can practice with greater understanding. Tracy suggested that nurses could examine Watson's carative factor of a humanistic altruistic value system in their personal views and growth experiences. This would increase nursing maturity, and the resulting insight would permit more altruistic behavior toward patients. Carative factors of faith and hope should permit nurture of faith and hope in chronically ill patients. Two strengths of this study are the discovery of the experience of growing up with a chronic illness and the close tie of the findings to the carative factors Watson suggested. The implication of this study is that caring nurses need to be sensitive to what is important to children growing up with a chronic illness.

Using Watson's conceptualization of human care as an orienting framework, Percy (1995) asked homeless children living in a shelter to take photographs to describe what was special or meaningful to them. By understanding what was meaningful, Percy hoped to uncover inner resources that could overcome health challenges. School-age children expressed that having fun was important. Playing, having toys, going fun places, and having people with whom to share fun were important. Special people, usually mothers or grandmothers that cared for the youngsters, were also important to school-age children. Preadolescents indicated that feeling cared for and having someone always there were of primary importance. Other important areas for preadolescents included a sense of belonging, trust in friends and others, fun, and relief from stress through play. The theme of always being there demonstrated the need for someone or something that provided support. Watson's theory offered a perspective in this study in that it calls for a commitment to preserving and enhancing the dignity of human beings. Percy linked preservation of dignity with actions that were facilitated by nurses' understanding of how homeless children derive meaning. Future studies should consider wholistic approaches that focus on the participants' perspectives. If nurses can better understand homelessness in children, they will be more sensitive to their needs and can design more effective interventions.

Using Watson's ten carative factors, Nyman and Lützen (1999) identified caring needs of patients with rheumatoid arthritis who sought acupuncture. An interesting finding in this study is the focus on individuals informing themselves rather than relying on the care provider for information. This finding may relate to the fact that these women were seeking acupuncture treatment for their rheumatoid arthritis. The carative factor of developing a trusting relationship was particularly difficult for the women because many had been disappointed by traditional medicine before seeking acupuncture. This study primarily provides insights for nurses treating patients who seek alternative therapies for a chronic problem.

Using Watson's proposal that perceiving can lead to caring behaviors, Weeks (1995) studied the educational needs of prospective family caregivers for newly disabled adults. The investigator proposed that the caregiver's sensitivity to family educational needs would help family members handle painful feelings, adapt to new roles, and gain confidence in providing care. Increasing nurses' understanding of family educational needs would facilitate caring behaviors toward family caregivers. Watson's carative factors suggest that a sensitivity to self and others must be cultivated and that nurses should promote interpersonal teaching and learning. Weeks found that family caregivers most wanted to know how to assist disabled adults and to learn about health and human resources. Family caregivers also wanted to learn how to maintain their own well-being. Although this information provides insight to nurses teaching caregivers for disabled adults, Weeks failed to tie the findings to Watson's Theory of Human Caring.

Andershed and Ternestedt (1999) took a different look at caring by examining how hospice nurses could guide family members to care for dying relatives. Investigators based their study on Leininger's suggestion (1988, 1991) that care practices are founded on values, beliefs, and social structures present in various cultures. Investigators also considered Watson's belief that human care is a demonstrable interpersonal process. Findings indicated that family members can be involved in a relative's dying in three different ways: knowing, being, and doing. Andershed and Ternestedt compared family involvement to that of professional caregivers. Although knowing was not part of Watson's theory, being was congruent with Watson's description of authentic presence. Doing was also consistent with Watson's carative factor of assisting persons in meeting basic needs while protecting dignity and wholeness. Researchers proposed that nurses guide relatives in providing care for their dying family members.

Many of the studies (Martin, 1991; Tracy, 1997; Percy, 1995; Weeks, 1995) investigated the needs of patients handling chronic problems. Carative factors associated with these patients included help seeking (Nyman & Lützen, 1999), a search for meaning (Nyman & Lützen, 1999; Tracy, 1997), and promotion of teaching and learning (Weeks, 1995). Although these studies were descriptive, they supported the aforementioned carative factors. Further exploration to discover the nature of needs of individuals experiencing other chronic health problems is needed. As needs become known, evaluation of interventions to resolve those needs should be completed.

Outcomes Studies. Although most research using Watson's concepts of transpersonal care are descriptive, a limited number of studies focus on outcomes. Four of these studies, found in Table 13-2 and described in the following paragraphs, are related to the Denver Nursing Project in Human Caring (DNPHC). An additional study by Duffy (1992) focuses on outcomes of medical or surgical patients. These studies represent the initial look at how nurse caring behaviors make a difference in patient outcomes. These studies approach outcomes from a qualitative perspective (Neil & Schroeder, 1992; Schroeder & Maeve, 1992) or descriptively explain costs (Schroeder, 1993; Leenerts, Koehler, & Neil, 1996). These are not experimental studies.

Nursing Care Partnerships at the DNPHC has been the source four studies (Neil & Schroeder, 1992; Schroeder & Maeve, 1992; Schroeder, 1993; Leenerts, Koehler, & Neil, 1996) that focus on the effects of interventions derived from Watson's work in transpersonal caring. The DNPHC is a nursing center grounded in Watson's philosophy of human caring. The Nursing Care Partnership model (NCP) emerged from an evaluation study and emphasizes collaborative connecting between nurse and patient to achieve mutual empowerment. Patients who use the Caring Center can access medically supportive nursing services and independent nursing services to promote health and healing. These services can include therapeutic touch, massage, counseling, education about care management, emotional support, and coordination of services.

Using focus groups to evaluate the caring program, Neil and Schroeder (1992) conducted the initial evaluation study for the DNPHC. Descriptive information derived from the focus groups of patients, significant others, and care providers identified the strengths and weaknesses of the DNPHC program (see Table 13-2). A positive outcome using the focus group method for evaluation was that participants felt valued by being able to tell their stories. Because of their sensitivity to others, focus groups were perceived to be discovery techniques congruent with Watson's theoretical perspectives.

Schroeder and Maeve (1992) further evaluated the DNPHC. The concept of NCPs was an outgrowth of findings from the initial evaluation focus groups conducted by Neil and Schroeder (1992). These partnerships enable the establishment of caring relationships between patients and nurses with the goal of mutual empowerment. This partnership is designed so that patient care will be facilitated throughout an illness. One strength of this study is the connection between the philosophical tenets of Watson's Theory of Human Caring and the practical realities of implementing a program based on those characteristics. All methods of evaluation—nurse focus groups, chart review, patient survey, and narrative accounts—support the value of nurse caring partnerships. This study determined that Watson's ideas about transpersonal caring can be implemented and that positive outcomes can be realized.

In a series of two studies, the cost-effectiveness of the DNPHC was estimated for the years 1991 and 1992 (Schroeder, 1993) as well as for 1993 (Leenerts, Koehler, & Neil, 1996). The partnership emphasized Watson's concept of a caring consciousness and the collaborative nurse-patient connecting process. These studies sought to demonstrate that theory-based caring models can improve both quality of care and patient use of healthcare services. Using estimated costs of care for HIV patients in Colorado, Schroeder (1993) estimated the savings in hospital charges for prevented hospital stays, shortened lengths of stay, complex medically supported treatments, and supported deaths at home.

Using Schroeder's cost-effectiveness evaluation for 1991 and 1992, Leenerts, Koehler, and Neil (1996) examined the cost-effectiveness of the DNPHC for 1993. Congruent with Schroeder's study (1993), significant cost savings were achieved once again. In these studies, nurse-patient partnerships prevented hospital stays, shortened length of stay when patients were hospitalized, and prevented readmissions. These factors resulted in significant cost savings over those not receiving services from the Caring Center. Patients expressed satisfaction with the wholistic nature of the care and preferred involving the nursing care partner in hospital care and discharge planning. These studies are an exciting example of how a nursing model driven by Watson's theory can impact patient outcomes in a cost-effective manner.

In an outcome study not related to the Denver project, Duffy (1992) focused on the relationship of caring behaviors to outcomes of health status, satisfaction, length of stay, and nursing care cost of hospitalized medical and surgical patients. As predicted, a significant relationship between nurse caring behaviors and patient satisfaction was present. As caring behaviors increased, so did patient satisfaction. However, no relationships between caring behaviors and patient health status, length of stay, and nursing care costs emerged. This study supports Watson's contention that nurse caring promotes patient satisfaction.

To summarize the outcome studies, the DNPHC studies demonstrated that Watson's theoretical model could be implemented in a primary care setting and that cost savings could be achieved while offering coordinated care. In Duffy's study (1992)—which examined caring behaviors for their relationship to health status, length of stay, nursing costs, and satisfaction of hospitalized medical and surgical patients—patients were more satisfied by nurses practicing from Watson's theory. However, unlike the studies by Schroeder (1993) and Leenerts, Koehler, and Neil (1996), cost savings were not demonstrated. Further investigation regarding specific caring factors that influence patient outcomes needs to be completed.

Research Summary. The research review of studies using Watson's theory revealed a number of published studies that were primarily descriptive. Only five studies were aimed toward nursing intervention and outcome evaluation. Four of these studies were related to the DNPHC (Duffy, 1992; Leenerts, Koehler, & Neil, 1996; Neil & Schroeder, 1992; Schroeder & Maeve, 1992; Schroeder, 1993), and in these studies a nursing care model based on Watson's philosophy of human caring clearly demonstrated positive, cost-effective outcomes. Duffy (1992) demonstrated increased patient satisfaction but could not demonstrate cost-effectiveness. Although descriptive information is valuable, these studies do not demonstrate the value of nurse caring behaviors. This factor is of critical consideration in nursing—a profession that prides itself on caring—but it has not yet substantiated the value of caring in practice. Research using Watson's philosophy reflects the presuppositions or gut instincts that caring is important, but more research that conclusively demonstrates the value of caring is needed. Although further description of caring can be useful, intervention studies are critically needed. In addition, studies that specifically address Watson's theory would be help to test the theoretical propositions. Many studies used a composite of several caring frameworks to lay the groundwork for their investigations.

PRAXIS AND THEORY UTILIZATION: DESIGNING NURSING PRACTICE PROGRAMS WITHIN WATSON'S THEORETICAL SYSTEM

Life is not a problem to be solved but a mystery to be lived. (Watson, 1985, p. ix)

Although in recent writings Watson (1999) describes her transpersonal caring-healing model as a transformative paradigm beyond nursing, the following discussion of application of this theory to practice is confined to nursing practice.

Watson (1994) states that her theory of caring provides practicing nurses with both a philosophy and theory based on the act of caring. From this perspective, at the heart of the nursing profession is a covenant "to develop with the other a trusting, caring-healing relationship that potentiates health and well-being, physical comfort, symptom management, and pain control and promotes meaning, growth, and harmony between provider and other" (Watson, 1994, p. 1). Watson does not view the theory as a rule for nursing practice but rather as a means for focusing on the human dimensions of practice. She views caring as a mode of being human and professional caring as a "special way of being in relation to self, other, and being in the world" (Watson, 1994, p. 3). The emphasis on the artistry of nursing, with being and knowing in relation to caring, is as important as doing.

Nurses are required to consider both personally and professionally what it means to be human. Characteristics of being human within this perspective include viewing the self and other as subjectively whole, accepting that being evolves and changes through greater consciousness of self and its relation to the world, and knowing that embodiment is more than physical. From a professional perspective, the nurse acknowledges a *caring moment—* that is, the moment in time when nurse and another individual engage in transpersonal caring (see Figure 13-1). These transpersonal caring relationships are mutual and reciprocal. The values and beliefs of both persons are equally significant. The contribution and perspective of each within the relationship may be different. The focus of the patient is self-directed; the focus of the nurse is other-directed. The patient seeks help, whereas the nurse's involvement is in terms of being and becoming in the relationship. The patient's immediate distress generates in the nurse a reflective process that leads to being with the patient, sharing the experience, and attempting to help through this spiritual union of two persons (Watson, 1985). The caring relationship between nurse and other can become an existential turning point. Significant healing possibilities may originate in this turning point (Watson, 1994). Watson (1994) explains that at this point,

> new levels of nursing competencies arise, such as authenticity of being, ability to be authentically present to self and other in reflective caring sense, ability to center one's consciousness and intentionality to promote caring-healing outcomes and wholeness. Responsivity, mutuality, intersubjectivity, and the full engagement and expressivity of the nurse as appropriate to the caring needs of the other are paramount" (p. 5).

The Variables of Concern for Practice

Variables of concern in practicing nursing from the perspective of Watson's theory include the ten carative components presented in Box 13-3; a moral commitment to protect, enhance and preserve human dignity; and nurses' respect for the subjective significance of the patient (Watson, 1985; Sourial, 1996). The carative components presuppose a technical knowledge base and clinical competence. Watson does not elaborate on the substance of the technical knowledge base nor on clinical competence. The carative components are not meant to be prescriptive but rather to guide practice philosophically. Although Watson states that the carative components direct assessment, charting, and engagement in caring practices and although the DNPHC has demonstrated their use, their substantive structure has not been developed. It presently depends on individual interpretation or group consensus.

Watson (1999) also has identified intentionality, nonlocal consciousness, and quantum ambiguity as factors significant in the practice of nursing. The meaning of these in relation to nursing needs to be explored further to facilitate translation into nursing practice.

Describing a Population for Nursing Purposes

At this stage of development, it is not appropriate to use the theory for describing populations for nursing purposes.

Expected Outcomes of Nursing

The outcomes identified in the DNPHC of practicing nursing from this perspective included "seeing the uniqueness and wholeness of the person-family, coming home, discovering a personal path for healing, and feeling the energy of love and compassion" (Smith, 1997, p. 56). The possible outcomes identified by Sourial (1996) include transcendence, harmony, and healing (see Figure 13-1). Watson (1988b) suggests that nurse-recipient interaction can facilitate the patient directing energy to his or her own healing process.

Process Models

The processes of nursing center on establishing and maintaining a subject-to-subject, human-to-human caring relationship. The nurse possesses an intentional caring-healing consciousness that, along with the caring acts, facilitates healing and wholeness. Sourial (1996) describes the process of nursing as a construction of human care transactions in relation to the actual caring occasion. When nurse and patient come together, an intersubjective caring occasion occurs in which the subjective worlds of the participants in the caring occasion meet in the transpersonal caring moment. Watson defines **transpersonal caring** as "the full actualisation of the carative factors in a human-to-human transaction" (1989, p. 232).

The DNPHC developed a model called *nursing care partnerships* that is based in Watson's theory of caring (Schroeder & Maeve, 1992). Unfortunately, this demonstration project has been discontinued. The goal of nursing at the center was "to help persons gain harmony within mind, body, and soul" (Schroeder & Maeve, 1992, p. 27). Fundamental to the model is the idea of intersubjective caring-healing. Mutual empowerment through authentic caring relationships is to be achieved through mutual consent partnerships between patients and nurses. The nurse, through interviews, strives to understand the lived experiences of the recipient of care. The nurse uses appropriate carative factors as organizers in the documentation process.

Watson (1999) emphasizes spiritual caring as the central process of nursing. Care is not a noun or a verb but a way of being. Caring is consciousness as energy. Through caring, the energy is shared and directed toward healing. This requires "regular spiritual, contemplative, meditative centering practice from the practitioner" (Watson, 1999, p. 179). The modalities of transpersonal caring are auditory, visual, olfactory, tactile, gustatory, mental-cognitive, being, and presence.

Practice Models

The state of development of this theory does not yet support development of nursing practice models within the frame of reference introduced in Chapter 3. Before such models can be developed, study and analysis of individual cases and nursing populations is required, as is additional research and specification of theoretical and operational variables. In addition to the carative components, caring behaviors have been identified in a number of research studies. These have primarily been identified from the patient's perspective. Further study and exploration may lead to the development of practice models associated with these caring behaviors. However, because Watson does not view the theory as prescriptive, it may not be appropriate to consider developing practice models.

Implications for Administration

Implementing caring theory within an organization requires a structure that promotes the development of nurse-patient relationships as well as caring behaviors in management-staff interactions. Such structures incorporate principles of autonomy, flexibility, and creativity. Primary nursing service delivery models are preferred to functional work assignments. Nyberg (1994) suggests that staff development associated with implementing Watson's theory of caring in practice should include the following:

- Emphasis on self-worth
- Committing to patients and their families rather than to the delivery system, emphasizing patients' whole needs, and assignments that provide for continuous care
- Encouraging openness to patients' and staff's communications
- Prioritizing caring
- Recognizing that all people have the potential to learn and to grow
- Teaching new modalities of care such as therapeutic touch, imaging, music, art, massage, and relaxation

Watson (1994) describes the following outcomes of her theory on a practice setting:

- Provision of a moral foundation that results in commitment "to preserving integrity and wholeness of self/other in relation to patients, families, communities" (p. 5).
- Attempts by the nurse to stay within the patient's frame of reference in order "to promote a mutual search toward meaning and wholeness of being, while honoring diversity and the inner cultural life world of the other" (p. 5).
- Preservation of the "humanity, dignity, and integrity of self and other(s)" by the nurse (p. 5).
- Nurses' use of modalities that include "compassionate listening to competencies required by complex medical technologies, to advanced caring-healing derived from the arts and humanities" (p. 5).

Thus the theory of caring would not only be evident in the interaction between the nurse and the patient, family, or community but also would be evident in relationships and interactions among all persons in the healthcare setting and potentially in the community at large. Watson suggests that agencies should use the language of human caring, including the ten carative components, to guide assessment, nursing acts, recording, quality assurance criteria, and research. Within this environment the contribution of all persons would be equal and necessary.

The DNPHC project demonstrated a structure of nursing practice from the caring perspective and carried this philosophy from the mission statement to individual nurse acts to recording in the patient record and evaluating effectiveness in terms of patient and economic outcomes. They established this project as an economically viable delivery of nursing services to a particular population—patients with human immunodeficiency virus (HIV) or acquired immunodeficiency syndrome (AIDS), their partners, and their families. Within this project, staff, clients, environment, and even their consciousnesses were considered interconnected, (Hecomovich, 1994).

Research in relation to caring behaviors could expand to performance appraisal guidelines that could guide implementation of caring practice–based nursing in an organization.

Implications for Education

Watson views knowledge development and the teaching-learning process as more than a cognitive rational process. It is a human process and activity (Watson, 1989). Nursing education should proceed using methods "that attend to the moral ideals and values that are relational, subjective inner experiences, while honoring intuition, personal, spiritual cognitive, and physical senses alike" (Watson, 1989). Caring and healing are linked. Educators within this perspective care for their students by enabling them to "know their own voice" (p. 53) and by encouraging students' self-affirmation and self-discovery. Modeling and dialogue are prime modalities of education from this perspective. The relationship of teacher and student in the clinical area would involve constant demonstration of caring behaviors and dialogue as students learned the processes associated with human care transactions.

Future Theory Developments Required to Facilitate Practice

The ten carative components can be used to estimate the state of caring-healing practices of individual nurses, and/or of an organization. As demonstrated in the DNPHC (Schroeder & Maeve, 1992; Watson, 1994), they can guide assessment, charting, and evaluation of patient-care decisions and outcomes. They can indicate quality outcome measures that are nursing- or patient-centered. They can clarify values to establish priorities and translate them into action. They specify caring practices for patient-identified populations. They can also provide a database for a broad spectrum of research that stems from the caring perspective. However, agencies that wish to use Watson's carative factors would first need to develop the substantive structure of each so that all nursing staff would clearly understand the meaning of each. For example, what is meant by "instilling of faith-hope"? How is this accomplished? What criteria would be used to indicate that this had been accomplished?

New caring modalities are required for practice from this perspective. What are these modalities? What is meant by "healing"? How is it accomplished? What are natural healing modalities? What is involved in the practice of knowing and being and doing in caring relationships? How does one develop/perfect caring behaviors? What are caring behaviors?

McCance, McKenna, and Boore (1999) raise the very practical question of whether it possible to use Watson's theory in practice without an extensive understanding of the existential-phenomenological-spiritual underpinnings of this theory.

NEXUS

In moving the caring-healing model beyond nursing, Watson obscures the object of nursing. How a nurse comes into a professional relationship with another person remains in question. The distinction between human caring as a general case and nursing as a particular case is not made. It seems that one must first be a nurse to understand Watson's concerns and to be able to transform oneself. Barker, Reynolds and Ward (1995) are concerned that the focus of nursing is not expressed in the literature on caring. They find it an "unnecessary distraction from the continued exploration of the boundaries of nursing" (p. 396) and from establishing the *raison d'etre* of nursing.

Watson noted that caring in nursing conveys bodily physical acts but emphasizes "authentic presencing of being in the caring moments, carrying an intentional caring-healing consciousness" (1999, p. 10). She concluded with the statement that "the hope is that academic nursing will transform its educational-practice models to prepare practitioners to practice the more complete paradigm of nursing, one that not only is able to integrate medical and technological aspects into its practices but also transforms them along with a totally new view of advanced nursing practice" (1999, p. 233).

REFERENCES

Andershed, B. & Ternestedt, B. (1999). Involvement of relatives in care of the dying in different care cultures: Development of a theoretical understanding. *Nursing Science Quarterly, 12*(1), 45-51.

Barker, P.J., Reynolds, W., & Ward, T. (1995). The proper focus of nursing: a critique of the caring ideology. *International Journal of Nursing Studies, 32*(4), 386-397.

Brown, L. (1986). The experience of care: Patient perspectives. *Topics in Clinical Nursing, 8*(2), 56-62.

Conway, M.E. (1985). Toward greater specificity in defining nursing's metaparadigm. *Advances in Nursing Science, 7*(4), 73-81.

Cronin, S. & Harrison, B. (1988). Importance of nurse caring behaviors as perceived by patients after myocardial infarction. *Heart-Lung, 17*(4), 374-380.

Dennis, P. (1991). Components of spiritual nursing care from the nurse's perspective. *Journal of Holistic Nursing, 9*(1), 27-42.

Dietrich, L. (1992). The caring nursing environment. In D. Gaut (Ed.), *The presence of caring in nursing.* New York: National League for Nursing.

Duffy, J. (1992). The impact of caring on patient outcomes. In D. Gaut (Ed.), *The presence of caring in nursing.* New York: National League for Nursing.

Hecomovich, K. (1994). Learning to work together in a way that nurtures our ability to care. In D. Gaut, (Ed.), *The presence of caring in nursing.* New York: National League for Nursing.

Jensen, K., Bäck-Pettersson, S. & Segesten, K. (1993). The caring moment and the green-thumb phenomenon among Swedish nurses. *Nursing Science Quarterly, 6*(2), 98-104.

Jensen, K., Bäck-Pettersson, S., & Segesten, K. (1996). Catching my wavelength: Perceptions of the excellent nurse. *Nursing Science Quarterly, 9*(3), 115-120.

Kerouac, S. & Rouillier, L. (1992). Reflections on the promotion of caring with head nurses. In D. Gaut (Ed.), *The presence of caring in Nursing.* New York: National League for Nursing.

Leenerts, M., Koehler, J., & Neil, R. (1996). Nursing care models increase quality while reducing costs. *Journal of the Association of Nurses in AIDS Care, 7*(4), 37-49.

Leininger, M. (1981). *Caring: An essential human* need. Thorofare, NJ: Charles B. Slack.

Leininger, M.M. (1988). Care: The essence of nursing and health. In M.M. Leininger (Ed.), *Care: The essence of nursing and health.* Detroit: Wayne State University Press.

Leininger, M.M. (1991). *Culture care diversity and universality: A theory of nursing.* New York: National League for Nursing.

Lemmer, C. (1991). Parental perceptions of caring following perinatal bereavement. *Western Journal of Nursing Research, 13*(4), 475-493.

Marini, B. (1999). Institutionalized older adults' perceptions of nurse caring behaviors: A pilot study. *Journal of Gerontological Nursing, 25*(5), 11-15.

Martin, L.S. (1991). Using Watson's theory to explore the dimensions of adult polycystic kidney disease. *ANNA Journal, 18*(5), 493-499.

McCance, T.V., McKenna, H.P., & Boore, J.R.P. (1999). Caring: theoretical perspectives of relevance to nursing. *Journal of Advanced Nursing, 30*(6), 1388-1395.

McNamara, S. (1995). Perioperative nurses' perceptions of caring practices. *AORN Journal, 61*(2), 377-382, 384-388.

Miller, B., Haber, J., & Byrne, M. (1992). The experience of caring in the acute care setting: Patient and nurse perspectives. In D. Gaut (Ed.), *The presence of caring in nursing.* New York: National League for Nursing.

Montgomery, C. (1992). The spiritual connection: Nurses' perceptions of the experience of caring. In D. Gaut (Ed.), *The presence of caring in nursing.* New York: National League for Nursing.

Neil, R. & Schroeder, C. (1992). Evaluation research within the human caring framework. In D. Gaut (Ed.), *The presence of caring in nursing.* New York: National League for Nursing.

Nyberg, J. (1994). Implementing Watson's theory of caring. In J. Watson (Ed.), *Applying the art and science of human caring.* New York: National League for Nursing.

Nyman, C. & Lützen, K. (1999). Caring needs of patients with rheumatoid arthritis. *Nursing Science Quarterly, 12*(2), 164-169.

Parsons, E., Kee, C., & Gray, D. (1993). Perioperative nurse caring behaviors: Perceptions of surgical patients. *AORN Journal, 57*(5), 1106-1114.

Percy, M. (1995). Children from homeless families describe what is special in their lives. *Holistic Nursing Practice, 9*(4), 24-33.

Running, A. (1997). Snapshots of experience: Vignettes from a nursing home. *Journal of Advanced Nursing, 25*(1), 117-122.

Ryan, P. (1992). Perceptions of the most helpful nursing behaviors in a home-care hospice setting: Caregivers and nurses. *American Journal of Hospice & Palliative Care, 9*(5), 22-31.

Schroeder, C. & Maeve, M. (1992). Nursing care partnerships at the Denver nursing project in human caring: An application and extension of caring theory in practice. *Advances in Nursing Science, 15*(2), 25-38.

Schroeder, C. (1993). Nursing's response to the crisis of access, costs, and quality in healthcare. *Advances in Nursing Science, 16*(1), 1-20.

Smith, M.C. (1997). Practice guided by Watson's theory: The Denver Nursing Project in human caring. *Nursing Science Quarterly, 10*(1), 56-58.

Sourial, S. (1996). An analysis and evaluation of Watson's theory of human care. *Journal of Advanced Nursing, 24*(2), 400-404.

Swanson-Kauffman, K. (1986). Caring in the instance of unexpected early pregnancy loss. *Topics in Clinical Nursing, 8*(2), 37-46.

Tracy, J. (1997). Growing up with chronic illness: The experience of growing up with cystic fibrosis. *Holistic Nursing Practice, 12*(1), 27-35.

Watson, J. (1979). *Nursing: The philosophy and science of caring.* Boston: Little, Brown.

Watson, J. (1985). *Nursing: Human science and human care. A theory of nursing.* Norwalk, CT: Appleton-Century-Crofts.

Watson, J. (1988a). New dimensions of human caring theory. *Nursing Science Quarterly, 1*(4), 175-181.

Watson, J. (1988b). *Nursing: Human science and human care. A theory of nursing.* Sudbury, MA: Jones and Bartlett.

Watson, J. (1989). Transformative thinking and a caring curriculum. In E.O. Bevis & J. Watson (Eds.), *Toward a caring curriculum: A new pedagogy for nursing.* New York: National League for Nursing.

Watson, J. (1994). *Applying the art and science of human caring.* New York: National League for Nursing.

Watson, J. (1997). The Theory of Human Caring: retrospective and prospective. *Nursing Science Quarterly, 10*(1), 49-52.

Watson, J. (1999). *Postmodern nursing and beyond*. Edinburgh: Churchill Livingstone.

Weeks, S. (1995). What are the educational needs of prospective family caregivers of newly disabled adults. *Rehabilitation Nursing, 20*(5), 256-260, 272, 298.

Wolf, Z. (1986). The caring concept and nurse identified caring behaviors. *Topics in Clinical Nursing, 8*(2), 84-93.

Wolf, Z., Giardino, E., Osborne, P., & Ambrose, M. (1994). Dimensions of nurse caring. *Image, 26*(2), 107-111.

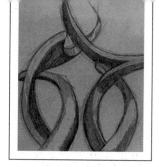

Epilogue

THE INTEGRATION of NURSING THEORY and RESEARCH for PRACTICE

USING THE PAST TO CREATE THE FUTURE: THE INTEGRATION OF NURSING THEORY AND RESEARCH FOR PRACTICE

The central metaphor for the integration of theory, research, and practice is the nexus. Unit 1 described the broad concept of the nexus. The integration within each theoretical system was the focus of Unit 2. Consideration should be given at this time to integrating current nursing theoretical systems into a few highly developed theoretical systems. There are two aspects to this work: (1) the evaluation and organization of existing work in nursing theoretical systems, and (2) a commitment to deriving further research and practice from existing nursing theoretical systems.

EXISTING THEORETICAL SYSTEMS
Nursing: A Practice Discipline with Practical Science

It is ultimately the knowledgeable practice of nursing in service of the public that must drive nursing scholars and practitioners. As the discipline develops, its knowledge must be applied to that service. Persons who provide a particular service to the public and use a particular and unique body of knowledge characterize a profession. The development of the discipline must be integrated with the development of the profession of nursing for knowledge to have meaning. The focus of knowledge development should come from and feed back into the general nursing theoretical systems. Developing research and knowledge within a theoretical system will expedite the progress of nursing as a discipline.

As a practice discipline, nursing is concerned with the development of knowledge and the use of that knowledge to structure and inform practice. Nurses can no longer be satisfied with describing their practice in terms of what tasks they perform. The focus on outcomes and quality demands that nurses be able to articulate knowledgeably and convincingly the reasons for what they do. To do this, nurses must first understand the *why* of what they are doing as well as what they could and should be contributing to healthcare. They need to be able to communicate this to a broader public—the other health professionals with whom they work, the policymakers whose decisions influence their profession, and, most importantly, the public they serve. Professional knowledge includes awareness of the conditions necessary for effective nursing; however, such knowledge development needs to be based in a clear understanding of the object of nursing.

The linking of theory and research to practice is accomplished through processes of development and diffusion. Development makes abstract knowledge useful in concrete ways. Using nursing research findings is not only significant in the individual nurse's practice. In a broader context, nursing practice improves as research findings and advances in nursing knowledge become the foundation for the development of practice procedures, protocols, and programs. These advances, when diffused to a broader public, impact the provision and structure of healthcare. The importance of formal development processes in integrating theory and research is illustrated in Figure 14-1. The development of practice models

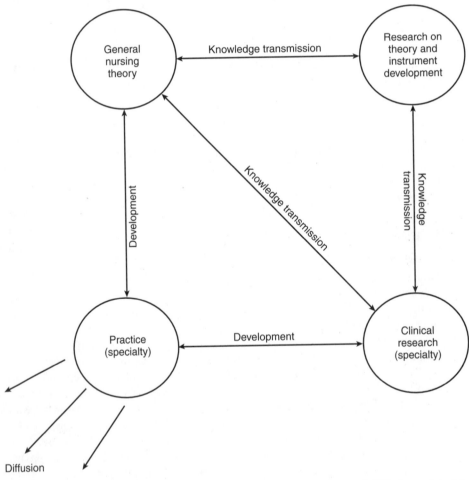

FIGURE 14-1 The linking processes of transmission, development, and diffusion related to theory, research, and practice.

should be a national or even international effort, not simply an institutional effort or the work of individual researchers. This is both an efficient and effective approach. This approach will also facilitate the development of policy initiatives relevant to the object of nursing. The efforts to identify nursing interventions and outcomes and to construct evidence-based nursing practice are examples of some broader initiatives.

Recognition of the Duality in the Ontology of the Discipline

The ontology of the discipline must include the nature of person and the nature of relationships. Some theoretical systems include progressive development of both, as in the work of Orem and Watson. Others have more high developed one side, as in Peplau's emphasis on relationships. Still others focus on only a single element within the ontology, such as in Pender's Health Promotion Model.

The ontology of person is necessary for understanding why a person needs or can benefit from nursing and for recognizing the characteristics or attributes of the nurse. Some theorists—notably Orem, Roy, Neuman, Pender, and Peplau—base their conceptualizations on persons who have a capacity for deliberate action and who can modify themselves or their environments to produce change. These theories more typically identify characteristics of persons than clarify the object of nursing. Others, such as Rogers, Parse, and Watson, are less specific about personal characteristics that engender change. The focus on mutual simultaneous interaction with the environment gives as much power to the environment as to the person.

Some theorists have identified the characteristics or dimensions of the patient but have not extended these same characteristics to the nurse. For example, Roy described the person as an adaptive system from the patient's perspective. She has yet to similarly describe the nurse. Nursing, then, is the interaction of two adapting systems within some broader system. Any change within one system must affect the other; this applies to both nurses and patients. Orem, Roy, and Pender explicitly call for nurses to be engaged with patients on that level.

An ontology of interaction is necessary to express the nurse-patient relationship. Nursing is, in essence and in existence, interpersonal. Some theorists, such as Peplau, focus primarily on the interpersonal interaction. Some, such as Rogers and Parse, focus on the interaction of person and environment. They hold strongly to the mutuality and simultaneity of the person-environment interaction. Parse described the relationship as subject-to-subject engagement, a "being with" that differs from an interaction (Huch, 1991). Others include the interaction as an integral element of their theories. This is most notable in Orem's and in Parse's work. Models built on general system theory, including those of King and Neuman, apparently assume that the nurse is a part of the system, but the nurse's role is not made explicit in their models. Watson describes the ontology of nursing as a relational ontology based in a transpersonal caring–healing model.

The Scope of Theoretical Systems

Nursing and nursing theoretical systems are located within a broader frame of reference. Orem placed her work in the broader frame of the world of humans and their affairs (1997). Neuman and Watson describe their work as useful to all health professions or as "beyond" nursing. Roy places her work in an explicit cosmology. The articulation of nursing knowledge with the broader domain of knowledge of the universe, human science, and healthcare is necessary to maintain the disciplinary identity of nursing.

This text examined some theoretical systems that include the whole of nursing. Although each theorist began with different philosophical or conceptual views, each intended to structure knowledge for the discipline of nursing. With established substantive content, these general models provide alternate views of nursing. Other theoretical systems explain particular aspects of nursing but not the entire discipline. These works can fit within those described as general or grand theoretical systems to the extent that the cosmology (if one exists) and ontology are compatible. For example, Peplau's work is congruent with the theories of all but Rogers and Parse described in this text. Hanucharurnkul (1989) compared Orem's and King's theories and discovered many similarities in the two works. The theories complement each other and "can be used together to make nursing theory more complete" (p. 371). Similarly, Comley (1994) compared Orem and Peplau. Her analysis suggests that the two are philosophically congruent and could be used together to further understand the nurse-patient relationship. Armstrong and Kelly (1995) compared Rogers and Peplau and concluded that both perspectives are needed. They raise the discrepancy between the two perspectives on causality and linear process and then dismiss it as nonessential. Further exploration of these differences is needed.

Some theoretical systems are limited to or include theories that are narrower in scope and are referred to as middle-range theories. From the perspective of the discipline of nursing, these theories are appropriately named when they are derived from or related to a grand or general theory of nursing. Many middle-range theories originated in existing belief systems about nursing and proceeded to conceptualize and formalize one or more aspects of that belief system. This type of work begins in the logical middle and progresses toward science, with limited if any movement toward philosophy. However, many middle-range theories are not connected to nursing theory. At some point, these developing bodies of knowledge should be articulated with or reconceptualized from a broader nursing disciplinary matrix.

As the nursing theoretical disciplines continue to develop, as they make explicit the philosophical basis of the work, and as major changes to the models or theories occur, nursing scholars must continue to evaluate previous work in light of the new. Roy's and Watson's 1999 modifications of their theories demonstrate this necessary type of change.

Practical Usefulness

Nursing theoretical systems may be useful for individual nurses as they develop personal concepts of nursing. For many, this occurs as part of professional education. Others restructure their existing knowledge when they first encounter a nursing theoretical system that illuminates their practice.

Although personal conceptualizations of nursing are important, the development of nursing practice programs from a nursing theoretical perspective is also important. Many opportunities for further development of practice from a theory-based perspective exist. Such programs not only help to highlight the unique contribution of nursing to public healthcare but are the basis for specifying expected outcomes of nursing activity, related information systems, and costs associated with delivery of nursing services.

Empirical Adequacy

According to Fawcett (1993), the empirical adequacy of theoretical models depends on the composite findings of research studies. Ideally, empirical evidence is congruent with the theoretical assertions, thus indicating support. Although the nature and adequacy of research varies, advances in using and supporting theoretical systems and models have been made in multiple studies. Theory has guided research, and in turn, research has provided supporting evidence. However, the research conducted to date is limited in that a preponderance of the studies have been descriptive and that far fewer have been theory-testing studies. Some studies have insufficiently connected the variables of study and the theory. Investigators have not always been careful about examining findings in the light of the related theoretical propositions. Because of the nature of grand theory, only a limited aspect of the theory can be tested at any given time.

Nevertheless, many studies have yielded support for selected aspects of theoretical systems. Research findings have generated conceptual changes in some models. For example, Pender changed her conceptualization of factors that directly influenced engagement in health-promoting activities because research indicated that those direct connections existed. Measuring instruments and research methods have continued to evolve. For example, the Self-Care Inventory is a more adequate measure than early instruments assessing self-care. Investigators using Rogers' Science of Unitary Human Beings have developed a number of creative methodologies for gathering data. Perhaps the most exciting aspect of nursing research is the emergence of some programs of research. Although many studies remain single and isolated, some investigators have begun to publish series of studies that build from findings of one initial study—for example, Duffy's work on the determinants of health promotion or the work of Fawcett, Tulman, and others on functional status. This discovery method is far more efficient than models that were used in the early years of nursing research.

THE FUTURE

The future of nursing as a discipline rests with those scholars and practitioners who understand the need for nursing discipline-specific perspectives. Although the discipline focuses on knowledge and use of knowledge to develop practice, it is through the profession of nursing that interactions with other persons are made. The nexus is completed when the knowledge developed through theory and research is made useful for practice.

In the early twentieth century scientists attempted to define a unified view of science. This work led to field theory, systems theory, and the theory of relativity. In the late twentieth century, the search continued. Physicists searched for a "Grand Unified Theory" that would unite all the forces and particles of nature into one coherent package (Gribbin, 1998). Likewise, nurses today desire a unified view of nursing. Decades have witnessed discussions on one theory or many theories for nursing. In 1999, a group of nurses put forth a "consensus statement on emerging nursing knowledge" (Boston College, 1999). The brief statement is limited to a values-based perspective and does not incorporate a science-based perspective of human being and human existence in a material world. Nursing as a discipline and a profession should integrate theory, research, and practice. But it is too early in the process of knowledge development to seek a unified view of nursing. As nurses in practice know, diversity is an important consideration. So too is diversity in knowledge development. Barring some major breakthrough in science, substantively different views of the human/person and person/environment relationship will continue to develop. Diverse views of the realities of nursing are useful in guiding research and practice.

Although no unified view of nursing exists, it may be possible to agree on the proper object of nursing. The medical profession demonstrates the fracture that results from lack of consensus on the proper object of the discipline. Although many agree that the object of the medical discipline is to cure disease or to make people well, numerous branches of medicine have emerged from differing beliefs on the causes of disease. These include allopathic, chiropractic, osteopathic, naturopathic, and other branches. One paradigm became predominant, in part because of the quality of science but also because of the politics of the profession. To avoid similar problems, nursing would be well advised to keep its focus on the science of nursing.

If nursing is to significantly impact the delivery of multidisciplinary healthcare, our knowledge base needs to be sufficiently defined so as to recognize the unique focus of nursing practice and value it for the substantive contributions it can make to advancing it. Gortner (2000) has suggested that nursing science has matured during the past 15 years. Nursing has made excellent strides in developing and applying nursing knowledge. As a discipline, nursing should appreciate the growth of its knowledge base and strengthen its resolve to develop it further. Opportunity awaits all nurses.

REFERENCES

Armstrong, M.A. & Kelly, A.E. (1995). More than the sum of their parts: Martha Rogers and Hildegard Peplau. *Archives of Psychiatric Nursing, 9*(1), 40-44.

Boston College. (1999). Consensus statement on emerging nursing knowledge. URL http://www.bc.edu/bc_org/avp/son/theorist/consensus2.html

Comley, A.L. (1994). A comparative analysis of Orem's self-care model and Peplau's interpersonal theory. *Journal of Advanced Nursing, 20*(4), 755-760.

Fawcett, J. (1993). *Analysis and evaluation of nursing theories*. Philadelphia: F.A. Davis.

Gortner, S. (2000). Knowledge development in nursing: Our historical roots and future opportunities. *Nursing Outlook, 48*(2), 60-67.

Gribbin, J.R. (1998). *The search for superstrings, symmetry, and the theory of everything*. Boston: Little, Brown.

Hanucharurnkul, S. (1989). Comparative analysis of Orem's and King's theories. *Journal of Advanced Nursing, 14*(5), 365-372.

Huch, M.H. (1991). Perspectives on health. *Nursing Science Quarterly, 4*(1), 33-40.

Orem, D.E. (1997). Views of human beings specific to nursing. *Nursing Science Quarterly, 10*(1), 26-31.

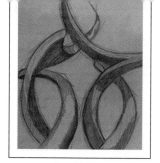

Appendix

RESEARCH INSTRUMENTS

Complete contact information for the developer(s) of each instrument is presented at the end of this section. Contact information is also provided for some instruments that could not be included in the book.

THE ETIQUETTE OF USING RESEARCH INSTRUMENTS

Instrument development plays a key role in theory-related research. It provides a mechanism for measuring phenomenon identified by the theory. Instrument development may be specifically guided by philosophical beliefs about the nature of knowing found within the theoretical framework. To facilitate better communication and continuity of research, this appendix presents research instruments derived from the various nursing theories discussed in earlier chapters. In some instances the complete instrument is presented for perusal; in other instances sample items from the instruments are provided. Sometimes only the name and contact information for the instrument developer is included. This information is crucial because an investigator planning to use an instrument developed by others must request permission. It also may be prudent to ensure that the author of the instrument agrees that the proposed use of the instrument is appropriate.

When using an already developed instrument, investigators should always consider reliability and validity. Reliability and validity reflect the research situation in which the instruments are tested. Although reliability is necessary to establish validity, the presence of reliability does not ensure validity. A reliable instrument that is used for purpose other than that evaluated in validity testing may not be valid for measuring a new purpose or population (Pedhazur & Schmelkin, 1991). An investigator who selects an instrument for a study should weigh carefully the previously established attributes of reliability and validity and then consider the nature of the proposed instrument use. Different circumstances may influence reliability and validity. Waltz, Strickland, and Lenz (1991) have suggested that validity be determined each time a measure is used, because random errors and individual differences can be factors in each administration of a test. Pretesting an instrument in a situation similar to that of the proposed study is an excellent mechanism to ensure adequate instrument reliability and validity for the major study.

When using an instrument developed by others, investigators should adhere to the following guidelines:

- *Never use an instrument without the written permission of the developer.* Investigators should always request permission, and they must note the permission in publications of their findings. Most developers are pleased when use of their instrument is sought. However, developers may refuse if they believe that their instrument may be used inappropriately. Most developers request information about the proposed use of the instrument before giving permission. Although many instruments can be used free of charge, sometimes a fee is attached. The developer also may limit duplication of the instrument.
- *Reliability and validity are characteristics of the research instrument in its inherent format.* This means that the instrument cannot be modified without further work to reestablish adequate levels of reliability and validity.
- *Do not modify instruments without the permission of the developer.* Although developers may be amenable to minor modifications to their instruments, they have the right to refuse any modifications. Investigators must consider how changes might influence the instrument's reliability and validity.

- *Send a report of findings back to the instrument developer.* Many developers make such a report a contingency of instrument use.
- *Publish findings, crediting the instrument developer for the instrument.* Making findings available to the scientific community transmits information about research instruments. The reliability and validity of a measuring instrument is an ongoing concern. One assessment of reliability and validity is not adequate. However, multiple published studies that include findings regarding reliability and validity can firmly establish those characteristics for a particular measuring instrument.

REFERENCES

Pedhazur, E. & Schmelkin, L. (1991). *Measurement, design, and analysis: An integrated approach.* Hillsdale, NJ: Lawrence Erlbaum Associates.

Waltz, C., Strickland, O., & Lenz, E. (1991). *Measurement in nursing research.* (2nd ed.). Philadelphia: F.A. Davis.

CONTACT INFORMATION
Instruments in the Appendix
Orem: Self-Care Deficit Theory of Nursing

Self-as-Carer Inventory
   Susan Taylor, PhD, FAAN
   7 Gipson Court
   Columbia, MO 65202
   email: taylors@health.missouri.edu

   Elizabeth A. Geden, PhD, RNC, FAAN
   Professor
   Sinclair School of Nursing
   University of Missouri—Columbia
   Columbia, MO 65211
   email: gedene@missouri.edu

DCA: Dependent Care Agent Instrument Questionnaire for Mothers
   Dr. Jean Burley Moore
   College of Nursing and Health Science
   George Mason University
   4400 University Drive
   Fairfax, VA 22030

Children's Self-Care Performance Questionnaire
   Dr. Jean Burley Moore
   College of Nursing and Health Science
   George Mason University
   4400 University Drive
   Fairfax, VA 22030

Mental Health Self-Care Agency Scale
Patricia West, PhD, RN
Director of Behavioral Science
St. John Family Medical Center
24911 Little Mack, Suite C
St. Clair Shores, Michigan 48080
(810) 447-9070

Rogers: Science of Unitary Human Beings

Power as Knowing Participation in Change
Elizabeth Ann Manhart Barrett, RN, PhD, FAAN
Professor and Coordinator, Center for Nursing Research
Hunter-Bellevue School of Nursing
Hunter College of the City University of New York
425 East 25th Street
New York, NY 10010
(212) 481-5079
or
415 East 85th Street, 9E
New York, NY 10028
(212) 861-8228

Temporal Experience Scales
Dr. Jeanne L. Paletta
3320 Perimeter Drive
Greenacres, FL 33467-2061
(407) 433-0608

Perceived Field Motion Scale
Adela Yarcheski, PhD, FAAN
Professor, College of Nursing
Rutgers, The State University of New Jersey
University Heights
Newark, NJ 07102
(973) 353-5326, ext 520
email: yarcheski@nightingale.rutgers.edu

Noreen E. Mahon, PhD, FAAN
Professor, College of Nursing
Rutgers, The State University of New Jersey
University Heights
Newark, NJ 07102
(201) 648-5388
email: mahon@nightingale.rutgers.edu

Human Field Rhythms
   Adela Yarcheski, PhD, FAAN
   Professor, College of Nursing
   Rutgers, The State University of New Jersey
   University Heights
   Newark, NJ 07102
   (973) 353-5326, ext 520
   email: yarcheski@nightingale.rutgers.edu

   Noreen E. Mahon, PhD, FAAN
   Professor, College of Nursing
   Rutgers, The State University of New Jersey
   University Heights
   Newark, NJ 07102
   (201) 648-5388
   email: mahon@nightingale.rutgers.edu

Human Field Image Metaphor Scale
   Linda W. Johnston, RN, PhD
   School of Nursing
   University of South Carolina—Aiken
   471 University Parkway
   Aiken, SC 29801
   (803) 641-3277
   email: lindaj@aiken.sc.edu

Assessment of Dream Experience
   Dr. Juanita Watson
   Sutton Towers A103
   Collingwood, NJ 08107
   (610) 499-4254
   email: juanita.watson@widener.edu

Index of Field Energy
   Sarah Hall Gueldner, DNS, RN, FAAN
   Director and Professor, School of Nursing
   Pennsylvania State University
   201 Health and Human Development East
   University Park, PA 16802-6096
   (814) 865-2940
   fax: (814) 865-3779
   email: shg9@psu.edu

Leddy Healthiness Scale
  Susan Kun Leddy, PhD, RN
  Professor, School of Nursing
  Widener University
  One University Place
  Chester, PA 19013-5792
    or
  609 Wilder Road
  Wallingford, PA 19086
  (610) 499-4207
  email: pasleddy@cyber.widener.edu

Person-Environment Participation Scale
  Susan Kun Leddy, PhD, RN
  Professor, School of Nursing
  Widener University
  One University Place
  Chester, PA 19013-5792
    or
  609 Wilder Road
  Wallingford, PA 19086
  (610) 499-4207
  email: pasleddy@cyber.widener.edu

Neuman: Neuman Systems Model
Levels of Cognitive Functioning Assessment Scale
  Jeanne Flannery, DSN, ARNP, CNRN, CRRN, CCH
  Florida State University
  School of Nursing
  Tallahassee, FL 32306-4310
  (850) 644-5626

Roy: Roy Adaptation Model
Inventory of Functional Status—Antepartum Period
  Dr. Lorraine Tulman
  School of Nursing
  University of Pennsylvania
  420 Guardina Drive
  Philadelphia, PA 19104-6096

  Jacqueline Fawcett, PhD, FAAN
  3506 Atlantic Highway
  P.O. Box 1156
  Waldoboro, ME 04572
  (207) 832-7398
  email: jacqueline.fawcett@umb.edu

Inventory of Functional Status After Childbirth
    Dr. Lorraine Tulman
    School of Nursing
    University of Pennsylvania
    420 Guardina Drive
    Philadelphia, PA 19104-6096

    Jacqueline Fawcett, PhD, FAAN
    3506 Atlantic Highway
    P.O. Box 1156
    Waldoboro, ME 04572
    (207) 832-7398
    email: jacqueline.fawcett@umb.edu

Inventory of Functional Status—Fathers
    Dr. Lorraine Tulman
    School of Nursing
    University of Pennsylvania
    420 Guardina Drive
    Philadelphia, PA 19104-6096

    Jacqueline Fawcett, PhD, FAAN
    3506 Atlantic Highway
    P.O. Box 1156
    Waldoboro, ME 04572
    (207) 832-7398
    email: jacqueline.fawcett@umb.edu

Inventory of Functional Status—Cancer
    Dr. Lorraine Tulman
    School of Nursing
    University of Pennsylvania
    420 Guardina Drive
    Philadelphia, PA 19104-6096

    Jacqueline Fawcett, PhD, FAAN
    3506 Atlantic Highway
    P.O. Box 1156
    Waldoboro, ME 04572
    (207) 832-7398
    email: jacqueline.fawcett@umb.edu

Inventory of Functional Status—Caregiver of Child in a Body Cast
    Diana M.L. Newman, RN, EdD
    P.O. Box 765
    Chadds Ford, PA 19317-0623
    email: dianaml@bellatlantic.net

Self-Consistency Scale
 Lin Zhan, PhD, RN
 Associate Professor, College of Nursing
 University of Massachusetts—Boston
 100 Morrissey Boulevard
 Boston, MA 02125
 (781) 646-1635
 email: lin.zhan@umb.edu

Peplau: Theory of Interpersonal Relations
The Relationship Form
 Cheryl Forchuk, RN, PhD
 Nurse Scientist
 London Health Science Centre Research, Inc.
 375 South Street, Room C205NR
 London, Ontario
 CANADA N6A 4G5
 (519) 685-8500

Watson: Transpersonal Nursing and the Theory of Human Caring
Caring Behaviors Inventory
 Dr. Zane Robinson Wolf
 School of Nursing
 LaSalle University
 1900 West Olney Avenue
 Philadelphia, PA 19141
 (215) 951-1432
 email: wolf@lasalle.edu
  or
 27 Haverford Road
 Ardmore, PA 19003
 (610) 642-8473

INSTRUMENTS NOT IN THE APPENDIX
Orem: Self-Care Deficit Theory of Nursing
Denyes Self-Care Agency Instrument
 Dr. M.J. Denyes
 College of Nursing
 Wayne State University
 Detroit, MI 48202

Denyes Self-Care Practices Inventory
 Dr. M.J. Denyes
 College of Nursing
 Wayne State University
 Detroit, MI 48202

Appraisal of Self-Care Agency
   Dr. Marjorie Isenberg
   College of Nursing
   Wayne State University
   Detroit, MI 48202

Rogers: Science of Unitary Human Beings
Diversity of Human Field Patterns Scale
   Dr. M. Hastings-Tolsma
   University of Southern Maine School of Nursing
   96 Falmouth Street
   Portland, ME 04103

Neuman: Neuman Systems Model
Spiritual Care Scale
   Pearson Education
   Maura Connor, Nursing Editor
   1 Lake Street
   Upper Saddle River, NJ 07458

King: King's Conceptual System and Theory of Goal Attainment
A Criterion-Referenced Measure of Goal Attainment: Assessment of Functional Abilities
and Goal Attainment Scales
   Springer Publishing Company
   Permissions Coordinator
   536 Broadway
   New York, NY 10012-3955

Pender: Health Promotion Model
Health Promotion Lifestyle Profile II
   Susan Noble Walker, RN, EdD
   University of Nebraska Medical Center.
   42nd and Dewey Avenue
   Omaha, Nebraska 68105-1065

Exercise Benefits and Barriers Scale
   Susan Noble Walker, RN, EdD
   University of Nebraska Medical Center.
   42nd and Dewey Avenue
   Omaha, Nebraska 68105-1065

Day of your birth/Last 4 digits of your social security number

_____ / _____
day   soc. sec. #

SELF-AS-CARER INVENTORY

Instructions: Below are a number of statements about caring for yourself. (The word "self-care" is used a lot. It means those things you do for yourself to maintain life, health, and well-being.)

Use a #2 pencil to mark the number that best describes how you take care of yourself. Marking the number "6" means the statement is a very accurate statement about how you care for yourself; marking number "1" means that the statement is not at all accurate.

	Very Inaccurate				Very Accurate	
1. My joints are flexible enough for me to take care of myself	1	2	3	4	5	6
2. I think about health information in choosing solutions to problems in caring for myself	1	2	3	4	5	6
3. The way I take care of myself fits in well with my family life	1	2	3	4	5	6
4. I try out new ways to take care of myself based on information from experts	1	2	3	4	5	6
5. My self-care routine fits in with other parts of my life	1	2	3	4	5	6
6. I watch for signs that tell me if I am taking good care of myself	1	2	3	4	5	6
7. I use different ways of thinking based on the kind of self-care problem I have	1	2	3	4	5	6
8. I watch for things around me that will make a difference in how I take care of myself	1	2	3	4	5	6
9. I am strong enough for the physical work of caring for myself	1	2	3	4	5	6
10. I pay attention to signs telling me to change the way I care for myself	1	2	3	4	5	6
11. I plan my self-care by how much energy I have	1	2	3	4	5	6
12. I am aware of things around me that affect how I take care of myself	1	2	3	4	5	6
13. I have the necessary skills to care for myself	1	2	3	4	5	6
14. I stick to my decisions about caring for myself even when I run into setbacks or problems.	1	2	3	4	5	6
15. I know what I need to take care of myself	1	2	3	4	5	6
16. If the doctor tells me to do something, I do it	1	2	3	4	5	6
17. I take care of myself because my health is important to me	1	2	3	4	5	6

Day of your birth/Last 4 digits of your social security number

_____ / _____

day   soc. sec. #

SELF-AS-CARER INVENTORY—cont'd

	Very Inaccurate					Very Accurate
18. I remember health care information about what I should do for myself	1	2	3	4	5	6
19. I know how much energy I need to take care of myself	1	2	3	4	5	6
20. To make a decision about my care, I look at both sides of my choices	1	2	3	4	5	6
21. It matters to me that I care for myself	1	2	3	4	5	6
22. I know when I have enough energy to take care of myself	1	2	3	4	5	6
23. I know where to find good information I need to help me take care of myself	1	2	3	4	5	6
24. I think about how all the things I do fit together to help me reach my health goals	1	2	3	4	5	6
25. I have the physical balance I need in order to take care of myself.	1	2	3	4	5	6
26. I fit new self-care actions into what I already do . . .	1	2	3	4	5	6
27. My hearing and vision are good enough to allow me to care for myself	1	2	3	4	5	6
28. The way I take care of myself fits in with what I consider important in my life	1	2	3	4	5	6
29. I do what I know is best in taking care of myself even though I may not like it	1	2	3	4	5	6
30. I do my self-care in several different ways	1	2	3	4	5	6
31. I follow through with decisions I make about caring for myself	1	2	3	4	5	6
32. I have a set routine for caring for myself	1	2	3	4	5	6
33. I think about how decisions I make will affect my health and self-care	1	2	3	4	5	6
34. I knowingly spend my energies on the most important self-care tasks	1	2	3	4	5	6
35. I use information from authorities to help me take better care of myself	1	2	3	4	5	6
36. I have enough muscle strength to perform my self-care	1	2	3	4	5	6
37. I think about several choices before I make a decision about my self-care	1	2	3	4	5	6
38. I know why I make the choices I do in order to care for myself	1	2	3	4	5	6

Continued

Day of your birth/Last 4 digits of your social security number

_____ / _____
day   soc. sec. #

SELF-AS-CARER INVENTORY—cont'd

	Very Inaccurate				Very Accurate	
39. I know which actions to do first to best accomplish my self-care	1	2	3	4	5	6
40. Once I begin to care for myself in a certain way, I check to see if it is working	1	2	3	4	5	6

	Unhealthy				Healthy	
1. Using a scale of 1 to 6, how would you rate your health at this moment?	1	2	3	4	5	6

	Unhealthy				Healthy	
2. Using a scale of 1 to 6, how would you rate your own health in general?	1	2	3	4	5	6

	None				All	
3. Using a scale of 1 to 6, how much of your own care are you providing?	1	2	3	4	5	6

PERSONAL INFORMATION

Age	☐ ☐
Gender	☐ Female
	☐ Male
Current living arrangement	☐ alone
	☐ with family in the same house
	☐ with others in the same house
Ethnic group	☐ American Indian/Alaskan Native
	☐ Asian/Pacific Islander
	☐ Hispanic
	☐ Black
	☐ White
	☐ Other_____

Day of your birth/Last 4 digits of your social security number

_____ / _____
day   soc. sec. #

SELF-AS-CARER INVENTORY—cont'd

Who assists you with your self-care?	☐	no one
	☐	me
	☐	other family member(s)
	☐	friend(s)
	☐	nurse(s)
	☐	housekeeper
	☐	other_____
Are you currently taking any prescription medications?	☐	yes
	☐	no

If yes, please list medications

Do you need help in taking your medication?	☐ Yes	☐ No

If yes, please describe the help given.

PERSONAL INFORMATION—cont'd

Are you on a special diet?	☐	yes
	☐	no
If yes, what is the name of that diet? Why are you on this diet?		
Last time seen by a health care professional (MD, nurse, Chiropractor, etc.)?	_____ Month	_____ Year

Continued

Day of your birth/Last 4 digits of your social security number

_____ / _____

day   soc. sec. #

SELF-AS-CARER INVENTORY—cont'd

If yes, please list the problem.

List your diagnoses, if known, and length of time you have had this health problem.

DCA: DEPENDENT CARE AGENT INSTRUMENT

Questionnaire for Mothers

This questionnaire is designed to identify activities that mothers perform with children. Please circle the number that indicates how frequently you do each activity with your child.

What is the age of the child for whom you are answering this questionnaire? _____

Key

5 = *Always*—what you consistently do all the time.
4 = *Frequently*—what you usually do.
3 = *Occasionally*—what you sometimes do.
2 = *Seldom*—what you rarely do.
1 = *Never*—what you never do at any time.

1. I take my child for regular health checkups.	Always	5	4	3	2	1	Never
2. I take action to insure that my child's home is a safe one.	Always	5	4	3	2	1	Never
3. I try to help my child have a healthy self-image.	Always	5	4	3	2	1	Never
4. I encourage my child to be in activities with others his/her own age.	Always	5	4	3	2	1	Never
5. I make sure that my child is provided with foods from each of the four basic food groups.	Always	5	4	3	2	1	Never
6. I encourage periods of rest in my child's day.	Always	5	4	3	2	1	Never
7. Before judging his/her performance, I take my child's limitations into consideration.	Always	5	4	3	2	1	Never
8. I see that my child receives immunizations on time.	Always	5	4	3	2	1	Never
9. I make sure my child has play opportunities.	Always	5	4	3	2	1	Never
10. I encourage my child to participate in family activities.	Always	5	4	3	2	1	Never
11. I make sure my child gets a good night's sleep.	Always	5	4	3	2	1	Never
12. I evaluate my child for signs of minor illness.	Always	5	4	3	2	1	Never
13. I remind my child to drink enough fluid.	Always	5	4	3	2	1	Never

Continued

DCA: DEPENDENT CARE AGENT INSTRUMENT—cont'd

Questionnaire for Mothers—cont'd

14. I help my child learn to get along with others.	Always	5	4	3	2	1	Never
15. When someone is smoking, I try to get my child out of the room.	Always	5	4	3	2	1	Never
16. I make sure my child develops an understanding of the nutritional value of food he/she eats.	Always	5	4	3	2	1	Never
17. When planning meals, I pay attention to my child's food preferences.	Always	5	4	3	2	1	Never
18. I teach my child to be aware of safety hazards.	Always	5	4	3	2	1	Never
19. I assist my child in coping with stressful events.	Always	5	4	3	2	1	Never
20. When the doctor orders a medication for my child, I follow the directions carefully.	Always	5	4	3	2	1	Never
21. I ask the doctor or nurse about complications of medical treatments my child is receiving.	Always	5	4	3	2	1	Never
22. I notice how often my child urinates.	Always	5	4	3	2	1	Never
23. I encourage social activities for my child.	Always	5	4	3	2	1	Never
24. I make judgments about whether my child is growing and developing normally.	Always	5	4	3	2	1	Never
25. I support my child's participation in group activities.	Always	5	4	3	2	1	Never
26. I praise my child.	Always	5	4	3	2	1	Never
27. I check places outside our home for potential hazards for my child.	Always	5	4	3	2	1	Never
28. I make sure my child uses safety restraints in the car.	Always	5	4	3	2	1	Never
29. I encourage my child to be increasingly independent.	Always	5	4	3	2	1	Never
30. I help my child learn new words.	Always	5	4	3	2	1	Never

DCA: DEPENDENT CARE AGENT INSTRUMENT—cont'd

Questionnaire for Mothers—cont'd

31. I evaluate the quality of the air my child breathes.	Always	5	4	3	2	1	Never
32. I help my child learn to communicate effectively.	Always	5	4	3	2	1	Never
33. I note how often my child has a bowel movement.	Always	5	4	3	2	1	Never
34. I teach my child to take care of other people's property.	Always	5	4	3	2	1	Never
35. I help my child adjust to changes.	Always	5	4	3	2	1	Never
36. I encourage my child to be a responsible family member.	Always	5	4	3	2	1	Never
37. I try to know what my child is doing in school.	Always	5	4	3	2	1	Never
38. I make sure that my child participates in physical exercise.	Always	5	4	3	2	1	Never
39. When the weather is hot or when my child has been active, I encourage him/her to drink more liquids.	Always	5	4	3	2	1	Never

CHILDREN'S SELF-CARE PERFORMANCE QUESTIONNAIRE

This questionnaire is designed to collect information about the activities children and teenagers perform to promote their own health. Please answer the questions honestly and carefully. All answers will be kept CONFIDENTIAL.

Directions

1. Please circle the number that best states how often you do the activity.

2. There are no right or wrong answers.

3. Please do not skip any items.

4. Feel free to write comments if you wish.

Number	Heading	Meaning
5	**Always:**	All of the time
4	**Often:**	Most of the time, frequently
3	**Sometimes:**	Some of the time, occasionally
2	**Rarely:**	Seldom, not much
1	**Never:**	None of the time

	Always 5	Often 4	Sometimes 3	Rarely 2	Never 1
Section I					
1. I smoke.	5	4	3	2	1
2. I drink beverages with caffeine in them (coffee, soda, tea, etc.)	5	4	3	2	1
3. I skip lunch.	5	4	3	2	1
4. I eat junk food.	5	4	3	2	1
5. I eat meals with food from the four food groups.	5	4	3	2	1
6. I eat candy or other sweets.	5	4	3	2	1
7. I eat too much food.	5	4	3	2	1
8. I skip breakfast.	5	4	3	2	1
9. I take a bath or shower every day.	5	4	3	2	1
10. I wash my hands after going to the bathroom.	5	4	3	2	1
11. I exercise every day.	5	4	3	2	1
12. I sleep at least eight hours at night.	5	4	3	2	1
13. I stay up so late on school nights that I am tired the next day.	5	4	3	2	1

CHILDREN'S SELF-CARE PERFORMANCE QUESTIONNAIRE—cont'd

	Always 5	Often 4	Sometimes 3	Rarely 2	Never 1
Section I—cont'd					
14. I do things with my friends.	5	4	3	2	1
15. I ride a bike safely.	5	4	3	2	1
16. I keep away from stray animals.	5	4	3	2	1
17. I drink alcohol.	5	4	3	2	1
18. I look before I cross the street or road.	5	4	3	2	1
19. I am careful around strangers.	5	4	3	2	1
20. I wear a seatbelt in the car.	5	4	3	2	1
Section II					
21. I hand in my work on time at school.	5	4	3	2	1
22. I play sports and games with others.	5	4	3	2	1
23. I spend money as soon as I get it.	5	4	3	2	1
24. I follow the rules at home.	5	4	3	2	1
25. I follow the rules at school.	5	4	3	2	1
26. I am honest with my parents.	5	4	3	2	1
27. I watch too much TV.	5	4	3	2	1
28. I tell a family member where I am going.	5	4	3	2	1
29. I do all of my homework.	5	4	3	2	1
30. I bully other children.	5	4	3	2	1
Section III					
31. I wash my hands before eating.	5	4	3	2	1
32. I follow my doctor's advice.	5	4	3	2	1
33. I tell a parent if I think I am getting sick.	5	4	3	2	1
34. I brush my teeth.	5	4	3	2	1
35. I clean my cuts well, if I cut myself.	5	4	3	2	1

MENTAL HEALTH SELF-CARE AGENCY SCALE

The Mental Health Self-Care Agency Scale (MH-SCA) was developed to measure individuals' mental health–related self-care capabilities. The development and initial testing is addressed in the paper "Instrument Development: The Mental Health Self-Care Agency Scale" (West & Isenberg, 1997).

Scoring Guidelines: The original instrument had 35 items. After initial testing, three items were determined to add nothing or very little to the reliability of the instrument, and therefore, were deleted. These are items 4, 26 and 28 of the original instrument. They should not be included in further analysis. Following the initial testing 9 items were stated in the negative to reduce response bias. These include items 3, 5, 8, 10, 11, 14, 17, 21, and 32.

To calculate a score on the MH-SCA, the investigators should eliminate items 4, 26, and 28, if they have an original draft. Then the investigator should reverse scoring of the negatively stated items. Points are given on the basis of the respondent's answers and totaled.

Reliability:
In preliminary testing (West, 1993) the reliability of the MH-SCA and its subscales were as follows:

MH-SCA
Affective Subscale/New	.76
Cognitive Subscale	.66/.73
Pattern of Activity	.83
Perceptual Subscale/New	.59/.66
Valuative Processes Subscales	.64
Total/New Total	.93/.94

Items by content domains (original items):
Affective	1, 11, 23, 27, 29, 33
Cognitive	4, 8, 14, 16, 21, 25, 30
Patterns of Activity	2, 5, 7, 10, 13, 15, 17, 19, 22, 24, 32, 34
Perceptual	3, 6, 26, 28, 31, 35
Valuative Processes	9, 12, 18, 20

ID#_____

MH-SCA SCALE

The following list of statements are used by people to describe themselves. Please read each statement and then circle the number to the right which indicates how much you agree or disagree with the statement as a description of you. There are no right or wrong answers.

	Totally Disagree	Disagree	Neither Disagree Nor Agree	Agree	Totally Agree
1) If I am stressed in my daily routine, I can usually handle it.	1	2	3	4	5
2) Over the years, I have been able to maintain at least one close relationship.	1	2	3	4	5
3) I experience a lot of confusion about who I am.	1	2	3	4	5
4) I lack the energy to let others know what I need from them.	1	2	3	4	5
5) I view my body pretty much as other people do.	1	2	3	4	5
6) As things change, I remain flexible.	1	2	3	4	5
7) I have trouble remembering things.	1	2	3	4	5
8) At times I examine my values to see if I need to change.	1	2	3	4	5
9) I don't have the energy to be concerned about other people.	1	2	3	4	5
10) I rarely enjoy my successes.	1	2	3	4	5
11) I find time to do the things which are important to me.	1	2	3	4	5
12) I have ways to work out problems with others.	1	2	3	4	5
13) I am easily distracted from doing things I need to do for myself.	1	2	3	4	5
14) I am able to laugh and enjoy myself.	1	2	3	4	5
15) I regularly evaluate the choices I make.	1	2	3	4	5
16) I seldom take time to relax.	1	2	3	4	5

Continued

MH-SCA SCALE—cont'd

	Totally Disagree	Disagree	Neither Disagree Nor Agree	Agree	Totally Agree
17) I look for ways to feel more in tune with life around me.	1	2	3	4	5
18) I know how to get the information I need, when confronted with a crisis.	1	2	3	4	5
19) I have found meaning or a purpose to my life.	1	2	3	4	5
20) I have trouble telling what's happening around me.	1	2	3	4	5
21) I am able to express my sexuality in ways which are comfortable for me.	1	2	3	4	5
22) I can express my feelings in a healthy way, so that others understand me.	1	2	3	4	5
23) I look for more useful ways to resolve problems with others.	1	2	3	4	5
24) I am usually comfortable in making decisions for myself.	1	2	3	4	5
25) I am able to wait for the things that are important to me.	1	2	3	4	5
26) In most situations, I experience the same feelings that other people do.	1	2	3	4	5
27) I look for better ways to solve problems.	1	2	3	4	5
28) When things change, I am able to decide how I am going to handle the situation.	1	2	3	4	5
29) I am overly dependent on others.	1	2	3	4	5
30) I look for better ways to handle my frustration.	1	2	3	4	5
31) I can set new priorities to meet my responsibilities in life.	1	2	3	4	5
32) I look for ways to feel good about myself.	1	2	3	4	5

POWER AS KNOWING PARTICIPATION IN CHANGE

Introduction to Barrett's PKPCT

The PKPCT is designed to help you describe the meaning of day-to-day change in your life. Four indicators of experiencing change are:

AWARENESS
CHOICES
FREEDOM TO ACT INTENTIONALLY
INVOLVEMENT IN CREATING CHANGE

It takes about 10 minutes to complete the PKPCT.

Instructions For Completing Barrett's PKPCT

For each indicator, there are 13 lines. There are words at both ends of each line. The meaning of the words are opposite to each other. There are 7 spaces between each pair of words which provide a range of possible responses. Place an "X" in the space along the line that best describes the meaning of the indicator (AWARENESS, CHOICES, FREEDOM TO ACT INTENTIONALLY, or INVOLVEMENT IN CREATING CHANGE) for you <u>at this time</u>.

For example:
Under the indicator CHOICES, if your CHOICES are quite closely described as "informed," your answer might look like this:

informed ____|_X_|____|____|____|____|____ uninformed

If your CHOICES are quite closely described as "uninformed," your answer might look like this:

informed ____|____|____|____|____|_X_|____ uninformed

If your CHOICES are equally "informed" and "uninformed," place an "X" in the middle space on the line. Your answer might look like this:

informed ____|____|____|_X_|____|____|____ uninformed

REMEMBER:
- There are no right or wrong answers.
- Record your first impression for **each** <u>pair of words.</u>
- You can place an "X" in any space along the line that best describes the meaning the indicator has for you <u>at this time.</u>
- Mark only one "X" for each pair of words.
- Mark an "X" for <u>every pair of words.</u>

PLEASE BEGIN TO MARK YOUR X'S ON BARRETT'S PKPCT

(Please go to NEXT PAGE and continue)

BARRETT PKPCT, VERSION II

Mark an "X" as Described in the Instructions

MY AWARENESS IS

profound ___|___|___|___|___|___|___ superficial

avoiding ___|___|___|___|___|___|___ seeking

valuable ___|___|___|___|___|___|___ worthless

unintentional ___|___|___|___|___|___|___ intentional

timid ___|___|___|___|___|___|___ assertive

leading ___|___|___|___|___|___|___ following

chaotic ___|___|___|___|___|___|___ orderly

expanding ___|___|___|___|___|___|___ shrinking

pleasant ___|___|___|___|___|___|___ unpleasant

uninformed ___|___|___|___|___|___|___ informed

free ___|___|___|___|___|___|___ constrained

unimportant ___|___|___|___|___|___|___ important

unpleasant ___|___|___|___|___|___|___ pleasant

Mark an "X" as Described in the Instructions

MY CHOICES ARE

shrinking ___|___|___|___|___|___|___ expanding

seeking ___|___|___|___|___|___|___ avoiding

assertive ___|___|___|___|___|___|___ timid

important ___|___|___|___|___|___|___ unimportant

orderly ___|___|___|___|___|___|___ chaotic

intentional ___|___|___|___|___|___|___ unintentional

unpleasant ___|___|___|___|___|___|___ pleasant

constrained ___|___|___|___|___|___|___ free

worthless ___|___|___|___|___|___|___ valuable

following ___|___|___|___|___|___|___ leading

superficial ___|___|___|___|___|___|___ profound

informed ___|___|___|___|___|___|___ uninformed

timid ___|___|___|___|___|___|___ assertive

(Please go to NEXT PAGE and continue)

BARRETT PKPCT, VERSION II, PART 2

Mark an "X" as Described in the Instructions

MY FREEDOM TO ACT INTENTIONALLY IS

timid ___|___|___|___|___|___| ___ assertive

uninformed ___|___|___|___|___|___| ___ informed

leading ___|___|___|___|___|___| ___ following

profound ___|___|___|___|___|___| ___ superficial

expanding ___|___|___|___|___|___| ___ shrinking

unimportant ___|___|___|___|___|___| ___ important

valuable ___|___|___|___|___|___| ___ worthless

chaotic ___|___|___|___|___|___| ___ orderly

avoiding ___|___|___|___|___|___| ___ seeking

free ___|___|___|___|___|___| ___ constrained

unintentional ___|___|___|___|___|___| ___ intentional

pleasant ___|___|___|___|___|___| ___ unpleasant

orderly ___|___|___|___|___|___| ___ chaotic

Mark an "X" as Described in the Instructions

MY INVOLVEMENT IN CREATING CHANGE IS

unintentional ___|___|___|___|___|___| ___ intentional

expanding ___|___|___|___|___|___| ___ shrinking

profound ___|___|___|___|___|___| ___ superficial

chaotic ___|___|___|___|___|___| ___ orderly

free ___|___|___|___|___|___| ___ constrained

valuable ___|___|___|___|___|___| ___ worthless

uninformed ___|___|___|___|___|___| ___ informed

avoiding ___|___|___|___|___|___| ___ seeking

leading ___|___|___|___|___|___| ___ following

unimportant ___|___|___|___|___|___| ___ important

timid ___|___|___|___|___|___| ___ assertive

pleasant ___|___|___|___|___|___| ___ unpleasant

superficial ___|___|___|___|___|___| ___ profound

THANK YOU

TEMPORAL EXPERIENCE SCALES

Instructions

Each person experiences the movement of events in an individual way. This personal experience cannot be measured by clocks or calendars, but can be compared with the movement represented by the metaphors listed in the Temporal Experience Scales.

Directions: Imagine the events, happenings or occurrences for each of the listed phrases. Place an "X" in the column which best represents how events move for you in your life.

Example: Imagine the metaphor, "a merry-go-round". Form an image in your mind of a merry-go-round in motion. Is this how events move for you in your life?

If you agree that this is representative, place an "X" in the <u>agree</u> (A) or <u>agree strongly</u> (AS) column; if you conclude that it has no relevance for you in your experience, place an "X" in the <u>disagree</u> (D) or <u>disagree strongly</u> (DS) column. If you cannot decide whether the metaphor image has any relevance in your life experience, then place an "X" in the <u>no opinion</u> (NO) column.

Thus, if you decided that the image did represent how events move in your life, your response would look like this:

Metaphor	AS	A	NO	D	DS
Merry-go-round	_____	__X__	_____	_____	_____

If you decided that the image was not at all representative of how events move in your life, you might respond like this:

Metaphor	AS	A	NO	D	DS
Merry-go-round	_____	_____	_____	_____	__X__

TEMPORAL EXPERIENCE SCALES—cont'd

Metaphors	AS	A	NO	D	DS
1. A GALLOPING HORSEMAN	____	____	____	____	____
2. A GULL MOTIONLESS IN MIDAIR	____	____	____	____	____
3. FLASH OF LIGHTNING	____	____	____	____	____
4. A SPEEDING TRAIN	____	____	____	____	____
5. ROLLING WAVES	____	____	____	____	____
6. SWINGING GATE	____	____	____	____	____
7. DRIFTING CLOUDS	____	____	____	____	____
8. SOARING KITE	____	____	____	____	____
9. FLAME SWIRLING UP	____	____	____	____	____
10. STATIC SERENITY	____	____	____	____	____
11. STREAM OF THOUGHT	____	____	____	____	____
12. QUIET, MOTIONLESS OCEAN	____	____	____	____	____
13. FLOATING DRIFTWOOD	____	____	____	____	____
14. EMPTINESS	____	____	____	____	____
15. SILENT STREAM	____	____	____	____	____
16. SPACE SHUTTLE	____	____	____	____	____
17. ENDURING	____	____	____	____	____
18. CARVED IN STONE	____	____	____	____	____
19. AUTOMOBILE CRUSHER	____	____	____	____	____
20. BUTTERFLIES HOVERING	____	____	____	____	____
21. FREE FALLING SKYDIVERS	____	____	____	____	____
22. FALLING ROCK	____	____	____	____	____
23. TORNADO	____	____	____	____	____
24. DASHING WATERFALL	____	____	____	____	____

PERCEIVED FIELD MOTION

Directions: Below you will find a series of adjective pairs, preceded by a concept. <u>To show how you feel about the concept, place an "X" between each of the adjective pairs in the series. The closer your "X" is to one adjective in the pair, the more you feel it describes the concept better than does its opposite.</u> Place the "X" in the middle space if you are neutral, unsure, or feel that neither adjective in the pair describes better how you feel about the particular concept. Let your initial reactions guide your responses.

FIRST, THINK OF YOURSELF AS A HUMAN ENERGY FIELD MOVING
IN AN ENVIRONMENTAL ENERGY FIELD

NOW, RESPOND TO THE CONCEPT

<u>MY "FIELD" MOTION</u>

FAST ____:____:____:____:____:____:____ SLOW

DARK ____:____:____:____:____:____:____ BRIGHT

CLEAR ____:____:____:____:____:____:____ DENSE

STRONG ____:____:____:____:____:____:____ WEAK

LIGHT ____:____:____:____:____:____:____ HEAVY

CALM ____:____:____:____:____:____:____ EXCITABLE

UNLIMITED ____:____:____:____:____:____:____ LIMITED

DEEP ____:____:____:____:____:____:____ SHALLOW

STATIC ____:____:____:____:____:____:____ DYNAMIC

ACTIVE ____:____:____:____:____:____:____ PASSIVE

DULL ____:____:____:____:____:____:____ SHARP

PERCEIVED FIELD MOTION—SCORING

<u>Directions:</u> Below you will find a series of adjective pairs, preceded by a concept. <u>To show how you feel about the concept, place an "X" between each of the adjective pairs in the series. The closer your "X" is to one adjective in the pair, the more you feel it describes the concept better than does its opposite.</u> Place the "X" in the middle space if you are neutral, unsure, or feel that neither adjective in the pair describes better how you feel about the particular concept. Let your initial reactions guide your responses.

FIRST, THINK OF YOURSELF AS A HUMAN ENERGY FIELD MOVING
IN AN ENVIRONMENTAL ENERGY FIELD

NOW, RESPOND TO THE CONCEPT

<u>MY "FIELD" MOTION</u>

FAST <u>_7_</u> : <u>_6_</u> : <u>_5_</u> : <u>_4_</u> : <u>_3_</u> : <u>_2_</u> : <u>_1_</u> SLOW

DARK ____ : ____ : ____ : ____ : ____ : ____ : ____ BRIGHT

CLEAR ____ : ____ : ____ : ____ : ____ : ____ : ____ DENSE

STRONG <u>_7_</u> : <u>_6_</u> : <u>_5_</u> : <u>_4_</u> : <u>_3_</u> : <u>_2_</u> : <u>_1_</u> WEAK

LIGHT ____ : ____ : ____ : ____ : ____ : ____ : ____ HEAVY

CALM ____ : ____ : ____ : ____ : ____ : ____ : ____ EXCITABLE

UNLIMITED <u>_7_</u> : <u>_6_</u> : <u>_5_</u> : <u>_4_</u> : <u>_3_</u> : <u>_2_</u> : <u>_1_</u> LIMITED

DEEP <u>_7_</u> : <u>_6_</u> : <u>_5_</u> : <u>_4_</u> : <u>_3_</u> : <u>_2_</u> : <u>_1_</u> SHALLOW

STATIC <u>_1_</u> : <u>_2_</u> : <u>_3_</u> : <u>_4_</u> : <u>_5_</u> : <u>_6_</u> : <u>_7_</u> DYNAMIC

ACTIVE <u>_7_</u> : <u>_6_</u> : <u>_5_</u> : <u>_4_</u> : <u>_3_</u> : <u>_2_</u> : <u>_1_</u> PASSIVE

DULL <u>_1_</u> : <u>_2_</u> : <u>_3_</u> : <u>_4_</u> : <u>_5_</u> : <u>_6_</u> : <u>_7_</u> SHARP

<u>Instructions for scoring the PFM scale:</u> The above seven (7) items comprise the PFM scale. Administer the entire scale, but use only the responses to the 7 items above to measure PFM. You can score the items as indicated above, or you can score all 7 items 7 to 1 and instruct the computer to reverse score Static-Dynamic and Dull-Sharp.

HUMAN FIELD RHYTHMS

Directions: Answer the question below by placing a vertical mark across the answer line at the point which BEST REFLECTS YOUR OPINION.

Example: HAPPY _____|_____ SAD

Answer the following question about your HUMAN FIELD RHYTHMS

LOW
FREQUENCY _____

HIGH
FREQUENCY

HUMAN FIELD IMAGE METAPHOR SCALE

Instructions: Please read each of the following metaphors and indicate how you feel at the moment. Check the box that best describes how you identify with each statement. If you do not identify with the statement, check the box under "Do Not Identify". If you identify strongly with the statement, check the box under "Strongly Identify". There are no right or wrong answers.

	Do Not Identify	Slightly Identify	Moderately Identify	Strongly Identify	Totally Identify
I FEEL					
1. Free as a bird.	[ ]	[ ]	[ ]	[ ]	[ ]
2. One with the universe.	[ ]	[ ]	[ ]	[ ]	[ ]
3. Like an eternal song.	[ ]	[ ]	[ ]	[ ]	[ ]
4. Like a melody.	[ ]	[ ]	[ ]	[ ]	[ ]
5. Like a tree in winter.	[ ]	[ ]	[ ]	[ ]	[ ]
6. Like a fenced in yard.	[ ]	[ ]	[ ]	[ ]	[ ]
7. Like a symphony.	[ ]	[ ]	[ ]	[ ]	[ ]
8. Like a ray of light.	[ ]	[ ]	[ ]	[ ]	[ ]
9. Like a bird in a cage.	[ ]	[ ]	[ ]	[ ]	[ ]
10. Like an ocean breeze.	[ ]	[ ]	[ ]	[ ]	[ ]
11. Like a kite with no wind.	[ ]	[ ]	[ ]	[ ]	[ ]
12. One with my world.	[ ]	[ ]	[ ]	[ ]	[ ]

Continued

HUMAN FIELD IMAGE METAPHOR SCALE—cont'd

I FEEL	Do Not Identify	Slightly Identify	Moderately Identify	Strongly Identify	Totally Identify
13. Like a ray of hope.	[ ]	[ ]	[ ]	[ ]	[ ]
14. Like a worn out shoe.	[ ]	[ ]	[ ]	[ ]	[ ]
15. Like I can touch the stars.	[ ]	[ ]	[ ]	[ ]	[ ]
16. Like a fragrance on the wind.	[ ]	[ ]	[ ]	[ ]	[ ]
17. Like I'm standing on the highest mountain.	[ ]	[ ]	[ ]	[ ]	[ ]
18. Like ripples on a pond.	[ ]	[ ]	[ ]	[ ]	[ ]
19. Like a free spirit.	[ ]	[ ]	[ ]	[ ]	[ ]
20. Like a new pair of skates.	[ ]	[ ]	[ ]	[ ]	[ ]
21. Like a tree in springtime.	[ ]	[ ]	[ ]	[ ]	[ ]
22. Like a garden in spring.	[ ]	[ ]	[ ]	[ ]	[ ]
23. Like an artist without a brush.	[ ]	[ ]	[ ]	[ ]	[ ]
24. Like I can see forever.	[ ]	[ ]	[ ]	[ ]	[ ]
25. Like my hands are tied.	[ ]	[ ]	[ ]	[ ]	[ ]

ASSESSMENT OF DREAM EXPERIENCE

<u>Directions:</u> Listed below are words which may be used to describe the experience of dreaming. Please consider what your dreams have been like <u>over the past two weeks.</u> Then, using the rating scale provided, indicate the extent to which each word describes what your dreams were generally like by placing an "X" in the appropriate space. There are no right or wrong answers. <u>Please be sure to rate each word.</u>

	Almost Always	Often	Sometimes	Almost Never
1. Constrained	____	____	____	____
2. Boring	____	____	____	____
3. Imaginative	____	____	____	____
4. Intense	____	____	____	____
5. Vivid	____	____	____	____
6. Exciting	____	____	____	____
7. Simple	____	____	____	____
8. Vague	____	____	____	____
9. Colorful	____	____	____	____
10. Energetic	____	____	____	____
11. Limited	____	____	____	____
12. Passive	____	____	____	____
13. Drab	____	____	____	____
14. Active	____	____	____	____
15. Complex	____	____	____	____
16. Dull	____	____	____	____
17. Clear	____	____	____	____
18. Dramatic	____	____	____	____
19. Expansive	____	____	____	____
20. Unimaginative	____	____	____	____

INDEX OF FIELD ENERGY

Last four numbers of your
Social Security #_____

Field Dynamics Index

Today's Date: Month _____

Day _____

Year _____

Your Birthday: Month _____

Day _____

Year _____

Sex: Male _____

Female _____

INSTRUCTIONS:

Look at the scale of points between each pair of pictures. Mark (X) the scale according to which picture best describes how you feel now.

Continued

DEMOGRAPHIC INFORMATION

<u>Directions:</u>   Kindly check the boxes that best describe you. Print other information that is requested.

1. Sex
   [ ] Female   [ ] Male

2. Age
   _____ years

3. Education
   [ ] No formal schooling
   [ ] Grade school (completed)
   ____Years attended (not completed)
   [ ] High school (completed)
   ____Years attended (not completed)
   [ ] Vocational training (completed)
   ____Years attended (not completed)
   College:
   ____ Years attended (no degree)
   College degree:
   [ ] Associate
   [ ] Bachelors
   [ ] Masters
   [ ] Doctorate
   [ ] Other _____

4. Occupation or Career
   (briefly describe)
   _____

5. Current Residence:
   State _____
   Population of city/town
   [ ] Less than 70,000
   [ ] 70,000 to 1,000,000
   [ ] More than 1,000,000

6. Check the country of your birth:
   [ ] U.S.A.
   [ ] Other: _____

7. Check the language that you read, write and speak best:
   [ ] American-English
   [ ] Other:_____

8. Check if you ingested or inhaled any stimulants, depressants or hallucinogens today:
   [ ] None
   [ ] Coffee or Tea
   [ ] Other:_____

9. Do you practice any form of meditation?
   [ ] Yes   [ ] No

10. Have you experienced a crisis during the past 6 months?
    [ ] Yes   [ ] No

11. Check the number of hours you slept last night:
    [ ] None
    [ ] 3-4
    [ ] 5-8
    [ ] 9 or more
    Was your sleep pattern last night normal for you?
    [ ] Yes   [ ] No

12. Check the time of day when you function best:
    [ ] Morning   [ ] Afternoon
    [ ] Evening   [ ] Night

Continued

SCORING KEY

INSTRUCTIONS:

Look at the scale of points between each pair of pictures. Mark (X) the scale according to which picture best describes how you feel now.

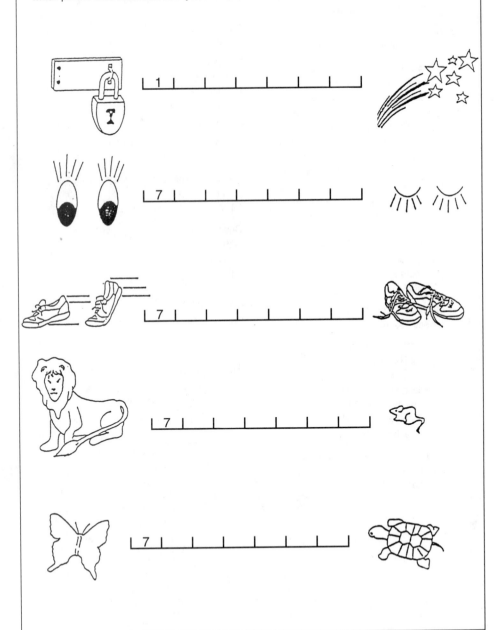

Continued

SCORING KEY—cont'd

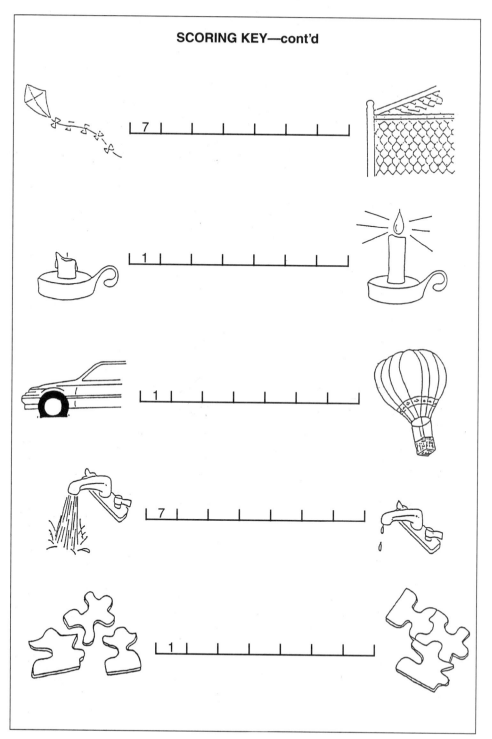

Continued

SCORING KEY—cont'd

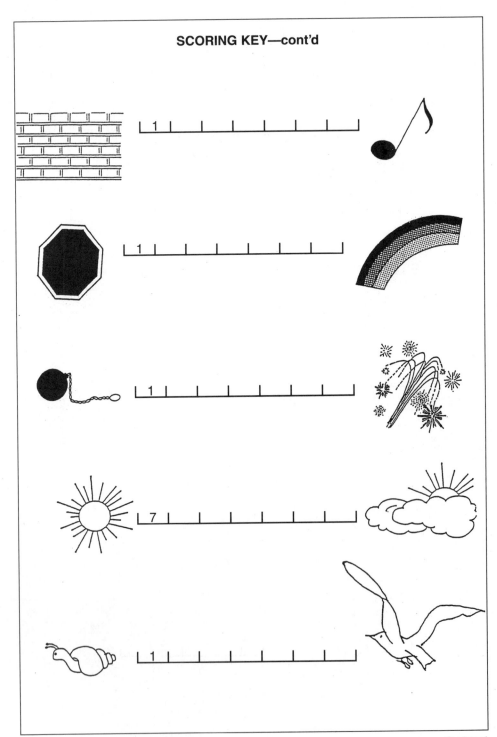

Continued

SCORING KEY—cont'd

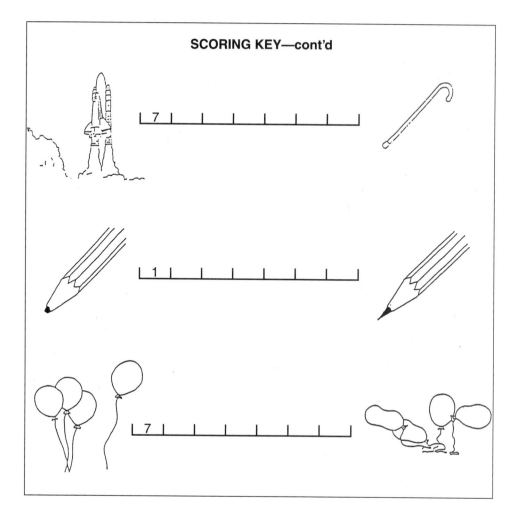

LEDDY HEALTHINESS SCALE (LHS)

Circle the number that best indicates your degree of agreement with each of the following statements. Please answer all of the questions the way you feel **right now.**

	Completely Agree	Mostly Agree	Slightly Agree	Slightly Disagree	Mostly Disagree	Completely Disagree
1. I think that I function pretty well.	6	5	4	3	2	1
2. I have goals that I look forward to accomplishing in the next year.	6	5	4	3	2	1
3. I am part of a close and supportive family.	6	5	4	3	2	1
4. I don't feel there is much that is meaningful in my life.	6	5	4	3	2	1
5. I have more than enough energy to do what I want to do.	6	5	4	3	2	1
6. I feel that I can accomplish anything I set out to do.	6	5	4	3	2	1
7. There is very little that I value in my life right now.	6	5	4	3	2	1
8. Having change(s) in my life makes me feel uncomfortable.	6	5	4	3	2	1
9. I have rewarding relationships with people.	6	5	4	3	2	1
10. I enjoy making plans for the future.	6	5	4	3	2	1
11. I feel free to choose actions that are right for me.	6	5	4	3	2	1
12. I feel like I've got little energy.	6	5	4	3	2	1
13. I am pleased to find that I am getting better with age.	6	5	4	3	2	1
14. I don't communicate much with family or friends.	6	5	4	3	2	1
15. I get excited thinking about new projects.	6	5	4	3	2	1
16. I feel good about my ability to influence change.	6	5	4	3	2	1

LEDDY HEALTHINESS SCALE (LHS)—cont'd

	Completely Agree	Mostly Agree	Slightly Agree	Slightly Disagree	Mostly Disagree	Completely Disagree
17. I'm not what you would call a goal oriented person.	6	5	4	3	2	1
18. I feel energetic.	6	5	4	3	2	1
19. I feel good about my freedom to make choices for my life.	6	5	4	3	2	1
20. I have a goal that I am trying to achieve.	6	5	4	3	2	1
21. I don't expect the future to hold much meaning for me.	6	5	4	3	2	1
22. I like exploring new possibilities.	6	5	4	3	2	1
23. I feel full of zest and vigor.	6	5	4	3	2	1
24. I feel fine.	6	5	4	3	2	1
25. I feel pretty sure of myself.	6	5	4	3	2	1
26. I feel isolated from people.	6	5	4	3	2	1

PERSON-ENVIRONMENT PARTICIPATION SCALE (PEPS)

Directions: Here are some questions about YOUR INTERACTION WITH YOUR ENVIRON-MENT. Each question has answers from 1 to 7. If the word(s) under 1 are right for you, circle 1; if the word(s) under 7 are right for you, circle 7. If you feel differently, circle one of the numbers inbetween. Answer the questions the way you feel **right now.**

MY INTERACTION WITH MY ENVIRONMENT FEELS:

1	2	3	4	5	6	7
Flexible						Inflexible
1	2	3	4	5	6	7
Integrated						Fragmented
1	2	3	4	5	6	7
Powerless						Powerful
1	2	3	4	5	6	7
Energetic						Lethargic
1	2	3	4	5	6	7
Laborious						Effortless
1	2	3	4	5	6	7
Empty						Full
1	2	3	4	5	6	7
Calm						Agitated
1	2	3	4	5	6	7
Dissonant						Harmonious
1	2	3	4	5	6	7
Flowing						Clogged
1	2	3	4	5	6	7
Connected						Separated
1	2	3	4	5	6	7
Passive						Active
1	2	3	4	5	6	7
Smooth						Turbulent
1	2	3	4	5	6	7
Discomforting						Comforting
1	2	3	4	5	6	7
Manageable						Unmanageable
1	2	3	4	5	6	7
Expanding						Shrinking

LEVELS OF COGNITIVE FUNCTIONING ASSESSMENT SCALE

Developed by Jeanne Flannery, D.S.N., A.R.N.P., CNRN, CRRN,
using Levels 1-5 from Rancho Los Amigos Scale

Date

Time

Initials

Level I. <u>NO RESPONSE</u>

A. Attention to the Environment: NONE

   1. Appears unaware of environment; eyes usually closed   1.

B. Response to Stimuli: NONE

   2. Completely unresponsive to tactile stimuli and position changes   2.

   3. Completely unresponsive to auditory stimuli   3.

   4. Completely unresponsive to visual stimuli (This not to be confused with papillary response to light, which is reflective.)   4.

   5. Completely unresponsive to painful stimuli   5.

   6. Completely unresponsive to gustatory stimuli   6.

C. Behavior Status: REFLEXIVE

   7. May have primitive responses such as snorting, chewing, blinking, eye opening, which are unrelated to specific stimuli   7.

D. Ability to Process Information: NONE

E. Ability to Follow Commands: NONE

F. Awareness of Person (Self):   NONE

G. Awareness of Time: NONE

H. Ability to Perform Self-Care: NONE

I. Ability to Converse: NONE

J. Ability to Learn New Information: NONE

Continued

LEVELS OF COGNITIVE FUNCTIONING ASSESSMENT SCALE—cont'd

Date

Time

Initials

Level II. GENERALIZED RESPONSE

    A. Attention to the Environment: **NONE**

    B. Response to Stimuli: **NONSPECIFIC, INCONSISTENT**

        8. May respond to external stimuli, such as position changes, with physiologic changes such as increased BP, P, or R, or increased perspiration   8.

        9. Responds to painful stimuli with generalized reflex action (nonpurposeful gross body movement, as decerebration or decortication)   9.

        10. Repetitive stimuli produce a change in the level of response, either dampening or heightening it (e.g. stroking may reduce physiologic changes or intensify response, which occurred initially)   10.

        11. Demonstrates nonpurposeful variations in responses to the same stimulus; delayed, limited response   11.

    C. Behavior Status: **AWAKE**

        12. May be awake but unaware of environment unless directly stimulated   12.

        13. Demonstrates inconsistent infrequent visual fixation; may have roving eye movements, but is incapable of visual tracking   13.

        14. Behavioral response may be the same regardless of stimulus (e.g. eye opening, startle, gross body movement, or decerebration upon tactile, painful, or auditory stimulus)   14.

    D. Ability to Process Information: **NONE**

    E. Ability to Follow Commands: **NONE**

    F. Awareness of Person (Self):   **STIMULI TO BODY PRODUCE GENERAL RESPONSE**

    G. Awareness of Time (Present):   **NONE**

    H. Ability to Perform Self-Care: **NONE**

    I. Ability to Converse: **NONE**

    J. Ability to Learn New Information: **NONE**

LEVELS OF COGNITIVE FUNCTIONING ASSESSMENT SCALE—cont'd

Date

Time

Initials

Level III. <u>LOCALIZED RESPONSE</u>

   A. Attention to the Environment: NONE

   B. Response to Stimuli: SPECIFIC, INCONSISTENT

   15. Tracks briefly a moving object in visual field when awake only if stimulus intensity gains attention; inconsistent response   15.

   16. Demonstrates withdrawal responses or facial grimacing to tactile stimuli (pressure, temperature, texture) but inconsistently   16.

   17. Responds specifically to the stimulus (e.g. resists restraints, swallows food, relaxes to stroking, pulls at NGT) but inconsistently   17.

   18. Responds inconsistently to same stimulus (e.g. turns toward or away from a sound)   18.

   C. Behavior Status: BEGINNING AWARENESS

   19. Awakens to stimuli; has sleep/wake cycles: awakens spontaneously   19.

   20. Demonstrates purposeful visual orientation and fixation   20.

   21. Moves body parts purposefully, if able   21.

   D. Ability to Process Information: NONE

   E. Ability to Follow Commands: INCONSISTENT, DELAYED

   22. Response to commands is delayed   22.

   23. Responds more consistently with some persons than with others (e.g. may look at regular caregiver when called, but may not do it with others)   23.

   24. Demonstrates inconsistent attention and language comprehension, but when there is a response it is unequivocally meaningful (e.g. may not respond to command "touch your nose" when it has been followed before)   24.

   F. Awareness of Person (Self):   VAGUE, NOT MEASURABLE

   G. Awareness of Time (Present):   VAGUE, NOT MEASURABLE

   H. Ability to Perform Self-Care: NONE

   I. Ability to Converse: INCONSISTENT

   25. May vocalize inconsistently to stimuli; but may be infrequent   25.

   26. May vocalize automatically with one or two-word response or just make loud noises   26.

   J. Ability to Learn New Information: NONE

Continued

LEVELS OF COGNITIVE FUNCTIONING ASSESSMENT SCALE—cont'd

Date ☐☐☐☐☐☐☐
Time ☐☐☐☐☐☐☐
Initials ☐☐☐☐☐☐☐

Level IV. <u>CONFUSED–AGITATED</u>

A. Attention to the Environment: BRIEF

27. Demonstrates fleeting general attention to surroundings; unable to concentrate   27. ☐☐☐☐☐☐☐

28. Selective attention may be nonexistent or so brief that is not acted upon; easily distractible   28. ☐☐☐☐☐☐☐

B. Response to Stimuli: SPECIFIC, INAPPROPRIATE

29. May respond consistently to a stimulus, but the response is inappropriate because of internal confusion   29. ☐☐☐☐☐☐☐

30. May become very agitated or yell in response to a mild stimulus and sustain response after stimulus removed; "sticks" in response; low tolerance for frustration or pain   30. ☐☐☐☐☐☐☐

31. Responds to presence of devices, attachments or anything confining with strong, persistent, purposeful attempt to remove; impatient; demanding   31. ☐☐☐☐☐☐☐

C. Behavior Status: AGITATED, CONFUSED

32. In a heightened state of activity related to internal agitation (environment may be quiet and nonstimulating); restless; pacing; rocking; rubbing; moaning   32. ☐☐☐☐☐☐☐

33. May demonstrate aggressive, hostile behavior; has explosive or unpredictable anger; may be self abusive   33. ☐☐☐☐☐☐☐

34. May show sudden changes in mood (e.g. crying, laughter, anger, or sleep)   34. ☐☐☐☐☐☐☐

35. Performs overlearned motor activities automatically, but may resist commands to do these same activities, such as "sit up"   35. ☐☐☐☐☐☐☐

D. Ability to Process Information: MINIMAL

36. Unable to understand or cooperate with treatment efforts; may be combative; resistant to care; will leave area, if able   36. ☐☐☐☐☐☐☐

E. Ability to Follow Commands: INCONSISTENT

37. May respond briefly or inconsistently to simple commands when agitation is lessened   37. ☐☐☐☐☐☐☐

F. Awareness of Person (Self):   ORIENTED X1

38. Is oriented to own name; aware of own body   38. ☐☐☐☐☐☐☐

G. Awareness of Time (Present):   NONE

39. Unaware of present events; responds primarily to own state of severe confusion   39. ☐☐☐☐☐☐☐

LEVELS OF COGNITIVE FUNCTIONING ASSESSMENT SCALE—cont'd

Date ☐☐☐☐☐☐☐

Time ☐☐☐☐☐☐☐

Initials ☐☐☐☐☐☐☐

Level IV. CONFUSED–AGITATED—cont'd

H. Ability to Perform Self-Care: MINIMAL

40. Performs self care activities for brief periods with maximum direction and cuing; cannot focus without redirection   40. ☐☐☐☐☐☐☐

I. Ability to Converse: PRESENT, INAPPROPRIATE

41. Verbalizes incoherently or with words unrelated to the current situation; talking may be rapid, loud, excessive   41. ☐☐☐☐☐☐☐

42. May confabulate (give incorrect answers to questions about the present from unrelated long-term memory stores); lacks short-term recall   42. ☐☐☐☐☐☐☐

43. Conversation reflects confusion and memory deficits   43. ☐☐☐☐☐☐☐

J. Ability to Learn New Information: NONE

Level V. CONFUSED—INAPPROPRIATE, NON-AGITATED

A. Attention to Environment: DISTRACTIBLE

44. Demonstrates gross attention consistently   44. ☐☐☐☐☐☐☐

45. Has difficulty sustaining selective attention; highly distractible; limited concentration   45.

46. Lacks ability to focus on a specific thing without frequent redirection   46. ☐☐☐☐☐☐☐

B. Response to Stimuli: VARIABLE

47. Responds readily to stimuli related to self, body comfort, family   47. ☐☐☐☐☐☐☐

48. Use of objects in environment often inappropriate, without direction   48. ☐☐☐☐☐☐☐

C. Behavior Status: INAPPROPRIATE

49. Unable to initiate functional tasks   49. ☐☐☐☐☐☐☐

50. May demonstrate frustration and negative, inappropriate behaviors in response to external stimuli, usually out of proportion to stimulus   50. ☐☐☐☐☐☐☐

51. Will tend to wander (on foot or in a wheel chair) from unit; will not remember a command to remain in a certain place; will not remember how to return from a strange area to a familiar place   51. ☐☐☐☐☐☐☐

D. Ability to Process Information: LIMITED TO SELF

52. May relate to conversation about own body comfort, personal needs, momentary concerns   52. ☐☐☐☐☐☐☐

Continued

LEVELS OF COGNITIVE FUNCTIONING ASSESSMENT SCALE—cont'd

Date

Time

Initials

Level V. <u>CONFUSED—INAPPROPRIATE, NON-AGITATED—cont'd</u>

E. Ability to Follow Commands:

53. Responds to single simple commands consistently   53.

54. Response to a complex command becomes fragmented, nonpurposeful, and unrelated to command; requires redirection to follow through   54.

F. Awareness of Person (Self):   ORIENTED X1

55. Oriented to self; knows name, special things about self, but not how the present self is different from past   55.

G. Awareness of Time (Present):   CONFUSED

56. Disoriented to time and place, confusing past and present; unaware of situation   56.

57. Demonstrates severe short-term memory deficit   57.

H. Ability to Perform Self-Care: REQUIRES MAXIMUM ASSISTANCE

58. Performs overlearned tasks with maximum structure and cuing, but does not initiate the activity   58.

I. Ability to Converse: SOCIAL-AUTOMATIC

59. May converse on a social-automatic level for short periods, as "I'm fine, how are you?", but responses are often unrelated to specific topics of conversation   59.

60. If not verbal, may use social-automatic gestures, as shoulder shrug, thumbs up   60.

J. Ability to Learn New Information: NONE

61. Unable to learn new tasks; even though tries, listens, follows commands, outcome not achieved.   61.

LEVELS OF COGNITIVE FUNCTIONING ASSESSMENT SCALE—cont'd

Date

Time

Initials

SUMMARY

62. Select a number from 1 to 5 which represents the highest Cognitive Level where most of the observed behaviors are checked at this time of observation.

62.

Signature	Title	Initials	Signature	Title	Initials

Continued

DIRECTIONS TO EXAMINER USING LEVELS OF COGNITIVE FUNCTIONING ASSESSMENT SCALE

1. Stamp record with Addressograph or write patient's name and birth date.

2. Enter diagnosis and date of injury and onset of cognitive deficits.

3. Record the date and time of examination and your initials at the top of the column to be used.

4. Record your legal signature with your initials on the back of the first page of the record.

5. After familiarizing yourself with the clustered behaviors in each level described on LOCFAS, begin to observe the patient without disturbing him/her for a few minutes (3-5). From this brief observation of his/her random interaction with uncontrolled environmental stimuli, you will have a general idea of what level to anticipate (Level I as opposed to Level V).

6. Proceed to observe and elicit responses and mark the box beside the observed behavior in the appropriate column. A single column is used for each assessment. Continue upward on the scale assessing for observable behaviors for each level. Cease assessment at the point that no expected behaviors for a whole level can be observed. The cognitive level is designated as the <u>highest</u> level at which the <u>preponderance</u> of matching behavioral responses occur. There is always a scatter of responses above and below this level. The next higher level in which two or more behaviors are checked is also recorded. The patient is assessed for his best effort since these behaviors indicate the patient's capacity to move up to a higher level. There is expected a certain amount of overlap between levels, since human behavior is not precise. Variation downward during the day, particularly in relation to distractions, fatigue, and stress, is expected to occur.

7. As the patient progresses up the Levels, the team may want to give three separate scores—cognitive, behavioral, and functional—since there can be such variations among these areas. For example, the patient may clearly respond cognitively to stimuli on a Level V and physically is able to execute most tasks, but behaviorally he chooses not to do them (without expressing these thoughts). A quick assessment without follow-up would lead the observers to believe the patient is on a lower cognitive level.

8. The assessment may take approximately fifteen minutes. It can be incorporated within other aspects of routine care and therefore no exact time frame is set. Observations begin with the caregiver's first encounter with the patient and may extend through whatever activities in which the patient and caregiver normally engage until adequate assessment data are gathered.

9. The LOCFAS has a grid that accommodates an ongoing assessment over time. The frequency of recording is relative to the stability of the patient's condition and the number of team members assessing the patient. It is appropriate for use by an interdisciplinary health team. Accumulated data from all sources over time provide an accurate assessment, generally discussed by the team on a weekly basis. Progression, or regression, if any, can readily be determined from the overall evaluation.

10. Absence of the opportunity to observe these behaviors does not affect the decision regarding the cognitive level. In certain situations the precipitating stimulus may be absent. For example in Level II, Behavior 10, referring to change in level of activity upon repeated stimuli, may not be observed because it was not possible to provide stimuli repetitively. However, if more behaviors were observed in Level II than in any other level, the patient would still be ranked Level II without Behavior 10.

SAMPLE ITEMS FOR THE INVENTORY OF FUNCTIONAL STATUS—ANTEPARTUM PERIOD (IFSAP)

DIRECTIONS: PLEASE THINK ABOUT THE TIME SINCE YOU BECAME PREGNANT, AND THEN RESPOND TO THE FOLLOWING ITEMS.

Personal Care Activities
Please respond to the following phrases by indicating whether the performance of an activity has decreased, remained the same, or increased during the past week or two.

	DECREASED	REMAINED THE SAME	INCREASED
29. Variety of foods and beverages eaten	1	2	3
30. Time spent on care of hair	1	2	3
32. Walking distances, climbing stairs, or exercising	1	2	3

Household Activities
Please check all the usual household activities you did prior to your pregnancy and then indicate to what extent you have continued these activities during this pregnancy.

Prior to my pregnancy,
my usual activities included:

I have continued this activity:

	NOT AT ALL	PARTIALLY	FULLY
3. ___ Doing laundry	1	2	3
4. ___ Ironing clothes	1	2	3
5. ___ Doing dishes	1	2	3

Continued

SAMPLE ITEMS FOR THE INVENTORY OF FUNCTIONAL STATUS—ANTEPARTUM PERIOD (IFSAP)—cont'd

Childcare Activities
IF YOU HAVE CHILDREN, PLEASE RESPOND TO THE ITEMS ON THIS PAGE.
IF YOU DO NOT HAVE CHILDREN, PLEASE TURN TO THE NEXT PAGE.
Please check all the usual childcare activities you did prior to your pregnancy and then indicate to what extent you have continued these activities since you became pregnant.

Prior to this pregnancy,
my usual activities
included:

I have continued this activity:

		NOT AT ALL	PARTIALLY	FULLY
18.	___ Feeding the child(ren)	1	2	3
23.	___ Playing with the child(ren)	1	2	3
25.	___ Helping with schoolwork/reading to the child(ren)	1	2	3

Occupational Activities
IF YOU ARE CURRENTLY EMPLOYED, PLEASE RESPOND TO THE ITEMS ON THIS PAGE.
IF YOU ARE NOT CURRENTLY EMPLOYED, PLEASE TURN TO THE NEXT PAGE.
Please respond to the following phrases by indicating whether an aspect of work has decreased, remained the same, or increased during the past week or two.

	DECREASED	REMAINED THE SAME	INCREASED
35. Quality of my relationships with work associates	1	2	3
37. Doing my job carefully and accurately	1	2	3
38. Participating in professional organization(s)/union	1	2	3

SAMPLE ITEMS FOR THE INVENTORY OF FUNCTIONAL STATUS—ANTEPARTUM PERIOD (IFSAP)—cont'd

Educational Activities
IF YOU ARE CURRENTLY GOING TO SCHOOL, PLEASE RESPOND TO THE ITEMS ON THIS PAGE.
Please respond to the following phrases by indicating whether an aspect of <u>school</u> has decreased, remained the same, or increased during the past week or two.

	DECREASED	REMAINED THE SAME	INCREASED
40. Attend classes	1	2	3
41. Complete assignments on time	1	2	3
42. Sit through classes without getting up	1	2	3

Social and Community Activities
Please check all the usual <u>social</u> and <u>community</u> activities you did <u>prior</u> to your pregnancy and then indicate to what extent you have continued these activities <u>since</u> you became pregnant.

Prior to this pregnancy,
my usual activities included:

I have continued this activity:

	NOT AT ALL	PARTIALLY	FULLY
15. ___ Socializing with friends/ neighbors/coworkers	1	2	3
16. ___ Socializing with relatives	1	2	3
17. ___ Participating in social clubs (e.g., cards, bowling, tennis, photography)	1	2	3

SAMPLE ITEMS FOR THE INVENTORY OF FUNCTIONAL STATUS AFTER CHILDBIRTH (IFSAC)

DIRECTIONS: PLEASE THINK ABOUT THE TIME SINCE THE BIRTH OF YOUR BABY, AND THEN RESPOND TO THE FOLLOWING ITEMS.

Personal Care Activities
Please respond to the following phrases based on how your life has been during the past week or two.

	NEVER	SOMETIMES	MOST OF THE TIME	ALL THE TIME
25. Spend much of the day lying down	1	2	3	4
26. Sit during much of my day	1	2	3	4
27. Spend much of the day sleeping or dozing	1	2	3	4

Household Activities
Please check all the usual household responsibilities you had prior to the baby's birth and then indicate to what extent you have resumed these responsibilities since the baby was born.

Prior to the baby's birth,
my usual responsibilities
included:

I have resumed this activity:

	NOT AT ALL	JUST BEGINNING	PARTIALLY	FULLY
7. ___ Household business (paying bills, banking, etc.)	1	2	3	4
8. ___ Grocery shopping	1	2	3	4
9. ___ Shopping, other than groceries	1	2	3	4

SAMPLE ITEMS FOR THE INVENTORY OF FUNCTIONAL STATUS AFTER CHILDBIRTH (IFSAC)—cont'd

Infant Care Responsibilities
Please circle the number that indicates to what extent you have assumed your part of the following aspects of the baby's care.

	NOT AT ALL	JUST BEGINNING	PARTIALLY	FULLY
20. Night feedings	1	2	3	4
21. Bathe the baby	1	2	3	4
22. Change diapers	1	2	3	4

Occupational Activities
IF YOU ARE CURRENTLY EMPLOYED, PLEASE RESPOND TO THE FOLLOWING ITEMS.
Please respond to the following phrases based on how your life at work has been during the past week or two.

	NEVER	SOMETIMES	MOST OF THE TIME	ALL THE TIME
34. Act irritable toward my work associates (give sharp answers, snap at them, criticize easily, etc.)	1	2	3	4
35. Am working shorter hours	1	2	3	4
36. Am doing my job as carefully and accurately as usual	1	2	3	4

Continued

SAMPLE ITEMS FOR THE INVENTORY OF FUNCTIONAL STATUS AFTER CHILDBIRTH (IFSAC)—cont'd

Social and Community Activities
Please check all the usual social and community activities you did prior to the baby's birth and then indicate to what extent you have resumed these responsibilities since the baby was born.

Prior to the baby's birth,
my usual responsibilities
included:

I have resumed this activity:

	NOT AT ALL	JUST BEGINNING	PARTIALLY	FULLY
15. ___ Religious organizations	1	2	3	4
16. ___ Socializing with friends	1	2	3	4
17. ___ Socializing with relatives	1	2	3	4

SAMPLE ITEMS FOR THE INVENTORY OF FUNCTIONAL STATUS–FATHERS (IFS-F)

DIRECTIONS: PLEASE THINK ABOUT THE TIME SINCE YOUR WIFE BECAME PREGNANT, AND THEN RESPOND TO THE FOLLOWING ITEMS.

Personal Care Activities
Please check all the usual personal care activities you did prior to your wife's most recent pregnancy and then indicate to what extent you have continued these activities during the past week or two.

Prior to my wife's pregnancy,
my usual activities
included:

		I have continued this activity:		
	NOT AT ALL	PARTIALLY	SAME AS BEFORE	MORE THAN BEFORE
35. ____ Exercising	1	2	3	4
36. ____ Eating more or different foods	1	2	3	4
37. ____ Listening to music	1	2	3	4

Household Activities
Please check all the usual household activities you had prior to your wife's pregnancy and then indicate to what extent you have continued these activities since the pregnancy.

Prior to my wife's pregnancy,
my usual activities included:

		I have continued this activity:		
	NOT AT ALL	PARTIALLY	SAME AS BEFORE	MORE THAN BEFORE
1. ____ Cleaning the house	1	2	3	4
5. ____ Doing dishes	1	2	3	4

Continued

SAMPLE ITEMS FOR THE INVENTORY OF FUNCTIONAL STATUS–FATHERS (IFS-F)—cont'd

	NOT AT ALL	PARTIALLY	SAME AS BEFORE	MORE THAN BEFORE
12. ___ Caring for pets	1	2	3	4

Infant Care Responsibilities
IF YOUR BABY HAS BEEN BORN, PLEASE RESPOND TO THESE ITEMS.
IF YOUR BABY HAS NOT YET BEEN BORN, PLEASE TURN TO THE NEXT PAGE.
Please circle the number that indicates to what extent you have assumed your desired part of the following aspects of the baby's care.

	NOT AT ALL	JUST BEGINNING	PARTIALLY	FULLY
18. Daytime feedings	1	2	3	4
19. Night feedings	1	2	3	4
23. Playing with the baby	1	2	3	4

SAMPLE ITEMS FOR THE INVENTORY OF FUNCTIONAL STATUS–FATHERS (IFS-F)—cont'd

Childcare Activities

IF YOU HAVE OTHER CHILDREN, PLEASE RESPOND TO THE ITEMS ON THIS PAGE.

IF YOU DO NOT HAVE OTHER CHILDREN, PLEASE TURN TO THE NEXT PAGE.

Please check all the usual childcare activities you did prior to your wife's most recent pregnancy and then indicate to what extent you have continued these activities since the pregnancy.

Prior to my wife's pregnancy,
my usual activities
included:

I have continued this activity:

	NOT AT ALL	PARTIALLY	SAME AS BEFORE	MORE THAN BEFORE
24. ___ Feeding the child(ren)	1	2	3	4
25. ___ Getting up with the child(ren)	1	2	3	4
26. ___ Bathing the child(ren)	1	2	3	4

Occupational Activities

IF YOU ARE CURRENTLY EMPLOYED, PLEASE RESPOND TO THE FOLLOWING ITEMS.

IF YOU ARE NOT EMPLOYED, PLEASE TURN TO THE NEXT PAGE.

Please respond to the following phrases based on how your life at work has been during the past week or two compared to before your wife became pregnant.

	NEVER	SOMETIMES	SAME AS BEFORE	MORE THAN BEFORE
42. Accomplished usual amount of work at my job	1	2	3	4
43. Achieved work goals	1	2	3	4
44. Worked usual number of hours	1	2	3	4

Continued

SAMPLE ITEMS FOR THE INVENTORY OF FUNCTIONAL STATUS–FATHERS (IFS-F)—cont'd

Educational Activities
IF YOU ARE CURRENTLY GOING TO SCHOOL, PLEASE RESPOND TO THE ITEMS ON THIS PAGE.
Please respond to the following phrases by indicating how your life <u>at school</u> has been during the <u>past week or two compared to before your wife became pregnant.</u>

	NEVER	SOMETIMES	SAME AS BEFORE	MORE THAN BEFORE
48. Completing assignments on time	1	2	3	4
49. Achieving goals/learning content	1	2	3	4
50. Participating in extracurricular activities	1	2	3	4

Social and Community Activities
Please check all the usual social and community activities you did <u>prior</u> to your wife's pregnancy and then indicate to what extent you have continued these activities <u>since</u> the pregnancy.

Prior to my wife's pregnancy,
my usual activities
included:

I have continued this activity:

	NOT AT ALL	PARTIALLY	SAME AS BEFORE	MORE THAN BEFORE
13. ___ Participating in community service organizations (e.g., political activities, Cub Scouts, volunteer fire companies)	1	2	3	4
14. ___ Participating in religious organizations	1	2	3	4
15. ___ Socializing with friends	1	2	3	4

SAMPLE ITEMS FOR THE INVENTORY OF FUNCTIONAL STATUS–CANCER (IFS-CA)

DIRECTIONS: PLEASE THINK ABOUT THE TIME SINCE YOU WERE DIAGNOSED WITH CANCER, AND THEN RESPOND TO THE FOLLOWING ITEMS.

Personal Care Activities

Please respond to the following phrases based on how your life has been during the past few weeks.

	NEVER	SOMETIMES	MOST OF THE TIME	ALL OF THE TIME
22. Rest or sleep more during the day	1	2	3	4
23. Spend most of the day in my pajamas/nightgown/bathrobe	1	2	3	4
24. Walk as much as usual	1	2	3	4

Household Activities

Please check all the usual household activities you did prior to your illness and then indicate to what extent you have continued doing these activities in the past few weeks.

Prior to my illness,
my usual activities
included:

		I have continued doing this activity:		
	NOT AT ALL	JUST BEGINNING	PARTIALLY	FULLY
1. ___ Care of children	1	2	3	4
2. ___ Care of (husband) (wife)	1	2	3	4
4. ___ Cleaning the house	1	2	3	4

Continued

SAMPLE ITEMS FOR THE INVENTORY OF FUNCTIONAL STATUS–CANCER (IFS-CA)—cont'd

Occupational Activities
IF YOU ARE CURRENTLY EMPLOYED, PLEASE RESPOND TO THE FOLLOWING ITEMS.
Please respond to the following phrases based on how your life at work has been during the past few weeks.

	NEVER	SOMETIMES	MOST OF THE TIME	ALL OF THE TIME
32. Accomplishing as much as usual in my job	1	2	3	4
33. Acting irritably toward my work associates (give sharp answers, snap at them, criticize easily, etc.)	1	2	3	4
34. Working fewer hours	1	2	3	4

Social and Community Activities
Please check all the usual social and community activities you did prior to your illness and then indicate to what extent you have continued doing these activities in the past few weeks.

Prior to my illness,
my usual activities
included:

		I have continued doing this activity:		
	NOT AT ALL	JUST BEGINNING	PARTIALLY	FULLY
16. ___ Community service organizations	1	2	3	4
17. ___ Religious organizations	1	2	3	4
18. ___ Socializing with friends	1	2	3	4

INVENTORY OF FUNCTIONAL STATUS—CAREGIVER OF CHILD IN BODY CAST (SAMPLE ITEMS)

PLEASE THINK ABOUT THE TIME SINCE YOU HAVE BEEN CARING FOR A CHILD IN A BODY CAST, AND THEN RESPOND TO THE FOLLOWING ITEMS.

Please check all the usual (household, social and community, care of child in body cast, care of other children, personal care, occupational) you did prior to your child's casting. Please circle the number that indicates the extent that you have continued these activities while caring for your child.

Prior to the child's
casting my usual activities included:
(please check activities that were done)

I have continued this activity
(please circle your response)

	NOT AT ALL	PARTIALLY	FULLY	MORE THAN BEFORE
HOUSEHOLD				
1. ____ Cleaning the house	1	2	3	4
SOCIAL AND COMMUNITY				
1. ____ Participating in community service organizations	1	2	3	4
CARE OF CHILD IN BODY CAST				
1. Bathing the child	1	2	3	4

Continued

INVENTORY OF FUNCTIONAL STATUS—CAREGIVER OF CHILD IN BODY CAST (SAMPLE ITEMS)—cont'd

Please circle the number that indicates the extent to which you do each activity

	NOT AT ALL	SOMETIMES	MOST OF THE TIME	ALL OF THE TIME
1. Clean the cast	1	2	3	4

CARING FOR OTHER CHILDREN

	NOT AT ALL	PARTIALLY	FULLY	MORE THAN BEFORE
1. Feed the child(ren)	1	2	3	4

PERSONAL CARE ACTIVITIES

	NOT AT ALL	SOMETIMES	MOST OF THE TIME	ALL OF THE TIME
1. ___ Eat the right amount of food	1	2	3	4

OCCUPATIONAL ACTIVITIES

1. ___ Maintain Employment	1	2	3	4

SELF-CONSISTENCY SCALE

Instructions:

People have some sense of self to be able to function as an individual in the world. Sometimes, people's sense of self is affected in different ways by having a hearing loss condition. Below are statements about people's sense of self. For each item please circle the number closest to how you personally feel this way:

1 = Never;   2 = Rarely;   3 = Sometimes;   4 = Always

When I think about myself lately, I

	Never	Rarely	Sometimes	Always
1. Spend time thinking about what I am like	1	2	3	4
2. Feel that I am a person of worth, at least on an equal with others	1	2	3	4
3. Think to myself about what I am like	1	2	3	4
4. Spend time thinking about who I am	1	2	3	4
5. Get nervous in a social gathering	1	2	3	4
6. Tend to think "I am no good"	1	2	3	4
7. Am able to do things as well as most other people	1	2	3	4
8. Understand who I am	1	2	3	4
9. Feel I am no good at all	1	2	3	4
10. Think how others are looking at me when I am talking to someone	1	2	3	4
11. Feel there is a lot wrong with me	1	2	3	4
12. Am sure that I know what kind of person I really am	1	2	3	4
13. Am bothered if I do not dress appropriately for an event	1	2	3	4
14. Spend time thinking about what kind of person I am	1	2	3	4

Continued

SELF-CONSISTENCY SCALE—cont'd

As I think about myself lately, I

	Never	Rarely	Sometimes	Always
15. Feel mixed up about myself	1	2	3	4
16. Feel I know just what I am like	1	2	3	4
17. Take a positive attitude toward myself	1	2	3	4
18. Feel mixed up about what I am really like	1	2	3	4
19. Feel changes like "Some days I am happy with the kind of person I am. Other days I am not happy with the kind of person I am"	1	2	3	4
20. Am satisfied with myself, on the whole	1	2	3	4
21. Certainly feel useless at times	1	2	3	4
22. Feel that I have a number of good qualities	1	2	3	4
23. Feel changes like "Some days I think I am one kind of person. Other days I am a different kind of person"	1	2	3	4
24. Am not much good at anything	1	2	3	4
25. Know for sure how nice I am	1	2	3	4
26. Feel I know just what I am like	1	2	3	4
27. Change ideas about who I am	1	2	3	4

SELF-CONSISTENCY SCALE—cont'd

The line below represents how people feel about their stability of sense of self from no change (at the bottom) to a great deal of change (at the top). Please place a mark X on the line to show how you feel about your sense of self since you have had a hearing loss.

THE SENSE OF SELF SCALE

A great deal of change

No change at all

THE RELATIONSHIP FORM**

Phases of the Nurse-Client Relationship*~

Date of Visit:

Name:

| Orientation | Identification | Exploitation | Resolution |

| **Orientation Phase** | **Working Phase** | | **Resolution Phase** |
| | Identification | Exploitation | |

Client:

Seeks assistance.	Participates in identifying problems.	Makes full use of services.	Abandons old needs.
Conveys educative needs.	Begins to be aware of time.	Identifies new goals.	Aspires to new goals.
Asks questions.	Responds to help.	Attempts to attain new goals.	Becomes independent of helping person.
Tests parameters.	Identifies with nurse.	Rapid shifts in behavior; dependent <---> independent.	Applies new problem-solving skills.
Shares preconceptions and expectations of nurse due to past experience.	Recognizes nurse as a person.	Exploitative behavior.	Maintains changes in style of communication and interaction.
	Explores feelings.	Realistic exploitation.	Positive changes in view of self.
	Fluctuates dependence, independence and interdependence in relationship with nurse.	Self-directing.	Integrates illness.
	Increases focal attention.	Develops skills in interpersonal relationships and problem solving.	Exhibits ability to stand alone.
	Changes appearance (for better or worse).	Displays changes in manner of communication (more open, flexible).	
	Understands purpose of meeting.		
	Maintains continuity between sessions (process and content).		

Nurse:

Respond to emergency	Maintain separate identity.	Continue assessment.	Sustain relationship as long as patient feels necessary.
Give parameters of meetings.	Exhibits ability to edit speech or control focal attention.	Meet needs as they emerge.	Promote family interaction.
Explain roles.	Testing maneuvers decrease.	Understand reason for shifts in behavior.	Assist with goal setting.
Gather data.	Unconditional acceptance.	Initiate rehabilitative plans.	Teach preventive measures.
Help patient identify problem.	Help express needs, feelings.	Reduce anxiety.	Utilize community agencies.
Help patient plan use of community resources and services.	Assess and adjust to needs.	Identify positive factors.	Teach self-care.
Reduce anxiety and tension.	Provide information.	Help plan for total needs.	Terminate nurse-client relationship.
Practice non-directive listening.	Provide experiences that diminish feelings of helplessness.	Facilitate forward movement of personality.	
Focus patient's energies.	Do not allow anxiety to overwhelm patient.	Deal with therapeutic impasse.	
Clarify preconceptions and expectations of nurse.	Help patient to focus on cues.		
	Help patient develop responses to cues.		
	Use word stimuli.		

NOTE: Phases Are Overlapping

Date Completed: _____   Signature: _____

*Peplau, H.E. *Interpersonal Relations in Nursing,* New York: G.P. Putnam's Sons 1952

Nordall, D., Seto, A. Peplau's Model Applied to Primary Nursing in Clinical Practice. In J. Riehl and C. Roy (ed.) *Conceptual Models for Nursing Practice.* New York: Appleton-Century-Crofts. 1980.

Peplau, H.E. audio-tape series. San Antonio, Texas: P.F.S. Productions. 1973.

**This form can be used to assess the phases of the therapeutic relationship by professions other than nursing, by reading the term "Nurse" as "Health Care Professional"

~ as published in: Forchuk, C., & Brown, B. (1989). Establishing a nurse-client relationship. *Journal of Psychosocial Nursing, 27*(2), 30-34.

CARING BEHAVIORS INVENTORY

<u>Directions:</u> Below is a list of the responses that represent nurse caring. For each item, rank the extent that a nurse or nurses made each response visible.

Please use the scale provided to select your answer. Circle the number you select after reading each item.

1 = never
2 = almost never
3 = occasionally
4 = usually
5 = almost always
6 = always

1. Attentively listening to the patient.	1	2	3	4	5	6
2. Giving instructions or teaching the patient.	1	2	3	4	5	6
3. Treating the patient as an individual.	1	2	3	4	5	6
4. Spending time with the patient.	1	2	3	4	5	6
5. Touching the patient to communicate caring.	1	2	3	4	5	6
6. Being hopeful for the patient.	1	2	3	4	5	6
7. Giving the patient information so that he or she can make a decision.	1	2	3	4	5	6
8. Showing respect for the patient.	1	2	3	4	5	6
9. Supporting the patient.	1	2	3	4	5	6
10. Calling the patient by his/her preferred name.	1	2	3	4	5	6
11. Being honest with the patient.	1	2	3	4	5	6
12. Trusting the patient.	1	2	3	4	5	6
13. Being empathetic or identifying with the patient.	1	2	3	4	5	6
14. Helping the patient grow.	1	2	3	4	5	6
15. Making the patient physically or emotionally comfortable.	1	2	3	4	5	6
16. Being sensitive to the patient.	1	2	3	4	5	6
17. Being patient or tireless with the patient.	1	2	3	4	5	6
18. Helping the patient.	1	2	3	4	5	6
19. Knowing how to give shots, IVs, etc.	1	2	3	4	5	6
20. Being confident with the patient.	1	2	3	4	5	6
21. Using a soft, gentle voice with the patient.	1	2	3	4	5	6

Continued

CARING BEHAVIORS INVENTORY—cont'd

1 = never
2 = almost never
3 = occasionally
4 = usually
5 = almost always
6 = always

	1	2	3	4	5	6
22. Demonstrating professional knowledge and skill.	1	2	3	4	5	6
23. Watching over the patient.	1	2	3	4	5	6
24. Managing equipment skillfully.	1	2	3	4	5	6
25. Being cheerful with the patient.	1	2	3	4	5	6
26. Allowing the patient to express feelings about his or her disease and treatment.	1	2	3	4	5	6
27. Including the patient in planning his or her care.	1	2	3	4	5	6
28. Treating patient information confidentially.	1	2	3	4	5	6
29. Providing a reassuring presence.	1	2	3	4	5	6
30. Returning to the patient voluntarily.	1	2	3	4	5	6
31. Talking with the patient.	1	2	3	4	5	6
32. Encouraging the patient to call if there are problems.	1	2	3	4	5	6
33. Meeting the patient's stated and unstated needs.	1	2	3	4	5	6
34. Responding quickly to the patient's call.	1	2	3	4	5	6
35. Appreciating the patient as a human being.	1	2	3	4	5	6
36. Helping to reduce the patient's pain.	1	2	3	4	5	6
37. Showing concern for the patient.	1	2	3	4	5	6
38. Giving the patient's treatments and medications on time.	1	2	3	4	5	6
39. Paying special attention to the patient during first times, as hospitalization, treatments.	1	2	3	4	5	6
40. Relieving the patient's symptoms.	1	2	3	4	5	6
41. Putting the patient first.	1	2	3	4	5	6
42. Giving good physical care.	1	2	3	4	5	6

CARING BEHAVIORS INVENTORY—cont'd

Please complete the following information:

Patient Profile:
    Patients are asked to complete this section.

1. Sex: 1. female _____   2. male _____

2. Age: _____

3. Marital Status: 1. single
                      2. married
                      3. divorced
                      4. widowed
                      5. separated

4. Race: 1. African American _____
          2. Asian _____
          3. Caucasian _____
          4. Hispanic _____
          5. Native American Indian _____
          6. Other, please specify _____

5. Educational Level: 1. 1-8 grade _____
                         2. 9-12 grade _____
                         3. 1-2 years college _____
                         4. 3-4 years college _____
                         5. 5 years college and over _____

6. Highest degree earned _____

7. Type of health care setting where you were cared for by nurses:
    1. university hospital _____
    2. suburban/community hospital _____
    3. long term care facility _____
    4. nursing home _____
    5. community health nursing agency _____
    6. senior citizen center _____
    7. other, please specify _____

8. Number of admissions to hospital or other health care setting in the last 5 years _____

9. Reason for last admission or need for health care services of nurse
    _____

10. Number of days in hospital or other health care setting during the last admission
    _____

Continued

CARING BEHAVIORS INVENTORY—cont'd

Nurse Profile:
 Nursing staff are asked to complete this section.

1. Sex: 1. female _____ 2. male _____

2. Age: _____

3. Marital Status: 1. single
                    2. married
                    3. divorced
                    4. widowed
                    5. separated

4. Race: 1. African American _____
          2. Asian _____
          3. Caucasian _____
          4. Hispanic _____
          5. Native American Indian _____
          6. Other, please specify _____

5. Educational Level: 1. 1-8 grade _____
                       2. 9-12 grade _____
                       3. 1-2 years college _____
                       4. 3-4 years college _____
                       5. 5 years college and over _____

6. Work place (for example, hospital, nursing home, home care): _____

7. Highest degree earned _____

8. Position in nursing: 1. NA—nursing assistant staff _____
                         2. LPN—staff nurse _____
                         3. RN—staff nurse _____
                         4. RN—nurse manager _____
                         5. RN—assistant nurse manager _____
                         6. RN—supervisor _____
                         7. RN—care coordinator _____
                         8. RN—director of nursing _____
                         9. RN—nursing faculty
                        10. Other, please specify _____

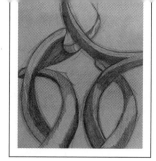

Glossary

The definitions offered in this glossary are intended to promote understanding of terms used within this text. Many of these terms are specific to the theorists and represent expressions of complex ideas. To better understand these terms, readers should consult the chapters within this text and the works of the theorists themselves.

adaptation "The process and outcome whereby the thinking and feeling person uses conscious awareness and choice to create human and environmental integration" (Roy, 1997, p. 44).

basic conditioning factors Factors that influence therapeutic self-care demand. For example, culture can be a basic conditioning factor in influencing sufficient food intake (Orem, 1995).

carative components Ten factors that serve as a basis for nursing practice founded on a transpersonal concept of caring. These factors are essential to satisfying certain human needs (Watson, 1979). (See Box 13-3 for a list of carative factors.)

caring An essential part of human life, caring represents a moral idea about the nature of nurse-patient relationships. The goal of caring relationships is to preserve human dignity and humanity. Caring can be practiced intrapersonally (within the self), interpersonally (the traditional relationship between the nurse and patient), and transpersonally (the relationship between the nurse and the patient, in which each party is influenced and changed by the relationship) (Watson, 1999).

client/client system The object of nursing, which may be an individual, family, group, or even a "social issue," within Neuman's theoretical system. The client/client system is described as "an open system in interaction and total interface with the environment" (1989, p. 23).

cocreating, coconstituting, cotranscending The prefix "co" refers to the mutuality of the human life process. It describes experiences of the person in the here and now (Parse, 1997).

cognator A coping subsystem that responds to information processed, learning, judgment, and emotion. Cognators are those processes that the individual uses through conscious awareness and choice to create the future.

cognitive perceptual factors Motivational mechanisms that influence decisions about whether to engage in health-promoting behaviors. Examples of cognitive perceptual factors are the following: importance of health, self-efficacy, and perceived control of health; health definition; health status; benefits of health-promoting behaviors; and barriers to health-promoting behaviors.

conceptual model "A network of concepts that accounts for broad nursing phenomena" (King & Fawcett, 1997, p. 93).

constructivism A research paradigm that considers reality knowable through individuals' mental constructions or interpretations. More than one relative consensus can exist at any given time (Guba & Lincoln, 1994).

contextual stimuli Environmental factors that are present in a situation; they are not the center of attention but contribute to the effect of the focal stimulus (Roy & Andrews, 1991).

cosmology The study of the whole universe, including theories about its origin, evolution, structure, and future, including the meaning and place of human beings within the universe.

critical theory A broad research paradigm holding that reality is shaped by social, political, cultural economic, ethnic, and gender-related factors. The aim of research is to critique and transform structures that permit human exploitation (Guba & Lincoln, 1994).

dependent-care agency The "capabilities of persons to know and meet the therapeutic self-care demands of persons socially dependent on them or to regulate the development or exercise of these person's self-care agency" (Orem, 1995, p. 457).

dependent-care deficit The relationship between the self-care deficit (the required assistance) and dependent-care agency (the capabilities of the care provider) (Orem, 1995).

dialectical interchange A dialogue between individuals that challenges accepted ways of thinking and promotes more informed ways of thinking (Guba & Lincoln, 1994).

dialogical engagement A process through which an investigator is truly present with participants and is open to discussion of the phenomenon of study (Parse, 1987).

dimensions of relations The nature, origin, function, mode, and integrations of interpersonal relations (Peplau, 1992).

discipline A structured body of knowledge about a particular segment of reality; each discipline has a distinctive outlook and style of thinking, distinctive organized ideas and concepts, methods of inquiry, and modes of understanding data.

energy field The "fundamental unit of the living and the nonliving. Field is a unifying concept. Energy signifies the dynamic nature of the field; a field is in continuous motion and is infinite" (Rogers, 1990, p. 7).

emic An ethnographic term that refers to an insider's view. An emic view is the goal of ethnography.

epistemology The study of knowledge itself—what it is, its properties, and why it has these properties. Epistemology seeks to answer questions about the properties of truth and falsity, the nature of evidence, and the certainty that evidence produces (Wallace, 1977).

ethnography A type of qualitative research concerned with the meaning of actions and events associated with cultural groups (Boyle, 1994).

etic An ethnographic term that refers to the outsider's perspective (such as that of the investigators) that scientifically views reality within a group under study.

flexible line of defense "A protective accordion-like mechanism that protects the normal line of defense from invasion by stressors" (Neuman, 1995, p. 46).

focal stimuli Internal or external factors that most immediately confront the person (Roy & Andrews, 1991).

general theory The dominant features and relationships that characterize a practice field.

grounded theory A method of qualitative research concerned with theory generation regarding social and psychological phenomena (Glaser & Strauss, 1967).

helicy The "continuous, innovative, unpredictable, increasing diversity of human and environmental field patterns" (Rogers, 1990, p. 8).

hermeneutics   The interpretation of phenomena in order to depict the context and better clarify the phenomenon of study.

homeodynamics   Three principles—resonancy, helicy, and integrality—that deal with the state of change.

human becoming   A "unitary construct referring to the human being's living health" (Parse, 1997, p. 32).

human interaction   A process between the nurse and patient that leads to transactions. Perception, judgment, and action on the parts of both the nurse and the patient lead to a reaction, then to interaction, and finally to transaction (King, 1981).

interpersonal systems   Component of King's dynamic interacting systems that are formed through the interaction of two or more people (King, 1995).

lines of resistance   "Protection factors activated when stressors penetrate the normal line of defense" (Neuman, 1995, p. 46).

meaning   Linguistic and imagined content and the interpretation one gives to something (Parse, 1998).

middle-range theory   Theory that explains conceptual models representative of a partial view of nursing practice and consisting of concepts, propositions, or relational statements from which testable hypotheses can be derived and empirically measured.

mindbodyspirit   The connected whole of persons (Watson, 1999).

model   Virtual or imagined systems that bear varying degrees of relevant similarity to aspects of the real world they represent. A model is a system of relations used to represent another system of relations.

modeling   The process of developing and providing and abstraction of reality (Wallace, 1994).

modifying factors   Demographical characteristics such as age, income, gender, education, and ethnicity, that affect health promotion and participation.

normal line of defense   "An adaptational level of health developed over time and considered normal for a particular individual or client system; it becomes a standard for wellness deviation determination" (Neuman, 1995, p. 46).

nurse-patient relationship   The center of nursing.

nursing agency   Nurses' empowerment to act and to know. Nursing agency reflects nurses' ability to regulate patients, assist patients in accomplishing self-care, and achieve self-care agency through legitimate interpersonal relationships (Orem, 1995).

nursing system   A system composed of the patient(s), the nurse, and the actions and interactions between the nurse and the patient(s) (Orem, 1995).

nursing theoretical system   An abstract system consisting of the following: (1) a general model and theory of nursing placed within a particular philosophical tradition and structuring the discipline of nursing; (2) the models, middle-range theories, and empirical referents; and (3) the models that direct that process.

object   The focus of a discipline, the object establishes the fields and boundaries, builds the center of professional endeavor, indicates the differences between scientific disciplines, provides the methods for investigating and exploring knowledge, and determines the conclusions in a discipline.

ontology   Specifications of the ways of identifying and marking boundaries or particulars for a purpose.

originating   Inventing or creating new ways of living with the paradoxes of daily living (Parse, 1998).

pandimensionality   A "nonlinear domain without spatial or temporal attributes" (Rogers, 1990, p. 7). The shift in terminology from *multidimensionality to pandimensionality* is discussed in Rogers (1992).

paradigms The "operating rules about the appropriate relationships among theories, methods, and evidence that constitute the actual practices of the members of a scientific community, research program, or tradition" (Alford, 1998, p. 2). Paradigms combine theoretical assumptions, methodological procedures, and standards of evidence.

pattern The "distinguishing characteristic of an energy field perceived as a single wave" (Rogers, 1990, p. 7).

personal systems A component of King's dynamic interacting systems in which individuals exist (King, 1995).

phenomenology A qualitative research method that focuses on individuals' experiential lives in terms of their views and interactions with the phenomenon of concern in their everyday lives (Holstein & Gubrium, 1994).

positivism An approach to science in which researchers assume that a discoverable reality exists. The goal of research is to discover reality in order to explain, predict, and control (Guba & Lincoln, 1994).

postpositivism A variation of positivist thought, postpositivism holds that reality can be only imperfectly understood. Research seeks to gain knowledge by falsifying hypotheses.

powering A "pushing-resisting process" (Parse, 1998, p. 47).

practice model A "design for nursing action" (Orem, 1995, p. 180).

praxiology The study of human conduct or of efficient action—that is, sets of actions coordinated toward a common end (Kortabinsky, in Orem, 1995).

primary prevention Intervention that occurs before a reaction to stressors (Neuman, 1995).

process model A representation of the relationship between nurse and patient variables. These models describe the actions, interactions, and interpersonal processes by which the goals of the relationship are achieved.

psychodynamic nursing The active, creative use of the self for the good of the patient.

regulator A coping subsystem that physiologically responds through neural, chemical, and endocrine processes (Roy & Andrews, 1991).

reliability A measure of the accuracy and dependability of an instrument.

residual stimuli Internal or external environmental factors, the effects of which are unclear (Roy & Andrews, 1991).

resonancy The "continuous change from lower to higher frequency wave patterns in human and environmental fields" (Rogers, 1990, p. 8).

rhythmicity The "patterning of human-universe mutual process" (Parse, 1998, p. 29).

sacred feminine archetype Watson's metaphor for nursing as the basis of reality (1999).

secondary prevention A treatment given after symptoms caused by a reaction to stressors (Neuman, 1995).

self-care The performance of sets of actions that regulate functioning and development in order to maintain or establish health (Orem, 1995).

self-care agency Persons' ability to know and meet their continuing requirements for self-care in order to regulate their own human functions and development (Orem, 1995).

self-care deficit A relational construct that expresses the disparity between therapeutic self-care demand and self-care agency when the self-care agency is inadequate (Orem, 1995).

self-care systems Sequences of action performed by individuals to meet their self-care requisites.

social systems A component of King's dynamic interacting systems that consists of groups that make up a society (King, 1995).

stressors Environmental factors—intrapersonal, interpersonal, and extrapersonal in nature—that can disrupt the system. Stressors may penetrate both the flexible and normal lines of defense (Neuman, 1995).

tertiary prevention The maintenance of optimal wellness after treatment (Neuman, 1995).

theory   The narrative that accompanies a conceptual model, including a description of the elements of the model and their relationships; a frame of reference that helps humans to understand their world and to function in it; a set of interrelated assumptions, principles, and/or propositions to guide action.

Theory of Nursing Systems   One of three constituent theories of the Self-Care Deficit Nursing Theory, this system describes the action systems through which nurses use their nursing agency to promote or assist with patients' self-care (Orem, 1995).

Theory of Self-Care   One of three constituent theories of the Self-Care Deficit Nursing Theory, this theory describes the purpose for taking care of self, the capacity for taking such action, and for being able to act on behalf of others (Orem, 1995).

Theory of Self-Care Deficit   One of three constituent theories of the Self-Care Deficit Nursing Theory, this theory is the center of the general theory and describes the conditions that are present when people need nursing (Orem, 1995).

theory-generating research   A process in which theories are derived from real world observations that involve the phenomenon of interest and suggest areas to be examined (Chinn & Kramer, 1995; Fawcett, 1999).

theory-testing research   A deductive operation in which hypotheses are derived from an existing theory and then tested. If outcomes are as predicted, the theory is supported (Acton, Irvin, & Hopkins, 1991).

therapeutic self-care demand   A summary of all the actions required over time to meet known self-care requisites (Orem, 1995).

transaction   Interactions that have temporal and spatial dimensions in which "human beings communicate with environment or achieve goals that are values" within a shared frame of reference that comprises facts, beliefs, experiences, and preferences (King, 1981, p. 82).

transcendence   Reaching beyond the ordinary boundaries of a situation (Parse, 1998).

transpersonal caring   The "full actualisation of the carative factors in a human-to-human transaction" (Watson, 1989, p. 232).

transforming   the human-universe process as the human coparticipates in change in a deliberate way (Parse, 1998).

validity   An indication of whether an instrument measures what it intends to measure.

wholism   The organization of parts or subparts of a system into an interrelating whole (Neuman, 1995).

REFERENCES

Acton, G.J., Irvin, B.L., & Hopkins, B.A. (1991). Theory-testing research: Building the science, *Advances in Nursing Science, 14*(1), 52-61.

Alford, R.R. (1998). *The craft of inquiry.* New York: Oxford University Press.

Boyle, J. (1994). Styles of ethnography. In J. Morse (Ed.), *Critical issues in qualitative research methods.* Thousand Oaks, CA: Sage.

Chinn, P.L. & Kramer, M.K. (1995). *Theory and nursing research: A systematic approach* (4th ed.). St. Louis: Mosby.

Fawcett, J. (1999). *The relationship of theory and research,* (3rd ed.). Philadelphia: Davis.

Glaser, B. & Strauss, A. (1967). *The discovery of grounded theory: Strategies for qualitative research.* Chicago: Aldine.

Guba, E.G., & Lincoln, Y.S. (1994). Competing paradigms in qualitative research. In E.K. Denzin & Y.S. Lincoln (Eds.), *Handbook of qualitative research.* Thousand Oaks, CA: Sage.

Holstein, J.A. & Gubrium J.F. (1994). Phenomenology, ethnomethodology, and interpretive practice. In E.K. Denzin & Y.S. Lincoln (Eds.), *Handbook of qualitative research.* Thousand Oaks, CA: Sage.

King, I. (1981). *A theory for nursing: Systems, concepts, process.* New York: John Wiley and Sons.

King, I. (1995). A systems framework for nursing. In M.A. Frey & C.L. Sielhoff (Eds.), *Advancing King's systems framework and theory of nursing.* Thousand Oaks, CA: Sage.

King, I. & Fawcett, J. (1997). *The language of theory and metatheory.* Indianapolis: Sigma Theta Tau.

Neuman, B.M. (1989). *The Neuman Systems Model.* (2nd ed.). Norwalk, CT: Appleton & Lange.

Neuman, B.M. (1995). *The Neuman Systems Model.* (3rd ed.). Norwalk, CT: Appleton & Lange.

Orem, D.E. (1995). *Nursing: Concepts of practice* (5th ed.). St. Louis: Mosby.

Parse, R.R. (1987). *Nursing science: Major paradigms, theories, and critiques.* Philadelphia: W.B. Saunders.

Parse, R.R. (1997). The Human Becoming Theory: The was, is, and will be. *Nursing Science Quarterly, 10*(1), 32-38.

Parse, R.R. (1998). *The Human Becoming school of thought.* Thousand Oaks, CA: Sage.

Peplau, H. (1992). Interpersonal relations: Theoretical framework for application in practice. *Nursing Science Quarterly, 5*(1), 13-16.

Rogers, M. (1990). Nursing: Science of unitary, irreducible human beings: Update 1990. In E.A.M. Barrett, (Ed.), *Visions of Rogers' science-based nursing.* New York: National League for Nursing.

Rogers, M. (1992). Nursing science and the space age. *Nursing Science Quarterly, 5*(1), 27-34.

Roy, C. (1997). Future of the Roy model: Challenge to redefine adaptation. *Nursing Science Quarterly, 10*(1), 42-48.

Roy, C. & Andrews, H. (1991). *The Roy Adaptation Model: The definitive statement.* Norwalk, CT: Appleton-Lange.

Wallace, W.A. (1977). *The elements of philosophy.* New York: Alba House.

Wallace, W.A. (1994). *Ethics in modeling.* Tarrytown, New York: Pergamon.

Watson, J. (1979). *Nursing: The philosophy and science of caring.* Boston: Little, Brown.

Watson, J. (1989). Transformative thinking and a caring curriculum. In E.O. Bevis & J. Watson (Eds.), *Toward a caring curriculum: A new pedagogy for nursing.* New York: National League for Nursing.

Watson, J. (1999). *Postmodern nursing and beyond.* Edinburgh: Churchill Livingstone.

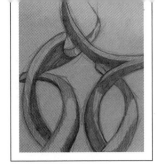

Index